Interventional Ultrasound

A Practical Guide and Atlas

Christoph F. Dietrich, MD
Professor and Head Physician
Medical Clinic 2
Caritas Hospital Bad Mergentheim gGmbH
Bad Mergentheim, Germany

Dieter Nuernberg, MD
Professor and Head Physician
Medical Clinic B
Ruppiner Hospitals GmbH
Neuruppin, Germany

380 illustrations

Thieme
Stuttgart • New York • Delhi • Rio

3.3 Documentation ... 33

3.4 Timing of the Consent Process ... 33

3.5 Special Situations ... 33

3.5.1 Implied Consent ... 33
3.5.2 Patients Lacking the Capacity to Consent ... 33
3.5.3 Minors ... 33
3.5.4 Language Barriers ... 34
3.5.5 Waiving of Informed Consent ... 34
References ... 34

4 Medications, Equipment, and Setup Requirements ... 35

D. Nuernberg, A. Jung

4.1 Medications ... 35

4.1.1 Premedication ... 35
4.1.2 Analgesia ... 35
4.1.3 Coagulation ... 36
4.1.4 Local Anesthesia ... 36

4.2 Equipment and Setup Requirements ... 37

4.2.1 Biopsy Equipment ... 37
4.2.2 Interventional Materials ... 37
4.2.3 Positioning, Preprocedure Examination, and Marking ... 37
4.2.4 Monitoring During the Procedure ... 37
4.2.5 Postprocedure Monitoring ... 37
4.2.6 Facilities (Procedure Room) ... 37
4.2.7 Functional and Design Requirements ... 38
4.2.8 Operational and Organizational Requirements ... 38
References ... 38

5 Pathology and Cytology ... 40

A. Tannapfel, C. F. Dietrich

5.1 Pathology ... 40

5.2 Biopsies ... 40

5.2.1 Types of Biopsy Procedure ... 40

5.3 Histology or Cytology? ... 40

5.3.1 Sources of Error ... 41

5.4 Typing, Grading, and Staging ... 41

5.4.1 Classification (Typing) ... 41
5.4.2 Grading ... 43

5.5 Specific Analysis ... 43

5.5.1 Lymph Nodes ... 43
5.5.2 Lymphomas ... 45

5.6 Hormone Growth Factor Receptor Analysis ... 47

References ... 48

6 Fine Needle Aspiration Cytology ... 49

C. Jenssen, T. Beyer

6.1 Specimen Collection ... 49

6.1.1 Ultrasound-Guided Biopsy ... 49
6.1.2 Needle Movement and Aspiration ... 49

6.2 Specimen Preparation ... 49

6.2.1 Fluid Aspirates ... 49
6.2.2 Centrifuging Effusions ... 49
6.2.3 Aspirates from Solid Lesions ... 50

6.3 Fixation and Staining ... 55

6.3.1 Basic Principles ... 55
6.3.2 Air Drying and Romanowsky Stains ... 55
6.3.3 Wet Fixation and Papanicolaou Staining ... 55
6.3.4 Ancillary Tests ... 56

6.4 Cytomorphologic Evaluation ... 58

6.4.1 Rapid On-Site Evaluation ... 58
6.4.2 Final Cytologic Diagnosis ... 63

6.5 Conclusions ... 64

References ... 64

Interventional Ultrasound

A Practical Guide and Atlas

Christoph F. Dietrich, MD
Professor and Head Physician
Medical Clinic 2
Caritas Hospital Bad Mergentheim gGmbH
Bad Mergentheim, Germany

Dieter Nuernberg, MD
Professor and Head Physician
Medical Clinic B
Ruppiner Hospitals GmbH
Neuruppin, Germany

380 illustrations

Thieme
Stuttgart • New York • Delhi • Rio

Library of Congress Cataloging-in-Publication Data

Interventioneller Ultraschall. English.

Interventional ultrasound : a practical guide and atlas / [edited by] Christoph F. Dietrich, Dieter Nuernberg ; translator, Terry C. Telger ; illustrator, Helmut Holtermann.

p. ; cm.

Includes bibliographical references and index.

ISBN 978-3-13-170821-2 – ISBN 978-3-13-170831-1 (eISBN)

I. Dietrich, Christoph Frank, editor. II. Nuernberg, Dieter, editor. III. Title.

[DNLM: 1. Ultrasonography, Interventional. WN 208]

RC78.7.U4

616.07'543–dc23

2014028919

This book is an authorized translation of the German edition published and copyrighted 2011 by Georg Thieme Verlag, Stuttgart. Title of the German edition: Interventionelle Ultraschall: Lehrbuch und Atlas für die Interventionelle Songraphie

Translator: Terry C. Telger, Fort Worth, TX, USA

Illustrator: Helmut Holtermann, Dannenberg, Germany

MIX
Papier aus verantwortungsvollen Quellen
FSC www.fsc.org FSC® C004592

Thieme Publishers Stuttgart
Rüdigerstrasse 14, 70469 Stuttgart, Germany
+49 [0]711 8931 421, customerservice@thieme.de

Thieme Publishers New York
333 Seventh Avenue, New York, NY 10001, USA
1-800-782-3488, customerservice@thieme.com

Thieme Publishers Delhi
A-12, Second Floor, Sector-2, Noida-201301
Uttar Pradesh, India
+91 120 45 566 00, customerservice@thieme.in

Thieme Publishers Rio,
Thieme Publicações Ltda.
Argentina Building, 16th Floor, Ala A,
228 Praia do Botafogo Rio de Janeiro
22250-040 Brazil
+55 21 3736-3631

Cover design: Thieme Publishing Group
Typesetting by Thomson Digital, India

Printed in Germany by Aprinta Druck, Wemding

ISBN 978-3-13-170821-2

Also available as an e-book:
eISBN 978-3-13-170831-1

Contents

Foreword ... xviii

Preface ... xix

Acknowledgments ... xx

Contributors ... xxi

Abbreviations ... xxiii

General Aspects of Interventional Ultrasound

1 Interventional Ultrasound: Introduction and Historical Background ... 2
H. Lutz

1.1 The Vienna Congress ... 2

1.2 The Introduction of Ultrasound into Routine Clinical Use ... 3

1.2.1 The Evolution of Ultrasound Imaging Techniques ... 3
1.2.2 Technical Evolution of Ultrasound-Guided Biopsies ... 4
1.2.3 Clinical Application ... 7
1.2.4 Risks of Interventional Ultrasound ... 9

1.3 Later Developments: Ultrasound-Guided Therapeutic Interventional Procedures ... 10

1.4 Outlook ... 10

References ... 11

2 Interventional Materials and Equipment ... 13

2.1 General Considerations on Interventional Procedures ... 13
U. Gottschalk, C. F. Dietrich

2.1.1 Brief Historical Introduction ... 13
2.1.2 Biopsy Principles and Techniques ... 13
2.1.3 Needle Systems ... 15

2.2 Therapeutic Interventions ... 20

2.2.1 Introduction ... 20
2.2.2 Brief Historical Review ... 20
2.2.3 Patient Preparation ... 21
2.2.4 Access Routes ... 21
2.2.5 Indications and Contraindications ... 21
2.2.6 Complications ... 22
2.2.7 Needle Techniques ... 23
2.2.8 Special Needle Types ... 23
2.2.9 Trocar Technique ... 23
2.2.10 Seldinger Technique ... 24
2.2.11 Peel Away Sheath ... 24
2.2.12 Anchor Systems, Suture Techniques ... 25
2.2.13 Guidewires ... 26
2.2.14 Dilators ... 27
2.2.15 Drainage Catheters ... 27
2.2.16 Other Drainage Systems ... 29
2.2.17 Accessories ... 29

References ... 31

3 Informed Consent ... 32
D. Nuernberg, A. Jung

3.1 What Should Be Disclosed? ... 32

3.1.1 Indication ... 32
3.1.2 Explaining the Procedure ... 32
3.1.3 Risks and Complications ... 32

3.2 Means of Disclosure ... 32

3.2.1 Consent Form ... 32
3.2.2 Informed Consent Discussion ... 32
3.2.3 Delegating Informed Consent ... 33

3.3 **Documentation** ... 33
3.4 **Timing of the Consent Process** ... 33
3.5 **Special Situations** ... 33
3.5.1 Implied Consent ... 33
3.5.2 Patients Lacking the Capacity to Consent ... 33
3.5.3 Minors ... 33
3.5.4 Language Barriers ... 34
3.5.5 Waiving of Informed Consent ... 34
References ... 34

4 **Medications, Equipment, and Setup Requirements** ... 35
D. Nuernberg, A. Jung

4.1 **Medications** ... 35
4.1.1 Premedication ... 35
4.1.2 Analgesia ... 35
4.1.3 Coagulation ... 36
4.1.4 Local Anesthesia ... 36
4.2 **Equipment and Setup Requirements** ... 37
4.2.1 Biopsy Equipment ... 37
4.2.2 Interventional Materials ... 37
4.2.3 Positioning, Preprocedure Examination, and Marking ... 37
4.2.4 Monitoring During the Procedure ... 37
4.2.5 Postprocedure Monitoring ... 37
4.2.6 Facilities (Procedure Room) ... 37
4.2.7 Functional and Design Requirements ... 38
4.2.8 Operational and Organizational Requirements ... 38
References ... 38

5 **Pathology and Cytology** ... 40
A. Tannapfel, C. F. Dietrich

5.1 **Pathology** ... 40
5.2 **Biopsies** ... 40
5.2.1 Types of Biopsy Procedure ... 40
5.3 **Histology or Cytology?** ... 40
5.3.1 Sources of Error ... 41
5.4 **Typing, Grading, and Staging** ... 41
5.4.1 Classification (Typing) ... 41
5.4.2 Grading ... 43
5.5 **Specific Analysis** ... 43
5.5.1 Lymph Nodes ... 43
5.5.2 Lymphomas ... 45
5.6 **Hormone Growth Factor Receptor Analysis** ... 47
References ... 48

6 **Fine Needle Aspiration Cytology** ... 49
C. Jenssen, T. Beyer

6.1 **Specimen Collection** ... 49
6.1.1 Ultrasound-Guided Biopsy ... 49
6.1.2 Needle Movement and Aspiration ... 49
6.2 **Specimen Preparation** ... 49
6.2.1 Fluid Aspirates ... 49
6.2.2 Centrifuging Effusions ... 49
6.2.3 Aspirates from Solid Lesions ... 50
6.3 **Fixation and Staining** ... 55
6.3.1 Basic Principles ... 55
6.3.2 Air Drying and Romanowsky Stains ... 55
6.3.3 Wet Fixation and Papanicolaou Staining ... 55
6.3.4 Ancillary Tests ... 56
6.4 **Cytomorphologic Evaluation** ... 58
6.4.1 Rapid On-Site Evaluation ... 58
6.4.2 Final Cytologic Diagnosis ... 63
6.5 **Conclusions** ... 64
References ... 64

7 **Infections and Diagnostic Microbiology** 68
T. Glueck, H. J. Linde, C. F. Dietrich

7.1 General Principles of Microbiological Testing 68

7.1.1 Microbiological Specimens 68
7.1.2 Prerequisites for Microbiological Testing 68

7.2 Microbiological Techniques 69

7.2.1 Stains 69
7.2.2 Culture Techniques 71
7.2.3 Nucleic Acid Amplification Techniques 71
7.2.4 Serology 71
7.2.5 When Are Microbiological Test Results Available? 72
7.2.6 Limitations of Microbiological Methods 72
7.2.7 Specimen Receipt during Off-hours (Nights, Weekends, Holidays) 72

7.3 Specific Guidelines for Microbiological Testing and Differential Diagnosis by Organ Systems and Syndromes 73

7.3.1 Investigation of Enlarged Lymph Nodes 73
7.3.2 Microbiological Testing and Antimicrobial Therapy for Suspected Tuberculosis 76
7.3.3 Liver Mass Suspicious for an Abscess (Including Amebic Abscess) 77
References 81

8 **Hygiene Management** 82
H. Martiny, D. Nuernberg

8.1 General Hygienic Requirements 82

8.1.1 Personal Protective Equipment and Coverings 82
8.1.2 Disposable Probe Covers 83
8.1.3 Ultrasound Gel 83

8.2 Hand Antisepsis and Skin Preparation 83

8.3 Ultrasound Probe and Accessories 84

8.3.1 Decontamination of the Ultrasound Probe 84
8.3.2 Decontamination of Ultrasound Accessories 85
References 85

9 **Contraindications, Complications, and Complication Management** 86
C. Jenssen, C. F. Dietrich

9.1 Interventional Risk 86

9.1.1 Complication Rates and Mortality 86
9.1.2 Factors that Influence Interventional Risk 86

9.2 Frequent Complications and Their Risk Factors 86

9.2.1 Pain and Vasovagal Reactions 86
9.2.2 Bleeding Complications 87
9.2.3 Needle Tract Seeding 88
9.2.4 Specific Complications 89

9.3 Prevention of Complications 89

9.3.1 Risk Assessment and Patient Selection 89
9.3.2 Modification of Risk Factors 90
9.3.3 Risk Reduction Techniques 92
9.3.4 Local Anesthesia and Intravenous Sedation 92
9.3.5 Prevention of Infection 93
9.3.6 Optimal Approach and Alternatives 93

9.4 Contraindications 93

9.4.1 Coagulopathies 93
9.4.2 Procoagulant Therapy and Antiplatelet Drugs 94
9.4.3 “Risky” Lesions and Access Routes 94

9.5 Management of Complications 95

9.5.1 Postinterventional Care and Detection of Complications 95
9.5.2 Treatment of Complications 95

9.6 Specific Biopsy Sites 95

9.6.1 Liver Biopsy 95
9.6.2 Renal Biopsy 99
9.6.3 Pancreatic Biopsy 99
9.6.4 Splenic Biopsy 100

9.6.5 Biopsy of Gastrointestinal Hollow Organs and Mesenteric Masses . . . 100
9.6.6 Adrenal Biopsy . . . 100
9.6.7 Lungs, Pleura, and Mediastinum . . . 101

9.7 Specific Interventions . . . 101

9.7.1 EUS-FNA, EUS-TCB, EBUS-TBNA . . . 101
9.7.2 EUS-Guided Therapeutic Interventions . . . 101
9.7.3 Transrectal Prostatic Biopsy . . . 102
9.7.4 Ultrasound-Guided Drainage (of Cysts, Pseudocysts, Abscesses, Cholecystitis) . . . 102
9.7.5 Ultrasound-Guided PTCD and Cholecystotomy . . . 103
9.7.6 Ultrasound-guided Tumor Ablation Therapy . . . 103
References . . . 104

10 Assistance in Ultrasound Interventions . . . 109
U. Gottschalk, C. F. Dietrich

10.1 Basic Principles . . . 109

10.2 Duties of Assisting Personnel . . . 109

10.3 Diagnostic Ultrasound . . . 110

10.4 Diagnostic Interventions . . . 110

10.5 Therapeutic Interventions . . . 111

10.6 Sedation . . . 111

10.7 Drain Placement . . . 111

10.8 Endosonography . . . 113

References . . . 113

11 Sedation in Interventions . . . 114
U. Gottschalk, C. F. Dietrich

11.1 Introduction . . . 114

11.2 Medications . . . 114

11.3 Personnel Requirements . . . 114

11.4 Monitoring Requirements . . . 115

11.5 Postprocedure Care . . . 115

11.6 Complications . . . 115

11.7 Summary . . . 115

References . . . 115

Specific Ultrasound-Guided Procedures: Abdomen

12 Indications for Diagnostic Interventions in the Abdomen and Thorax (Liver, Pancreas, Spleen, Kidneys, Lung, Other Sites) . . . 120
H. Kinkel, D. Nuernberg

12.1 Liver . . . 120

12.1.1 Diffuse Liver Diseases . . . 120
12.1.2 Focal Liver Lesions . . . 121

12.2 Pancreas . . . 123

12.3 Spleen . . . 123

12.4 Kidneys . . . 124

12.5 Lung . . . 125

12.6 Adrenal Gland . . . 125

12.7 Lymph Nodes . . . 125

12.8 Other Lesions . . . 126

References . . . 126

13 Diagnostic and Therapeutic Paracentesis of Free Abdominal Fluid 128

D. Nuernberg

13.1 Peritoneal Cavity 128

13.2 Sites of Predilection for Intra-abdominal Fluid 128

13.3 Pathogenesis and Differential Diagnosis of Ascites 129

13.4 Specific Indications 129

13.4.1 Transudate 129
13.4.2 Exudate 129
13.4.3 Cirrhosis 130
13.4.4 Heart Failure 130
13.4.5 Hypoalbuminemia 130
13.4.6 Peritonitis 130
13.4.7 Peritoneal Carcinomatosis 130
13.4.8 Hemoperitoneum 130
13.4.9 Pancreatitis 131
13.4.10 Other Rare Abdominal Fluid Collections .. 131

13.5 Differentiating a Localized Fluid Collection from Ascites 133

13.6 Practical Issues: How and Where to Aspirate? 133

13.7 Diagnostic Paracentesis: Laboratory Tests 134

13.8 Indications for Therapeutic Paracentesis 134

13.8.1 Treatment of Ascites in Hepatic Cirrhosis: Paracentesis for Symptom Relief in Hepatic Cirrhosis (and Pancreatitis)...... 134
13.8.2 Palliative Paracentesis for Peritoneal Carcinomatosis 135
13.8.3 Cytostatic Therapy of Peritoneal Carcinomatosis (Intraperitoneal Chemotherapy) 135
13.8.4 Drainage (with Irrigation) for Bile Leakage (For Example in a Palliative Setting)...... 135

13.9 Materials 136

13.10 Contraindications, Complications, and Postprocedure Care 136

References 137

14 Fine Needle Aspiration Biopsy and Core Needle Biopsy 138

J.-C. Kaemmer, D. Nuernberg

14.1 Historical Background 138

14.2 Description of Biopsy Techniques 138

14.2.1 What Type of Needle Should Be Used? ... 138

14.3 Biopsy Technique for Specific Needle Types 141

14.3.1 Biopsy with the Chiba Needle 142
14.3.2 Cutting Biopsy with an Otto or Franseen Needle 142
14.3.3 Autovac and BioPince Biopsy Systems 142
14.3.4 Biomol Biopsy System.................. 143
14.3.5 Trucut Needles 143

14.4 Summary 143

References 143

15 Abscess Drainage 144

C. F. Dietrich, A. Ignee, U. Gottschalk

15.1 Historical Considerations 144

15.2 Preliminary Remarks, Etiology 144

15.3 Selection of Imaging Modality 144

15.3.1 Ultrasound 144
15.3.2 Conventional Radiographic Drainage..... 146
15.3.3 Computed Tomography 146
15.3.4 Magnetic Resonance Imaging 146

15.4 Devices 146

15.4.1 Drainage Catheters 146

15.5 Indications 147

15.6 Contraindications 147

15.7 Patient Preparation 147

15.8 Treatment Options 148

15.8.1 General 148
15.8.2 Medical Treatment Options 148
15.8.3 Surgical Treatment Options 148

15.9 Technique of Percutaneous Abscess Drainage 148

15.9.1 Preparation 148
15.9.2 Initial Needle Insertion 149
15.9.3 Trocar Technique 151
15.9.4 Irrigation 154
15.9.5 Drain Removal 154
15.9.6 Specimen Processing 154

15.10 Postprocedure Care 154

15.11 Specific Diseases 154

15.11.1 Pyogenic Liver Abscess 154
15.11.2 Abscesses in Appendicitis, Peridiverticulitis 155
15.11.3 Liver Abscess in Biliary Disease 155
15.11.4 Abscess in Pancreatitis 156
15.11.5 Liver Abscess in Amebiasis 156
15.11.6 Protozoan Infections with Liver Involvement 157
15.11.7 Septic (Pyogenic) Abscess with Associated Diseases (Sepsis, Coagulopathies, Ascites) 157
15.11.8 Infection of Necrotic Tumor Components 158
15.11.9 Liver Abscess after Liver Transplantation 158

15.12 Complications 158

15.13 Irrigation 159

15.14 Sequelae 159

15.15 Ultrasound-Guided Gallbladder Drainage and Other Indications 159

References 160

16 Percutaneous Sclerotherapy of Cysts 163

C. F. Dietrich, B. Braden

16.1 Percutaneous Sclerotherapy of Liver Cysts 163

16.1.1 Epidemiology and Etiology 163
16.1.2 Symptoms 163
16.1.3 Indications 163
16.1.4 Contraindications 163
16.1.5 Interventional Materials and Equipment 163
16.1.6 Sclerosing Agents 163
16.1.7 Treatment Options 163
16.1.8 Technique for Percutaneous Sclerotherapy of a Liver Cyst 163

16.2 Sclerotherapy Technique 164

16.2.1 Follow-up Care 164
16.2.2 Prognosis 164

16.3 Percutaneous Sclerotherapy of Renal Cysts 164

16.3.1 Summary of the Literature 164
16.3.2 Epidemiology, Differential Diagnosis, and Classification 165
16.3.3 Technique 166
16.3.4 Sclerosing Agents 166

16.4 Alternative Procedures 167

16.5 Special Issues Relating to Splenic Cysts 167

16.6 Special Issues Relating to Pancreatic Cysts 167

References 167

17 Interventional Treatment of Echinococcosis 168

C. F. Dietrich, M. Hocke

17.1 Echinococci: Types and Epidemiology 168

17.1.1 *Echinococcus granulosus* 168
17.1.2 *Echinococcus multilocularis* 169

17.2 Clinical Manifestations 169

17.3 Diagnosis 169

17.3.1 Three Main Diagnostic Criteria 169

17.3.2 Laboratory Parameters 169
17.3.3 Serologic and Molecular Biologic Tests ... 169

17.4 Imaging Studies, Staging of Disease ... 169

17.4.1 Historical Background 169
17.4.2 Morphologic and Functional Classification Systems 171
17.4.3 WHO Classification 171

17.5 Treatment 173

17.5.1 Surgical Treatment Options 174
17.5.2 Drug Treatment Options 174
17.5.3 Local Ablative Procedures: PAIR 175
17.5.4 Endoscopic Retrograde Cholangiography 177
References 177

18 Local Ablative Procedures; Percutaneous Ethanol and Acetic Acid Injection 179

C. F. Dietrich, B. Braden, M. Hocke

18.1 Basic Considerations 179

18.1.1 What Tumors Are Suitable for Local Ablative Procedures? 179
18.1.2 Radiofrequency Ablation or Percutaneous Ethanol Injection? 179
18.1.3 Ethanol or Acetic Acid Injection? 179
18.1.4 Single or Multiple Sessions? 179

18.2 Indications 179

18.2.1 Considerations on Hepatocellular Carcinoma 180

18.3 Contraindications 180

18.4 Practical Aspects 180

18.4.1 Materials and Equipment 180
18.4.2 Preparations 180
18.4.3 Technique 180

18.5 Follow-up Care, Complications, and Prognosis 182

18.5.1 Follow-up Care 182
18.5.2 Complications 182
18.5.3 Monitoring of Treatment Response 182
18.5.4 Factors That Determine Prognosis 183

18.6 Summary 183

References 183

19 Local Ablative Procedures for Liver Tumors, Radiofrequency Ablation 185

C. F. Dietrich, T. Albrecht, T. Bernatik, A. Iqnee

19.1 Concepts (Curative, Palliative, Multimodal) 185

19.1.1 Hepatocellular Carcinoma 185
19.1.2 Colorectal Carcinoma 185

19.2 Selection of Imaging Modality (Ultrasound, CT, MRI) 186

19.3 Indications 186

19.3.1 Number of Tumors 186
19.3.2 Tumor Size 186
19.3.3 Tumor Location 186

19.4 Contraindications 187

19.5 Preparations 187

19.5.1 Antibiotic Prophylaxis 187
19.5.2 Local Anesthesia, Sedation, Sedation/Analgesia, and General Anesthesia 187
19.5.3 Treatment Planning 187

19.6 Materials 187

19.6.1 Standard Materials 187
19.6.2 Basic Principle 188
19.6.3 Monopolar versus Bipolar and Multipolar Systems 188
19.6.4 Needle Applicators 189
19.6.5 Control and Temperature Measurement 189
19.6.6 Flow Rate of Needle Perfusion 189

19.7 Technique 189

19.7.1 Patient Positioning 189
19.7.2 (Local) Anesthesia 190
19.7.3 Probe Insertion 190
19.7.4 Techniques for Specific Systems 191

19.8 Assessing the Efficacy of Treatment ... 192

19.9 Complications and Aftercare 193

19.9.1 Complications 193

19.9.2 Postinterventional Care 196

19.9.3 Clinical Aftercare and Follow-up......... 196

References 196

20 Percutaneous Transhepatic Cholangiodrainage 198

C. F. Dietrich, B. Braden, X. W. Cui, A. Ignee

20.1 Basic Principles 198

20.2 Indications 198

20.2.1 Endoscopic Retrograde or Percutaneous Approach 199

20.2.2 Rendezvous Technique................. 199

20.3 Contraindications 199

20.4 Materials and Equipment............. 200

20.4.1 Description of Materials................ 200

20.5 Technique 201

20.5.1 Patient Positioning 202

20.5.2 Needle Insertion and Drainage 202

20.5.3 Procedure Time....................... 207

20.6 Success Rate......................... 207

20.6.1 Results with Plastic Endoprostheses 207

20.6.2 Results with Metal Endoprostheses 208

20.7 Complications 208

20.7.1 Incidence 208

20.7.2 Management of Complications 208

20.8 Aftercare 208

20.9 Use of Intracavitary Ultrasound Contrast Agents 209

20.10 Analysis of the Literature 210

20.10.1 Present Authors' Data.................. 210

20.10.2 Comparison of Endoprostheses.......... 210

References 212

21 Percutaneous Gastrostomy 215

A. Ignee, G. Schuessler, C. F. Dietrich

21.1 Indications 215

21.2 Contraindications 215

21.3 Materials and Equipment............. 215

21.4 Types of Gastrostomy 215

21.4.1 Percutaneous Endoscopic Gastrostomy.......................... 215

21.4.2 Percutaneous Sonographic Gastrostomy .. 216

21.5 Advantages and Disadvantages of Different Methods 216

21.6 Success Rates of Different Gastrostomy Techniques 216

21.7 Complication Rates of Different Gastrostomy Techniques 216

21.8 Role of Ultrasonography.............. 217

21.8.1 General.............................. 217

21.8.2 Ultrasound-Assisted PEG............... 218

21.8.3 Technique of Percutaneous Sonographic Gastrostomy.......................... 219

21.9 Questions Relevant to Percutaneous Sonographic Gastrostomy 220

21.9.1 Use of a Spasmolytic Agent 220

21.9.2 Prophylactic Antibiotics................ 220

21.9.3 Use of a Guidewire 220

21.9.4 Need for Gastropexy................... 220

21.9.5 Type of Drainage 221

21.10 Summary............................ 222

References 223

22 **Interventional Endosonography** 224
C. F. Dietrich, M. Hocke, C. Jenssen

22.1 **Cost–Benefit Analysis** 224

22.2 **Historical Introduction** 224

22.3 **Materials and Equipment** 224

22.3.1 Requirements of the Endoscopy Unit 224
22.3.2 Which Endosonography Systems Have Become Established? 225
22.3.3 Which Biopsy Needles and Techniques Have Become Established? 225
22.3.4 Guidewires 227
22.3.5 Fixed-Diameter Dilators 228
22.3.6 Balloon Dilators 229
22.3.7 Plastic Stents (Pigtail) 230
22.3.8 Metal Stents 231
22.3.9 Diathermy Devices, Cystotome 232
22.3.10 Retrievers 233
22.3.11 Supplementary Techniques in EUS-guided Biopsy 234

22.4 **Procedure** 234

22.4.1 Sedation 234
22.4.2 Other Medications 234
22.4.3 Orientation 234
22.4.4 General Rules for Needle Insertion 234
22.4.5 Biopsy Technique 235
22.4.6 Suction 235
22.4.7 Specimen Processing 235

22.5 **Diagnostic Interventions** 236

22.5.1 Indications 236
22.5.2 Risk of Complications 237
22.5.3 Contraindications 238

22.6 **Therapeutic Interventions, General Aspects** 238

22.6.1 Therapeutic EUS-Guided Interventions 238
22.6.2 Endoscopes and Needle Types 238
22.6.3 General Rules for Needle and Wire Handling 239
22.6.4 Indications 239
22.6.5 Contraindications 239

22.7 **Drainage of Peripancreatic Fluid Collections** 239

22.7.1 History 239
22.7.2 Basic Anatomical Considerations 239
22.7.3 Pathophysiologic Considerations 239
22.7.4 Diagnostic Workup 239
22.7.5 Indications 240
22.7.6 Timing of the EUS Intervention 240
22.7.7 Selection of Procedure 240
22.7.8 Technique 240
22.7.9 One-Step Systems 240
22.7.10 Treatment of Nonpancreatic Fluid Collections 242
22.7.11 Surgical Options 243

22.8 **EUS-Guided Cholangiodrainage** 243

22.8.1 Introduction 243
22.8.2 Indications and Treatment Goals 244
22.8.3 Equipment 244
22.8.4 Preparatory Measures 244
22.8.5 Technique 244
22.8.6 Assessing the Result, Postinterventional Care, Complications 246

22.9 **EUS-Guided Pancreatic Duct Drainage** 246

22.9.1 Indications and Treatment Goals 246
22.9.2 Technique 246
22.9.3 Assessing the Result, Postinterventional Care, Complications 246

22.10 **Celiac Plexus Neurolysis and Celiac Plexus Blockade** 246

22.10.1 Indications and Treatment Goals 246
22.10.2 Materials 247
22.10.3 Technique 247
22.10.4 Assessing the Result, Postinterventional Care, Complications 247

22.11 **Tumor Ablation with Alcohol** 247

22.12 **EUS-Guided Vascular Interventions** 248

22.12.1 Indications and Treatment Goals 248
22.12.2 Materials 248
22.12.3 Technique 248
22.12.4 Assessing the Result, Postinterventional Care, Complications 248

22.13 **Complications** 249

22.14 **Postinterventional Care** 250

References 251

23 Special Issues Regarding Interventions in the Spleen ... 254
C. F. Dietrich

23.1 Diffuse Splenic Changes ... 254

23.2 Specific Disorders ... 254

23.2.1 Splenic Rupture ... 254
23.2.2 Splenic Infarction ... 254
23.2.3 Focal Splenic Changes ... 255

23.3 Procedures ... 255

23.3.1 Clinical Scenarios ... 255
23.3.2 Anatomical Considerations in Splenic Interventions ... 255
23.3.3 Procedures for Specific Applications ... 256

23.4 Abscess Drainage ... 256

23.5 Indications ... 256

23.6 Contraindications ... 256

23.7 Indications for Splenic Biopsy Drawn from Case Data ... 256

23.8 Postinterventional Care ... 257

23.9 Complications ... 257

23.10 Preinterventional Vaccinations ... 257

References ... 257

Specific Ultrasound-Guided Procedures: Thorax

24 Thoracic Interventions ... 260
W. Blank, A. Heinzmann

24.1 Advantages of Ultrasound-Guided Interventions ... 260

24.2 Indications ... 261

24.3 Contraindications ... 261

24.4 Selection of Materials ... 261

24.4.1 Ultrasound Technology ... 261
24.4.2 Biopsy Devices ... 262

24.5 Preparations ... 263

24.6 Technique ... 264

24.6.1 Chest Wall Lesions ... 264
24.6.2 Pleural Space ... 264
24.6.3 Subpleural Lung Lesions ... 265
24.6.4 Pulmonary Abscesses ... 268
24.6.5 Mediastinum ... 268

24.7 Steps in the Procedure ... 269

24.7.1 Preparations ... 269
24.7.2 Technique ... 269
24.7.3 Postprocedure Care ... 269

24.8 Problems and Complications ... 269

24.8.1 Postbiopsy Pneumothorax ... 269

24.9 Postprocedure Care and Follow-Up ... 270

References ... 271

Specific Ultrasound-Guided Procedures: Urogenital System

25 Percutaneous Renal Biopsy ... 274
U. Goettmann, B. K. Kraemer

25.1 Indications ... 274

25.2 Contraindications ... 274

25.3 Materials and Equipment ... 275

25.4 Preparations ... 275

25.5 Procedure ... 276

25.5.1 Native Renal Biopsy ... 276
25.5.2 Review of the Procedure Steps ... 277
25.5.3 Biopsy of a Renal Allograft ... 277

25.6 Complications ... 277

25.7 **Postbiopsy Care** 278

25.8 **List of Materials and Equipment** 278

References 278

26 Interventional Urology 280

D. Brix, A. Ignee, C. F. Dietrich

26.1 **Transrectal Ultrasonography of the Prostate** 280

26.1.1 Introduction 280
26.1.2 Equipment Requirements 280

26.2 **Diseases of the Prostate** 280

26.2.1 Prostate Cancer 280
26.2.2 Prostatic Abscess 281

26.3 **Prostate Biopsy** 281

26.3.1 Introduction 281
26.3.2 Indications 281
26.3.3 Informed Consent and Preparation 281
26.3.4 Complications and Their Management 281
26.3.5 Transperineal Biopsy 282

26.4 **Percutaneous Nephrostomy** 282

26.4.1 Introduction 282
26.4.2 Indications 282
26.4.3 Relative Contraindications 282
26.4.4 Complications 282
26.4.5 Preparations 282
26.4.6 Materials and Equipment 282
26.4.7 Technique 282
26.4.8 Anesthesia 283
26.4.9 Procedure 283
26.4.10 Postoperative Care 284
References 285

Specific Ultrasound-Guided Procedures: Other Organ Systems

27 Interventional Thyroid Ultrasound 288

B. Braun, T. Mueller

27.1 **Diagnostic Interventions** 288

27.1.1 Indications 288
27.1.2 Contraindications 288
27.1.3 Methods 288
27.1.4 Complications 290
27.1.5 Materials and Equipment 290
27.1.6 Preparation 291
27.1.7 Procedure 292
27.1.8 Problems 293
27.1.9 Pitfalls in Thyroid Biopsy 294

27.2 **Therapeutic Interventions** 295

27.2.1 Evacuation Procedures 296
27.2.2 Ablative Procedures 296
References 301

28 Musculoskeletal Interventions 304

W. Hartung, T. Weigand

28.1 **Indications and Contraindications** 304

28.1.1 Indications 304
28.1.2 Contraindications 304

28.2 **Materials and Equipment** 304

28.3 **Procedure** 305

28.3.1 Preparations 305
28.3.2 Overview of Technique 306
28.3.3 Details of Technique 306
28.3.4 Rotator Cuff (Supraspinatus Muscle) 309

28.4 **Pitfalls and Complications** 312

28.5 **Postprocedure Care** 313

References 313

29 Neurologic Interventions, Ultrasound-Guided Regional Anesthesia 315
H. H. Wilckens, A. Ignee, M. Kaeppler, H. Boehrer, C. F. Dietrich

29.1 History and Development 315

29.2 Indications 315

29.3 Contraindications 315

29.3.1 Patient Refusal 315
29.3.2 Clinically Overt Coagulopathy and Anticoagulant Medication 315
29.3.3 Infections at the Puncture Site 316
29.3.4 Neurologic Deficit 316

29.4 Needle Insertion Techniques 316

29.4.1 Out-of-Plane versus In-Plane Technique 316

29.5 Ultrasound Imaging of Nerves and Muscles 316

29.5.1 Nerves 316
29.5.2 Muscles 317

29.6 Materials and Equipment 317

29.6.1 Ultrasound Machines 317
29.6.2 Anesthesia Needles and Catheters 317

29.7 Regional Anesthesia at Specific Sites: Upper Limb 318

29.7.1 Brachial Plexus 318
29.7.2 Infraclavicular Brachial Plexus Block 320
29.7.3 Axillary Brachial Plexus Block 321

29.8 Regional Anesthesia at Specific Sites: Lower Limb 322

29.8.1 Lumbosacral Plexus 322
29.8.2 Femoral Nerve Block 323
29.8.3 Obturator Nerve Block 323
29.8.4 Sciatic Nerve Block 325
29.8.5 Saphenous Nerve Block 326
29.8.6 Lateral Femoral Cutaneous Nerve Block 326

29.9 Summary 327

References 328

30 Ultrasound-Guided Emergency and Vascular Interventions 330
T. Mueller, C. Jenssen

30.1 Emergency Interventions 330

30.1.1 Indications 330
30.1.2 Contraindications 331
30.1.3 Materials and Equipment 331
30.1.4 Antisepsis 332
30.1.5 Problems and Complications 332
30.1.6 Intra-abdominal Free Fluid 332
30.1.7 Intrathoracic Free Fluid 333
30.1.8 Pneumothorax 333
30.1.9 Pericardial Fluid 334

30.2 Percutaneous Vascular Interventions 335

30.2.1 Vascular Access 335
30.2.2 Ultrasound-Guided Treatment of Pseudoaneurysms 341

30.3 Endosonographically Guided Vascular Interventions 345

30.3.1 Indications and Treatment Goals 345
References 348

Specific Ultrasound-Guided Procedures: Other Applications of Interventional Ultrasound

31 Extravascular Use of Ultrasound Contrast Agents 354
A. Ignee, G. Schuessler, C. F Dietrich

31.1 Approved Indications 354

31.2 Contraindications and Complications 354

31.3 Technique ... 354

31.4 Use of Ultrasound Contrast Agents in Physiologic Body Cavities ... 355

31.4.1 Voiding Sonography for the Detection of Vesicoureteral Reflux ... 355
31.4.2 Contrast-Enhanced Ultrasound for Evaluating Tubal Patency ... 355
31.4.3 Imaging the Peritoneal Cavity with UCAs (for Detection of Ascites) ... 355
31.4.4 Biliary Tract ... 356
31.4.5 UCAs in Enterography ... 356
31.4.6 CEUS Gastrography—Percutaneous Injection of UCA into the Stomach to Assess Gastrostomy Placement ... 356

31.5 Use of Ultrasound Contrast Agents in Nonphysiologic Body Cavities ... 356

31.5.1 Ultrasound Fistulography ... 356
31.5.2 Percutaneous Injection of UCAs for Abscess Imaging ... 357
31.5.3 UCAs for Demonstrating Pancreatitis-Associated Cystic Lesions after EUS-Guided Biopsy ... 357

31.6 Summary ... 357

References ... 358

32 Volume Navigation ... 359

C. F Dietrich, A. Ignee, M. Hoepfner

32.1 How Tracking Works ... 359

32.2 Position Marking ... 359

32.3 Fusion with CT, MRI, or PET Volume Data Sets ... 359

32.4 Fusion with Archived Ultrasound Volume Data ... 362

32.5 Magnetic Field–Assisted Needle Tracking and Guidance ... 362

32.6 Illustrative Images and Case Reports ... 362

32.6.1 Case Report 1 ... 362
32.6.2 Case Report 2 ... 362
References ... 363

33 Palliative Interventions and the Role of Ultrasonography in Palliative Care ... 364

D. Nuernberg

33.1 Content and Goals of Palliative Care ... 364

33.2 Ultrasound in Palliative Staging, Follow-Up, and Palliative Treatment Monitoring ... 364

33.3 Ultrasound-Guided Palliative Interventions ... 365

33.3.1 Palliative Diagnostic Interventions ... 365
33.3.2 Specific Palliative Therapeutic Interventions ... 366

33.4 Portable Ultrasound in Specialized Ambulatory Palliative Care ... 367

33.5 Palliative Ultrasound in Caring Medicine ... 367

33.6 Conclusions ... 368

References ... 368

Index ... 369

Foreword

Surprisingly, no comprehensive textbook has been written on the topic of ultrasound guidance of interventional procedures. This may be because ultrasound use in different specialties or subspecialties is so broad and is expanding that is difficult to complete a comprehensive and timely text on the subject matter. Ultrasound is now used to guide interventional techniques by practitioners in nearly every specialty, including cardiology, radiology, intensive care, anesthesiology, gastroenterology, and others. For this reason it is difficult to collect all of the relevant knowledge and information into a single text. Fortunately, Christoph Dietrich and Dieter Nuernberg have undertaken to do this. Their joint skills as clinicians, teachers, and authors have produced an important textbook of interventional ultrasound. The coauthors of each chapter were carefully chosen to reflect their discipline with expertise in their particular field of interest. Together they have completed a comprehensive text on traditional methods of ultrasound guidance of interventional techniques and have included newer and more advanced use of ultrasound in guiding other techniques. They have also reviewed more recent advances in interventional ultrasound including the use of contrast agents that help identify, guide, and assess the success of different interventional procedures. Certainly ultrasound has been shown to have various advantages over other modalities such as CT in guiding interventional procedures. Ultrasound transducers have been adapted for endoscopic use and are now routinely used in biopsy of the thorax and the gastrointestinal tract. Many percutaneous biopsy aspiration or drainage techniques are now performed with ultrasound instead of CT because of the real-time capabilities, lack of ionizing radiation, and precision of sonographic needle placement. Furthermore, advanced ablative techniques can be guided by sonography, and the use of modern ultrasound contrast agents allows assessment of the adequacy of tumor ablation after treatment.

The authors first take us back in time with a historical perspective of the use of interventional ultrasound, then deal comprehensively with current technologies, and take us forward to future applications of ultrasound in different subspecialties.

I am very pleased to have been asked to write the foreword for this work because I believe this textbook on interventional ultrasound will be used as a standard reference text in this field. It gives both historical perspectives and up-to-date information on the use of ultrasound in guidance of different interventional techniques. The authors and the editors deserve congratulations for the completion of this important work.

John P. McGahan, MD
Professor and Vice Chair of Academic Affairs
Director of Abdominal Imaging
Department of Radiology
University of California, Davis, USA

Preface

Interventional ultrasound procedures have revolutionized clinical practice in recent decades. The advantages of ultrasound-guided interventions include an unsurpassed sharpness of detail and excellent controllability due to the real-time visual display, the wide availability of ultrasound equipment, and a simple and straightforward practical technique. This makes it all the more surprising that a standard textbook of interventional ultrasound has not previously been published.

The editors have accessed a wealth of experience from their expert contributors, who present the subject matter as concretely as possible and offer vivid descriptions of practical techniques. Particular attention is given to clinical significance.

The practice-oriented approach may have caused some instruments to be emphasized over other tested and proven devices, with the result that some reputable companies and their products were not given due attention.

The experience presented here, while proven, is often highly individualized. In future editions, it is intended that the content will be enhanced by input from ultrasound interventionalists who have not contributed to this book so that we may achieve a fuller and more balanced presentation. The advantage of a concrete, detailed chapter format is obvious, and the editors hope to see this work used as a "cookbook" in the everyday practice of interventional ultrasound.

The book consists of two main parts. Part I deals with general aspects of interventional ultrasound, Part II with specific ultrasound-guided procedures. Part I begins with a historical review, which is necessary for the understanding of some current techniques. Next come chapters that present essential basic information on interventional materials, issues of informed consent, equipment requirements, on-site material processing, microbiological aspects, and issues relating to hygiene and management of complications. The importance of assisting personnel is too often overlooked: this is addressed in a separate chapter and under specific subheads. Particularly in oncology, histologic (and/or cytologic) confirmation is essential for planning a highly specialized and differentiated modern treatment strategy. Up-to-date immunohistochemical and immunocytologic staining methods and proliferation indices are essential aids to directing the treatment of gastrointestinal stromal tumors and other lesions. Lymphomas are classified hematologically as low-grade, aggressive, or highly aggressive lesions, with each type having its own therapeutic implications. The knowledge of contraindications, complication management, and how to weigh risks against benefits forms the basis for the chapters presented.

Part II deals with pulmonary biopsy techniques and thoracic interventions as well as diagnostic and therapeutic interventions involving the thyroid gland, urogenital tract, and musculoskeletal system. Endosonographic interventions are described in detail. Other topics relate to combined radiologic and sonographic interventions as well as critical-care and emergency-room interventions including cardiologic and anesthesiologic procedures. Part II also explores interventions in children and takes a look at new techniques and future perspectives. Symptom-oriented palliative care interventions represent a very topical issue that rounds out the chapter. Therapeutic abscess drainage, interventional tumor ablation techniques, and interventional treatments for parasitic diseases (PAIR [puncture, aspiration, injection, reaspiration] for echinococcosis) enrich our daily practice, as do established therapeutic procedures such as percutaneous transhepatic cholangiography and drainage (PTCD), nephrostomy, and the drainage of pancreatic pseudocysts. In the matter of interventional guidance and approach, it is often necessary to decide between the competing modalities of CT guidance and other imaging techniques, which in some case can and should be used to complement or supplement one another. The role of ultrasound contrast agents in the preparation, support, and guidance of interventional procedures is also addressed.

This book is an expression of interdisciplinary and multiprofessional viewpoints, some of which represent different approaches; this reflects reality in all its diversity. The principle of "do no harm" is expressed in repeated urgings to apply the techniques judiciously in everyday practice and not to become fascinated with technology for its own sake. The decision to proceed with an intervention is always an individual one and should be measured by its benefit for the patient.

Professor Christoph F. Dietrich, MD
Professor Dieter Nuernberg, MD

Acknowledgments

Many experts had a hand in the creation of this book. This is evident from the list of distinguished authors. While the chapters were being written all contributions were subject to intense critical discussion by our circle of colleagues who contributed many important and very helpful suggestions and reviews on specific chapters. Some of these colleagues were outside the circle of our authors, and we wish to thank them by name for their extremely valuable feedback and commitment:

Ana Paula Barreiros, MD
Professor Joerg Bleck, MD
Bettina Fiedler, MD
Professor Christian Goerg, MD
Professor Martin Krueger, MD
Birgitt Lucke
Professor Juergen F. Riemann, MD
Christiane Schieferstein, MD
Professor Wolf Burkhardt Schwerk, MD
Professor Hanns M. Seitz, MD
Jochen Selbach, MD
Stephan Wagner, MD
Professor Till Wehrmann, MD
Matthias Woenchkaus, MD
Kriztina Zels

In addition, we thank Dr. Thomas Riebel and Dr. Holger Strunk for their valuable contribution to the orginal German edition.

We express our sincere thanks to Mrs. Kerstin Siehr, Dr. Michael Weber, Dr. Katrin Gottloeber, Dr. Stefanie Eylert, and Dr. Tiberius Maros for their tireless support whenever a little help was needed. We thank Dr. Lilian Chiorean for her proofreading and bright ideas. We also thank the team at Thieme Publishers Stuttgart, particularly acknowledging Dr. Brands for his swift decisions as well as Dr. Tegude, Mrs. Holzer, Joanne Stead, Stephan Konnry, and Gabriele Kuhn-Giovannini for their friendly and efficient work in project management and production.

Contributors

Thomas Albrecht, MD
Professor
Department of Radiology and Interventional Therapy
Vivantes Hospital Neukölln
Berlin, Germany

Thomas Bernatik, MD
Professor and Director
Department of Internal Medicine, Gastroenterology
Specialist in Internal Medicine and Diabetology
Ebersberg County Hospital
Ebersberg, Germany

Thomas Beyer, MD
Ballenstedt-Harz Lung Clinic GmbH
Ballenstedt, Germany

Wolfgang Blank, MD
Supervising Physician and Deputy Head Physician
Medical Clinic 1
Klinikum am Steinenberg Hospital
Reutlingen, Germany

Hubert Boehrer, MD
Professor
Department of Anesthesiology and Critical Care Medicine
Caritas Hospital Bad Mergentheim gGmbH
Bad Mergentheim, Germany

Barbara Braden, MD
Professor
Consultant Gastroenterologist
Translational Gastroenterology Unit
John Radcliffe Hospital
Oxford, UK

Bernd Braun, MD
Professor and former Head Physician
Medical Clinic 1
Klinikum am Steinenberg Hospital
Reutlingen, Germany

David Brix, MD
Department of Urology
Caritas Hospital Bad Mergentheim gGmbH
Bad Mergentheim, Germany

Xin Wu Cui
Medical Clinic 2
Caritas Hospital Bad Mergentheim gGmbH
Bad Mergentheim, Germany

Christoph F. Dietrich, MD
Professor and Head Physician
Medical Clinic 2
Caritas Hospital Bad Mergentheim gGmbH
Bad Mergentheim, Germany

Thomas Glueck, MD
Professor
Department of Internal Medicine
Trostberg District Hospital – Kliniken SO-Bayern
Trostberg, Germany

Uwe Goettmann, MD
Professor
Consultant Nephrologist
Medical Clinic V
University Medical Center Mannheim
Mannheim, Germany

Uwe Gottschalk, MD
Center for Liver Diseases at Checkpoint
Berlin, Germany

Wolfgang Hartung, MD
Department of Rheumatology and Clinical Immunology
Asklepios Hospital Bad Abbach
Regensburg University Care Network
Bad Abbach, Germany

Alexander Heinzmann, MD
Chief Physician
Medical Clinic I
Klinikum am Steinenberg Hospital
Reutlingen, Germany

Michael Hocke, MD
Department of Internal Medicine II
Meiningen Hospital GmbH
Meiningen, Germany

RCC	renal cell carcinoma
RFA	radiofrequency ablation
RFITT	radiofrequency-induced thermotherapy
RFTA	radiofrequency thermoablation
ROSE	rapid on-site evaluation
SAPV	specialized ambulatory palliative care
SBP	spontaneous bacterial peritonitis
SDMS	Society of Diagnostic Medical Sonography
SIRT	selective internal radiotherapy
SLE	systemic lupus erythematosus
SMA	smooth muscle actin
TACE	transarterial chemoembolization
TB	tuberculosis
THI	tissue harmonic imaging
TIA	transient ischemic attack
TIPS	transjugular intrahepatic portosystemic shunt
TIPSS	transjugular intrahepatic portosystemic stent shunt
TPCD	transpapillary cholangiodrainage
TPHA	Treponema pallidum hemagglutination
TRUS	transrectal ultrasonography
TSH	thyroid-stimulating hormone
TTF-1	thyroid transcription factor 1
TURP	transurethral resection of the prostate
UCA	ultrasound contrast agent
UICC	Union for International Cancer Control/Union Internationale Contre le Cancer
US-FNA	ultrasound-guided FNA
VAH	Association for Applied Hygiene
VaIN	vaginal intraepithelial neoplasia
VDRL	Venereal Disease Research Laboratory [test for syphilis]
VEGFR	vascular endothelial growth factor receptor
VIN	vulval intraepithelial neoplasia
VKA	vitamin K antagonist
VRE	vancomycin-resistant enterococci
VTE	venous thromboembolism
WBC	white blood cell count

General Aspects of Interventional Ultrasound

1 Interventional Ultrasound: Introduction and Historical Background ... 2

2 Interventional Materials and Equipment ... 13

3 Informed Consent ... 32

4 Medications, Equipment, and Setup Requirements ... 35

5 Pathology and Cytology ... 40

6 Fine Needle Aspiration Cytology ... 49

7 Infections and Diagnostic Microbiology ... 68

8 Hygiene Management ... 82

9 Contraindications, Complications, and Complication Management ... 86

10 Assistance in Ultrasound Interventions ... 109

11 Sedation in Interventions ... 114

1 Interventional Ultrasound: Introduction and Historical Background

H. Lutz

1.1 The Vienna Congress

The "First World Congress on Ultrasonic Diagnostics in Medicine" was held in Vienna in 1969. It marked the end of the pioneering age of diagnostic ultrasound that began after World War II. By that time ultrasonography had already found applications in ophthalmology as well as neurology (echoencephalography using A-mode ultrasound to detect intracranial hemorrhage, for example) and cardiology (TM-mode echocardiography for diagnosing valvular disease). Especially for the fields of obstetrics, gynecology, and internal medicine, the Congress marked the start of a burgeoning period of clinical research.

The Vienna Congress began as the Third International Symposium on Ultrasonic Diagnostics in Ophthalmology (SIDUO III) headed by Viennese ophthalmologists J. Böck, who served as president, and K. Ossoinig, who served as scientific secretary. The original symposium was changed to an interdisciplinary world conference when it was recognized that, for the first time, comprehensive reports on diagnostic ultrasound were available from a number of other specialties. A total of 190 papers were presented—48 in ophthalmology, 29 in neurology, 20 in cardiology, 19 in obstetrics and gynecology, and 23 in internal medicine.

Only two papers dealt with the capabilities of ultrasound-guided needle procedures, and both reflected the full spectrum of possible procedures and future diagnostic applications. A. Kratochwil[1] reported on ultrasound-guided amniocentesis using a specially designed biopsy transducer (▶ Fig. 1.1).

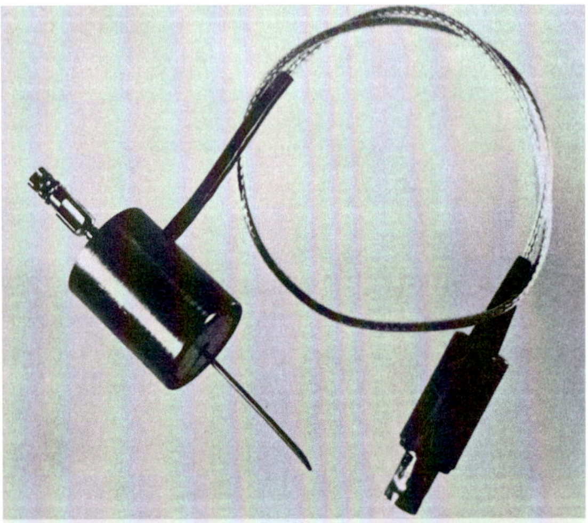

Fig. 1.1 A mode transducer with a central aperture for guiding the (amniocentesis) needle, introduced by Kratochwil in Vienna in 1969. (Source: With kind permission of the Vienna Medical Academy.[1])

U. W. Blauenstein used ultrasound to localize tumor nodules in the liver and puncture them percutaneously, aided by markings drawn on the skin (▶ Fig. 1.2).[2]

To appreciate the significance of these reports, we must recall the conventional diagnostic tools that were available at that time. The relatively simple percutaneous drainage of relatively large fluid collections was traditionally guided by anatomical landmarks (e.g., for draining ascites) or percussion (e.g., for thoracentesis). But these methods were difficult or impossible to use in patients with small fluid collections, adhesions, or septations. A relatively large organ like the liver could be sampled to investigate presumed diffuse disease using a standard technique following localization by percussion. The development of the Menghini needle in 1958 had made percutaneous liver biopsy a simple procedure.[3] On the other hand, a suspected tumor was considered at least a relative contraindication to needle biopsy, so that technique could not be used for the selective sampling of tumor nodules in the liver.

The only imaging modality available at that time for the percutaneous biopsy of nonpalpable organs and structures was classical radiography. But this method was problematic for several reasons. First, the relationship of the intended target (e.g., the inferior renal pole) to anatomical landmarks like the spinal column was measurable but the distance from skin to target (i.e., the second plane) was not. Moreover, the kidney had to have sufficient residual function that it could be opacified by intravenous contrast medium. Radiographic imaging also required costly radiation safety measures for the patient and staff.

Kratochwil described in his paper how ultrasound guidance could make standard needle procedures easier and safer (here, by avoiding the placenta), even in unusual situations. The sectional images produced by ultrasonography enable the target site to be visualized and localized in all three dimensions. As early as 1961, G. M. Berlyne[4] suggested that the two-dimensional pyelogram obtained before percutaneous renal biopsy could be supplemented by an A-mode scan to measure the depth from skin to target. In 1970, G. Rettenmaier noted the advantages of using two-dimensional real-time ultrasound to track the respiratory movements of the kidney and provide a third localizing dimension.[5]

Martin and Ellis[6] were the first authors to report on the aspiration biopsy of suspected neoplasms. Traditionally, however, a targeted aspiration biopsy could be used only

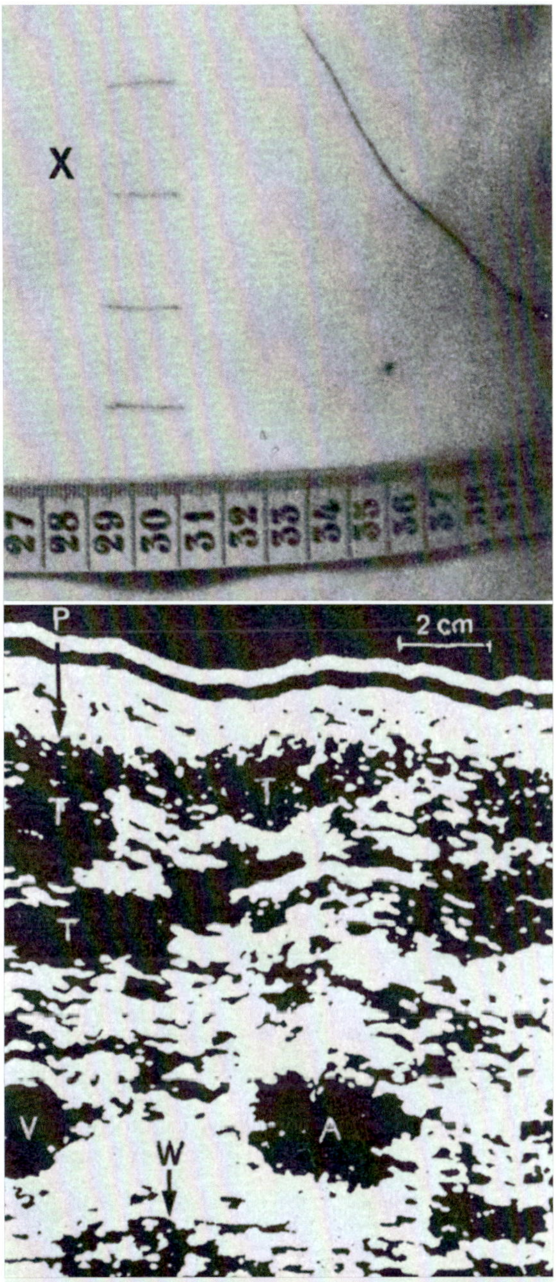

Fig. 1.2 Example of an ultrasound-guided percutaneous liver biopsy. Same-scale views of the skin site and ultrasound image as presented by Blauenstein in Vienna in 1969. X marks the skin entry site over the enlarged hepatic left lobe. (Source: With kind permission of the Vienna Medical Academy.[2])

for palpable masses, thoracic tumors accessible to radiographic guidance, or during (exploratory) laparotomy.

Blauenstein was the first author to show that ultrasound could be used not only to identify suspicious lesions in organs but also to biopsy them selectively for further differentiation. Thus began the development of a relatively simple diagnostic method for the detection and differentiation of even small, nonpalpable suspected neoplasms. By that time authors had already reported positive experience with the cytologic analysis of material sampled by percutaneous aspiration (e.g., from lymph nodes, the thyroid gland, the breast, or lung tumors) and of tumor lesions (e.g., of the pancreas) sampled by intraoperative needle biopsy.

Meanwhile, both Kratochwil and Blauenstein had demonstrated the two main options available for performing ultrasound-guided punctures. Blauenstein used a kind of freehand technique in which he first measured the location of the intended target and marked it on the skin, then advanced the needle to the target without observing it directly (▶ Fig. 1.2). Kratochwil used a special biopsy transducer (▶ Fig. 1.1), which provided an A-mode display of the structures (in this case the placenta) previously defined by a slow B-mode scan.

1.2 The Introduction of Ultrasound into Routine Clinical Use

1.2.1 The Evolution of Ultrasound Imaging Techniques

Over the next 10 to 15 years, two-dimensional sectional imaging with ultrasound was increasingly implemented in almost all medical specialties. At first the bistable compound scan was still the (international) standard and was supplemented by A-mode scanning for "structural" analysis. The introduction of gray-scale technology in 1974 significantly improved the images generated by this type of system. Even so, the slow compound scan was increasingly superseded by fast (real-time) B-mode scanning, which replaced it completely by about 1980. As early as 1965, R. Soldner of the Siemens company[7] had developed the Vidoson 635 as the first mechanical fast B-mode scanner. This device was widely used starting in 1970 and became especially popular in internal medicine and obstetrics. An electronic linear-array scanner was produced by ADR in 1974. By 1980 at the latest, all major ultrasound companies had developed mechanical or electronic real-time scanners. Real-time B-mode imaging was the technical prerequisite for the increasingly rapid implementation of diagnostic ultrasound during this period.

Some more theoretically oriented scientists believed that technical advances in ultrasonography would make it possible to discriminate among different tissue types, thus enabling a reliable benign–malignant differentiation. As a result, "tissue characterization" became a key topic of discussion at international conferences, which were now being held at regular intervals. Meanwhile, further technical advances in ultrasound-guided biopsy were pursued initially at centers of diagnostic ultrasound.

Clinical ultrasound specialists favored that modality as a simple, low-risk method for establishing a morphologic diagnosis. Hans Henrick Holm stated this viewpoint succinctly in his book, *Interventional Ultrasound*[8]:

When considering the difficulties frequently encountered with conventional microscopy, it does not seem likely that tissue characterization with ultrasound or with any other imaging modality will make it possible, with clinically acceptable accuracy, e.g. routinely to distinguish between a benign and a malignant intra-abdominal lesion.

1.2.2 Technical Evolution of Ultrasound-Guided Biopsies

From a technical standpoint, Kratochwil's concept of using a single transducer with a central aperture on a compound scanner was easily moved from the design stage to practical reality (▶ Fig. 1.3). Biopsy transducers for compound scanners became available commercially only a short time after the Vienna Congress.[9,10] These devices were used in many early studies.

On the other hand, this technique was still somewhat laborious for percutaneous biopsies: First, an image of the intended target was acquired slowly with a bistable compound scanner (this took at least several seconds), and the image was stored in memory. After the desired puncture site had been marked on the skin, a sterilized biopsy transducer was fastened to the scanner arm and applied to the marked skin site. Next, the biopsy transducer was swept through a sector arc to redefine the desired plane. The only orientation guide available beyond this point was the static (frozen) B-mode image. The target and needle path could be directly observed during the biopsy itself only by viewing an A-mode display (▶ Fig. 1.4).

Needle insertion with the fast B-mode Vidoson system was done using freehand technique: The intended target was first defined in the B-mode image. The most favorable entry site in the second plane was located and marked on the skin by noting the acoustic shadow cast by a small wooden stick placed between the skin and transducer (▶ Fig. 1.5). The depth from skin to target was measured on the monitor screen and could be preset on the needle with a set screw. Whenever possible, the cumbersome (transducer placed in a water bag!) Vidoson was positioned next to the entry site so that the intended target and needle could be monitored directly in the B-mode image.[11] Other authors used a needle guide mounted on the side of the Vidoson. This design was available as a prototype developed by Siemens in about 1974,[12] or users could create their own homemade version[13] (▶ Fig. 1.6).

This principle was adopted in the easier-to-use handy sector scanners (with direct contact to the skin) that were developed later. In 1978, Saitoh and Watanabe worked

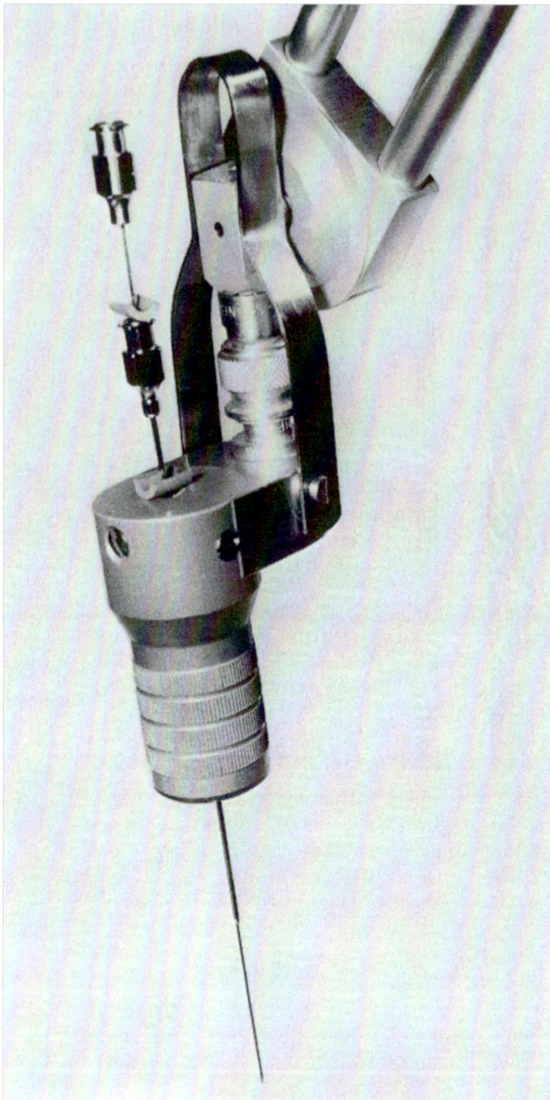

Fig. 1.3 Commercially available biopsy transducer (A-scan) with a central needle aperture, mounted on a compound scanner arm circa 1972.

with the Aloka company to develop an adapter for a sector scanner (▶ Fig. 1.7),[14] which was then marketed commercially. At about the same time, Kretz Ultrasound also developed an adapter for their Combison 100, which was widely used in Europe at that time.

A relatively simple, homemade linear array transducer with a central aperture (▶ Fig. 1.8) was first used by H. H. Holm in 1974 for applications such as amniocentesis. Under favorable conditions, the needle could be identified in the image. In 1976, Pedersen introduced the alternative design of a linear array device with a side-mounted needle guide,[15] which featured an adjustable needle angle (▶ Fig. 1.9). In 1980 Toshiba developed a special biopsy transducer with a triangular needle channel (▶ Fig. 1.10) for its SAL 20 linear array scanner. The

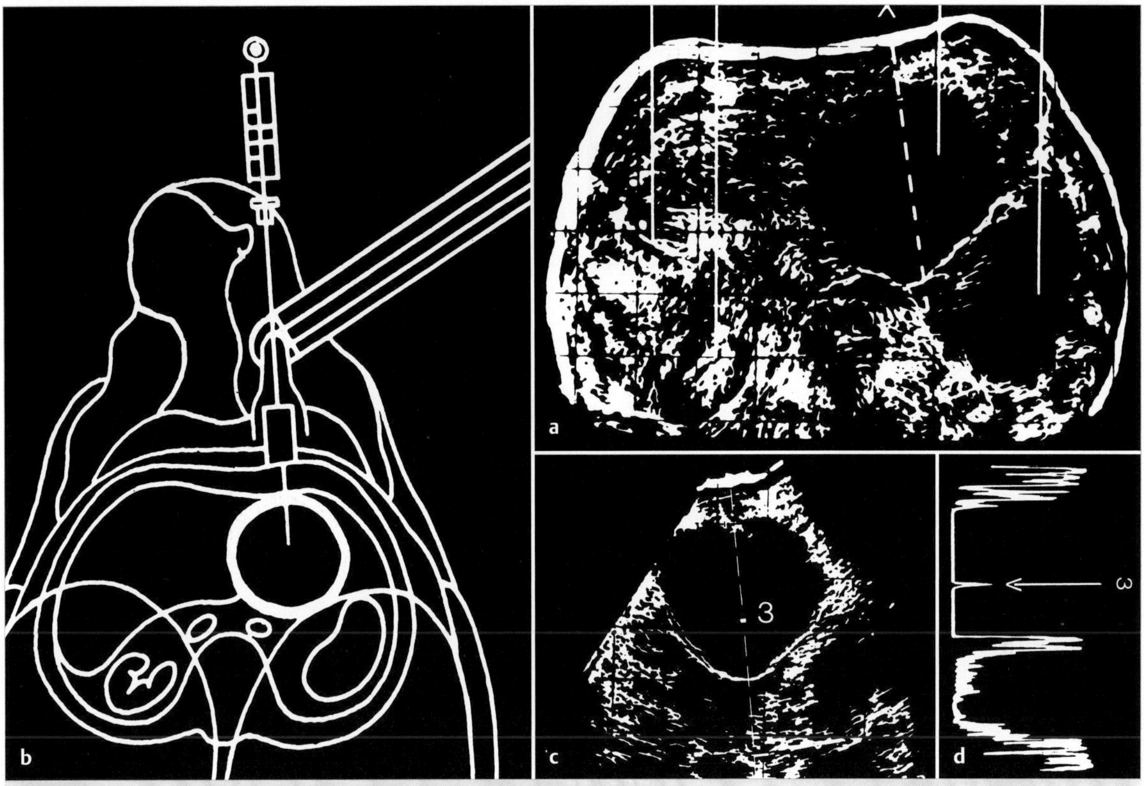

Fig. 1.4 Biopsy technique with a compound scanner.
a The intended target is displayed on a storage cathode-ray tube with a slow B-mode scan.
b The transducer is replaced with a (sterile) biopsy transducer (schematic illustration) (▶ Fig. 1.3).
c The intended target is again visualized in a sector-shaped scan (3 – needle tip).
d Direct observation of the biopsy needle in A-mode (← signal of the needle tip).

channel was open on one side for introducing the needle guide and needle and allowed the needle to be inserted at an oblique angle to the ultrasound beam.[16] This principle was advanced further by the development of disposable, plastic needle guides. The transducer could be placed within a sterile sheath and the sterile needle guide could be introduced from the side. In both systems, the needle path predefined by the needle guide was displayed in the image as an electronic line (▶ Fig. 1.11).

As special biopsy transducers were being developed and used, many examiners continued to use freehand technique for percutaneous biopsies (and many still do so today). This was facilitated by the development of smaller, lighter transducers that could be placed next to the puncture site. The needle could be observed as clearly as with a side-mounted adapter.[17] Freehand technique also simplified hygiene (transducers did not always have to be sterilized or placed in a sterile wrapper), and it was often possible to use shorter, less expensive needles.

Initially, material for cytologic analysis was aspirated from solid tumors with thin (≤0.7 mm), flexible Chiba-type needles using the technique described by Franzen.[18] A special syringe holder (Cameco, Sweden) was often used that allowed aspirations to be performed with one hand. Scandinavian authors in particular reported positive early experience with the cytologic analysis of well-preserved aspirated cells.[19–22] The basic equivalence between aspiration cytology and histologic biopsy had already been demonstrated in earlier studies, such as the study on liver biopsies published by Sheila Sherlock in 1967.[23] Later comparative studies confirmed these initial results, even showing a slight superiority of aspiration cytology with regard to the rate of nondiagnostic biopsies, for example.[24]

As the ultrasound-guided aspiration of solid tumors became more widely practiced, there was also a growing desire to obtain thin-needle core tissue samples for histologic examination. This desire arose mainly from pathologists, who generally preferred to work with histologic material or at least found it easier to identify malignant tumor types from histologic samples. Isler et al subsequently introduced a 22 gauge cutting needle in 1981.[25] The following year a commercially available modification of the Menghini needle called the Surecut needle[26] came into widespread use. The cutting edge at the needle tip excises a tissue core that is retained in the needle lumen by aspiration. Later the Trucut needle was also widely used. This needle slices off the tissue specimen in a side

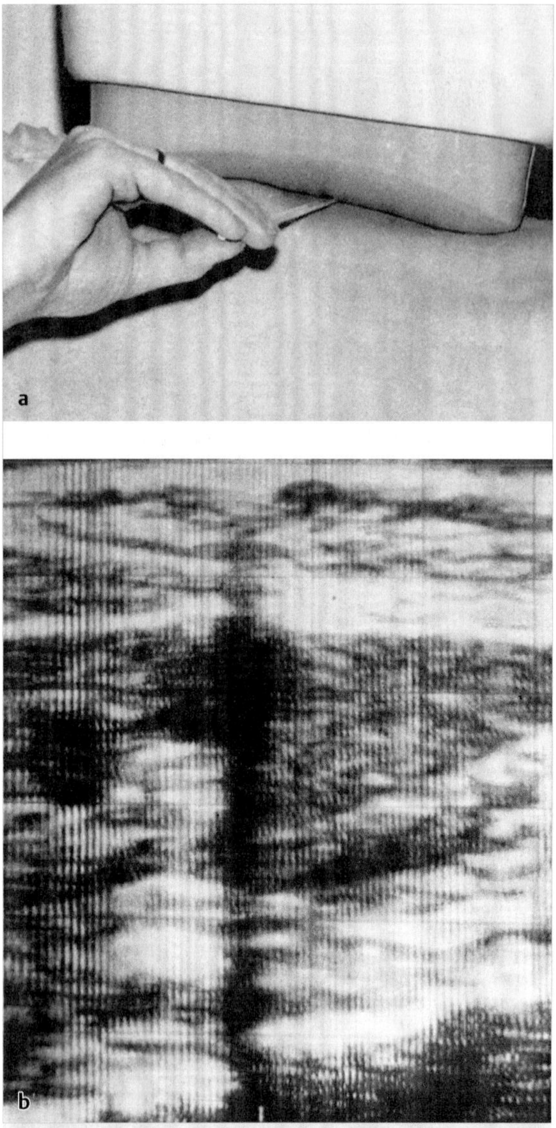

Fig. 1.5 Needle guidance with fast B-mode ultrasound (Siemens Vidoson). A small wooden stick placed between the transducer and skin (a) casts an acoustic shadow (b), which provides orientation in the second plane. The depth from skin to target is measured in the image. (Source: With kind permission from Springer Science + Business Media B.V.[77])

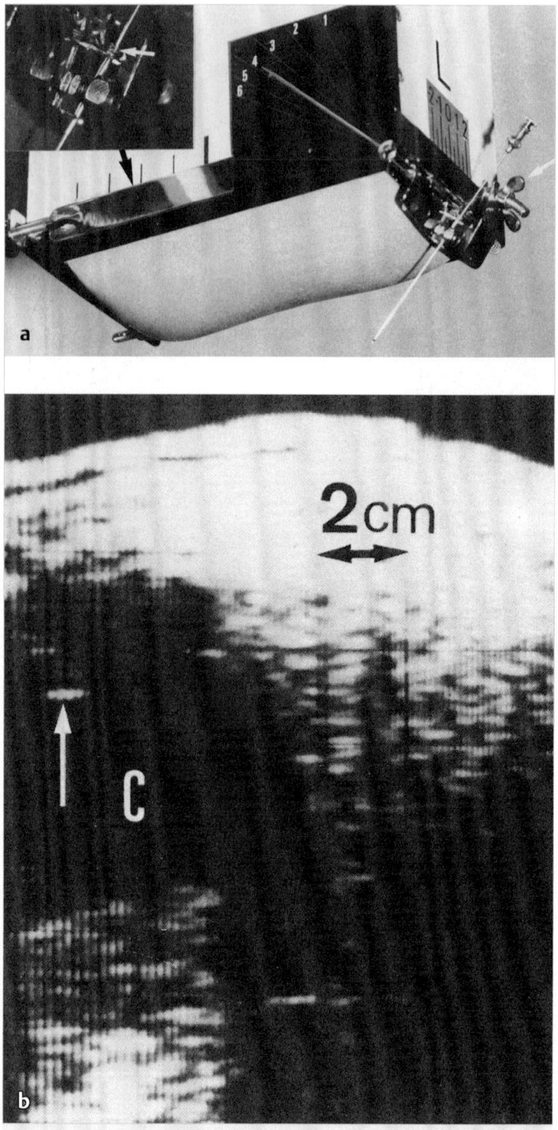

Fig. 1.6
a Vidoson (fast B-mode) with needle guide.
b Needle echo in a renal cyst (↑). (Source: Presented by Afschrift at the World Congress of Ultrasound in San Francisco in 1975. With kind permission from Springer Science + Business Media B.V.[13])

notch, allowing the tissue core to be removed within a sealed chamber. Cutting-needle biopsy was facilitated by the subsequent development of biopsy guns. These spring-loaded devices have an automated cutting action and are set to a specified biopsy depth before firing.

It could be difficult to detect the needle tip in the tissue, especially when a liner-array scanner was used. The ultrasound pulse travels parallel to the needle shaft and is not backscattered by the smooth needle surface, resulting in the absence of a definite tip echo on the screen. This prompted the development of special needles with transverse grooves at the tip. These grooves cause considerable (back)scattering of the sound, analogous to the reflector on a bicycle, giving rise to conspicuous echoes. But these needles were relatively expensive and more traumatizing than needles with a smooth surface. Examiners with good mechanical skills could score the needle tip themselves with a small file, producing a similar effect. Needles with a plastic sheath had better echogenicity but created a higher (frictional) resistance during insertion. Heckemann reported the results of comparative studies on the detectability of different needles in 1982.[27]

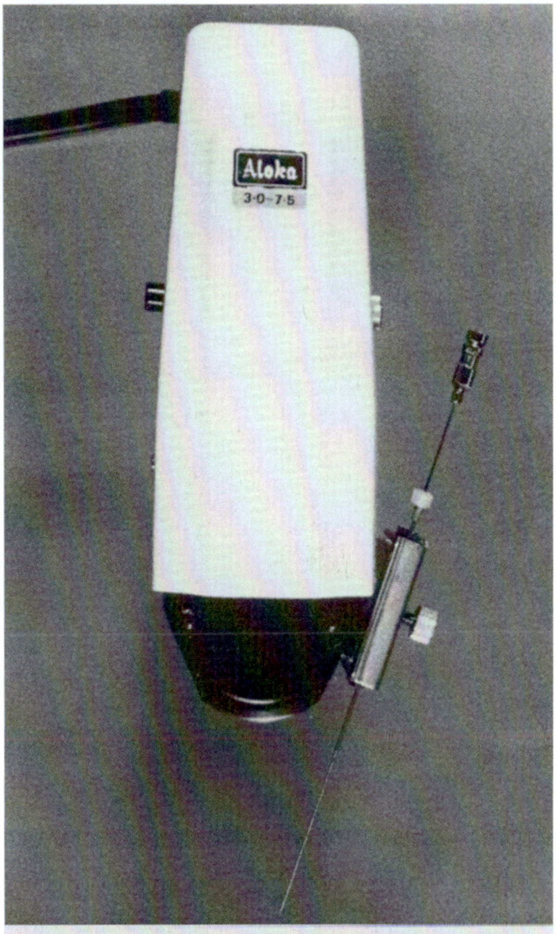

Fig. 1.7 Transducer with side-mounted needle holder and guide manufactured by Aloka. Developed in Japan by Saitho in 1978.[14]

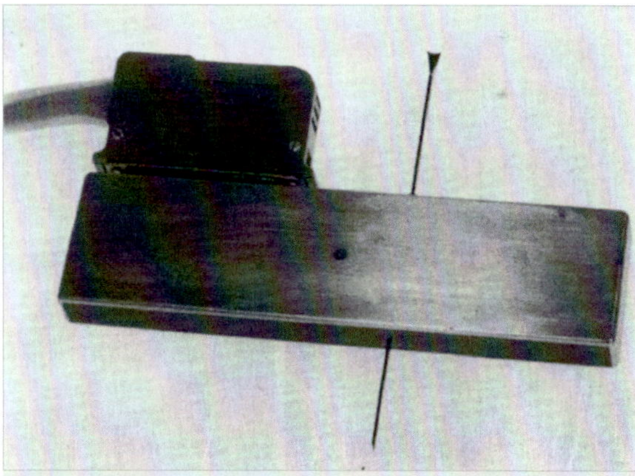

Fig. 1.8 Simple electronic linear array scanner with a central aperture for a biopsy needle, "homemade" in the ultrasound laboratory at Gentofte Hospital (H. H. Holm; first used in 1974).

1.2.3 Clinical Application

The clinical application of ultrasound guided percutaneous biopsies preceded technical developments. In other words, the rapid acceptance and implementation of this simple diagnostic (initially!) technique stimulated the development of special needles, guides, and biopsy transducers, not the other way around. Meanwhile, the expansion of ultrasound-guided biopsies to ever new and smaller target sites was dependent on advances in image quality, i.e., improvements in the resolution of ultrasound scanners.

At first, the organs of greatest interest were the liver and kidneys. Starting in 1972, initial studies based on small case numbers already revealed benefits from the ultrasound-guided fine needle biopsy of suspicious hepatic lesions, with a rate of nondiagnostic biopsies up to 10% and no false-positive results or serious complications.[11,28] Kristensen et al[29] reported on the fine needle biopsy of solid renal tumors in 1972, and Goldberg[30] described the diagnostic aspiration of renal cysts in 1973.

In 1974, Pedersen[31] reported on the ultrasound-guided percutaneous puncture of the (obstructed) renal pelvis for cytologic and microbiologic analysis as well as antegrade pyelography and nephrostomy (▶ Fig. 1.11).

In 1975, Hancke[32] and Smith[33] reported on the fine needle biopsy of suspicious solid pancreatic lesions using a compound scanner with a biopsy transducer. In 1976, Hancke[34] additionally reported on the puncture of pancreatic pseudocysts, initially for diagnostic reasons. This was followed in 1977 by reports from Makuuchi on the puncture of the dilated pancreatic duct (▶ Fig. 1.12) and antegrade cholangiography, followed in each case by radiographic visualization of the duct system.[16,35] Finally, advances in ultrasound equipment and resolution led to scores of reports and case studies up until 1985 dealing with the ultrasound-guided needle biopsy of suspected neoplasms in all abdominal regions.

In the field of cardiology, Goldberg[36] performed the first ultrasound-guided percutaneous aspirations of the pericardial sac as early as 1972. He used the biopsy transducer of the compound scan system with A-mode imaging of pericardial effusions and TM-mode imaging of cardiac pulsations. The fine needle biopsy of peripheral lung lesions under real-time ultrasound guidance was described by Schwerk in 1982.[37]

Ultrasound-guided vascular access for angiographic studies was first attempted with Doppler probes in 1973.[38] Catheter placement in the subclavian vein or internal jugular vein under ultrasound guidance was described in 1975.[39] B-mode image quality was constantly improved and was recommended for vascular localization in later studies.[40]

Ultrasound guidance in obstetrics and gynecology was used primarily to improve the safety of amniocentesis,[41] as was reported at the Vienna Congress. The percutaneous biopsy of gynecologic tumors, on the other hand, was not advocated because of a lack of indications as well as concerns about the intraperitoneal seeding of

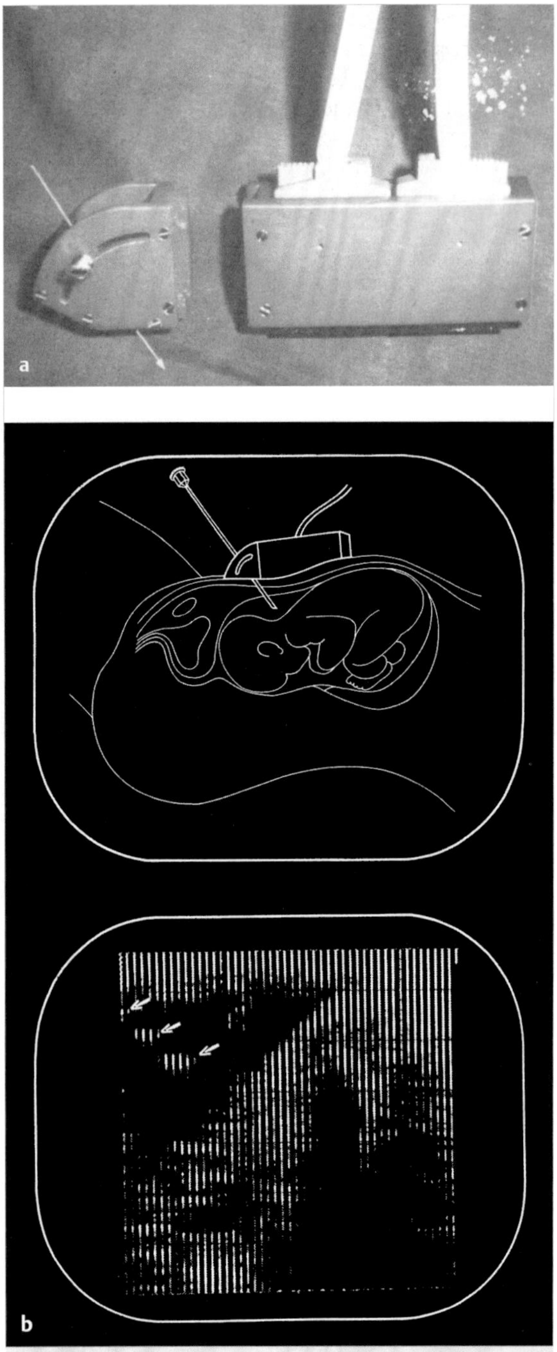

Fig. 1.9
a Electronic linear array scanner with side-mounted needle guide, "homemade" in the ultrasound laboratory at Gentofte Hospital.
b Original image obtained during amniocentesis, and corresponding drawing. The arrows indicate the needle echoes.

tumor cells. Needle biopsies were limited mainly to postoperative settings[42] such as the aspiration biopsy of suspicious retroperitoneal lymph nodes.[43] The ultrasound-guided biopsy of suspicious lesions in the breast was not introduced until after 1990.[44]

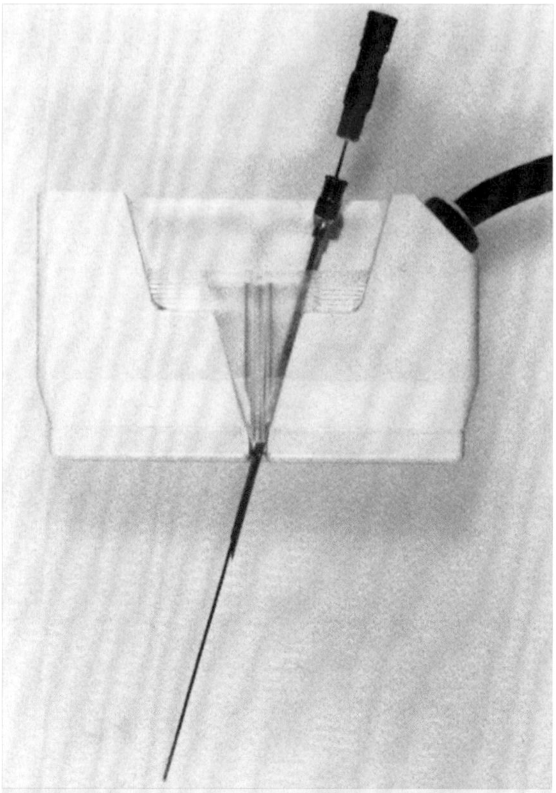

Fig. 1.10 Linear array transducer. Prototype of the Toshiba biopsy transducer made for the SAL 20, first available in 1978.

The "epicenter" at this stage in the development of interventional ultrasound was the ultrasound laboratory of Gentofte Hospital (later Herlev Hospital) in Copenhagen, Denmark, directed by H. H. Holm. Starting in 1978, this hospital began to host a series of international conferences on interventional ultrasound. Holm and Kristensen published their first book on ultrasound-guided

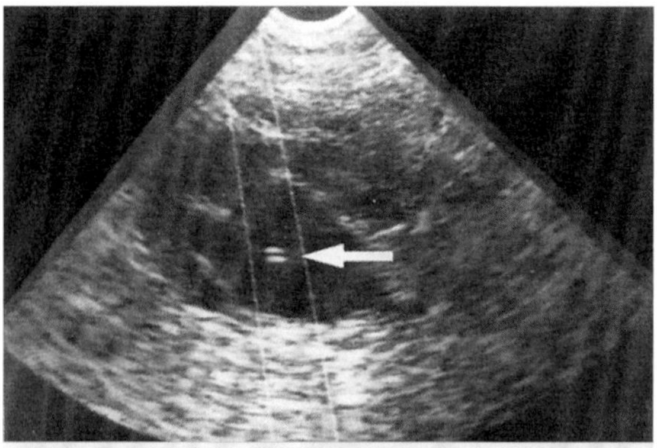

Fig. 1.11 Nephropyelostomy performed with a mechanical sector scanner and lateral needle guide. The needle path is marked electronically in the image. The needle tip (←) is clearly visible inside the cyst.

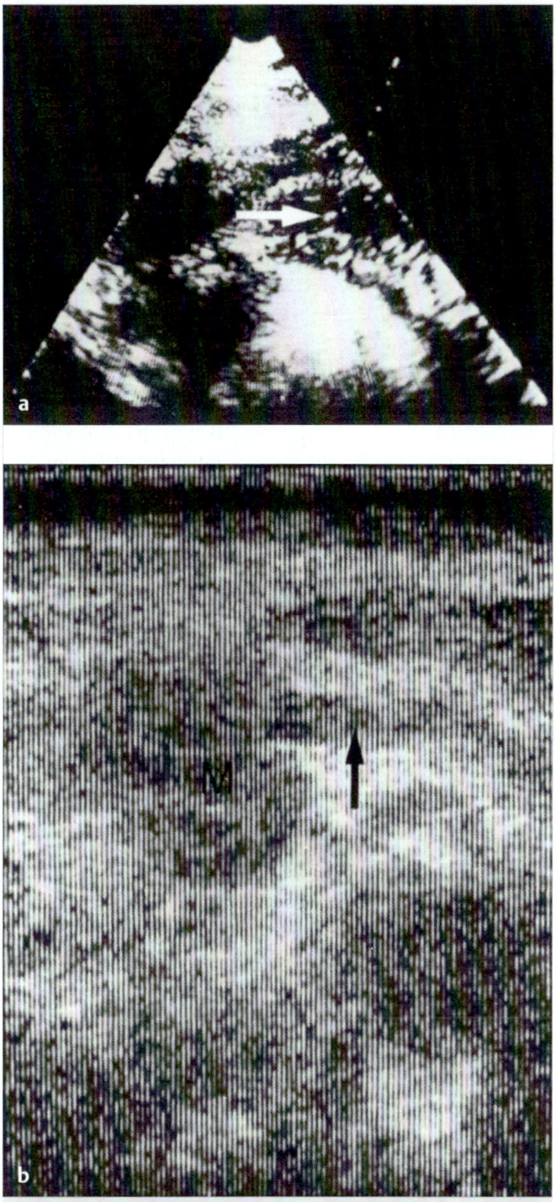

Fig. 1.12 Ultrasound-guided puncture of the dilated pancreatic duct in the presence of a pancreatic head tumor.
a Appearance of the needle tip in a compound scan.
b Real-time image with an electronic linear-array transducer (like that shown in ▶ Fig. 1.10). Note the discrepancy between equipment quality at that time and the availability of highly differentiated puncture techniques.

needle procedures in 1980. This was followed in 1985 by the book *Interventional Ultrasound*,[8] which reviews the development of interventional ultrasound during the 15 years after the Vienna Congress. This does not mean that important studies and discoveries were not made at many other centers and by many other clinicians. On the contrary, this branch of diagnostic ultrasound had what may be called a "multicentric" development. Interventional ultrasound was practiced very widely in German-speaking countries after about 1980, and some authors were able to report their experience in very large case numbers.[45] Ultrasound-guided needle biopsies were very often regarded as and performed as an integral component in the ultrasound investigation of suspected tumors, comparable to forceps biopsies in endoscopic examinations. It should be noted, however, that a biopsy turns a noninvasive ultrasound examination into an invasive procedure with associated risks that, while small, must still be taken into consideration.

1.2.4 Risks of Interventional Ultrasound

The risks of percutaneous biopsies were known and had been described in principle even before the age of interventional ultrasound.[46] Today they are still an important consideration in the development and practice of interventional sonography.

While initial studies showed no serious side effects associated with the use of needles less than 1 mm in diameter, publications over the years documented repeated instances of serious complications and even deaths, mostly in individual case reports.[47,48] Significant hemorrhages and bile leaks were described in association with liver biopsies, necrotizing pancreatitis after pancreatic biopsies, and the inadvertent transfer of infectious material leading to sepsis. Subsequent doctor surveys and reviews of the literature indicated a mortality rate between 0.001% and 0.096% with complication rates up to 0.9%.[47–52]

The risk of seeding tumor cells into the needle tract is a potentially serious problem. Reports of inoculation metastases from various tumors were published even before the era of ultrasound-guided biopsies.[47,48,50] As a precaution against needle-track seeding, Holm recommended introducing the actual biopsy needle through an outer needle that had been advanced to the biopsy site or target organ. A guide needle was also used for multiple sampling.[8] Holm believed that the Trucut needle was advantageous in this regard because it "sealed off" the tissue core prior to needle extraction. While some isolated case reports were published and analyzed in detail,[47] statistical data from very large case numbers indicated a risk of inoculation metastasis of less than 0.017%. Despite these low numbers, the debate on needle-tract seeding continued to be (and remains) controversial and emotionally charged. Grundmann was the first author, in 1979, to take a stand on this issue in the journal *Deutsches Ärzteblatt*,[53] and one year later the scientific advisory board of the Association of German Physicians issued a formal statement affirming that needle biopsies do not promote the spread of tumor cells.[54]

1.3 Later Developments: Ultrasound-Guided Therapeutic Interventional Procedures

By the mid-1980s, or about the time H. H. Holm published his book, ultrasound-guided needle biopsies had become an accepted and widely used method for establishing a rapid, definitive diagnosis at low risk.[8] New target sites were being added as the resolution of ultrasound images improved. The debate regarding cytologic versus histologic biopsy was continued in large clinical series,[55] with neither method showing a definite superiority. Discussions on the risk of needle-track seeding also continued.

Ambitious technical innovations such as superimposing a magnetic field over the B-mode image to allow "live" tracking of needle position or mounting an ultrasound transmitter on the needle tip were presented but were not widely adopted.

An important innovation, however, was the development of biopsy devices that could be used in conjunction with endosonography, which was being practiced on a growing scale. One of the first endosonographic techniques was transrectal imaging of the prostate. Ultrasound guidance enabled the prostate to be biopsied percutaneously by the transperitoneal route.[56] But flexible endoscopic ultrasound like that used in the digestive tract required biopsy needles that were integrated into the endoscope, and this technology was available by about 1990.

This later phase was marked by the development of therapeutic interventions, with Italian authors playing a leading role, especially in the treatment of solid tumors. In truth, therapeutic measures were already a part of interventional ultrasound from the beginning. For example, ultrasound-guided amniocentesis provided a safe means for performing intrauterine transfusions, first described by Hansmann in 1972,[57] using real-time imaging guidance. This in turn laid the groundwork for further advances in interventional intrauterine therapy.

From the outset, ultrasound-guided needles were used not only to detect and evaluate fluid collections but also, where necessary, to evacuate the fluid. Ultrasound guidance facilitated the percutaneous therapeutic aspiration of simple fluid collections such as ascites or pleural effusions and was sometimes an essential tool, as in cases complicated by adhesions. The "therapeutic" value of ultrasound guidance was already recognized during the early 1970s when applied to pericardiocentesis,[36] nephropyelotomy,[31] and the drainage of postoperative fluid collections such as lymphoceles.[58] Percutaneous cholangiography could also be followed by ultrasound-guided drainage if required.[35]

The diagnostic aspiration of intra-abdominal abscesses proved to be a low-risk procedure, like fine needle biopsies in general. It was a logical next step to evacuate and irrigate the abscess through the needle as a one-time procedure or to establish percutaneous catheter drainage, generally using Seldinger technique.[59–62] The biggest challenge circa 1974 lay in convincing surgical colleagues that these procedures were safe and effective.

In the early years of interventional ultrasound, the fine needle aspiration of cysts was still done for diagnostic reasons in selected cases to positively exclude a malignancy or confirm an abscess. Again, frequent efforts were also made to apply the procedure therapeutically. This was successfully accomplished in selected patients with pancreatic pseudocysts.[34] Often the pseudocysts still communicated with the duct system and tended to recur after evacuation. This led Hancke to develop a procedure for the internal gastric drainage of pancreatic pseudocysts by combining an ultrasound-guided percutaneous gastrostomy with gastroscopy. He published this technique in 1985.[63] At about the same time, a special percutaneous technique for the treatment of echinococcal cysts began to be developed in Tunisia and Italy.[64,65] After preliminary testing in sheep, the treatment, known by the acronym PAIR (puncture–aspiration–injection of alcohol–reaspiration), was finally incorporated into WHO guidelines for the treatment of cystic echinococcosis in 1996.[66]

Attempts to treat cysts definitively by a single aspiration were usually disappointing since a defining feature of cysts is the presence of a secretory epithelial lining. This suggested the idea of obliterating the epithelium with concentrated alcohol or other sclerosing agents. Reports on this treatment were first published in 1981 for renal cysts[67] and in 1989 for hepatic cysts.[68,69]

Solbiati reported in 1985 on the successful obliteration of enlarged parathyroid glands in secondary hyperparathyroidism by percutaneous ethanol injection (PEI).[70] This technique was later applied in the treatment of toxic thyroid nodules.[71,72]

Livraghi began to treat hepatocellular carcinomas and metastases by PEI in 1986[73] and by 1995 was able to report long-term results in 746 patients.[74] Buscarini and his group first reported on the percutaneous radiofrequency thermoablation (RFA) of liver tumors in 1991[75] and published long-term results in 2001.[76] Since that time, these treatment modalities have been adopted at many tumor centers and are also being tried on malignancies in other organs.

1.4 Outlook

The development of ultrasound-guided therapeutic interventions is not yet complete by any means. Positive experiences with guided needle placements for administering local anesthetics, as in carpal tunnel syndrome and other orthopedic problems, are but one example of this trend.

Fine needle aspirations and biopsies have become a well-established tool in the diagnostic armamentarium of many specialties. The statement by H. H. Holm quoted earlier in this chapter is still true today. Even at its current level of quality, diagnostic ultrasound cannot replace a microscopic tissue analysis because an ultrasound image simply maps the acoustic properties of tissues. On the other hand, given the remarkable development of the modality itself, it may be possible in some cases to determine the malignant or benign nature of an organ lesion within the clinical context by close scrutiny of the B-mode image, a color Doppler assessment of vascular architecture, dynamic flow analysis with contrast-enhanced ultrasound, and tissue strain analysis by elastography. This approach may eliminate the need for an invasive puncture, despite its minimal risks, in growing numbers of patients. Today it is unclear whether and to what extent the guided application of micro bubbles targeted to specific markers can complement or even replace ultrasound-guided punctures.

References

[1] Kratochwil A, Lim-Rachmat F. Ultraschallplazentalokalisation. In: Böck J, Ossoinig K, eds. Ultrasonographia Medica. Vol. III. Vienna: Verlag der Wiener Medizinischen Akademie; 1969:275–284

[2] Blauenstein W, Engelhart GJ, Müller HR. Sonographie und stereotaktische Biopsie von Lebertumoren. In: Böck J, Ossoinig K, eds. Ultrasonographia Medica. Vol. III. Vienna: Verlag der Wiener Medizinischen Akademie; 1969:93–99

[3] Menghini G. One-second needle biopsy of the liver. Gastroenterology 1958; 35: 190–199

[4] Berlyne GM. Ultrasonics in renal biopsy: an aid to determination of kidney position. Lancet 1961; 2: 750–751 (preliminary communication)

[5] Rettenmaier G. Tiefenortung der Niere und Bestimmung der Parenchymstärke mit einem Ultraschall-schnittbildverfahren vor der perkutanen Nierenbiopsie. In: Otto P, ed. Fortschritte auf dem Gebiet der Röntgenstrahlen und der Nuklearmedizin. Stuttgart: Thieme; 1970:76–77

[6] Martin HE, Ellis EB. Biopsy by needle puncture and aspiration. Ann Surg 1930; 92: 169–181

[7] Krause W, Soldner R. Ultraschallbildverfahren (B-scan) mit hoher Bildfrequenz für medizinische Diagnostik. Electro-medica 1967; 4: 8–12

[8] Holm HH, Kristensen JK, eds. Interventional Ultrasound. Copenhagen: Munksgaard; 1985

[9] Goldberg BB, Pollack HM. Ultrasonic aspiration transducer. Radiology 1972; 102: 187–189

[10] Holm HH, Kristensen JK, Rasmussen SN, Northeved A, Barlebo H. Ultrasound as a guide in percutaneous puncture technique. Ultrasonics 1972; 10: 83–86

[11] Lutz H, Weidenhiller S, Rettenmaier G. Ultrasonically guided fine-needle biopsy of the liver [Article in German]. Schweiz Med Wochenschr 1973; 103: 1030–1033

[12] Soldner R. Personal communication

[13] Afschrift M, Colardyn F, Verdonk G. Ultrasonic guidance of percutaneous punctures by means of real time echography. In: White D, Brown RE, eds. Ultrasound in Medicine. 3rd ed. New York: Plenum; 1977:363–370

[14] Saitoh M, Watanabe H, Oho H, Tanaka S, Itakura Y, Date S. Ultrasonic real-time guidance for percutaneous puncture. J Clin Ultrasound 1979; 7: 269–272

[15] Pedersen JF. Percutaneous puncture guided by ultrasonic multitransducer scanning. J Clin Ultrasound 1977; 5: 175–177

[16] Makuuchi M, Bandai Y, Ito T, Wada T. Ultrasonically guided percutaneous transhepatic cholangiography and percutaneous pancreatography. Radiology 1980; 134: 767–772

[17] Jakobeit C. Ultrasound-controlled puncture procedures: free-hand puncture versus transducer biopsy puncture. 5 years' experience [Article in German]. Ultraschall Med 1986; 7: 290–292

[18] Franzén S, Giertz G, Zajicek J. Cytological diagnosis of prostatic tumours by transrectal aspiration biopsy: a preliminary report. Br J Urol 1960; 32: 193–196

[19] Conn HO, Yesner R. A re-evaluation of needle biopsy in the diagnosis of metastatic cancer of the liver. Ann Intern Med 1963; 59: 53–61

[20] Esposti PL, Franzén S, Zajicek J. The aspiration biopsy smear. In: Koss G, ed. Diagnostic Cytology and Its Histopathologic Basis. 2nd ed. Philadelphia: JB Lippincott; 1968

[21] Lundquist A. Fine-needle aspiration biopsy for cytodiagnosis of malignant tumour in the liver. Acta Med Scand 1970; 188: 465–470

[22] Soderstrom N. Fine Needle Aspiration Biopsy. Orlando: Grune & Stratton; 1966

[23] Sherlock P, Kim YS, Koss LG. Cytologic diagnosis of cancer from aspirated material obtained at liver biopsy. Am J Dig Dis 1967; 12: 396–402

[24] Torp-Pedersen S, Vyberg M, Juul N, Sehested M. Fine needle histological sampling. In: Holm HH, Kristensen JK, eds. Interventional Ultrasound. Copenhagen: Munksgaard; 1985

[25] Isler RJ, Ferrucci JT, Jr, Wittenberg J et al. Tissue core biopsy of abdominal tumors with a 22 gauge cutting needle. AJR Am J Roentgenol 1981; 136: 725–728

[26] Torp-Pedersen S, Juul N, Vyberg M. Histological sampling with a 23 gauge modified Menghini needle. Br J Radiol 1984; 57: 151–154

[27] Heckemann R, Seidel KJ. In vitro and in vivo imaging of puncture instruments in the real-time ultrasound image. 1. Puncture needles [Article in German]. Ultraschall Med 1982; 3: 18–23

[28] Rasmussen SN, Holm HH, Kristensen JK, Barlebo H. Ultrasonically-guided liver biopsy. BMJ 1972; 2: 500–502

[29] Kristensen JK, Holm HH, Rasmussen SN, Barlebo H. Ultrasonically guided percutaneous puncture of renal masses. Scand J Urol Nephrol 1972; 6: 49–56

[30] Goldberg BB, Pollack HM. Ultrasonically guided renal cyst aspiration. J Urol 1973; 109: 5–7

[31] Pedersen JF. Percutaneous nephrostomy guided by ultrasound. J Urol 1974; 112: 157–159

[32] Hancke S, Holm HH, Koch F. Ultrasonically guided percutaneous fine needle biopsy of the pancreas. Surg Gynecol Obstet 1975; 140: 361–364

[33] Smith EH, Bartrum RJ, Jr, Chang YC et al. Percutaneous aspiration biopsy of the pancreas under ultrasonic guidance. N Engl J Med 1975; 292: 825–828

[34] Hancke S, Pedersen JF. Percutaneous puncture of pancreatic cysts guided by ultrasound. Surg Gynecol Obstet 1976; 142: 551–552

[35] Makuuchi M, Kamiya K, Beppu T. Percutaneous transhepatic cholangiography under ultrasonic guidance. Acta Hepat Jpn 1977; 18: 435–440

[36] Goldberg BB, Pollack HM. Ultrasonically guided pericardiocentesis. Am J Cardiol 1973; 31: 490–493

[37] Schwerk WB, Dombrowski H, Kalbfleisch H. Ultrasound tomography and guided fine needle biopsy of intrathoracic space occupying lesions [Article in German]. Ultraschall Med 1982; 3: 212–218

[38] Mozersky DJ, Olson RM, Coons HG, Hagood CO, Jr. Doppler-controlled needle director: a useful adjunct to angiography. Radiology 1973; 109: 221–222

[39] Petzoldt R, Kresse H. Punktion von Venen und Arterien mittels Ultraschall. Biomedizinische Technik 1975; 20: 345–346

[40] Metz S, Horrow JC, Balcar I. A controlled comparison of techniques for locating the internal jugular vein using ultrasonography. Anesth Analg 1984; 63: 673–679

[41] Bang J, Northeved A. A new ultrasonic method for transabdominal amniocentesis. Am J Obstet Gynecol 1972; 114: 599–601

[42] Jensen F. Puncture of gynecological masses. In: Holm HH, Kristensen JK, eds. Interventional Ultrasound. Copenhagen: Munksgaard; 1985

[43] Berkowitz RS, Leavitt T, Jr, Knapp RC. Ultrasound-directed percutaneous aspiration biopsy of periaortic lymph nodes in recurrence of cervical carcinoma. Am J Obstet Gynecol 1978; 131: 906–908
[44] Parker SH, Jobe WE, Dennis MA et al. US-guided automated large-core breast biopsy. Radiology 1993; 187: 507–511
[45] Otto R. Ultraschallgeführte Biopsie. Berlin: Springer; 1985
[46] Lindner H. Limitations and hazards of percutaneous liver biopsy with the Menghini needle. Experiences with 80,000 liver biopsies [Article in German]. Dtsch Med Wochenschr 1967; 92: 1751–1757
[47] Buscarini E, Di Stasi M. Complications of Abdominal Interventional Ultrasound. Milan: Poletto Edizione; 1996
[48] Smith EH. Fine-needle aspiration biopsy: are there any risks? In: Holm HH, Kristensen JK, eds. Copenhagen: Munksgaard; 1985
[49] Gebel M, Horstkotte H, Köster C, Brunkhorst R, Brandt M, Atay Z. Ultrasound-guided fine needle puncture of the abdominal organs: indications, results, risks [Article in German]. Ultraschall Med 1986; 7: 198–202
[50] Livraghi T, Damascelli B, Lombardi C, Spagnoli I. Risk in fine-needle abdominal biopsy. J Clin Ultrasound 1983; 11: 77–81
[51] Weiss H, Düntsch U, Weiss A. Risks of fine needle puncture—results of a survey in West Germany (German Society of Ultrasound in Medicine survey) [Article in German]. Ultraschall Med 1988; 9: 121–127
[52] Weiss H, Düntsch U. Complications of fine needle puncture. DEGUM survey II [Article in German]. Ultraschall Med 1996; 17: 118–130
[53] Grundmann E. Keine Metastasenförderung durch Biopsien. Dtsch Arzteblatt 1979; 7; 9: 699–702
[54] Wissenschaftlicher Beirat der Bundesärztekammer. Metastasenförderung durch diagnostische Gewebsentnahme (Biopsie)? Dtsch Arztebl 1980; 22: 1460–1467
[55] Buscarini L, Fornari F, Bolondi L et al. Ultrasound-guided fine-needle biopsy of focal liver lesions: techniques, diagnostic accuracy and complications. A retrospective study on 2091 biopsies. J Hepatol 1990; 11: 344–348
[56] Holm HH, Gammelgaard J. Ultrasonically guided precise needle placement in the prostate and the seminal vesicles. J Urol 1981; 125: 385–387
[57] Hansmann M, Lang N. Intrauterine transfusion controlled by ultrasound [Article in German]. Klin Wochenschr 1972; 50: 930–932
[58] Spigos D, Capek V. Ultrasonically guided percutaneous aspiration of lymphoceles following renal transplantation: a diagnostic and therapeutic method. J Clin Ultrasound 1976; 4: 45–46
[59] Braun B, Dormeyer HH. Ultrasonically guided fine needle aspiration biopsy of hepatic and pancreatic space-occupying lesions and percutaneous abscess drainage. Klin Wochenschr 1981; 59: 707–712
[60] Grønvall S, Gammelgaard J, Haubek A, Holm HH. Drainage of abdominal abscesses guided by sonography. AJR Am J Roentgenol 1982; 138: 527–529
[61] Smith EH, Bartrum RJ, Jr. Ultrasonically guided percutaneous aspiration of abscesses. Am J Roentgenol Radium Ther Nucl Med 1974; 122: 308–312
[62] vanSonnenberg E, Mueller PR, Ferrucci JT, Jr. Percutaneous drainage of 250 abdominal abscesses and fluid collections. Part I: Results, failures, and complications. Radiology 1984; 151: 337–341
[63] Hancke S, Henriksen FW. Percutaneous pancreatic cystogastrostomy guided by ultrasound scanning and gastroscopy. Br J Surg 1985; 72: 916–917
[64] Ben Amor N, Gargouri M, Gharbi HA, Golvan YJ, Ayachi K, Kchouck H. Trial therapy of inoperable abdominal hydatid cysts by puncture [Article in German]. Ann Parasitol Hum Comp 1986; 61: 689–692
[65] Filice C, Pirola F, Brunetti E, Dughetti S, Strosselli M, Foglieni CS. A new therapeutic approach for hydatid liver cysts. Aspiration and alcohol injection under sonographic guidance. Gastroenterology 1990; 98: 1366–1368
[66] WHO informal Working Group on Echinococcosis. Guidelines for treatment of cystic and alveolar echinococcosis in humans. Bull World Health Organ 1996; 74: 213–242
[67] Bean WJ. Renal cysts: treatment with alcohol. Radiology 1981; 138: 329–331
[68] Andersson R, Jeppsson B, Lunderquist A, Bengmark S. Alcohol sclerotherapy of non-parasitic cysts of the liver. Br J Surg 1989; 76: 254–255
[69] vanSonnenberg E, Wroblicka JT, D'Agostino HB et al. Symptomatic hepatic cysts: percutaneous drainage and sclerosis. Radiology 1994; 190: 387–392
[70] Solbiati L, Giangrande A, De Pra L, Bellotti E, Cantù P, Ravetto C. Percutaneous ethanol injection of parathyroid tumors under US guidance: treatment for secondary hyperparathyroidism. Radiology 1985; 155: 607–610
[71] Braun B, Blank W. Color Doppler sonography-guided percutaneous alcohol instillation in the therapy of functionally autonomous thyroid nodules [Article in German]. Dtsch Med Wochenschr 1994; 119: 1607–1612
[72] Livraghi T, Paracchi A, Ferrari C et al. Treatment of autonomous thyroid nodules with percutaneous ethanol injection: preliminary results. Work in progress. Radiology 1990; 175: 827–829
[73] Livraghi T, Festi D, Monti F, Salmi A, Vettori C. US-guided percutaneous alcohol injection of small hepatic and abdominal tumors. Radiology 1986; 161: 309–312
[74] Livraghi T, Giorgio A, Marin G et al. Hepatocellular carcinoma and cirrhosis in 746 patients: long-term results of percutaneous ethanol injection. Radiology 1995; 197: 101–108
[75] Buscarini L, Fornari F. Rossi P. Interstitial radiofrequency hyperthermia in the treatment of small hepatocellular carcinoma: percutaneous sonography-guidance of electrode needle. In: Anderegg A, Despland PA, Otto R, Henner H, eds. Ultraschall Diagnostik 1992;91:218–222
[76] Buscarini L, Buscarini E, Di Stasi M, Vallisa D, Quaretti P, Rocca A. Percutaneous radiofrequency ablation of small hepatocellular carcinoma: long-term results. Eur Radiol 2001; 11: 914–921
[77] Lutz H. Ultraschalldiagnostik (B-scan) in der Inneren Medizin. Berlin, Heidelberg, New York: Springer; 1978

2 Interventional Materials and Equipment

2.1 General Considerations on Interventional Procedures

U. Gottschalk, C. F. Dietrich

2.1.1 Brief Historical Introduction

Ultrasound-guided interventional procedures may be performed for diagnostic as well as therapeutic reasons. The goal of diagnostic procedures is to collect tissue or fluid samples for analysis, using percutaneous needles of various sizes and designs. One drawback of using large-caliber needle systems was already noted in an article published over 60 years ago[1]: "When we consider that percutaneous drainage rates need to be limited, it is pointless to use very large needles or trocars since the outflow must often be interrupted by clamping the tube so that fluid is not evacuated too rapidly." In the age before adequate imaging techniques were available, necessary drain size could usually be determined only by percutaneous aspiration, prompting an early policy statement that percutaneous drainage should never be attempted without prior needle aspiration.[2] An empyema, for example, required the placement of a drain approximately 15 to 20 mm in diameter. Milestones in the development of biopsy techniques are summarized in ▶ Table 2.1.

2.1.2 Biopsy Principles and Techniques

Freehand Biopsy, Needle Guide Attachments, and Biopsy Transducers

The most widely practiced ultrasound-guided biopsy techniques are a "blind" biopsy performed at a marked skin site after ultrasound localization, the freehand technique with one hand holding the transducer and the other guiding the needle, and the use of a needle guide or special biopsy transducer (▶ Table 2.2).

In the freehand technique, the needle is guided freely by the operator's hand. The challenge is to keep the needle at a proper angle to the imaging plane so that it is visible at all times. The main advantage of this technique is its flexibility. This makes it easier, for example, to interpose a

Table 2.1 Milestones in the development of biopsy techniques

Year	Procedure	Localization	First describer	Source
1851	Percutaneous tumor biopsy	Palpation, percussion	Lebert	3
1853	Breast tumor biopsy	Palpation, percussion	Paget	4
1883	Lung biopsy, identify infecting organism in pneumonia	Palpation, percussion	Leyerden	5
1883	Liver biopsy	Palpation, percussion	Ehrlich	6,7
1925	Special technique for fine needle biopsy	Palpation, percussion	Martin, Ellis	8
1930/1931	Bone marrow aspiration and biopsy	Palpation, percussion	Martin, Coley	9
1935	Vertebral body needle biopsy	Palpation, percussion	Robertson, Ball	10
1939	Lung tumor biopsy	Radiography	Blady	11
1951	Percutaneous pancreatic biopsy	Radiography	Kistland	12
1952	Thyroid biopsy	Palpation	Söderström	13
1952	Percutaneous renal biopsy	Radiography	Lindblom	14
1958	One-second liver biopsy	Percussion	Menghini	15
1967/1977	Lymph node biopsy, transperitoneal	Radiographic guidance	Nordenström, Zornoza	16
1972	Percutaneous liver biopsy	Ultrasound	Rasmusen	14
1975	Percutaneous pancreatic biopsy	Ultrasound	Hancke	16

Table 2.2 Comparison of different biopsy techniques

Technique	Advantage	Disadvantage
Freehand	Flexible angles, free guidance	Needle may move out of the image plane
Needle guide	Routine transducer can be used Better targeting Good needle tip visualization	Needle may deviate from desired biopsy path Longer pathway through the tissue Blind spot in the first 2–4 cm
Biopsy transducer	Short path to target	Needle tip may be more difficult to see because it is parallel to the ultrasound beam and cannot reflect sound waves Local infiltration anesthesia may obscure vision

sufficient rim of normal liver tissue between a superficial lesion and the liver capsule to minimize bleeding. Using a side-mounted needle guide has the advantage of providing the same image quality as without a biopsy attachment. Most guides are adjustable to two different needle angles (▶ Fig. 2.1, ▶ Fig. 2.2). Biopsy can be performed from the right and left sides by rotating the display.

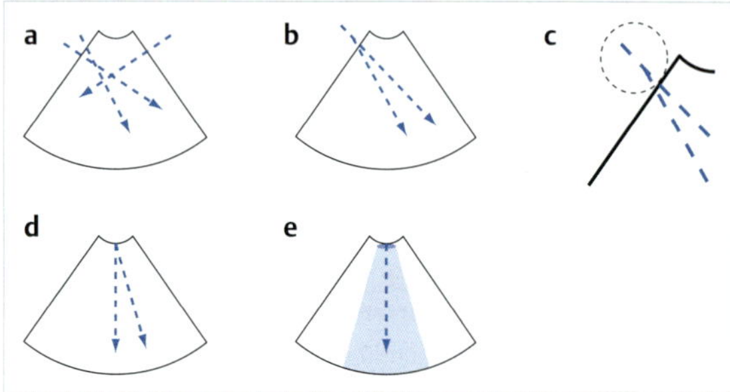

Fig. 2.1 Biopsy techniques.
a Freehand technique allows for multiple, variable needle paths.
b A separate needle guide mounted on the transducer can usually be adjusted for several angles of needle insertion.
c The first 2–4 cm cannot be visualized with this technique.
d The needle is introduced through a biopsy transducer.
e Visualization may sometimes be obscured by local infiltration anesthesia. (Source: reference[17].)

Biopsy Transducers

With a biopsy transducer, the needle can be introduced through the transducer at various angles by means of a sterilizable insert. Usually the insert has channels that determine the angle of needle insertion, and the prospective needle path is displayed as a virtual line on the ultrasound screen. This line can also be displayed with transducers that have a screw-on biopsy attachment. In this case the angle of insertion is defined by a stop on the needle guide. Only the biopsy inserts or detachable

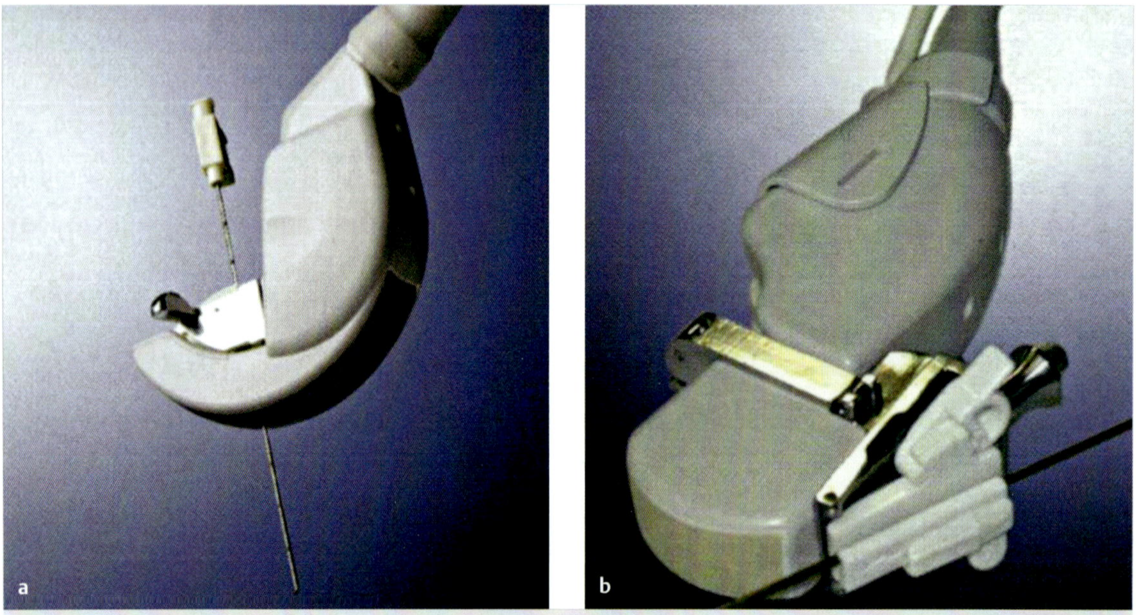

Fig. 2.2 Devices manufactured by Hitachi.
a Biopsy transducer.
b Ultrasound transducer with a detachable needle guide. (Source: reference[17].)

Table 2.3 Biopsy transducers produced by Hitachi Medical Systems, Wiesbaden, Germany (examples).

Designation	Frequency range	THI and CHI	Remarks
EUP B514	2–5 MHz	Yes	Needle is inserted through a sterilizable insert in a normal-size convex transducer
EUP B512	2–5 MHz	Yes	Sterilizable needle guide attaches externally to a small-footprint convex transducer

Abbreviations: THI, tissue harmonic imaging. CHI, contrast harmonic imaging.

needle guides require sterilization. The advantage of using a biopsy transducer with an integrated guide channel is that it permits accurate needle monitoring even with a limited acoustic window or long biopsy path. One disadvantage is a slight loss of image resolution in the area of the biopsy insert, which is devoid of piezoelectric crystals. A side-mounted needle guide creates a superficial blind spot, making it more difficult to sample lesions close to the transducer. This is not a problem in practice, however, because high-frequency transducers are usually used for superficial lesions and the needle can be guided without difficulty owing to the short pathway next to the probe. Since high-performance transducers are expensive, most biopsy transducers are offered in the low-frequency range (▶ Table 2.3).

2.1.3 Needle Systems

Needle Technology

Biopsy needles have a sharp, beveled tip that cuts the tissue when the needle is advanced. They enter the body more easily than a sharp-pointed needle without a cutting edge, which would damage the tissue and cause considerably more pain. Needles with an outer diameter < 1 mm are classified as "fine" needles; larger-caliber needles with an outer diameter of 1 mm or more are classified as "coarse."[18] Biopsy needles are manufactured from medically approved stainless steel alloys composed of iron, chromium, nickel, molybdenum, or manganese that are resistant to corrosion, acids, and alkalis. Chromium (at least 13%) imparts rust resistance, while nickel makes the alloy resistant to acids. For example, the designation chromium–nickel steel 18/10 means that the alloy consists of 18% chromium, 10% nickel, and 72% steel. Some needles are also coated to make their insertion as painless as possible. Silicone is often used as a biocompatible coating material. The increasing use of magnetic resonance imaging (MRI) has prompted the development of compatible needles made of carbon-fiber–reinforced plastics. These needles have the high stiffness of the composite material, a high strain to fracture, and excellent chemical stability. Current needles of this type are up to 20 cm long and are typically 1.2 mm in diameter. They are stiffer and stronger than metallic needles. A triple-lumen needle with an outer diameter of 1.2 mm and a biocompatible surface coating may contain three working channels with inner diameters of, say, 272 µm, 312 µm, and 612 µm.

Various systems are available for designating needle size. Needle diameters are most often stated in terms of millimeters or gauge. Other options are the Pravaz system (Gr) introduced by the French orthopedist Charles G. Pravaz (1791–1853) and the Charrière (Ch) or French (F) systems. The most popular unit for designating outer needle diameter is gauge, which is based on the America Wire Gauge (AWG) system. It was originally used to designate wire thickness and indicated the number of drawing operations needed to reduce a wire to the desired diameter (▶ Table 2.4). Thus, the higher the gauge number, the

Table 2.4 Size and color coding of biopsy needles

Size in gauge	14	15	16	17	18	19	20	21	22	23	25
Outer diameter (mm) based on ISO/DIN 9626	2.1	1.8	1.6	1.4	1.2	1.1	0.9	0.8	0.7	0.6	0.5
Charrière/French (Ch, F)	6.3	5.4	4.8	4.2	3.6	3.3	2.7	2.4	2.1	1.8	1.5
Pravaz system (Gr)							1	2	12	16	23
Color code based on ISO 6009 or DIN 13095	Light green	Blue-gray	White	Purple	Pink	Cream, ivory	Yellow	Dark green	Black	Dark blue	Orange

thinner the needle. For example, a 19-gauge needle is classified as "coarse" while a typical "fine" needle would be 22-gauge. There is no fixed linear relationship between the individual gradations, but the following formula gives a good approximation:

$$D_{mm} = 25.4 \times 10^{-(AWG+96954)/19.8578} \tag{2.1}$$

It is common to see both the millimeter and gauge systems used in everyday practice.

The gauge system was introduced by J. R. Brown in 1857 and was known initially as the Brown & Sharp (B&S) gauge. In accordance with ISO and DIN specifications, the hub for connecting a biopsy needle to a handle or syringe is color-coded to provide a clear indication of needle size (▶ Table 2.4).

In the manufacture of biopsy needles, sheet steel is wrapped around an arbor, welded, and drawn out into fine, thin-walled tubing, which is then cut to the necessary lengths and ground to the desired tip configuration.

Needle Length and Size

The length of a biopsy needle depends on the distance to the target site and, when a biopsy transducer is used, on the necessary needle length outside the body. The same considerations apply to the use of a needle guide, which is also associated with a longer needle path. Needle lengths from 10 to 22 cm are most commonly used.[19] In principle, an excessive needle length is unfavorable only if the target site is only 1 to 2 cm deep, as this would make the long needle unstable. In all other cases it is best to add a certain reserve length to make sure the needle will be long enough.

The selection of needle size is always a trade-off. In the biopsy of parenchymal organs, the pathologist requires a tissue sample with sufficient architectural organization, implying the use of a large-caliber needle. For example, it is desirable in liver biopsies to obtain 8 to 15 portal fields. Although it has been reported in the literature that complication rates increase with needle size,[20] published results to date are contradictory and inconclusive.[21,22] In the case of focal hepatic lesions, however, available data do appear to indicate that the risks of fine needle biopsy (< 1 mm) are less than with larger needles.[23,24] On the other hand, practical experience has shown that 1.2-mm (18-gauge) core-biopsy or Trucut needles provide good diagnostic accuracy with minimal hemorrhagic complications. This is consistent with our own technique, which permits even rare entities to be diagnosed with a high degree of confidence.

The retrieved specimen length also has an important bearing on diagnostic accuracy. In the case of liver biopsies, for example, it has been found that tissue cores < 1 cm long do not permit an accurate evaluation of viral hepatitis (grading and staging) and that the analysis of shorter cores may underestimate the severity of disease.[25]

Multiple tissue sampling improves the chance of obtaining representative material but also increases the complication rate, requiring that a reasonable trade-off be made. This compromise depends on the organ biopsied and on the access route and is an important consideration in organ biopsies. In the biopsy of circumscribed liver lesions, tissue samples should be taken from the edge and center of the lesion. In biopsies using an ultrasound contrast agent, it is easy to distinguish vascularized tissue from necrotic. This is important because the biopsy of a necrotic area would yield a nonrepresentative sample.

The question whether the risk of needle track seeding correlates with the size or type of needle is unresolved and will probably remain so in the future due to the extremely small case numbers. There is similar uncertainty regarding the complication rates associated with different needle types.

A 22-gauge needle is sufficient for aspirating watery exudates or transudates, while an 18-gauge or larger needle should be used for pus.[26,27] Tissue can be sampled by aspiration biopsy or by a cutting or core biopsy technique.[28,29]

Needle Tip Configurations

Chiba-type needles with a short beveled tip are used for the aspiration of fluids. The lumen size, and thus the outer needle diameter, should conform to the consistency of the aspirated fluid. Other tip configurations are shown in ▶ Fig. 2.3 and ▶ Table 2.5.

The most widely used tip configurations for biopsy needles are the short beveled tip and trocar tip. Neither is inherently superior, and technical considerations will usually guide the selection of a particular needle tip geometry. With the cannulas used for aspiration and core biopsies, a central trocar point can provide a tip with uniform circumferential sharpness. With needles for collecting cytologic material and Trucut needles (see below), a beveled tip is technically easier to produce, provides high needle sharpness, and makes for a smooth transition between the outer cannula and inner stylet. But if the needle will be rotated on its long axis during the biopsy, a central point is advantageous for fixation of the needle tip. This principle is illustrated by the triple-crown tip (Jamshidi needle) used for iliac crest biopsy.

Manufacturers use various methods of roughening the surface of the distal needle shaft to facilitate needle tip tracking in the ultrasound image. In most cases this is done by sandblasting the distal 10 to 15 mm but is uncertain whether this actually does improve needle visualization. A needle that is oblique to the image plane is almost always clearly visible. Visualization is a problem only if the needle is not angled relative to the beam, in

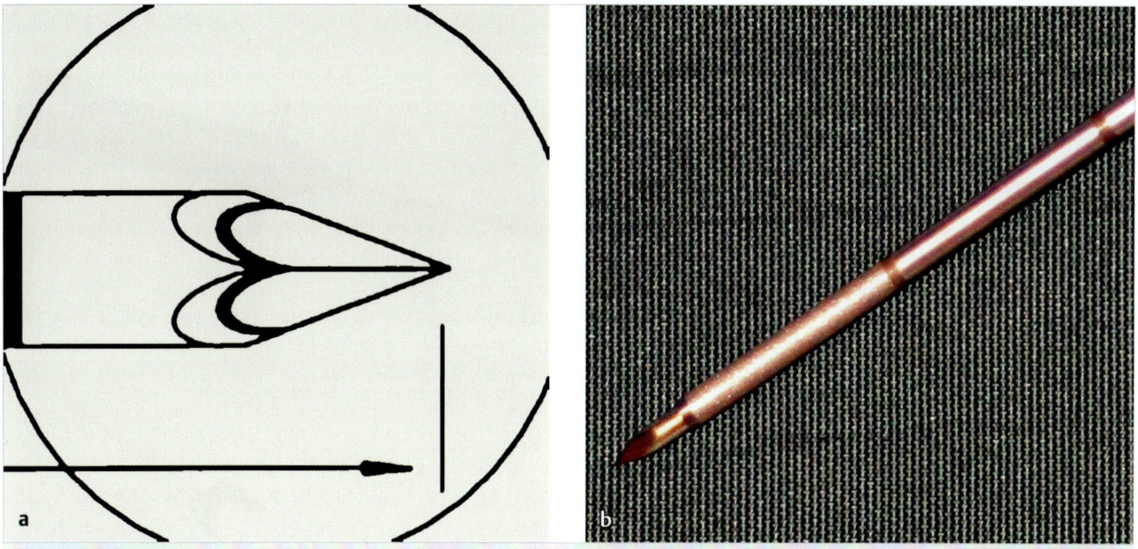

Fig. 2.3 Biopsy needles.
a Crown-point needle with a trocar-tip stylet.
b Needle with a beveled tip, sandblasted distal segment, and centimeter depth markings. (Source: reference[17].)

which case the operator must often rely on indirect signs for needle localization, such as concomitant tissue movements. One disadvantage of surface roughening is the potentially higher risk of needle track seeding, although there is no hard evidence at present to support this concern.

As a general rule, only needles with a stylet should be used to obtain representative organ tissue (e.g., in a percutaneous renal or liver biopsy). This prevents tissue contamination from the needle tract that might cause an erroneous diagnosis. The Luer lock connector has become standard for all hollow needle systems.

If a therapeutic agent is to be administered through the indwelling needle, a syringe with a screw-on attachment should be used to prevent accidental hub separation that could spray caustic material onto the patient and staff. The Luer lock connector has become standard for all hollow needle systems. A complete table setup is shown in ▶ Fig. 2.4. An example is percutaneous ethanol injection for hepatocellular carcinoma. The agent is injected through 20- to 22-gauge needles that are sealed at the end and have side holes over a length of 1 to 2 cm at the distal end. These side holes provide a more uniform, and thus more effective, dispersion of the alcohol into the tumor tissue.

Suction Biopsy Systems

Suction Needle without a Stylet

If the lesion is superficial and there is little danger of aspirating foreign material during needle insertion, a cannula without a stylet can be used. This applies mainly to thyroid and lymph node biopsies. Advancing the plunger slightly on reaching the biopsy site to clear the needle of any extraneous material is problematic for hygienic and other reasons and cannot be recommended. It could cause cellular contamination that would hamper later evaluation by the pathologist, and it might also degrade image quality. It is better to describe the needle pathway to the pathologist so that he or she can identify any extraneous cellular material, which often consists of skin particles. The tissue material is retained in the cannula by suction applied to an attached syringe (▶ Fig. 2.5).

Table 2.5 Selection of various needle tips and their recommended use

Tip configuration	Characteristics	Recommended use
Trocar	Three-sided point	Suitable for almost all applications
Single bevel (faceted, US bevel, MS bevel)	Oblique bevel with a fitted stylet at the tip	Suitable for almost all applications
V bevel	Noncoring with five cutting surfaces	Spinal anesthesia
Pencil point	Noncoring, inflow and outflow through a side hole	Spinal anesthesia
Huber tip	Angled (10%) behind the heel	Used for filling ports
Quincke point	Faceted tip similar to lancet point	Spinal anesthesia
Triple-sharpened point	Atraumatic	Bone marrow biopsy

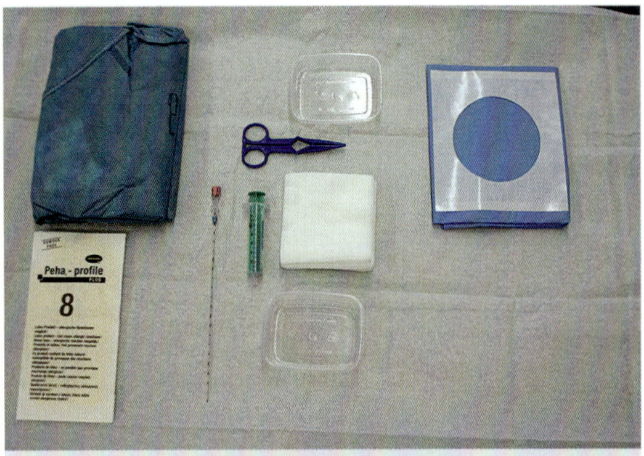

Fig. 2.4 Table setup for a Chiba fine needle biopsy.

Usually the suction is maintained by a syringe with a locking mechanism. Another option is to use a handle that mounts on the syringe and allows the operator to vary the negative pressure with one hand as needed (e.g., Aspir-Gun by Helmuth Industries, UK).

Caution

It is important to stop the suction before removing the needle from the biopsy site. Otherwise the aspirated tissue will be sucked into the syringe, making it extremely difficult to process, and additional tissue may be aspirated from the biopsy tract during needle removal.

Menghini Needle and Other Suction Needles with a Stylet

The classic representative of the suction biopsy needle is the Menghini needle (Surecut needle[30,31]). The Menghini needle is filled with saline solution to prevent aspiration of foreign material as the needle is advanced. The tissue is cored with a sharp cannula, and the specimen is retained in the cannula by a slight negative pressure ("one-second liver biopsy"[32]). With manual systems, the operator draws back on the plunger to create suction and retain the tissue core. This technique does not entirely preclude specimen loss, however, and there is still a very small risk of needle track seeding. The original technique for a "Menghini biopsy" consisted of advancing the needle to the biopsy site, applying suction with a locking syringe, and then inserting and withdrawing the needle quickly with a jabbing motion of the wrist.

Because this manual technique requires some experience and gives an imprecise penetration depth in focal lesions, automated suction biopsy devices were developed.[33] The Vim–Silverman needle, once widely used, functions by the suction biopsy principle but is rarely used today. In all cases the core needle should be rotated after insertion to help detach the tissue core from its bed.

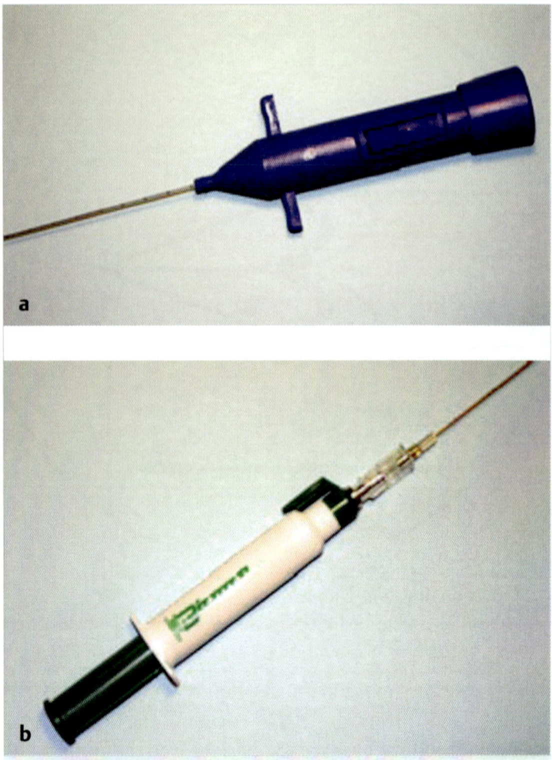

Fig. 2.5
a Fully automated core biopsy needle (Autovac, Bard GmbH).
b Semiautomated vacuum needle (Biomol, Pflugbeil GmbH).
(Source: reference[17].)

Retention mechanisms have been developed that occlude the distal needle opening to prevent specimen loss. One such mechanism has a small leaf spring that secures the tissue core within the cannula. In the BioPince needle manufactured by Peter Pflugbeil GmbH, a spring clip automatically hooks into a slot near the needle tip after the instrument is fired, trapping the core sample within the cannula without a vacuum system.[34,35] The specimen is then safely extracted within the closed system. Everyday experience has shown, however, that the standard automated and semiautomated systems almost always retain the tissue core with no real need for a complicated needle design.

After the needle is removed from the body, the stylet is advanced to expel the collected material. At the end of the procedure, a syringe can also be used to force air through the cannula to recover any residual particles left in the needle. For more information about specimen processing and pitfalls in cytologic analysis, we refer the reader to the detailed publications of Jenssen et al.[36,37] The needle should not be flushed with sodium chloride solution or water, as this might cause changes in the cellular material.

Cutting Biopsy Systems

Cutting needle biopsies employ either an end-cutting or side-notch (Trucut) technique for sampling tissue.

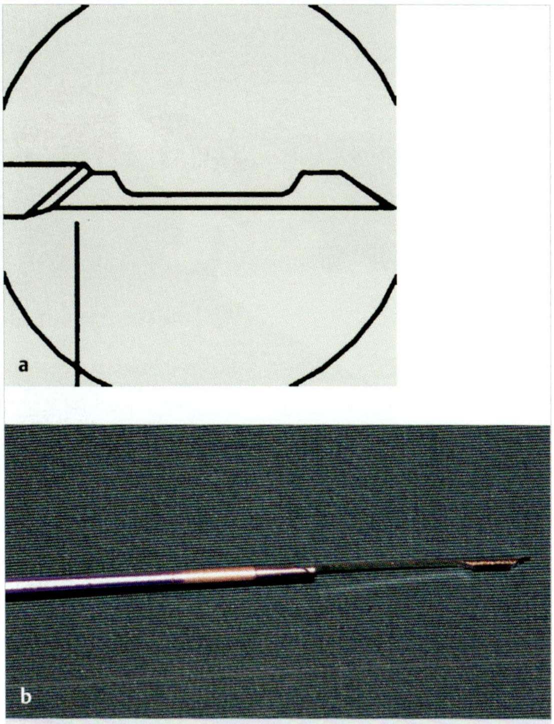

Fig. 2.6 Trucut needle with the notched inner stylet deployed.
a Schematic drawing.
b Photograph.

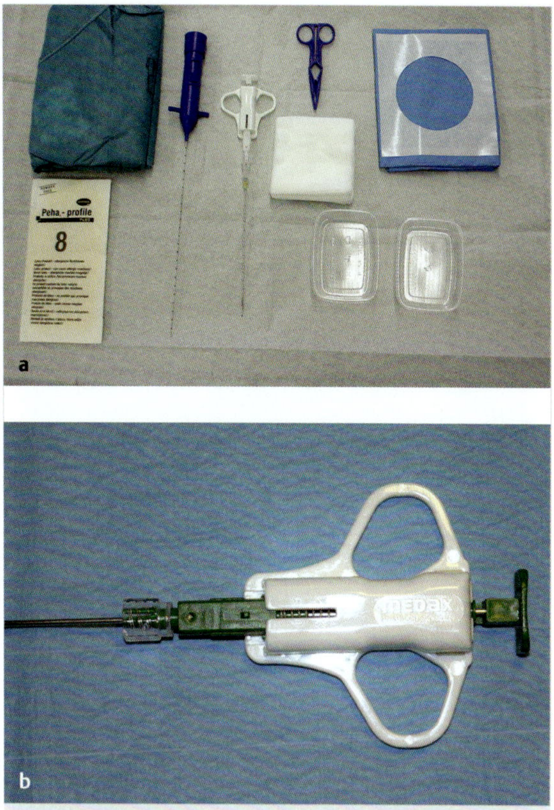

Fig. 2.7 Table setup for a percutaneous biopsy.
a With an automated core biopsy needle and Trucut needle.
b Close-up view of the semiautomated coaxial device.

End-Cutting Needles

Examples are the Franseen needle and the Otto needle, which are distinguished by the geometry of the cutting edges at the cannula tip. The first end-cutting needle was the Otto needle, available in fine and coarse sizes with two cutting teeth at the tip.[38] Because these needles must be simultaneously rotated and advanced at the biopsy site, practitioners rarely use them today, and they do not merit further discussion here.

Trucut Needle

Although the Trucut needle harvests only a semicylindrical tissue core, this technique offers a decisive advantage (▶ Fig. 2.6, ▶ Fig. 2.7, ▶ Fig. 2.8). The inner stylet, which has a side notch 10 to 20 mm long (throw), is advanced into the lesion. After tissue has entered the notch, the outer cutting cannula is advanced over the stylet to slice off and secure the specimen within the cannula. This mechanism protects the specimen and prevents seeding of the needle track with tumor cells. The main disadvantage is that Trucut biopsies require larger-caliber needles than other techniques to obtain specimens of equal quality. The side-cutting technique was introduced by Lindgren in the early 1980s.[39] There are devices on the market in which the cannula and stylet can be controlled by hand, making the puncture and cutting actions a purely manual process. An example is the Uni-Core biopsy needle (14–21 gauge, 11.5–20 cm length). First the closed needle is advanced to the lesion. Then the stylet is pushed manually into the lesion, and the cannula is slid manually over the stylet, cutting and trapping the tissue specimen. One disadvantage is that the needle must be operated with two hands, and so a second examiner is needed to hold the ultrasound transducer. In semiautomated systems, the stylet is advanced manually but the cannula is spring-loaded and is fired at the touch of a button, cutting off the tissue in the specimen notch (▶ Fig. 2.6). The instrument is cocked before the procedure. Various disposable models of these needles are available commercially. Also available are biopsy guns made of metal that can be reused for many years as they are easy to clean and sterilize. The only disposable component is the needle. The throw length of the needle is preset to the desired biopsy depth before use.

If multiple tissue cores are to be harvested from the same area, a biopsy device can be used in which the cannula is left in the body while the stylet is withdrawn. The sample is collected, and the empty stylet is reintroduced for another pass (coaxial technique). Despite the theoretical advantage that vulnerable structures in the biopsy path are traversed only once, this technique requires

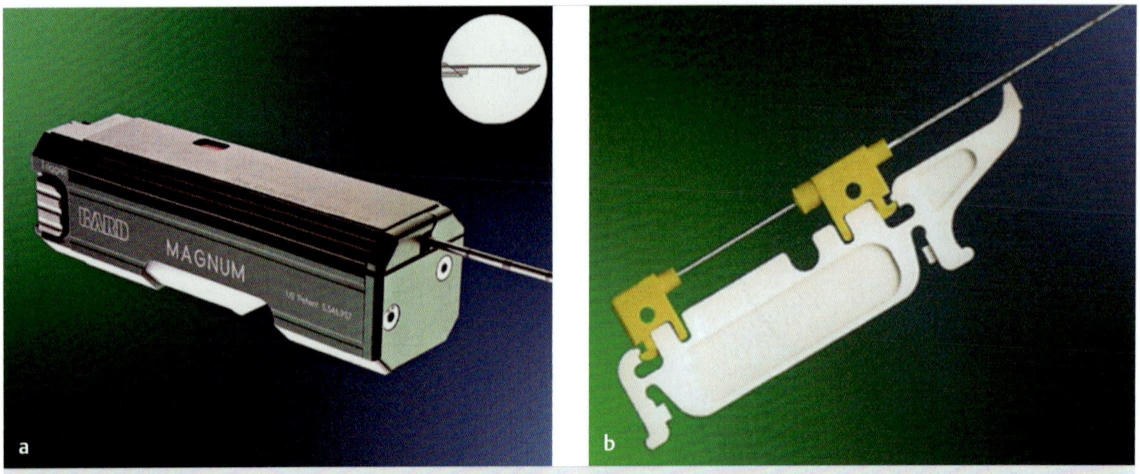

Fig. 2.8 Biopsy devices manufactured by Bard, Murray Hill, New Jersey, USA.
a Fully automated.
b Trucut needle.

larger-gauge needles that increase the complication rate and the cost.

In terms of the yield of diagnostic tissue, there is no definite evidence that fully automated systems are better. In fact, the data tend to show superiority of semiautomated core biopsy systems over fully automated devices.[40] One study, available only as an abstract, showed that the use of high-speed biopsy devices (1.3 mm) could yield compete, unfragmented tissue cores more often than manual biopsies.[41]

The theoretical advantage of fully automated systems is that the trocar is advanced at high speed, which may be advantageous for movable targets such as exophytic tumors and hard tumors embedded in very soft tissue like the breast. In experienced hands, semiautomated needles can also be safe and effective for this type of biopsy.

The Trucut technique described above is particularly suitable for soft tissue that can enter and fill the specimen notch. An end-cutting core needle on a suction syringe may be better for sampling very firm tissue.

2.2 Therapeutic Interventions

2.2.1 Introduction

Ultrasound-guided interventions have been standard procedures in clinical practice for many years. A distinction is made between diagnostic procedures[17] and therapeutic interventions.[42] For example, percutaneous abscess drainage (PAD) has become an indispensable therapeutic tool in everyday practice and is performed routinely at many hospitals and clinics. Often a one-stick trocar technique is used to evacuate the fluid collection and, if necessary, instill a therapeutic agent. It may also be necessary to place one or more drains for a prolonged period to establish access for continuous drainage and/or regular irrigation. These interventions may also be part of a larger procedure, such as a rendezvous procedure combining endoscopic and percutaneous techniques. Major advances have been made in minimally invasive procedures in recent years. Our emphasis in this chapter will be on interventional materials and issues relating to specific organs.[42]

2.2.2 Brief Historical Review

The drainage of body fluids has been practiced since antiquity. Understandably, the materials available for those procedures were quite limited in the ancient world. For example, lead was often used as a catheter material because it was easily bent to the desired shape. In accordance with the classical rule of *ubi pus ibi evacua* ("where there is pus, evacuate it"), the practice of opening and draining abscesses was introduced very early in medical history. Physicians also learned that intraperitoneal abscesses could initially be treated conservatively for a time before proceeding with successful surgical drainage.[43] The development of modern materials was a decisive step in the development of effective drainage systems that could remain indwelling for extended periods. Polyethylene, for example, was discovered by the chemist Hans von Pechlmann in 1898, but it was not until 1933 that Reginald Gibson and Eric Fawcett began the industrial production of polyethylene at laboratories in England. Since then, polyethylene has become the most widely manufactured plastic in the world, accounting for 29% of all plastic production. Detailed descriptions of percutaneous procedures have been published in the medical-surgical literature for many years, even appearing in the German textbook *Manual of Surgery* published in 1830.[44] This work included critical appraisals, such as that regarding the percutaneous drainage of intra-abdominal fluid collections: "In most cases this is merely a palliative measure, inasmuch as the fluid will soon collect again after the procedure." As techniques improved, however, contraindications became a less serious concern and gradually faded in importance. H. Kalk urged a more cautious policy in 1943: "Needle specimens should be taken only during surgery!"[19] In the years since then, the percutaneous aspiration of abscesses has achieved a diagnostic accuracy of nearly 100%. The success rate of drain placement is 98%, and the therapeutic success rate is 88%.[45]

2.2.3 Patient Preparation

Because all percutaneous interventions are invasive procedures, they require prior informed consent that should include full disclosure of the benefit of the procedure and potential complications (risk), which are documented in written form. In emergency situations such as with a septic patient, it may be necessary to deviate from this policy. Informed consent on the examination table is inadequate. The patient may not fully understand the need for the intervention. Consequently, time for explanations should be allotted in the preprocedure protocol.

2.2.4 Access Routes

Access to the intended target (abscess, tumor, etc.) is established at the start of the interventional procedure. Two different methods are available for this: the trocar technique ("direct puncture," "one-stick") and the Seldinger technique. The technique of choice depends on the degree of difficulty in traversing vulnerable tissue structures, the length of the approach, the experience of the examiner, and the necessary diameter of the drain that is to be placed. Navigation systems may allow for more accurate targeting in the future, but at present they are still too costly for practical use.[46] Compared with needle aspiration alone, the placement of a drain makes the selection of an access route much more difficult because it requires larger-caliber instruments and because drains will be left indwelling for some time, and injury to other organs must be avoided. With this in mind, a posterior approach should be considered for retroperitoneal lesions.[47] Multiple liver abscesses may require drainage at multiple sites,[48,49] and it may be necessary to combine percutaneous and transpapillary approaches. The question of whether to perform repeated needle aspirations of an abscess cavity or proceed with longer-term catheter drainage must be decided on a case-by-case basis.[50–52] Key considerations are not only the size of the abscess but also the sensitivity of the target organ, such as the breast.[53]

Meanwhile, various endosonographic techniques have made it possible to perform aspiration or drainage via the upper and lower gastrointestinal tract and by the transvaginal route.[54] These approaches are beyond our present scope, but it should be noted that as interdisciplinary procedures become more common in the future, there will be increasing use of combined techniques such as percutaneous and endoscopic approaches.[55]

Percutaneous decompression may be indicated in rare cases. An abdominal compartment syndrome following a spontaneous perforation or, more commonly, after endoscopy may create a life-threatening situation that calls for swift action. A variety of sites of access to the abdominal cavity are available, and the operator should select the pathway with the lowest risk. Of course, this assessment should include abdominal ultrasound to look for possible collateral vessels in the abdominal wall.[56]

2.2.5 Indications and Contraindications

Indications

Typical indications are as follows:

- Abscesses (after perforation, anastomotic leak, Crohn disease, tuberculosis, etc.)
- Empyemas
- Effusions
- Hematomas
- Biliomas and biliary obstructions
- Parasitisms
- Tumor ablation
- Urinary diversion

Contraindications

In listing contraindications, a clear distinction should be made between percutaneous needle aspiration and the placement of a drain. Whereas percutaneous aspiration with a fine needle can be performed safely through sensitive organ structures such as the gastrointestinal tract, this violation cannot be tolerated in placing a drain. Percutaneous procedures have the following contraindications:

- Uncooperative patient
- Quick value < 50%
- Platelet count < 50×10^9/L (50,000/μL)

Additionally, the partial thromboplastin time should not be prolonged.

Coagulation Testing

The Quick value is the measured prothrombin time expressed as a percentage of the coagulation time in a healthy person. The prothrombin time is the time it takes plasma to clot after addition of tissue factor. The rule that the Quick value be > 50% before an interventional procedure is based on an assessment of multiple risk factors.

The reported normal range is between 70% and 120%. In the range of 50 to 70%, it may be assumed that the hemostatic potential with a normal aPTT (activated partial thromboplastin time) and thrombin time is still essentially normal and is adequate for hemostasis. Other factor deficiencies or impaired coagulation factor synthesis in the liver should also be considered, however. If the Quick value is between 30% and 50%, there will not be a high risk of spontaneous hemorrhage if only the extrinsic coagulation pathway is affected, i.e., if the patient has a normal aPTT. On the other hand, the puncture of a parenchymal organ or a surgical procedure is generally not a reasonable option in the 30 to 50% range and is therefore contraindicated.[57] The cutoff values will naturally be adjusted upward in cases where multiple risk factors are present.[21,58] This also means that Quick values in the borderline range should prompt further diagnostic investigation.

The partial thromboplastin time (PTT) and the activated partial thromboplastin time (aPTT) assess the endogenous coagulation system as a whole and can therefore detect approximately 95% of congenital coagulopathies.[59] An exception is factor VII. Given the numerous variables and their varying degrees of importance, the aPTT cannot be interpreted in isolation and, when abnormal, calls for a detailed analysis. A prolongation of the aPTT (normal range is 18 to 40 seconds) should not be present before an intervention. A decline in factor VIII: C activity and factor IX activity to values between 0.3 and 0.5 U/mL is evidenced by a prolonged aPTT and leads to a markedly increased peri-interventional bleeding tendency. For this reason, the upper normal limit should be considered the cutoff value in deciding whether to perform an interventional procedure.[60] Aside from life-threatening cases, these findings should warrant further investigation. A prolongation of the aPTT to > 50 seconds already suggests the presence of a severe coagulation disorder. Patients with a congenital deficiency of factor XII, prekallikrein or HMWK (high–molecular weight kininogen) are assumed to have normal hemostasis despite an extremely prolonged aPTT. Heparin therapy must also be taken into account, of course. While the platelet count generally does not affect the aPTT, this situation is different in heparinized blood.

Empirical values also underlie the principle that when platelet function is normal and platelet counts are higher than 50×10^9/L (50,000/μL), the bleeding tendency should not be increased and, on the basis of current guidelines, there is no need to administer platelets before an interventional procedure.[61] If the counts are between 20×10^9/L and 50×10^9/L, interventions are permissible only if compression can produce hemostasis. With counts below 20×10^9/L, platelets should always be administered before an interventional procedure. In high-risk situations such as procedures on the CNS, the counts should be higher than 70×10^9/L.[62] One should also consider the possibility of platelet dysfunction due to uremia, for example, or following treatment with antiplatelet drugs.

Since the placement of a drain requires dilation of the access tract, several other contraindications should be noted:

- Nonvisualization of the drain site
- Uncertain access route along injured structures

If the goal of the procedure is pharmacologic obliteration (e.g., PAIR, see below), these additional contraindications should be noted:

- A cyst communicating with the biliary tract
- Cysts in the CNS, lung, or urogenital tract
- A calcified cyst

2.2.6 Complications

As in all invasive procedures, there is a possibility of hemorrhage, perforations, pleural and colon injuries, secondary abscess formation, empyema, and other complications. A well-organized regimen of postprocedure care is essential. Complications are classified into two broad groups: early and late. Hemorrhage due to large-vessel injury and hollow viscus injuries with air leak can usually be detected at once by sonographic imaging.[63] On the other hand, an oozing hemorrhage or retroperitoneal injuries are difficult to image with ultrasound and may go undetected until the appearance of clinical manifestations or laboratory abnormalities (hemoglobin/hematocrit, serum WBC, C-reactive protein, etc.). Besides direct injuries from drain placement, complications may also result from improper postprocedure care. For example, good aftercare should include regular irrigation of the drains. Drains should be flushed with physiologic saline solution until clear aspirate is returned. This may be necessary several times a day, depending on the fluid consistency and drain site. Because abscesses usually have viscous contents, continuous irrigation will not produce sufficient flow to dissolve and evacuate the material. A better result can be achieved by manual irrigation. In these cases it is better to place a large, single-lumen drainage catheter than a multilumen drain with smaller inner diameters.

If it is uncertain whether the drain has been correctly positioned, its placement can be assessed on the B-mode image. Some air can be injected through the drain to aid accurate localization of the catheter tip. A small amount of instilled fluid is also visible and can be clearly visualized by color duplex sonography (CDS). If proper drain placement is still uncertain, contrast material can be instilled under fluoroscopic control to provide additional information. A recent study reported good results with the use of diluted contrast material (1:10, 1 mL).[64]

In addition to accurate drain placement, catheter irrigation, and monitoring any drain suction and output, wound care is a critical factor in the success of the procedure. If it is not handled properly, even a procedure that has been well executed technically may still result in failure. The catheter position should also be checked daily by the physician or a trained assistant.

2.2.7 Needle Techniques

A needle with an outer diameter of 0.7 to 0.9 mm is usually sufficient for injecting low-viscosity agents at the treatment site. The classic needle for this application is the Chiba needle. Special needles with side holes near the tip can be used for percutaneous ethanol injection in the treatment of hepatocellular carcinoma or, less commonly, thyroid adenoma. The side holes allow for better dispersion of the alcohol in the tissue (see above). If viscous material is to be aspirated, the needle size should conform to the expected consistency of the aspirate. In the case of putrid material, the needle size should be at least 18 gauge (1.2 mm). The needle tip configuration may be highly variable, and selection will depend on the target area and technique. The variety of available needle designs was reviewed earlier in this chapter.[17] It is always best to use a two-part needle assembly consisting of an outer cannula and inner stylet to reduce needle track seeding.

Needle aspirations alone are almost always performed without prior incision of the skin. Generally this is not possible in drain placements, depending on the size of the drain, and a sharp-pointed scalpel should be used. Drains should be placed under adequate local anesthesia. The patient should lie quietly on the examination table to help prevent malpositioning or displacement of the drain before it is secured. Suitable local anesthetics are 1% lidocaine or 2% mepivacaine. Anxious patients may require sedation with midazolam, propofol, etc. (noting applicable surveillance standards). Besides patient comfort, it is important to weigh the risk of sedation against the risk of catheter malposition in a restless patient.

2.2.8 Special Needle Types

The injection of highly concentrated alcohol is a technically simple treatment option for selected neoplasms (▶ Fig. 2.9). Very good results have been reported, especially in the treatment of hepatocellular carcinoma (Chapter 18). A feared complications is malignant seeding along the needle track.[65]

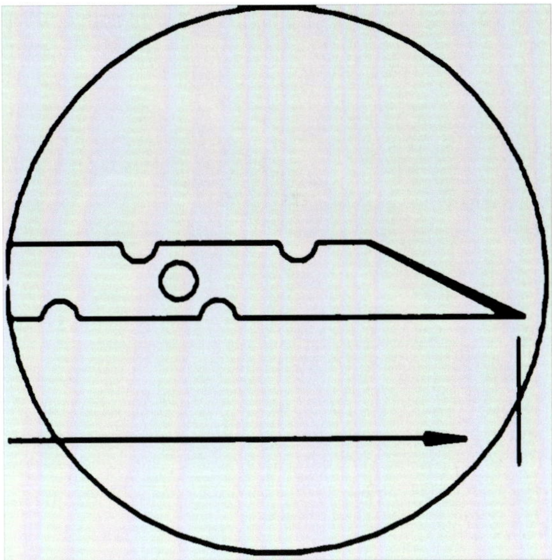

Fig. 2.9 Needle with a beveled tip and distal side holes for percutaneous ethanol injection.

2.2.9 Trocar Technique

In the trocar technique, the drainage catheter is mounted on a needle assembly and both are advanced together to the target site. This may be done directly, or a thin "pilot needle" of 18 to 22 gauge may be introduced first to establish access (tandem trocar technique, tandem needle biopsy technique[66]). Reported technical results are excellent, with success rates of 100% and a drain placement rate of 98%. The placement of a drain always carries higher risks than needle insertion alone, so it is best to maintain a safety margin of 5 to 10 mm with respect to vessels, bowel, ureters, and nerves.[67] It has been proven that percutaneous abscess drainage (PAD) can either avoid surgery or at least allow patients to improve enough for elective surgery. An impressive example in recent years is the increased use of PAD in patients with acute diverticulitis.[68] Even recurrences of surgically treated abdominal wall abscesses can be successfully treated by percutaneous catheter drainage, with one Boston study showing that PAD avoided a second operation in 56% of cases.[50]

Drains are available in various forms. They are stiffened for insertion by sliding them over a cannula (▶ Fig. 2.10, ▶ Fig. 2.11).

In a two-part system, a catheter made of kink-resistant material is mounted directly on the stylet. Upon its reaching the cavity, the catheter is advanced. The stylet remains in place as a guide and is not removed until the end of the procedure. But it is more common to use three-part drainage sets in which the cannula contains a

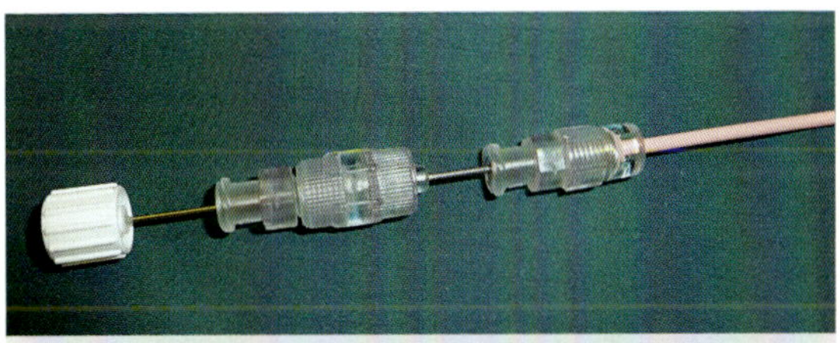

Fig. 2.10 The catheter is stiffened by a cannula and stylet for direct insertion.

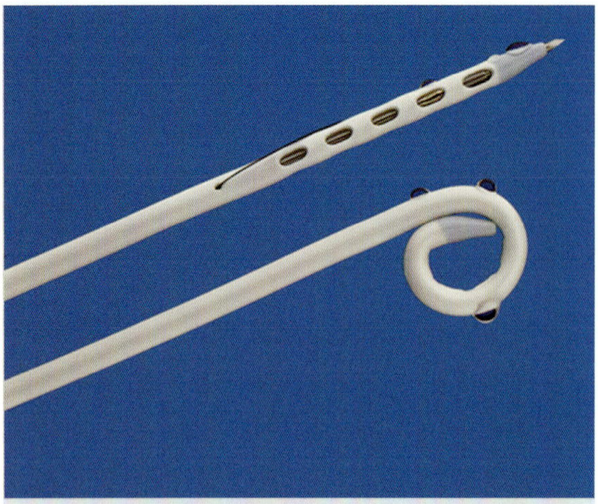

Fig. 2.11 Pigtail catheter in the coiled state and stiffened with a trocar-tip needle for direct insertion.

removable trocar stylet. After the stylet is withdrawn, the catheter is advanced over the cannula into the target area.

2.2.10 Seldinger Technique

The Seldinger technique was developed in 1953 by the Swedish radiologist Sven-Ivar Seldinger (1921–1998). It was originally devised as a means for introducing angiographic catheters into blood vessels.[69] After an initial needle puncture, a guidewire is advanced into the target area, and further manipulations are performed over the guidewire. The main advantage of this technique is that the target site can be located with a thin needle, establishing safe access for dilation and drain placement. As with other techniques, numerous variations have been devised. In most cases a Chiba needle is used for the initial puncture (▶ Fig. 2.12), and a compatible guidewire is advanced through the needle. For example, a 0.7-mm needle will accommodate a guidewire only 0.018 inch in diameter, which cannot withstand large shear forces. An obturator is used to exchange the thinner guidewire for a thicker one. It consists of two parts: a stiff inner cannula made of metal or Teflon, and a softer outer catheter. The stiff inner cannula, which has a blunt edge at its distal end, is advanced over the thin guidewire. Its stiffness enables the operator to control its direction from the outside and prevent looping of the guidewire. Next the outer catheter is advanced and the inner cannula is removed. It is now possible to place a thicker guidewire through the catheter (e.g., 0.035 inch), dilate the tract, and advance the actual drainage catheter over the thicker wire.

In a modified version, the drainage catheter is advanced directly over the very long, thin-lumen puncture needle as it would be over a guidewire. This requires a three-part introducer set consisting of a stylet, cannula, and catheter. On reaching the target site, the stylet is removed and a guidewire (0.018 to 0.038 inch, depending on the inner diameter of the cannula) is placed through the very long cannula, with the drainage catheter mounted on the outer half of the cannula. Finally, while the cannula is left in place or retracted slightly, the drainage catheter is advanced into place directly over the cannula and guidewire.

Methods

The trocar technique appears to be superior in experienced hands, owing mainly to its speed, simplicity, and modest material requirements.[70] The Seldinger technique is advantageous in regions difficult to access and in cases where a very large drain will be placed.

2.2.11 Peel-Away Sheath

If the goal is to place a relatively large-bore drainage catheter made of soft material, the use of a "peel-away sheath" is advised. Either the trocar or Seldinger technique is used

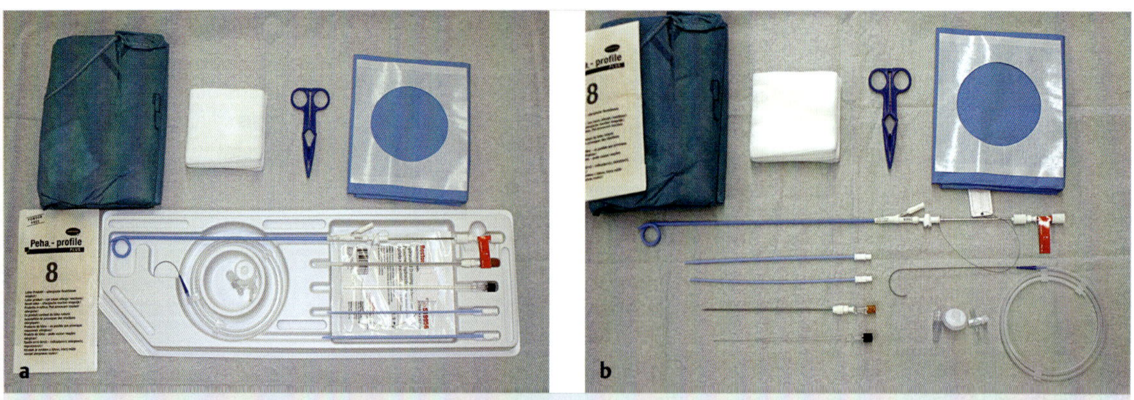

Fig. 2.12 Complete set for Seldinger access and drain placement (Boston Scientific, Natick, Massachusetts, USA).
a As supplied.
b Set ready for use.

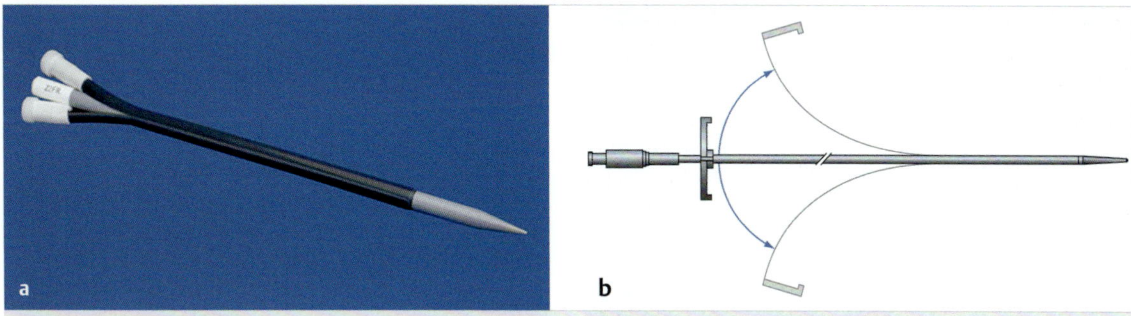

Fig. 2.13 Peel-away sheath.
a Complete sheath.
b Diagram.

to advance a stiff dilator-catheter into the target structure. Mounted on it is a thin-walled catheter that is subsequently advanced over the dilator. Once the sheath is in place, the dilator is removed and the actual drainage catheter is introduced into the target area. The sheath is withdrawn along the drainage catheter and removed by peeling it apart, similarly to opening a zipper (▶ Fig. 2.13).

2.2.12 Anchor Systems, Suture Techniques

When a large-caliber needle is used, for example, to puncture the stomach wall for an ultrasound-guided percutaneous gastrostomy, the large needle may have a tendency to push the target aside rather than pierce it cleanly. Special fixation systems have been developed for this purpose. The simplest of these devices are tissue anchors—small metal bars with a suture attached at the center that are introduced into the cavity with a special needle and released there. The metal bar is placed into a side slot at the distal end of the introducer needle, and the suture runs along the outside of the needle as the metal anchor is introduced (▶ Fig. 2.14, ▶ Fig. 2.15).

When all metal anchors have been deployed, the trailing sutures may be tied together to appose the stomach to the abdominal wall, or each suture can be fixed indi-

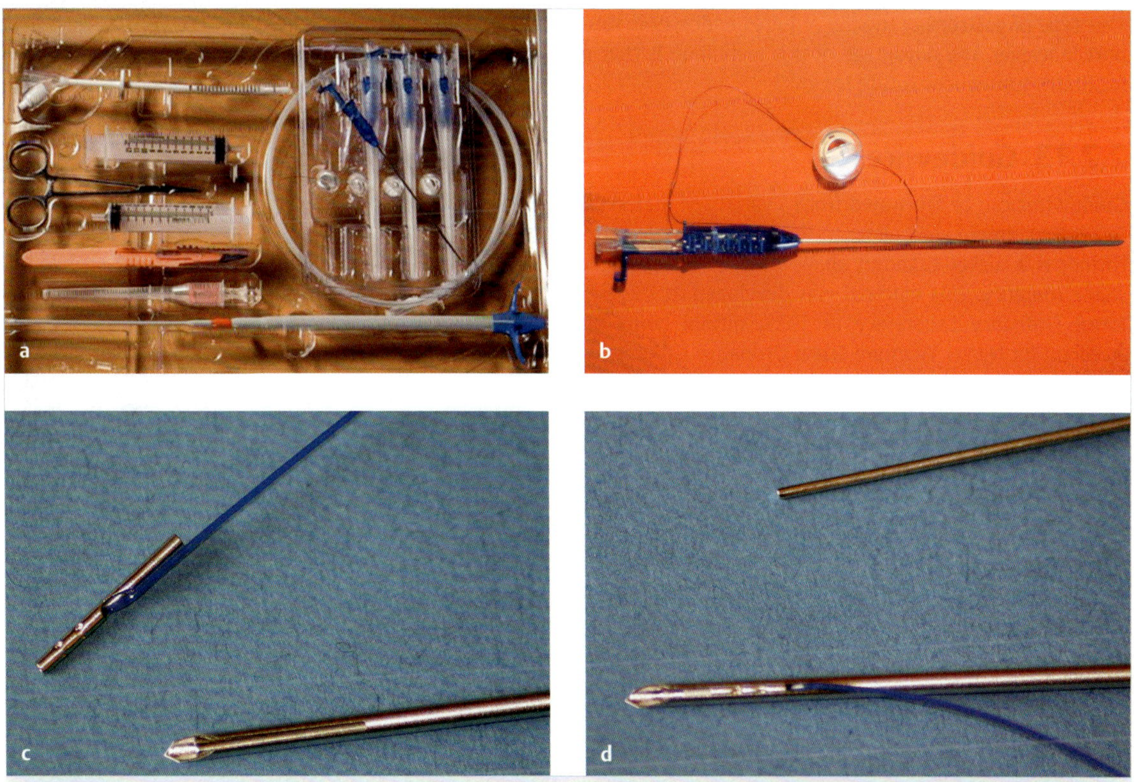

Fig. 2.14 Anchor systems manufactured by Kimberly-Clark, Roswell, Georgia, USA with locking disk (a, b) and by the firm MTW Medizintechnik, Rheinstetten, Germany (c, d).

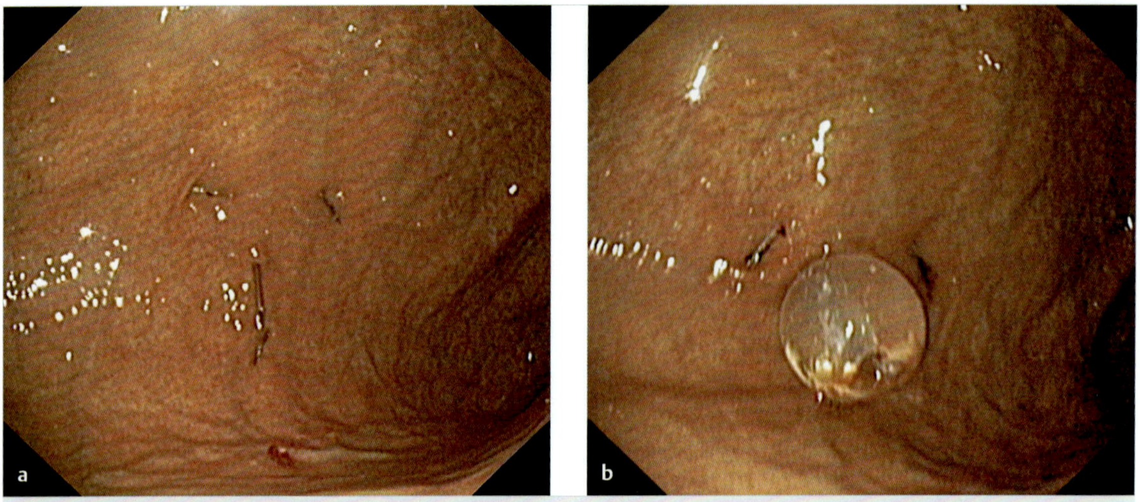

Fig. 2.15 Percutaneous gastrostomy, endoscopic view.
a Metal fixation anchors in the stomach.
b PEG (percutaneous endoscopic gastrostomy) retention balloon placed by direct puncture.

vidually against the skin with a small locking disk (▶ Fig. 2.14b).

A somewhat more complicated solution is the Freka Pexact system (Fresenius Kabi AG), which consists of two needles. A suture is passed through one needle into the cavity, where it is grasped with a wire loop passed through the other needle and brought out for fixation. This type of gastropexy usually requires endoscopic support, however. The advantage of this technique is that it facilitates subsequent suture removal.

2.2.13 Guidewires

Guidewires can be fabricated from a variety of materials. As well as simple steel alloys, nitinol is commonly used. Nitinol is a nickel–titanium allow with the property of shape memory. This material was developed at the U.S. Naval Ordnance Laboratory in 1958, nitinol being an acronym for Nickel Titanium Naval Ordnance Laboratory. This material is corrosion-resistant and can tolerate up to 8% deformation owing to its pseudoelastic behavior (memory effect). Common guidewire diameters are 0.018 and 0.035 inch (1 inch = 25.4 mm; see ▶ Table 2.6). Diameters of 0.025 and 0.038 inch are also available but are less commonly used. The very thin 0.018-inch wire will pass through a 0.7-mm Chiba needle and can secure access along a difficult tract, as in transhepatic biliary drainage.

The tip configuration at the flexible end of a guidewire may be straight, angled, J-curved (e.g., Schüller catheter exchange wire), or curled (pigtail). A small handle can be screwed onto the end of an angled guidewire to aid in crossing a tight stenosis. Practically all wires available today have a torque-stable design. Gold- or platinum-plated tips are available to reduce friction in difficult placements. If the only function of the wire is to serve as a guide for dilation and drain placement, there is no need for precious-metal plating, and a plain steel wire or coil-wrapped steel wire can be used (▶ Fig. 2.16).

But to negotiate stenotic areas as required in percutaneous transhepatic cholangiography and drainage (PTCD), the guidewire should have a highly flexible tip and minimal surface friction. This provides good tactile feel for precise wire manipulation and the crossing of tight stenoses. Manufacturers have developed a variety of wire systems for these applications. An example is the Terumo guidewire, which has an elastic nitinol-alloy core with a distal hydrophilic-coated M-polyurethane jacket that forms a smooth transition with the soft tip. This tip is highly flexible and has an atraumatic conical shape. The one-part design allows for good pushability and torque control. The wire structure is radiopaque. If the guidewire will need to transmit significant lateral forces, a number of suppliers offer more stable wire designs for that purpose. A polytetrafluoroethylene (PTFE) or Teflon coating is another common feature on guidewires.

Table 2.6 Wire diameters in millimeters and inches

Unit of measure	Corresponding values					
Diameter in mm	0.25	0.41	0.46	0.64	0.89	0.97
Diameter in inches	0.011	0.016	0.018	0.025	0.035	0.038

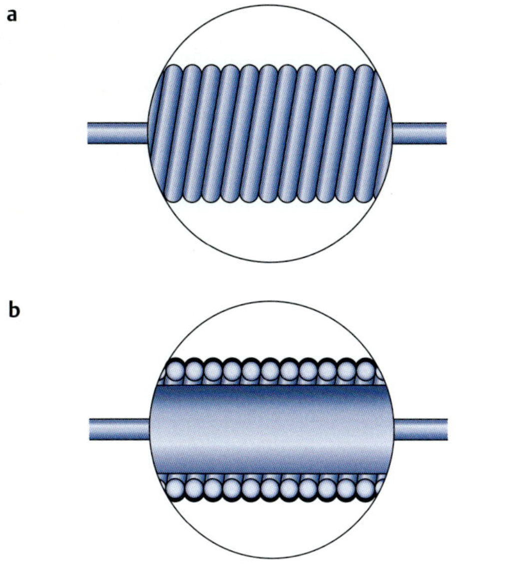

Fig. 2.16 Guidewire with a coil-wrapped core (**a**). Viewed in longitudinal section (**b**).

Surface coatings are not always advantageous, however. In cases where a long drain is to be placed, the presence of a coating on the drain and wire may cause increased friction, and considerable force may be needed to remove the wire following drain placement. The stability of a guidewire results in part from the thickness of the wire itself and from special design features. "Barber pole" movement markers are helpful for indicating relative wire position so that any slippage or displacement can be quickly recognized. An important criterion in guidewire selection is a smooth taper between the flexible tip and stiffer shaft. Questions of whether the hydrophilic coating covers the distal 5 cm or 10 cm of the wire tip, whether the conical part is 17 or 21 cm long, and whether the floppy part is 3 cm long or only 1 cm long will certainly contribute to the success of the placement in any given case but are not generally regarded as quality criteria (compare the Dreamwire and Jagwire from Boston Scientific).

Meanwhile, special wires have been developed that combine a soft hydrophilic tip with advanced features such as fluoroscopic length markings, a fluorine coating to reduce friction, and almost 1:1 torque control (e.g., VisiGlide, Olympus, Medical Systems Europe GmbH, Hamburg, Germany). Along with the excellent quality of these devices, however, their higher cost is an important consideration in selecting a particular type of wire.

The Lunderquist wire is rarely used now because of its very high stiffness. Spannguide wires have a simple mechanism for maintaining their shape and are useful for device delivery. There is little if any need for these wires today, however, owing to the high kink resistance of other guidewires available on the market.

Table 2.7 Criteria for selecting a suitable dilator

Property	Description
Material	Material should be stiff for good transmission of pushing and shear forces, also kink-resistant
Length	Depends on target site. Examples: 17 cm for a liver abscess, 60 cm for transhepatic papillary dilation
Diameter	Depends on proposed drainage catheter; usually 2F more than the catheter
Guidewire	Primary access with a 0.7-mm Chiba needle is followed by an uncoated 0.018-inch wire or a standard 0.035-inch wire (see below)

2.2.14 Dilators

Where stiffness is needed, as in the case of dilators, a common material of choice is Teflon (TFE or PTFE, polytetrafluoroethylene). This material is kink-resistant and provides good force transmission. A variety of lengths, diameters, and material characteristics are available on the market. Most suppliers offer lengths from 17 to 60 cm and outer diameters of 4F to 16F (▶ Table 2.7). A dilator length of 35 cm has proven most favorable for percutaneous dilatations of the biliary tract. Small dilators in the range of 4F to 6F, introduced over a 0.018-inch uncoated primary guidewire, are most commonly used for percutaneous biliary dilation. A typical dilation set would include a hollow needle (cannula) made of metal or Teflon with an outer 6F catheter. This assembly is advanced over a 0.018-inch wire, the inner cannula is removed, and a 0.035-inch wire is introduced through the catheter (e.g., Di Plus dilator from Peter Pflugbeil GmbH). Further dilators are usually advanced over a 0.035-inch or 0.038-inch wire. The proximal end should have a Luer lock connector so that contrast material can be instilled intermittently to assess the progress of a serial dilation.[71]

Polyurethane is also used. An example is the Nimura dilator. Since biliary dilation requires dilators of considerable length, the dilators should be radiopaque with outer centimeter markings. A stenosis can be crossed with a graduated catheter (e.g. Plus-Step dilator from Peter Pflugbeil GmbH). This technique saves time and reduces costs.

2.2.15 Drainage Catheters

A variety of drainage catheters made by various manufacturers are available on the market. They are sold separately or as part of a complete placement set. Single-lumen or multilumen types may be used, depending on the structure that requires drainage. With a single-lumen catheter, irrigation can alternate with suction. Multilumen catheters allow simultaneous or continuous irrigations to be performed. Most catheter systems are made of polyurethane or polyethylene (soft polyethylene is resistant to clogging). While polyethylene offers higher rigidity, polyurethane has greater flexibility. Polyethylene is a thermoplastic polymer of the polyolefin class. It is produced by the polymerization of ethene (CH_2=CH_2). Three main types of polyethylene are distinguished based on the manufacturing process: low-density (LDPE), high-density (HDPE), and linear low-density (LLDPE). These differ with respect to crystallinity, elastic modulus, and durability.

A special type of polyurethane is Ultrathane, which is highly resistant to degradation by mechanical, chemical and thermal effects. Recent innovations are C-Flex (Concept Polymer Technologies Inc.) and Silitec (Medical Engineering Corporation), which are silicone-based polymers. Percuflex (Boston Scientific) is an olefinic block copolymer.

As well as homogeneous materials, catheters made of mixed materials are also available. They are used mainly in cases where the drain will remain indwelling for some time and it is important to combine shape stability, for example, with a soft, tissue-compatible surface. This principle is illustrated by a catheter with a polyamide core, which provides excellent stiffness and smooth tracking, covered by a soft polyurethane outer layer, which has good blood compatibility and softens at body temperature. Raumedic Medical Industry is among the companies that manufacture and distribute these products.

Because most drainage catheters are curled at the end, good shape memory is essential. Kink resistance and smooth tracking are other key material properties. Because a thin wall can optimize the ratio of outer diameter to inner lumen, special wall structures have been created. The Navarre universal drainage catheter is nitinol-reinforced to produce a thinner wall that is still resistant to kinking and pressure.

Catheter position is often checked radiographically, so the catheter should be visible on radiographic images. One way this can be accomplished is by adding barium sulfate to the catheter material. Another option is a radiopaque filament embedded in the drain wall or a metal ring placed at the distal end. These markings are insufficient for assessing catheter position in some situations, however, and there are times when contrast material must be instilled through the catheter to define the radiographic extent of an abscess and localize the drain. This may be necessary with extensive pancreatic pseudocysts, for example, in order to determine whether all portions of the pseudocyst are being drained.[72–75]

An important factor in drain selection is the arrangement of the drainage holes. For percutaneous abscess drainage, all the holes should be in the pigtail portion of the catheter. A biliary drain, on the other hand, should have side holes along the catheter shaft to promote fluid collection.[32] Pigtail catheters are preshaped and must be straightened with a stiffener when introduced. Once the distal end of the drain is inside the cavity, the introducer is removed and the drain returns to its curled shape. Some catheters have a locking drawstring to stabilize the pigtail and prevent dislodgement. It is interesting to note that the bore size of a drain does not correlate directly with its performance. On the other hand, the consistency of the fluid will require a certain minimum drain size. Larger catheters are not generally advisable, however, and are much more difficult to place than smaller catheters.[76] Hydrophilic catheter coatings are helpful in that they facilitate tube advancement through the tissue and possible simultaneous dilation of the tract. The tip is usually conical and may have a short or long taper. Long tapered tips are best in cases where the catheter is also intended to function as a dilator (e.g., biliary Plus-Drain from Peter Pflugbeil GmbH).

For smoother tracking, the distal portion of the catheter can also be given a hydrophilic coating to reduce friction during advancement. This "AQ" (aqueous) coating provides a very slippery catheter surface that greatly reduces frictional resistance.

Many products come with centimeter length markings on their outer surface. This can be helpful in deep placements and makes it easier to assess insertion depth in the ultrasound image. Because drains are usually placed in a darkened room, funnel-shaped Luer lock connectors are helpful in facilitating the insertion.

Pigtail catheters can be advanced directly over a hollow needle, or they may be mounted on a metal introducer so that their tendency to assume their preformed shape will not curl the guidewire. When the catheter is mounted on the introducer, a sleeve already on the catheter shaft is usually advanced to straighten the catheter and prevent damage to its inner wall (▶ Fig. 2.17).

Basket-tipped catheters like the Malecot catheter are less commonly used and are not widely available for purchase. Malecot catheters are straightened with an introducer for insertion. When it is removed the basket expands, creating a large distal opening area that provides effective drainage and allows for 360° irrigation. The catheter is also self-retained by the expanded basket. Placement follows the technique described above.

Drainage catheters are available individually and in complete sets. We personally prefer to use individually packaged materials. This allows us to assemble our own sets for specific procedures and eliminates the need to open a new set when an extra part is needed. Our standard assortment includes a range of drainage catheters with outer diameters of 6F to 16F.

In principle, almost any hollow needle can be used for the drainage of ascites and pleural effusions. Drainage obstruction due to kinking can be avoided by using the

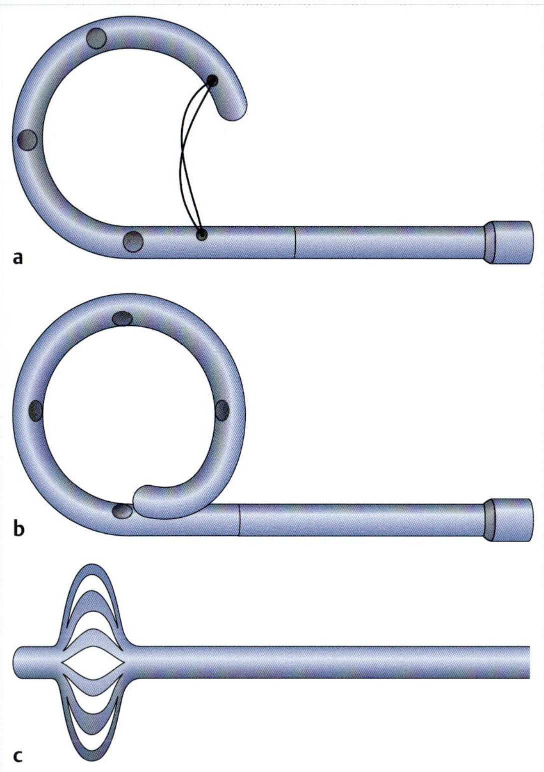

Fig. 2.17 Drainage systems.
a Pigtail catheter with drawstring.
b Pigtail system.
c Basket system.

Schlottmann paracentesis needle (Peter Pflugbeil GmbH), which is fixed to the skin with a retention plate. The needle has a 6F diameter, is available in 7 to 15 cm lengths, and has variable side hole lengths to prevent occlusion. The needle is placed by a direct trocar technique.

Because the percutaneous aspiration and external drainage of pancreatic pseudocysts is often associated with late complications, a drainage system was developed in which the pseudocyst was aspirated with a transgastric needle followed by the placement of a double-pigtail drainage stent with one end in the pseudocyst and one end in the stomach.[77] Since then, this technique has been largely abandoned since transgastric pseudocyst drainage can be performed far more easily by endosonography.

2.2.16 Other Drainage Systems

The variety of complete drainage systems available on the market has led to an "interdisciplinary" use of these devices. For example, the Cystofix system (for suprapubic cystostomy) and the Pneumocath device (for pleural drainage) can also be used for the placement of superficial and large-bore drains (▶ Fig. 2.18) even though they are not specifically approved for that indication.

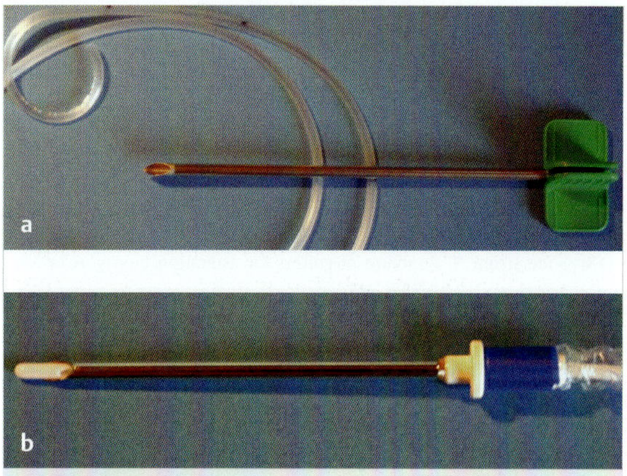

Fig. 2.18
a Cystofix catheter (Braun Melsungen AG, Germany).
b Pneumocath catheter (Intra Special Catheters GmbH, Germany). (Source: reference[42].)

Especially in patients with chronic abscesses, large-bore catheter systems are essential for flushing necrotic material and debris from the abscess cavity.[78] These systems are introduced by direct puncture with a very large-gauge cannula, through which the drainage catheter is then advanced. This technique may pose a high risk of injury when targeting deeper structures, however.

2.2.17 Accessories

Drains are fitted with 2- and 3-way stopcocks for occlusion. Again, a variety of designs are available. Device options include "high-flow" 3-way stopcocks and hemostatic valves. Drainage tubing is available in various lengths with collecting bags of various sizes. If a syringe with a Luer lock fitting is not to be placed at the proximal end of the catheter, an adapter is needed (rotating adapter). Industry offers funnel adapters in a variety of lengths and sizes. The same applies to drainage bags, which must be sterile. Negative-pressure systems are used for smaller fluid collections or in situations where fluid may reaccumulate after drainage.

References

[1] Stursberg H. Technik der wichtigsten Eingriffe in der Behandlung innerer Krankheiten. Berlin: A. Marcus & E. Weber's Verlag; 1949
[2] Kalk H. Die Therapie an den Berliner Universitäts-Kliniken. Berlin Vienna: Urban & Schwarzenberg; 1943
[3] Lebert H. Traite pracique des maladies cancereuses et des affections eurables confondues avec le caner. Paris: Baillière; 1935
[4] Bocking A. Perkutane diagnostische Punktion: Aspekte der Zytologie und Histologie. In: Günther RW, Thelen M, eds. Stuttgart: Thieme; 1996: 596–605
[5] Vogel H, Renk C. Punktion der Hals- und Brustorgane: Risiken der Röntgendiagnostik. Munich: Urban & Schwarzenberg; 1986
[6] Frerichs FT. Über den Diabetes. Berlin: Hirschwald; 1884
[7] Baron E. Aspiration for removal of biopsy material from the liver. Arch Intern Med 1939; 63: 276–289
[8] Martin HE, Ellis EB. Biopsy by needle puncture and aspiration. Ann Surg 1930; 92: 169–181

[9] Coley B, Sharp G, Ellis E. Diagnosis of bone tumors by aspiration. Am J Surg 193 1; 13: 21: 4–224

[10] Robertson R, Ball R. Destructive spine lesions: diagnosis by needle biopsy. J Bone Joint Surg 1935; 17: 749–75-8

[11] Blady J. Aspiration biopsy of tumors in obscure or difficult location under roentgenoscopic guidance. AJR Am J Roentgenol 1939; 42: 515–524

[12] Kirtland HB. A safe method of pancreatic biopsy; a preliminary report. Am J Surg 1951; 82: 451–457

[13] Soderstrom N. Puncture of goiters for aspiration biopsy. Acta Med Scand 1952; 144: 237–244

[14] Rasmussen SN, Holm HH, Kristensen JK, Barlebo H. Ultrasonically-guided liver biopsy. BMJ 1972; 2: 500–502

[15] Menghini G. One-second needle biopsy of the liver. Gastroenterology 1958; 35: 190–199

[16] Gebel M, Horstkotte H, Köster C, Brunkhorst R, Brandt M, Atay Z. Ultrasound-guided fine needle puncture of the abdominal organs: indications, results, risks [Article in German]. Ultraschall Med 1986; 7: 198–202

[17] Gottschalk U, Ignee A, Dietrich CF. Ultrasound guided interventions, part 1, diagnostic procedures [Article in German]. Z Gastroenterol 2009; 47: 682–690

[18] Swobodnik W, Janowitz P, Kratzer W et al. Comparison of ultrasound-controlled fine needle and coarse needle puncture of defined lesions in the abdomen [Article in German]. Ultraschall Med 1990; 11: 287–289

[19] Jakobeit C. Ultrasound-controlled puncture procedures: free-hand puncture versus transducer biopsy puncture. 5 years' experience [Article in German]. Ultraschall Med 1986; 7: 290–292

[20] Mathis G, Bitschnau R, Gehmacher O, Dirschmid K. Ultrasound-guided transthoracic puncture [Article in German]. Ultraschall Med 1999; 20: 226–235

[21] Glaser J, Mann O, Siegmüller M, Pausch J. Prospective study of the incidence of ultrasound-detected hepatic hematomas due to percutaneous Menghini needle liver biopsy and laparoscopy-guided Silverman needle biopsy. Ital J Gastroenterol 1994; 26: 338–341

[22] Haage P, Piroth W, Staatz G, Adam G, Günther RW. CT-guided percutaneous biopsies for the classification of focal liver lesions: a comparison between 14 G and 18 G puncture biopsy needles [Article in German]. Rofo 1999; 171: 44–48

[23] Piccinino F, Sagnelli E, Pasquale G, Giusti G. Complications following percutaneous liver biopsy. A multicentre retrospective study on 68,276 biopsies. J Hepatol 1986; 2: 165–173

[24] Weiss H, Düntsch U, Weiss A. Risks of fine needle puncture: results of a survey in West Germany (German Society of Ultrasound in Medicine survey) [Article in German]. Ultraschall Med 1988; 9: 121–127

[25] Colloredo G, Guido M, Sonzogni A, Leandro G. Impact of liver biopsy size on histological evaluation of chronic viral hepatitis: the smaller the sample, the milder the disease. J Hepatol 2003; 39: 239–244

[26] Schaeberle W. Interventionelle Sonographie. Berlin, Heidelberg, New York: Springer Verlag; 2000

[27] Giorgio A, de Stefano G, Di Sarno A, Liorre G, Ferraioli G. Percutaneous needle aspiration of multiple pyogenic abscesses of the liver: 13-year single-center experience. AJR Am J Roentgenol 2006; 187: 1585–1590

[28] Nürnberg D. Ultrasound of adrenal gland tumours and indications for fine needle biopsy (uFNB) [Article in German]. Ultraschall Med 2005; 26: 458–469

[29] Ojalehto M, Tikkakoski T, Rissanen T, Apaja-Sarkkinen M. Ultrasound-guided percutaneous thoracoabdominal biopsy. Acta Radiol 2002; 43: 152–158

[30] Rigamonti C, Fraquelli M, Francesca Donato M, Colombo M. Liver biopsy techniques: automated aspiration needles provide adequate tissue samples. Am J Gastroenterol 2007; 102: 2608–2609

[31] Menghini G. The needle biopsy of the liver, an effective technical progress. Sci Med Ital (Engl Ed) 1957; 6: 212–229

[32] Roschlau G. Patho-histological liver diagnostics-yesterday and today [Article in German]. Zentralbl Allg Pathol 1985; 130: 477–480

[33] Riemann B, Menzel J, Schiemann U, Domschke W, Konturek JW. Ultrasound-guided biopsies of abdominal organs with an automatic biopsy system. A retrospective analysis of the quality of biopsies and of hemorrhagic complications. Scand J Gastroenterol 2000; 35: 102–107

[34] Diederich S, Padge B, Vossas U, Hake R, Eidt S. Application of a single needle type for all image-guided biopsies: results of 100 consecutive core biopsies in various organs using a novel tri-axial, end-cut needle. Cancer Imaging 2006; 6: 43–50

[35] Diederich S, Padge B, Hake R, Vossas U, Eidt S. Ergebnisse der perkutanen Schneidbiopsie mit einem neuartigen vollautomatischen triaxialen Biopsiesystem in verschiedenen Organen. Fortschr Roentgenstr 2005; 177: PO-176

[36] Jenssen C, Dietrich CF. Endoscopic ultrasound in chronic pancreatitis [Article in German]. Z Gastroenterol 2005; 43: 737–749

[37] Dumonceau J-M, Polkowski M, Larghi A et al. European Society of Gastrointestinal Endoscopy. Indications, results, and clinical impact of endoscopic ultrasound (EUS)-guided sampling in gastroenterology: European Society of Gastrointestinal Endoscopy (ESGE) Clinical Guideline. Endoscopy 2011; 43: 897–912

[38] Otto RC, Wellauer J. Ultraschallgeführte Biopsie. Berlin: Springer; 1985

[39] Lindgren PG. Percutaneous needle biopsy. A new technique. Acta Radiol Diagn (Stockh) 1982; 23: 653–656

[40] Sittek H, Schneider P, Perlet C, Baudrexel C, Reiser M. Minimally invasive surgical procedures of the breast: comparison of different biopsy systems in a breast parenchymal model [Article in German]. Radiologe 2002; 42: 6–10

[41] Becker D, Strobel D, Niedobitek G, Steininger H, Kirchner T, Hahn EG. Sonographisch gezielte Leberparenchympunktion: Vergleich von zwei verschiedenen Nadeltypen, erste Ergebnisse. 22. Dreiländertreffen, 1998

[42] Gottschalk U, Ignee A, Dietrich CF. Ultrasound-guided interventions and description of the equipment [Article in German]. Z Gastroenterol 2010; 48: 1305–1316

[43] Nather K, Ochsner A. Der linksseitige Abszeß bei Appendicitis. Langenbecks Arch Surg 1924; 188: 114–123

[44] Chelius MJ. Handbuch der Chirurgie. Stuttgart: Bei Eberhard Friedrich Wolters; 1830

[45] Gray R, Leekam R, Mackenzie R, St Louis EL, Grosman H. Percutaneous abscess drainage. Gastrointest Radiol 1985; 10: 79–84

[46] Birth M, Iblher P, Hildebrand P, Nolde J, Bruch HP. Ultrasound-guided interventions using magnetic field navigation. First experiences with Ultra-Guide 2000 under operative conditions [Article in German]. Ultraschall Med 2003; 24: 90–95

[47] Dahami Z, Sarf I, Dakir M et al. Treatment of primary pyogenic abscess of the psoas: retrospective study of 18 cases [Article in French]. Ann Urol (Paris) 2001; 35: 329–334

[48] Men S, Akhan O, Köroğlu M. Percutaneous drainage of abdominal abcess. Eur J Radiol 2002; 43: 204–218

[49] Liu CH, Gervais DA, Hahn PF, Arellano RS, Uppot RN, Mueller PR. Percutaneous hepatic abscess drainage: do multiple abscesses or multiloculated abscesses preclude drainage or affect outcome? J Vasc Interv Radiol 2009; 20: 1059–1065

[50] Gervais DA, Ho CH, O'Neill MJ, Arellano RS, Hahn PF, Mueller PR. Recurrent abdominal and pelvic abscesses: incidence, results of repeated percutaneous drainage, and underlying causes in 956 drainages. AJR Am J Roentgenol 2004; 182: 463–466

[51] Zerem E, Hadzic A. Sonographically guided percutaneous catheter drainage versus needle aspiration in the management of pyogenic liver abscess. AJR Am J Roentgenol 2007; 189: W138–W142

[52] Tan YM, Chung AY, Chow PK et al. An appraisal of surgical and percutaneous drainage for pyogenic liver abscesses larger than 5 cm. Ann Surg 2005; 241: 485–490

[53] Kägeth CJ, Ricklin ES, Schöll B, Saurenmann E. Conservative treatment of puerperal breast abscesses with repeated sonographically guided aspirations and oral antibiotic administrations [Article in German]. Z Geburtshilfe Neonatol 2004; 208: 170–173

[54] vanSonnenberg E, D'Agostino HB, Casola G, Goodacre BW, Sanchez RB, Taylor B. US-guided transvaginal drainage of pelvic abscesses and fluid collections. Radiology 1991; 181: 53–56
[55] Chung YF, Tan YM, Lui HF et al. Management of pyogenic liver abscesses - percutaneous or open drainage? Singapore Med J 2007; 48: 1158–1165, quiz 1165
[56] Vikrama KS, Shyamkumar NK, Vinu M, Joseph P, Vyas F, Venkatramani S. Percutaneous catheter drainage in the treatment of abdominal compartment syndrome. Can J Surg 2009; 52: E19–E20
[57] Barthels M, von Epka M. Hämostaseologische Therapie – Plasmatisches System. In: Barthels M, von Depka M, eds. Das Gerinnungskompendium. Stuttgart, New York: Thieme; 2003
[58] Glaser J, Pausch J. The risk of liver biopsy [Article in German]. Z Gastroenterol 1995; 33: 673–676
[59] Suchman AL, Griner PF. Diagnostic uses of the activated partial thromboplastin time and prothrombin time. Ann Intern Med 1986; 104: 810–816
[60] Hellstern P, Oberfrank K, Kohler M, Heinkel K, Wenzel E. Die aktivierte partielle Thromboplastinzeit als Screeningtest für leichte Gerinnungsfaktorenmängel – Untersuchungen zur Sensitivität von verschiedener Reagenzien. Lab Med 1989; 13: 83–86
[61] Contreras M. Final statement from the consensus conference on platelet transfusion. Transfusion 1998; 38: 796–797
[62] García-Erce JA, Muñoz M, Bisbe E et al. Predeposit autologous donation in spinal surgery: a multicentre study. Eur Spine J 2004; 13 Suppl 1: S34–S39
[63] Dietrich CF, Muller G, Ignee A. Acute abdomen, gastroenterologists view [Article in German]. Praxis (Bern 1994) 2007; 96: 645–659
[64] Ignee A, Baum U, Schuessler G, Dietrich CF. Contrast-enhanced ultrasound-guided percutaneous cholangiography and cholangiodrainage (CEUS-PTCD). Endoscopy 2009; 41: 725–726
[65] Almeida J, Mesquita M, Ferraz J et al. Hepatocellular carcinoma developing at the puncture site after percutaneous ethanol injection. J Clin Ultrasound 2008; 36: 105–107
[66] Schäberle W, Eisele R. Percutaneous ultrasound controlled drainage of large splenic abscesses [Article in German]. Chirurg 1997; 68: 744–748
[67] Kos S, Jacob L. Perkutane Abszessdrainagen. Radiologie up2date 2008; 8: 107–131
[68] Seitz K. Sonographic diagnosis of diverticulitis: the burdensome way to acceptance [Article in German]. Ultraschall Med 2004; 25: 335–336
[69] Seldinger SI. Catheter replacement of the needle in percutaneous arteriography; a new technique. Acta Radiol 1953; 39: 368–376
[70] Moll R, Knupffler J, Fruhwald P, Range R, Schindler G. Vergleich der Trokar- und der Seldingertechnik bei CT-gesteuerten Abszessdrainagen. Ro Fo 2003: VO60.3
[71] Overdeck DL, Lynch JL, Gervais DA. Percutaneous abdominal and pelvic abscess drainage techniques. Part I: Tools of the trade. Semin Intervent Radiol 2003; 20: 177–184
[72] Habashi S, Draganov PV. Pancreatic pseudocyst. World J Gastroenterol 2009; 15: 38–47
[73] Seifert H, Biermer M, Schmitt W et al. Transluminal endoscopic necrosectomy after acute pancreatitis: a multicentre study with long-term follow-up (the GEPARD Study). Gut 2009; 58: 1260–1266
[74] Seifert H, Faust D, Schmitt T, Dietrich C, Caspary W, Wehrmann T. Transmural drainage of cystic peripancreatic lesions with a new large-channel echo endoscope. Endoscopy 2001; 33: 1022–1026
[75] Seifert H, Dietrich C, Schmitt T, Caspary W, Wehrmann T. Endoscopic ultrasound-guided one-step transmural drainage of cystic abdominal lesions with a large-channel echo endoscope. Endoscopy 2000; 32: 255–259
[76] Bruennler T, Langgartner J, Lang S et al. Outcome of patients with acute, necrotizing pancreatitis requiring drainage-does drainage size matter? World J Gastroenterol 2008; 14: 725–730
[77] Bilbao JI, Alejandre PL, Longo JM et al. Percutaneous transgastric cystoduodenostomy in the treatment of a pancreatic pseudocyst: a new approach. Cardiovasc Intervent Radiol 1995; 18: 422–425
[78] vanSonnenberg E, Wittich GR, Casola G, Cabrera OA, Gosink BB, Resnick DL. Sonography of thigh abscess: detection, diagnosis, and drainage. AJR Am J Roentgenol 1987; 149: 769–772

3 Informed Consent

D. Nuernberg, A. Jung

When a physician has determined that a certain procedure is indicated for the diagnosis or treatment of a disease, that procedure may be undertaken only with the informed consent of the patient.[1] For this consent to be informed, the physician must explain the diagnostic or therapeutic procedure to the patient in a *comprehensive*, *understandable*, and *timely* manner prior to the proposed intervention. This disclosure must take place in an individual, face-to-face discussion between the physician and patient.

3.1 What Should Be Disclosed?

Before the patient can give written informed consent to proceed, he or she must be fully informed about the goal and necessity of the procedure, what the procedure will entail, potential risks and complications, and possible alternatives. The patient must be informed as to the nature, significance, and scope of the proposed test or treatment in its basic elements.

3.1.1 Indication

The proposed procedure is *indicated* if it is the best method available for investigating or treating the disease with an acceptable risk-to-benefit ratio. There may be no reasonable alternatives, or if such alternatives exist, they should be explained. Any therapeutic implications of the procedure should also be disclosed.[1]

3.1.2 Explaining the Procedure

The physician outlines the typical steps involved in the proposed test or treatment, with the aid if necessary of small drawings. If alternatives exist, they are also briefly explained. The patient must also be informed about any medications (sedatives, local anesthetics, analgesics) that will be administered. Necessary preliminary tests and follow-up care are also described.

3.1.3 Risks and Complications

The patient should be informed about risks and complications, regardless of the likelihood of their occurrence. Disclosing the risks of complications is an essential part of the informed consent process.

It should be noted that the more urgent a procedure is, the less stringent the requirements for informed consent. By the same token, the more dangerous or risky a procedure is, the greater the need to provide a detailed disclosure.[2]

Risks may be patient-related or procedure-related. Patient-related risks result from the history, laboratory data (e.g., coagulation), and available findings. The condition of the patient may also affect the risk. Procedure-related complications can be reduced by suitable preparation (see Chapter 9). They depend on the materials and instruments used and on the competence of the operator. Attention to guidelines, sound procedural technique, and follow-up measures after the intervention can reduce the incidence of complications.

The patient should be informed about typical risks of the procedure, regardless of the complication rate. Atypical risks may or may not be disclosed, depending on the complication rate. Rare risks should be disclosed only if they would adversely affect the patient's quality of life.[3]

3.2 Means of Disclosure

There are no laws defining the exact way in which information about a procedure must be provided to the patient. But, in all cases, necessary information should be disclosed and discussed individually in a conversation between the doctor and patient.

3.2.1 Consent Form

In most countries, physicians are obligated to document informed consent. This means that, as a rule, physicians employ patient consent forms that can be ordered or downloaded online. In Germany for example:

- www.perimed.de (click on Innere Medizin, Gastroenterologie).
- www.diomed.de (click on Innere Medizin, Gastroenterologie).
- www.thieme-compliance.com

3.2.2 Informed Consent Discussion

Consent forms provide the physician with a helpful guide in preparing to discuss the proposed test or treatment with the patient. They should never replace a verbal conversation between the physician and the patient (▶ Fig. 3.1). The doctor should describe the procedure using language that a lay person can understand. The scope of the informed consent discussion will depend on the nature, urgency, and extent of the procedure, on its consequences, and on the patient's level of education and knowledge. The patient is given an opportunity to ask any questions that he or she might have. The physician is obligated to answer those questions truthfully and completely, again using language that is easily understood. A small drawing or handwritten note by the physician on the consent form provides additional documentation of the face-to-face discussion, and we strongly recommend that this be done routinely.

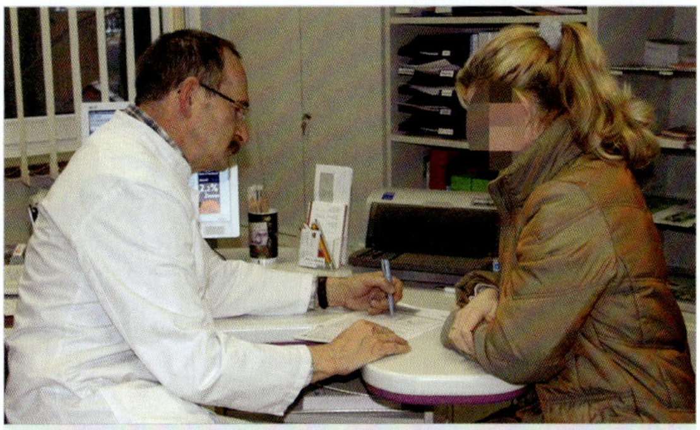

Fig. 3.1 Before the consent form is signed the physician explains the procedure to the patient in a calm and relaxed atmosphere.

Having been allowed adequate time to consider their decision, patients confirm their understanding and agreement by signing the consent form.

3.2.3 Delegating Informed Consent

The responsibility for patient education lies with the physician and should not be delegated to a nonphysician. On the other hand, the informing physician does not have to be the physician who will carry out the procedure. He or she may be a family practitioner or ward physician, for example. Nevertheless, the physician performing the intervention must see to it that the patient has been fully informed by a competent physician. A department head or supervising physician who delegates risk disclosure to a subordinate physician must take whatever steps are necessary to ensure and confirm that the patient has been properly informed.[3,4]

3.3 Documentation

Preprinted consent forms in which patients merely confirm that they have received necessary information, but with no details on the scope of the disclosure, are worth little in a court of law. Thus, even when standard consent forms are used, a personal handwritten entry as to the content of the discussion, the timing of the patient's signature, and possible explanatory drawings (no entries after the fact!) may be essential for documenting valid informed consent.

3.4 Timing of the Consent Process

Patients must be allowed sufficient time to reflect on the purported benefits and risks of the test or treatment before giving their consent. Patients should make their decision for or against the procedure of their own free will, without pressure or coercion, and should be able to seek further advice if needed. In the case of minor ambulatory or diagnostic procedures, such as paracentesis for ascites, thoracentesis, or fine needle biopsy of the thyroid gland, it may be acceptable to obtain informed consent on the day of the procedure.[2] In the case of major outpatient procedures such as the percutaneous biopsy of hepatic or pancreatic lesions, informed consent should be obtained before the day of the procedure. A hospitalized patient will generally provide informed consent on the day before the procedure.[2–6] In Germany for example, informed consent obtained the evening before the procedure is not considered adequate under the law. The obligation to secure informed consent on the day before the procedure is waived in an emergent or life-threatening situation, but the nature of the emergency should be clearly documented. A premedicated patient cannot legitimately participate in the informed consent process.

3.5 Special Situations

3.5.1 Implied Consent

The consent given by a patient initially applies only to measures that were included in the informed consent discussion. If the physician recognizes at the time of the consultation that the procedure will have to be extended, this fact should be noted during the informed consent discussion (e.g., the need to place a drain because the percutaneous aspiration of a presumed tumor yielded pus). If it is discovered during the intervention that the procedure will have to be altered or extended, the physician must first weigh the risk of discontinuing and repeating the procedure against the risk of proceeding with an extended procedure. **Implied consent** is present if it may be assumed that a reasonable patient in the same situation would have consented to the extended procedure if he or she had been properly informed. In a legal sense, however, implied consent can provide a valid justification only if withholding the procedure would have posed a significant danger to the life or health of the patient (e.g., the development of sepsis).

3.5.2 Patients Lacking the Capacity to Consent

In cases where patients lack the capacity to give informed consent, any further actions should conform to their wishes as expressed in an advance directive, health care power of attorney, or living will. If an individual is designated as the decision-maker (e.g., parents, caregivers, or health care proxy), his or her decisions will be final.

3.5.3 Minors

Patients who are not of legal age to give informed consent are represented by both parents.[7] The treating physician may assume consent from both parents when one parent presents with the minor for treatment or makes the appointment. In the case of difficult procedures in which complications may arise that could seriously impair the minor's quality of life, informed consent should be obtained from both parents whenever possible.[7]

Minors themselves have the authority to give consent if they are capable of understanding the significance and implications of the procedure. If a patient is near the legal age of consent, that person cannot be forced to undergo a medical procedure against his or her will (see Chapter 32).

3.5.4 Language Barriers

In obtaining informed consent from foreign language speakers, it is important to make sure that the patient can follow the explanations of the informing physician. Whenever possible, someone who speaks the patient's language (a family member, interpreter, or multilingual hospital staff member) should be called in. Information and consent forms in the patient's native language are also helpful and will be available from online sources.

Similar considerations apply to patients who have impaired speech comprehension, such as stroke patients and hearing-impaired persons.

3.5.5 Waiving of Informed Consent

In the case of patients who elect to give "uninformed" consent without receiving a formal explanation of the proposed test or treatment, the usual informed consent process may be waived. These patients must confirm that they have full confidence in their physician to make all diagnostic and therapeutic decisions on their behalf, and this waiver must be documented.

If a patient refuses a procedure despite a detailed explanation of the consequences of withholding treatment, the physician is obliged to respect that decision.[4]

References

[1] Lutz H. Patient Information and Informed Consent. Paper presented at the Interventional Ultrasound Conference in Berlin, May 27–20, 2010

[2] Teubel A. Aufklären, aber richtig. Deutsches Ärzteblatt 2010; 107: A951–A952

[3] Arbeitshilfen der DKG. Empfehlungen zur Aufklärung der Krankenhauspatienten über vorgesehene ärztliche Maßnahmen. 6th ed. Deutsche Krankenhaus Verlagsgesellschaft: 2012

[4] Schara J, Brandt L. Provision of information to patients - legal and humanitarian requirements [Article in German]. Schmerz 2008; 22: 91–98

[5] Baur U. Aufklärung und Einwilligung des Patienten. Arzt Krankenhaus 1991; 64: 222–226

[6] Schreiber H-L. Patient education from the legal viewpoint [Article in German]. Internist (Berl) 1983; 24: 185–189

[7] Laum HD, Smentkowski U. Ärztliche Behandlungsfehler – Statut der Gutachterkommission, ÄK NR. Köln: Deutscher Ärzteverlag; 2006

4 Medications, Equipment, and Setup Requirements

D. Nuernberg, A. Jung

4.1 Medications

Chapters 7, 8, and 9 may be consulted for further information on medications for endocarditis prophylaxis and on dealing with and correcting coagulopathies prior to interventional procedures.

4.1.1 Premedication

Sedation

Interventional procedures often require sedation as well as adequate patient monitoring. The risk of serious side effects depends on the type of procedure, the individual risk profile of the patient, and the spectrum of side effects associated with the sedative agent. Whether to use sedation (and analgesia) is always decided on an individual basis. Individual criteria are the patient, the operator/examiner, and the planned procedure. Thus, minor procedures (e.g., thoracentesis, paracentesis, percutaneous liver biopsy) and procedures that require patient cooperation (e.g., deep inspiration to aid lesion visualization) can often be performed successfully without sedation. On the other hand, sedation-analgesia is essential for longer and potentially painful procedures (e.g., abscess drainage, PTCD, nephrostomy, local tumor therapy) (see Chapter 11).

Risk Factors

The risk profile depends on the type of procedure and the health status of the patient. The individual patient risk should be assessed before any interventional procedure is performed. The ASA (American Society of Anesthesiologists) classification is helpful in assessing patient risk.[1–4]

The following factors are associated with an **increased risk** (ASA class III to V):

- Decompensated heart failure
- NYHA class III to IV
- Coronary heart disease
- Valvular heart disease
- Liver and renal failure
- Pulmonary diseases
- Coagulopathies

Thus, a detailed history and clinical examination should be performed before every interventional procedure. The physician performing the intervention should be aware of any comorbid conditions so that preventive care measures (e.g., endocarditis prophylaxis) can be instituted to prevent complications.

Since interventions may be unpleasant as well as painful, the patient may express a desire for sedation and the physician may recommend it in advance of the procedure. Interventional procedures, especially those of a difficult nature (percutaneous transhepatic cholangiography and drainage [PTCD], abscess drainage, endoscopic ultrasonography with fine-needle biopsy [EUS-FNB]), require an immobilized patient. Sedation facilitates and expedites this goal and also results in higher patient satisfaction.[5]

4.1.2 Analgesia

The following interventional procedures often require sedation with analgesia:

- Abscess drainage (Chapter 15)
- Percutaneous therapy of liver tumors (Chapters 18 and 19)
- PTCD (Chapter 20)
- Pancreatic interventions (Chapters 12 and 22)

Sedation is withheld if the procedure will require active cooperation from the patient such as deep inspiration or a short breath-hold to aid localization. Propofol is indicated in cases where patient cooperation is not required, when the patient is very anxious, when the patient expressly desires procedural sedation, or in patients with a prior history of poor or paradoxical response to other sedatives (▶ Table 4.1).

Benzodiazepine and opioid antagonists should always be immediately accessible (▶ Table 4.2). The routine use of antagonists is not recommended.

Table 4.1 Sedatives and analgesics used in interventional procedures

Agent	Brand name	Dosage
Benzodiazepines		
Midazolam	Dormicum	2–5 mg IV; up to 10 mg in rare cases (bolus of 30–80 mg/kg BW[1,6–8])
Propofol	Disoprivan	Intermittent bolus injection[1]: 40/60 mg bolus (for < 70 kg BW, 60 mg for > 70 kg BW), then 10–20 mg boluses while monitoring depth of sedation
Analgesics		
Pethidine	Dolantin	25–50 mg IV

Table 4.2 Sedative antagonists

Agent	Brand name	Dosage
Benzodiazepine antagonist		
Flumazenil	Anexate	0.2–0.5 mg IV (bolus)
Opioid antagonist		
Naloxone	Narcanti	0.4–2 mg IV

Intravenous sedation requires secure intravenous access throughout the procedure and recovery period. Intravenous access is necessary even in patients not receiving primary sedation, as it will permit a rapid response to any complications that arise. Medication doses are adjusted for individual body weight and titrated to response. Resuscitation drugs and equipment should be immediately accessible. Pulse oximetry is routinely employed. Nasal oxygen supplementation is optional but should be available whenever propofol is used[1,9–12] (▶ Table 4.3).

4.1.3 Coagulation

Laboratory values for blood count and coagulation should be available before every interventional procedure. Iatrogenic hemorrhage is an ever-present risk. There are various ways of assessing this risk. On the one hand, it is determined by patient-dependent factors such as a bleeding diathesis due to congenital, acquired, or pharmacologically induced coagulopathies. It also depends critically on the nature of the procedure (Chapter 9).

Table 4.3 Recommendations on sedation and monitoring for interventional procedures[1]

Procedure	Recommendation
1. Monitoring	Monitoring by qualified personnel
	Pulse oximetry should always be used
	Suitable rooms and monitoring equipment should be available for postinterventional monitoring
2. Sedation	Sedative dosage should be adjusted for each patient individually, and antagonists should be accessible
	The use of propofol means more stringent monitoring requirements: a pulse oximeter and BP monitor, or preferably an ECG and BP monitor should be available. Oxygen administration should be available if required[13–16]
	Intravenous sedation requires secure intravenous access, patient monitoring, and immediate accessibility to resuscitation drugs and equipment. It should be noted that procedural sedation with propofol significantly reduces pain sensation
3. Individual risk assessment	Individual patient risk should be determined in advance of the procedure based on ASA criteria

In preparation for the intervention, we generally recommend obtaining a bleeding history and determining the platelet count and activated partial thromboplastin time (PTT) and thromboplastin time (Quick value). A drug history should also be obtained (oral anticoagulants, antiplatelet drugs, heparin) (Chapter 3).

Discontinuing Antiplatelet Therapy (Anticoagulation)

The decision whether to discontinue antiplatelet therapy in the perioperative period will depend on three questions:

1. What is the urgency of the planned procedure?
2. How important is antiplatelet therapy to the patient?
3. What is the bleeding risk of the planned procedure?

The final decision whether to continue or withdraw antiplatelet drugs rests with the physician. There are growing numbers of physicians who are even willing to operate on patients taking ASA (aspirin) or clopidogrel. Nevertheless, caution is advised in patients scheduled for a liver or renal biopsy. Percutaneous renal and liver biopsies are classified as procedures with a high bleeding risk, whereas biopsies of other organs and endoscopic biopsies are not considered to have a high bleeding risk. There is the possibility to bridge platelet inhibition on patients with high stroke risks by the administration of Aggrastat (tirofiban, a reversible GPIIb/IIIa inhibitor; Merck) periinterventionally. After discontinuing ASA and clopidogrel (e.g., 5 days preoperatively), Aggrastat may be given intravenously 3 days before intervention. This is a common practice, although it represents an off-label use of Aggrastat. Afterwards, the inhibition of platelet aggregation can be restarted postoperatively, depending on the risk of rebleeding.

4.1.4 Local Anesthesia

Interventional procedures generally require local anesthesia. Following ultrasound localization and marking of the puncture site, the skin is prepped and then infiltrated with a local anesthetic. The most commonly used agents are 1% or 2% lidocaine and procaine. Local anesthetic may be infiltrated into the superficial and deeper tissues and even down to the peritoneum, depending on the location of the target lesion. Peritoneal infiltration should always be done under ultrasound guidance. Local anesthesia is administered with the thinnest possible needle size (e.g., a 23-gauge disposable hypodermic needle of adequate length). For superficial targets (e.g., a thyroid biopsy or lymph node biopsy), 2 to 3 mL of a 2% lidocaine solution should be sufficient. Deeper targets (kidney, liver, pancreas, organ abscess) will require a larger dose (8–10 mL). Thus, the necessary dose of local anesthetic depends on the depth and location of the intended target. Effective local anesthesia may eliminate the need for sedation. Initial local anesthesia should always be administered in cases where it cannot be predicted in advance whether one or multiple needle passes will be required during the procedure.

4.2 Equipment and Setup Requirements

4.2.1 Biopsy Equipment

The main prerequisite is an ultrasound scanner with a suitable transducer. Localization techniques are described in Chapters 2 and 14.

4.2.2 Interventional Materials

The various biopsy needles and catheters are described in Chapter 2 and under specific headings elsewhere in the text. Assisting personnel lay out the equipment needed for a particular procedure after first checking the expiration dates, since most interventional materials are single-use items. Different surgeons may have considerably different setup preferences. Catheters should be stored in proximity to the procedure room so that additional materials can be quickly accessed if needed.

4.2.3 Positioning, Preprocedure Examination, and Marking

Good patient positioning is essential for a successful procedure that is well tolerated by the patient. Correct positioning should:

- Provide optimum access for the procedure
- Ensure patient comfort and tolerance, taking into account the anticipated procedure time
- Allow for optimum monitoring, which is usually handled by assisting personnel

Positioning aids are a perfectly valid tool that is helpful in certain situations. A thorough preprocedure examination will not only determine the optimum patient position but will also confirm the site of the lesion, assess its movement with respirations, indicate where the skin should be marked (cross-hairs), and define the overall extent of the interventional field (in case multiple or alternative access routes will be needed). The skin marker should have non–water-soluble ink so that the skin prep will not eradicate the marking. The skin marking also defines the optimum area for infiltration with local anesthetic. Skin marking should be done after the patient has been positioned for the procedure.

4.2.4 Monitoring During the Procedure

Monitoring is handled mainly by assistants and the physician. Monitoring devices are simply aids to patient surveillance. The operator should have only an indirect role in monitoring since he or she must concentrate on performing the procedure swiftly and accurately. This circumstance requires the constant presence of qualified nursing staff during the intervention. Recommendations on monitoring are listed in ▶ Table 4.3.[1]

The use of propofol requires the presence of a second physician experienced in emergency medicine or a second, specially trained and qualified individual who is responsible for monitoring the patient.[1]

4.2.5 Postprocedure Monitoring

The effect of the sedatives will persist for some time after the procedure is completed. This creates the need for postprocedure monitoring, preferably in a dedicated recovery room where machine monitoring and pulse oximetry will be continued. Ambulatory patients should be released only when accompanied by a companion who can observe the patient for several hours. Patients should not drive a motor vehicle or drink alcohol for 24 hours. These rules also apply to cases in which reversal agents have been used, since these agents are shorter-acting than the sedatives themselves. It is good practice to discharge patients with a procedure information sheet that indicates any sedatives that were used and lists possible complications (Chapter 3). The telephone number of the department should also be sent home with the patient in the event that questions or postinterventional problems arise. Some procedures require special follow-up scheduling for ultrasound, laboratory testing, etc.

4.2.6 Facilities (Procedure Room)

Different interventions require different facilities. More demanding and complex procedures require a more spacious procedure room. Simple, uncomplicated procedures are generally performed in an ordinary examination room. For patients who cannot be transported, some of these procedures (e.g., the percutaneous aspiration of effusions) can be performed at bedside in the patient's room. Patients who cannot be transported from the ICU pose a special challenge. In these cases, procedures such as a fine needle lymph node biopsy or a drain placement may be done at the bedside if the risk of intrahospital transport is deemed too high (e.g., in ventilated patients). The risks and benefits for a patient should always be weighed on a case-by-case basis.

More challenging procedures such as a complex drain insertion or percutaneous tumor therapy should be performed in procedure rooms. These rooms must meet well-defined technical and hygienic standards (Chapter 8).

Invasive procedures are classified into three groups on the basis of their extent and the level of patient risk:

- Operations
- Minor invasive procedures
- Invasive examinations and comparable measures

4.2.7 Functional and Design Requirements

Examination Rooms

Examination and treatment rooms should be designed such that the activities intended for those areas can be carried out in a technically proficient manner. These rooms should not be used for performing operations or other invasive procedures. The rooms should be equipped with scrub sinks and supplies for disinfecting the hands. Personnel should wear protective clothing and gloves for examinations, dressing changes, and comparable actions.

Procedure Room for "Minor Invasive Procedures"

The following rooms or areas are necessary for conducting (minor) invasive procedures, which include interventional procedures in internal medicine and radiology as well as more complex ultrasound-guided interventions that may require a combination of modalities:

- Procedure room
- Staff changing area (including means for hand disinfection and a disposal container)
- Area for the storage, disposal, and preparation of equipment and supplies
- Facilities may include a patient changing room
- A holding area may be provided for patients waiting for their procedure

As a general rule, invasive examinations should also be performed in procedure rooms. Invasive examinations are considered to include thorough clinical examinations, the probing of natural and artificial body orifices, endoscopies, injections, extensive dressing changes, the placement of certain intravascular catheters, and ultrasound-guided interventions.

Facilities

The layout and equipment of treatment and recovery rooms must meet the needs of patients with significant comorbid conditions. Accordingly, the treatment room should be equipped with monitoring devices (pulse oximetry, BP and ECG monitoring), appropriate emergency medications, oxygen, suction, resuscitation equipment (emergency kit), and a patient trolley.

4.2.8 Operational and Organizational Requirements

Personnel should remove ward attire and disinfect their hands in a designated staff changing room. Next, in the procedure room, they put on a protective gown and, if necessary, sterile gloves. A hair cover and a mask that covers the nose and mouth should additionally be worn for minor operative procedures that have an increased risk of infection. Also, a sterile surgical gown and sterile gloves are donned following surgical hand disinfection. Gloves, masks, and gowns are changed after every procedure (Chapter 8).

Ambulatory Procedures

Ambulatory procedures should not pose an increase of infection for patients. As in other settings, invasive procedures are classified as "operations" or "minor invasive procedures" and are subject to the same spatial, technical, and organizational requirements as inpatient procedures. Ultrasound-guided services for outpatients include percutaneous liver biopsy and pancreatic biopsy.

References

[1] Riphaus A, Wehrmann T, Weber B et al. Sektion Enoskopie im Auftrag der Deutschen Gesellschaft für Verdauungs- und Stoffwechselerkrankungen e.V. (DGVS). Bundesverband Niedergelassener Gastroenterologen Deuschlands e. V. (Bng). Chirurgische Arbeitsgemeinschaft für Endoskopie und Sonographie der Deutschen Gesellschaft für Allgemein- und Viszeralchirurgie (DGAV). Deutsche Morbus Crohn/Colitis ulcerosa Vereinigung e. V. (DCCV). Deutsche Gesellschaft für Endoskopie-Assistenzpersonal (DEGEA). Deutsche Gesellschaft für Anästhesie und Intensivmedizin (DGAI). Gesellschaft für Recht und Politik im Gesundheitswesen (GPRG). S3-guidelines—sedation in gastrointestinal endoscopy [Article in German]. Z Gastroenterol 2008; 46: 1298–1330

[2] Practice guidelines for sedation and analgesia by non-anesthesiologists. A report by the American Society of Anesthesiologists Task Force on Sedation and Analgesia by Non-Anesthesiologists. Anesthesiology 1996; 84: 459–471

[3] American Society of Anesthesiologists Task Force on Sedation and Analgesia by Non-Anesthesiologists. Practice guidelines for sedation and analgesia by non-anesthesiologists. Anesthesiology 2002; 96: 1004–1017

[4] Cohen LB, Delegge MH, Aisenberg J et al. AGA Institute. AGA Institute review of endoscopic sedation. Gastroenterology 2007; 133: 675–701

[5] Jung M, Hofmann C, Kiesslich R, Brackertz A. Improved sedation in diagnostic and therapeutic ERCP: propofol is an alternative to midazolam. Endoscopy 2000; 32: 233–238

[6] Carlsson U, Grattidge P. Sedation for upper gastrointestinal endoscopy: a comparative study of propofol and midazolam. Endoscopy 1995; 27: 240–243

[7] Christe C, Janssens JP, Armenian B, Herrmann F, Vogt N. Midazolam sedation for upper gastrointestinal endoscopy in older persons: a randomized, double-blind, placebo-controlled study. J Am Geriatr Soc 2000; 48: 1398–1403

[8] Patterson KW, Casey PB, Murray JP, O'Boyle CA, Cunningham AJ. Propofol sedation for outpatient upper gastrointestinal endoscopy: comparison with midazolam. Br J Anaesth 1991; 67: 108–111

[9] Dumonceau JM, Riphaus A, Aparicio JR et al. NAAP Task Force Members. European Society of Gastrointestinal Endoscopy, European Society of Gastroenterology and Endoscopy Nurses and Associates, and the European Society of Anaesthesiology Guideline: Non-anesthesiologist administration of propofol for GI endoscopy. Endoscopy 2010; 42: 960–974

[10] Riphaus A, Wehrmann T. Sedation, surveillance and preparation. Endoscopy 2007; 39: 2–6

[11] Riphaus A, Lechowicz I, Frenz MB, Wehrmann T. Propofol sedation for upper gastrointestinal endoscopy in patients with liver cirrhosis as an alternative to midazolam to avoid acute deterioration of minimal encephalopathy: a randomized, controlled study. Scand J Gastroenterol 2009; 44: 1244–1251

[12] Wehrmann T, Riphaus A. Sedation with propofol for interventional endoscopic procedures: a risk factor analysis. Scand J Gastroenterol 2008; 43: 368–374

[13] Practice guidelines for sedation and analgesia by non-anesthesiologists. A report by the American Society of Anesthesiologists Task Force on Sedation and Analgesia by Non-Anesthesiologists. Anesthesiology 1996; 84: 459–471

[14] Society of Gastroenterology Nurses and Associates, Inc. SGNA position statement: Statement on the use of sedation and analgesia in the gastrointestinal endoscopy setting. Gastroenterol Nurs 2003; 26: 209–211

[15] Society of Gastroenterology Nurses and Associates. SGNA position statement. Statement on the use of sedation and analgesia in the gastrointestinal endoscopy setting. Gastroenterol Nurs 2004; 27: 142–144

[16] SGNA Practice Committee. Statement on the use of sedation and analgesia in the gastrointestinal endoscopy setting. Gastroenterol Nurs 2008; 31: 249–251

5 Pathology and Cytology

A. Tannapfel, C. F. Dietrich

5.1 Pathology

Pathology deals with the diagnosis and classification of pathologic changes in organs and tissues.

Pathology has become an essential tool for intravital diagnosis. Pathologists examine biopsies, surgical specimens, and intraoperative frozen sections. Their services include the cytopathologic evaluation of cells and smears collected from mucous membranes and aspirated fluids. This subject is explored more fully in Chapter 6.

5.2 Biopsies

Despite the capabilities of modern imaging and interventional techniques and biochemical methods, a histologic diagnosis based on the biopsy of a suspected malignancy is still the fastest, safest, most reliable, and most cost-effective method for establishing a precise diagnosis. The histologic evaluation of tumors is essential not only for initial diagnosis but also in the follow-up care of patients who develop recurrent or metastatic disease.

5.2.1 Types of Biopsy Procedure

Excisional Biopsy

An excisional biopsy is a large tissue specimen removing the entire lesion. In the case of complete excision the biopsy is surrounded by adjacent connective tissue, muscles, nerve tissue, and blood vessels. Excisional biopsy with complete removal of the entire lesion is recommended for melanocytic lesions or skin tumors.

Incisional Biopsy

In an incisional biopsy, only a portion of the suspicious lesion is surgically removed.

Endoscopic Biopsy

In endoscopic biopsy, tissue samples are taken with an instrument introduced through the working channel of an endoscope during an endoscopic examination. Ulcerated lesions in the stomach or bladder are sampled with a small forceps (punch biopsy). A raised lesion can be completely excised with an electrocautery loop.

Smear Cytology (Exfoliative Cytology)

Individual, loosely adherent cells can be collected with a small brush and transferred to a glass slide for cytologic evaluation. The procedure is completely painless, although a small tissue sample may still have to be removed if the pathologist finds abnormal cells in the smear.

Curettage

This is a procedure in which material is carefully scraped from a mucosal lining using a spoonlike instrument.

Fine Needle Biopsy

Fine needles with an outer diameter of 1.0 mm or less are used for "partial biopsies." Fine needle biopsies that collect mostly cytologic material (needle diameter < 1 mm) are known by various terms in everyday practice. Common synonyms for fine needle biopsy (FNB) are

- Fine needle aspiration (FNA)
- Fine needle aspiration biopsy (FNAB)
- Fine needle aspiration cytology (FNAC)
- Fine needle cytology (FNC)

It is understandable that fine needle biopsies have an inherently high "sampling error," especially in the case of focal lesions. Thus, fine needle biopsy has an error rate of approximately 40% in focal liver lesions but is more than 90% accurate in the diagnosis of diffuse tissue processes.[1]

For this reason, blind biopsies should be performed only when there is suspicion of a diffuse process (such as hepatitis or an autoimmune disease). In practice we try to avoid the term "blind," since most "blind biopsies" nowadays are actually performed with ultrasound guidance (e.g., a Menghini liver biopsy). Focal lesions should always be biopsied under imaging guidance (ultrasound, fluoroscopy, CT, MRI) to reduce the rate of false-negative diagnoses.[2,3]

A special technique is the fine needle aspiration biopsy, in which a fine needle, introduced percutaneously or after thoracotomy or laparotomy, collects material that is then smeared onto glass slides like blood[4] (see Chapter 6).

5.3 Histology or Cytology?

Generally speaking, the same basic principle applies to histology as to cytologic analysis: close cooperation between the clinician and pathologist is essential for establishing a precise diagnosis. Cytology is not a substitute for histology. The parallel application of both techniques is needed for diagnostic accuracy. Thus, the question of "histology or cytology?" should be answered "cytology *and* histology!" since a cytologic examination will necessarily provide a lower degree of confidence. For example, cytology alone usually cannot distinguish between carcinoma in situ and a more advanced cancer. Consequently, sound treatment planning would require a histologic examination.[1,5] We cannot offer a general recommendation as to when cytology is adequate and, more importantly, when it can provide an adequate degree of certainty. A valid cytologic diagnosis cannot be made for certain tumor entities such as Hodgkin and non-Hodgkin lymphomas. Although immunocytologic testing can be done to distinguish between small-cell and non–small-cell lung cancers, the specimen volume is generally inadequate to allow for ancillary tests (epidermal growth factor receptor [EGFR] mutations, ALK-EML4 translocations).

5.3.1 Sources of Error

Potential sources of error that may cause misinterpretations include obtaining an inadequate specimen volume. Also, a biopsy taken from a necrotic area will make tissue classification impossible. Inadequate tissue processing and crush artifacts are other possible factors that can hamper histopathologic evaluation. Of course, the biopsy should always be taken from the disease focus itself and not from, say, an inflammatory area surrounding a tumor (▶ Table 5.1).

5.4 Typing, Grading, and Staging

Histology is concerned with determining the histologic type of a tumor (typing) and its histologic grade of malignancy (grading). Both determinations can also be applied clinically to make a biological and/or prognostic assessment. These kinds of information cannot be consistently or reliably determined from cytologic specimens.[6] By providing this information, pathology assumes a key role in oncologic diagnosis. Histologic evaluation is based on the classification, grading, and staging of neoplasms. At organ centers, pathology findings are often correlated with clinical and radiologic findings to establish a definitive tumor stage, which can then help to direct further treatment decisions and recommendations. The histologic evaluation is based on classification and grading.

5.4.1 Classification (Typing)

Classification is based on the evaluation of clinical behavior (benign/malignant) and assigning the neoplasm to a tissue of origin (histogenesis). A definite benign–malignant differentiation can be made for most neoplasms based on pathoanatomical findings. Malignant tumors, with their capacity for metastasis, often exhibit "atypias" relative to the original tissue. These changes present microscopically as variable cell sizes and shapes and abnormal nuclear morphology. The latter is marked by anisonucleosis with variable nuclear shapes, nuclear pleomorphism, nuclear hyperchromasia with increased nuclear chromatin staining, atypical nuclear divisions, and a shift in the nuclear–cytoplasmic ratio in favor of nuclear size, all of which reflect a more aggressive biological behavior. Benign tumors have pushing margins and

Table 5.1 Possible causes of histologic misinterpretation

Procedural step	Purpose	Possible errors
Step 1: Specimen collection	Needle biopsy, excision, resection, extirpation: collecting an adequate amount of representative tissue in good condition	Tissue not sampled from the "pathology" itself but from its surroundings (e.g., when sampling a liver nodule)
Step 2: Specimen fixation	Tissue preservation (interruption of autolysis and decomposition), preparation for further processing; usually fixed in formalin (4% aqueous formaldehyde solution)	Failure to perform fixation or using an improper fixative solution Fixation time too long or too short Formalin concentration too high or too low Inadequate volume of fixative solution (recommended: 1 part tissue in 10 parts liquid) Impaired diffusion (organs with thick fibrous capsule, hollow viscus with thick muscular layer)
Step 3: Specimen submission to the pathologist	Every surgically removed specimen must be submitted in its entirety Compliance with submission requirements	Delayed or faulty submission Submission container or requisition improperly labeled
Step 4: Gross examination by the pathologist Gross preparation	Assess the size, shape, consistency, appearance, and weight of the submitted tissue Take representative samples for histologic examination	Removal of unsuitable, unrepresentative tissue samples Incomplete preparation and/or inadequate sampling
Step 5: Microscopic evaluation and pathology report	In conjunction with gross examination and clinical findings: typing, grading, staging, R classification (resection status)	Inexperienced pathologist Careless working technique Misinterpretation or incomplete classification through not taking all findings into account

undergo a local, circumscribed, nonmetastasizing type of growth. This contrasts with the destructive, invasive growth of malignant tumors, which may undergo metastasis.

Besides invasive neoplasms, precursor lesions are also identified and classified. Studies of premalignant lesions have revealed a typical progression from potential to obligate precancerous lesions and then to (micro)invasive cancer.

The relevant genetic changes associated with the various stages of lesion progression have been well investigated for some malignancies such as colorectal cancer. The changes follow a sequence from normal epithelium to a small adenoma (< 10 mm with subtle architectural changes and minor cellular and nuclear atypias). Next come larger adenomas (> 10 mm) often showing moderate atypias, followed by adenomas with high-grade atypias. The sequence culminates in invasive adenocarcinoma, which may also metastasize. A similar progression of changes has been described for the squamous epithelium of the uterine cervix, for example. Mild, moderate, or severe dysplasia of the cervical epithelium may progress to carcinoma in situ, then microinvasive carcinoma, and finally grossly invasive cancer that may undergo metastasis. In the endometrium, simple hyperplasia without atypias signifies a potentially precancerous change, whereas complex hyperplasia with atypias indicates an obligate precancerous lesion. In between are various grades of dysplasia ranging to in situ neoplasia, described as intraepithelial neoplasia (low-grade for mild or moderate dysplasia and high-grade for severe dysplasia). The cervical form is called cervical intraepithelial neoplasia (CIN, grades I–III), and similar terms exist for the vulva (VIN), vagina (VaIN), prostate (PIN), and pancreas (PanIN). Testicular in situ lesions have a precursor described in the WHO nomenclature as intratubular germ cell neoplasia, unclassified (IGCNU).

The tissue diagnosis provides the first subdivision of the various types of tumor that may occur in an organ. The appearance of the tumor is compared with normal tissue to appreciate similarities or differences with regard to cell type and structure. It is not enough to classify a tumor by its primary site as a gastric, colon, or bronchial carcinoma, for example, because neuroendocrine tumors and many other less common neoplasms may also occur at those sites. Once a benign/malignant determination has been made, the tumor must be assigned to a tissue of origin. Most tumors can be classified by light microscopy alone as an epithelial, mesenchymal, neuroectodermal, embryonal, or germ cell tumor. Mixed tumors with epithelial and mesenchymal elements are distinct rarities.

Epithelial neoplasms are subdivided into papillomas (squamous cell, transitional cell, or urothelial) and adenomas (cylindrical cell). Malignant epithelial tumors are carcinomas (squamous cell, urothelial, adenocarcinoma, etc.). These terms are further characterized by a descriptive adjective or prefix to indicate distinctive structural features. Examples are villous, tubular, and tubulovillous adenomas of the colon and follicular adenoma of the thyroid gland. Adenocarcinomas of parenchymal organs are described as hepatocellular, cholangiocytic, renal-cell, or thyroid carcinoma. If no morphologic or immunohistochemical differentiating features can be found, the carcinoma is described as undifferentiated (anaplastic) with respect to its growth pattern. Another category of epithelial neoplasms is neuroendocrine tumors, which, like most tumors of endocrine organs, exhibit distinctive features relating to their benign–malignant differentiation. Definitely malignant neoplasms are called neuroendocrine carcinomas.

Note

The comparison of malignant epithelial tumors with normal tissue has given rise to the terms "squamous cell carcinoma," "adenocarcinoma," and "transitional cell carcinoma," which account for more than 90% of all malignancies.

Mesenchymal tumors are classified by distinguishing features that they share with a differentiated tissue. The suffix "-oma" indicates a benign tumor, while "-sarcoma" (from the Greek *sarx* = "flesh") indicates a malignant tumor. Lipoma, for instance, is distinguished from liposarcoma and leiomyosarcoma, and angioma from angiosarcoma, to name just a few examples. If no differentiating features are found, the tumor is an undifferentiated sarcoma, which is classified by its cellular morphology as round cell, spindle cell, or pleomorphic (having cells of variable shape).

Tumors of blood-forming and lymphatic cells, which include the leukemias and lymphomas, also have a mesenchymal origin but are classified separately.

Neuroectodermal tumors include tumors of the supportive cells of the central nervous system (CNS)—gliomas, astrocytomas, oligodendrogliomas, etc.—and tumors of the CNS coverings such as meningiomas.

Neuroectodermal tumors also include melanocytic tumors such as melanocytic nevi and malignant melanoma.

Embryonal tumors exhibit tissue patterns like those occurring in organogenesis. These tumors are often given the suffix "-blastoma" to indicate their origin from primitive organ cells, such as nephroblastoma, neuroblastoma, retinoblastoma, medulloblastoma, pulmoblastoma, and hepatoblastoma.

Germ cell tumors are another entity that may be differentiated in various ways and may exhibit germ cell–specific features as well as features of extraembryonal tissues derived from all three germ layers. The sex and age of the patient and the maturity of these tissue elements are important factors in determining whether these tumors are benign or malignant.

Difficulties may arise when a tumor displays several different structural features or its histogenetic origin cannot be identified. Various rules are applied in the classification of these tumors. They may be classified by

1. The structures predominantly present in the tumor
2. The most highly differentiated structures, regardless of their quantity
3. The least differentiated (most malignant) structures, regardless of their quantity

A general rule cannot be stated, however, so it is necessary to establish a relevant histologic classification for each organ tumor, applying clear definitions and detailed classification principles. The WHO classifications define the individual tumors occurring in various organ systems and illustrate them with color plates. In the interest of international cooperation and comparability, it is generally recommended that the WHO classification be applied to all tumor diagnoses.[6] When the classification principles in that system are rigorously followed, they will ensure a high degree of reproducibility in diagnosis and a high level of agreement among different pathologists. Most discrepancies result from the heterogeneity of tumors. Since a tumor may present different histologies at different sites, there is a danger that a single, small tissue sample will not be representative of all structures present in the tumor.

5.4.2 Grading

The differentiation of tumor tissue refers to its morphologic and functional similarity to the tissue of origin. The grading of tumors is based on specific histologic and cytologic criteria. As well as comparing the tumor with its tissue of origin, examiners make use of specific semi-quantitative methods. The number of mitoses per high-power field, the prominence of glandular formation (in breast and colorectal cancers), and the size and stainability of cell nuclei are all considered in assessing the degree of tumor differentiation.

The WHO employs a three-tiered grading system. Some authors add a fourth grade for completely undifferentiated tumor forms. With some organ tumors, especially those in the gastrointestinal tract, G1 and G2 lesions (well differentiated and moderately differentiated) are both placed in the low-grade category while G3 and G4 lesions (poorly differentiated or undifferentiated) are both considered to be high-grade. Note that the degree of differentiation and degree of malignancy are inversely proportional to each other: the poorer the differentiation, the more malignant and aggressive the tumor and the faster its rate of growth. For example, if a colorectal adenocarcinoma closely resembles normal mucosa, it is classified as a well-differentiated (G1) tumor. But if the tumor tissue bears no more than a vague resemblance to its tissue of origin, it is classified as poorly differentiated (G3). Tumors with intermediate features are diagnosed as moderately differentiated (G2). A G4 tumor is undifferentiated.

For many organ tumors, G3 and G4 tumors are, on average, more advanced at the time of diagnosis than G1 and G2 lesions.

While the cells of benign tumors closely resemble the cells of the fully differentiated tissue of origin on cytologic examination, and the nuclei have the same size and same nuclear–cytoplasmic ratio, malignant tumors show a significant degree of nuclear atypia. A tumor is graded by examining the neoplastic tissue, which will sometimes show a heterogeneous pattern of differentiation, and evaluating those elements that deviate most sharply from the tissue of origin and thus show the highest grade of dedifferentiation.

As in histologic classification (typing), grading is subject to organ-specific differences that should be applied in a generally valid and comparable way. With this goal in mind, the UICC (Union for International Cancer Control, formerly Union Internationale Contre le Cancer) has issued guidelines for every organ tumor based on the four-part grading system (G1–G4) described above. These guidelines should definitely be followed in the grading of tumors.[7] For example, the grading of prostate cancer is based on the loss of normal glandular tissue architecture as defined in the Gleason scoring system. Similarly, breast cancers have their own grading system, the Elson–Ellis score, in which the degree of tubular differentiation, nuclear aplasia, and number of mitoses per 10 high-power fields are summed to yield a total score. Other organ tumors such as thyroid carcinoma are grossly subdivided into differentiated (follicular and papillary), insular, and anaplastic carcinomas, but there is no specific grading for follicular or papillary cancers. Malignant testicular tumors are also graded by their tissue components without using more specific grading criteria for those components (▶ Fig. 5.1, ▶ Fig. 5.2).

Tumors and their marker antibodies are summarized in ▶ Table 5.2. Antibody selection for investigating an "undifferentiated malignant tumor" and immunoreactivity patterns is summarized in ▶ Table 5.3.

5.5 Specific Analysis

5.5.1 Lymph Nodes

Lymphadenopathy is investigated to determine whether the lymph node enlargement is due to reactive inflammatory changes or neoplasia (▶ Fig. 5.3).

If neoplasia is present, it may represent a primary lymphatic tumor (non-Hodgkin lymphoma) or nodal metastasis. Differential diagnosis is aided by reference to clinical, microbiological, and histologic findings.

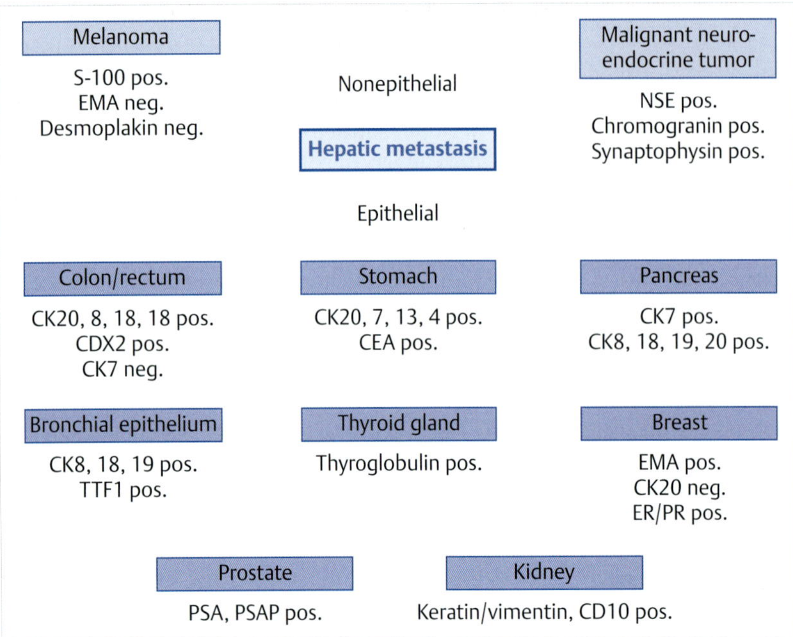

Fig. 5.1 Immunohistochemical investigation of indeterminate liver tumors. NSE, neuron-specific enolase; CEA, carcinoembryonic antigen; CK, cytokeratin; EMA, epithelial membrane antigen; ER, estrogen receptor; PR, prostate-specific antigen; PSAP, prostate-specific acid phosphatase; TTF-1, thyroid transcription factor 1.

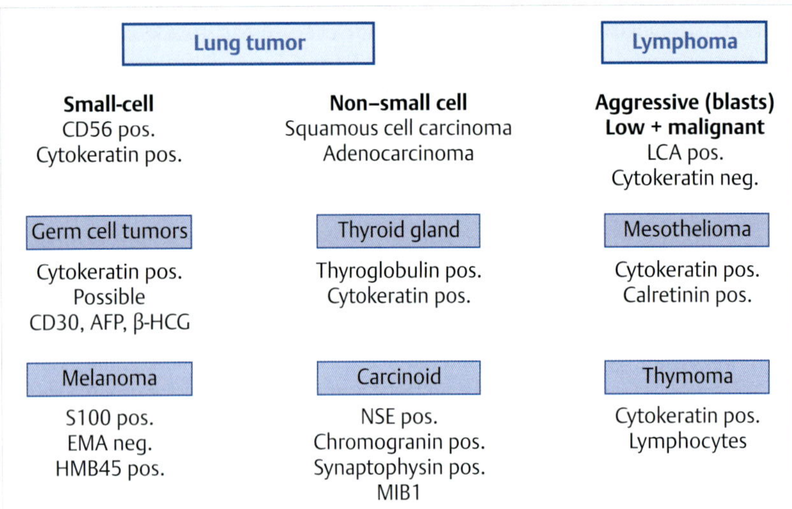

Fig. 5.2 Immunohistochemical investigation of indeterminate ("undifferentiated") lung tumors. AFP, α-fetoprotein; β-HCG, β human chorionic gonadotropin; EMA, epithelial membrane antigen; LCA, leukocyte common antigen; MIB-1, monoclonal antibody against Ki-67; NSE, neuron-specific enolase.

Table 5.2 Tumors and their marker antibodies

Tumor type	Antibodies
Epithelial tumors	Cytokeratins (keratin), EMA (epithelial membrane antigen), CEA (carcinoembryonic antigen), desmoplakins
Lymphoreticular and hematopoietic neoplasms	LCA (leukocyte common antigen, CD45), B-cell differentiation antigens, immunoglobulins, histiocyte/granulocyte differentiation antigens (e.g., lysozyme), vimentin
Melanomas	Vimentin, S-100, melanoma-specific antigen (MSA), HMB-45
Sarcomas	Vimentin, desmin, actin, myoglobin, S-100
Gastrointestinal stromal tumors (GIST)	c-Kit (CD117), CD34
Germ cell tumors	Keratins (exception: seminomas, dysgerminomas), β-HCG (human chorionic gonadotropin), α-fetoprotein, CD30, alkaline phosphatase
Tumors of neuroendocrine origin	NSE (neuron-specific enolase), chromogranin, synaptophysin
Tumors of glial tissue	GFAP (glial fibrillary acidic protein), S-100

Table 5.3 Antibody selection for investigating an "undifferentiated malignant tumor" and immunoreactivity patterns

Tumor	Keratin	LCA	S-100	Vimentin	Desmin
Carcinoma	+	–	±	±	–
Lymphoma	–	+	–	±	–
Sarcoma	±	–	±	+	±
Melanoma	–	–	+	+	–

In principle, histologic evaluation is required for any lymph node enlargement that is present for more than 3 weeks, does not respond to antibiotics, and lacks a discernible cause. Infectious causes can be excluded by looking for (rare) causative organisms (toxoplasmosis, brucellosis), especially in children, migrants, and patients with a suggestive history (farmers, hunters).

Anatomically, a "normal" lymph node consists of lymph follicles, which in turn are composed of germinal centers that may be sonographically visible under certain circumstances. Lymph node metastasis presents initially with circumscribed infiltration and (central) necrosis or other structural irregularities. Lymphomas present clinically with marked lymph node enlargement that may sometimes show a relatively homogeneous internal echo pattern. Destruction of the lymph node architecture may occur with the further progression of disease.

Lymph node removal for the diagnosis of lymphoma is justified if it will have diagnostic, therapeutic, or prognostic implications or if the patient is to be enrolled in a study. A core needle biopsy may be adequate for the diagnosis of high-grade lymphoma. The aspiration cytology of lymphomas usually yields no more than a "suspicious" finding of monomorphic or blastic lymphocytes, which may also be found in normal germinal centers.

Lymph node metastases can be diagnosed by core needle biopsy if the affected nodes are permeated by tumor cells. But if the metastases are small and circumscribed or are confined to the marginal sinus of the node, they may elude biopsy, resulting in a false-negative report (e.g., in early follicular lymphomas). Elastography during the ultrasound-guided biopsy of circumscribed lymph node changes has proven helpful in detecting these small metastases and supporting the use of neoadjuvant therapy. This particularly applies to the endosonography of esophageal, gastric, and rectal cancers.

The principal types of lymphoma are described below.

5.5.2 Lymphomas

Non-Hodgkin lymphoma (NHL) is classified as nodal or extranodal, depending on whether the tumor originates in lymph nodes or in extranodal structures. With extranodal lymphoma, the main tumor mass that will require treatment is located outside the lymph node. Note that this strict definition does not clearly distinguish extranodal lymphoma from primary nodal NHL with secondary organ involvement, which occurs in approximately 25% of cases (see ▶ Table 5.4).

Studies on the pathogenesis of primary extranodal lymphomas have shown that these tumors are closely related to mucosa-associated lymphatic tissue (MALT). Permeable mucous membranes that are in direct contact with the environment, as in the stomach, are the most likely sites to develop this specialized lymphatic tissue as a defense against possible disease-causing agents. MALT

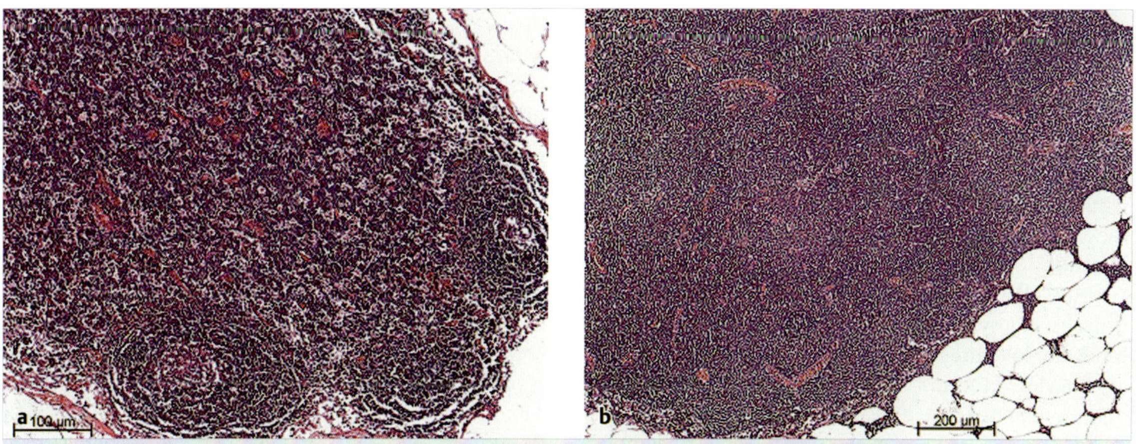

Fig. 5.3 Comparison of normal lymph node tissue with tissue infiltrated by non-Hodgkin lymphoma (NHL).
a Normal lymph node with lymph follicles.
b NHL has infiltrated this lymph node and spread diffusely into perinodal fat. Lymph follicles can no longer be identified (H&E; original magnification × 20).

Table 5.4 Immunohistochemistry of B-cell lymphomas

Entity	ICD-0-M	CD20	CD79α	CD5	CD43	CD10	BCL6	BCL2	Ki-67	Cyclin D1
MALT lymphoma	9699/3	+	+	–	±	–	–	+	5–20	–
Follicular lymphoma	9690/3	+	+	–	–	+	+	+	15–50	–
Mantle cell lymphoma	9673/3	+	+	+	+	–	–	+	15–50	+
Diffuse large cell B-cell lymphoma	9680/3	+	+	–	–	±	±	±	>50	–
Burkitt lymphoma	9687/3	+	+	–	+	+	+	–	100	–
Germinal centers in follicular dysplasia (reactive)		+	+	–	–	+	+	–	>60	–

differs from lymph nodes in its proximity to glandular surface epithelium and its relatively wide marginal zone.

The marginal zone cells, which are differentiated as post-germinal center memory B cells, are small to medium-sized lymphocytes. In the MALT, these cells may extend to the surface of the mucosa and become interspersed among the epithelial cells, appearing as intraepithelial clusters of B cells and forming "lymphoepithelial lesions." They express typical B-cell antigens (CD20, CD21, CD79α) and immunoglobulins (IgM).

Approximately 40% of all NHLs develop at extranodal sites, i.e., outside of lymph nodes. The region most commonly affected by extranodal NHL is the gastrointestinal tract. It is estimated that approximately 4 to 18% of all NHLs in the Western world and up to 25% of cases in the Middle East involve the gastrointestinal tract. In the Western world, the majority of gastrointestinal NHLs occur in the stomach. In the Middle East, the small intestine is most commonly affected. Approximately 10% of all gastric malignancies are non-Hodgkin lymphomas, and the overall incidence of this disease appears to be rising.

MALT lymphomas belong to the category of small-cell, extranodal marginal zone lymphomas. These are low-grade B-cell lymphomas that develop in response to the proliferation-inducing effect of a *Helicobacter pylori* infection.

MALT lymphomas have fairly characteristic histologic features. Biopsy usually reveals a dense, diffuse lymphatic infiltrate, sometimes occurring between reactive secondary follicles. If the specimen is large enough, lymphocytes may be identified in the submucosa or even in deeper wall layers (▶ Fig. 5.4). Conceptually, neoplastic lymphocytes infiltrate preexisting lymph follicles and initially enter the marginal zone, which is outside the follicular mantle zone. As the tumor progresses, the neoplastic B cells colonize the lymph follicles and form a diffuse lymphocytic infiltrate. Generally the tumor cells are of moderate size and have a thin rim of cytoplasm and an irregularly shaped nucleus. They are called "centrocyte-like cells" because of their resemblance to centrocytes. Monocytoid or plasmacytoid differentiation is usually present. The centrocyte-like cells destroy the gastric glands, creating the typical picture of lymphoepithelial lesions. The criteria for diagnosing a lymphoepithelial lesion should be applied rigorously. Unmistakable infiltration of the gastric epithelium by cluster-forming neoplastic lymphocytes should be associated with destruction of the glandular architecture. The centrocyte-like cells have a similar immunophenotype to marginal-zone B cells (▶ Table 5.1). Thus they express B-cell markers, and the lymphoma cells are negative for CD10. Bcl-2 is often detectable as well. Immunoglobulins, most commonly IgM and occasionally IgA or IgG with monoclonal expression of light chains (light-chain restriction), can be demonstrated. Cytokeratin is a useful immunohistochemical marker for the diagnosis of poorly differentiated or undifferentiated carcinoma.

Mantle cell lymphomas show a diffuse, monotonic infiltration of B cells that have a thin cytoplasmic rim and irregularly shaped nuclei. These B cells express CD5 and cyclin D1 in addition to the usual B cell markers. A mantle cell lymphoma in the gastrointestinal tract may present as "lymphomatous polyposis."

Diffuse large-cell B-cell lymphomas (DLCL) cause the complete destruction of lymph node structures. The tumor cells are large and have a vesicular nucleus with prominent nucleoli. Immunophenotyping demonstrates B cell markers (CD19, CD20, CD22, CD79α). The proliferation fraction, defined as the percentage of MIB-1 (Ki67)-positive cells, is greater than 50%.

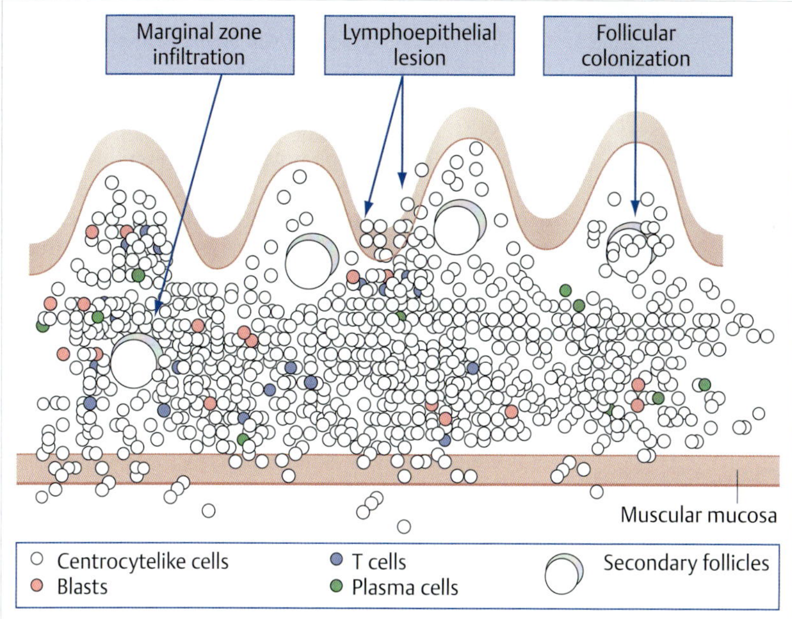

Fig. 5.4 Diagrammatic representation of the growth pattern of NHL, illustrated for MALT lymphoma. (Source: reference[8], with kind permission of Springer Science + Business Media.)

Follicular lymphomas (formerly called centroblastic-centrocytic NHL) exhibit a follicular growth pattern, meaning that the tumor cells are arranged in follicles. As a result, these tumors may be difficult to distinguish from reactive follicular hyperplasia. The lymphoma cells show immunohistochemical expression of CD10.

Primary T-cell lymphomas are relatively rare and require a histologic (rather than cytologic) diagnosis.

It can be difficult to distinguish between aggressive lymphomas and small cell undifferentiated tumors (▶ Fig. 5.5). The differential diagnosis is aided by immunohistochemistry.

Hodgkin lymphoma is distinguished by (usually) CD30-positive and CD15-expressing Hodgkin and Sternberg Reed cells. The lymph node architecture may be fully intact, so a cytologic diagnosis cannot be made. It is very difficult to identify the six different subtypes of Hodgkin lymphoma defined by the WHO, each having its own therapeutic implications. Differentiation from reactive lymphadenopathies due to toxoplasmosis, cat scratch disease, or *Yersinia* infection is sometimes difficult, even when immunohistochemical and molecular biological methods are applied. A second opinion from a reference pathologist is recommended in these cases.

5.6 Hormone Growth Factor Receptor Analysis

The spectrum of tumors that respond to hormonal therapy includes carcinomas of the breast, uterus, prostate, and thyroid gland. A number of tumors, such as colorectal and hepatocellular carcinomas, have receptors for estrogen or progesterone but are not responsive to hormonal therapy. The hormones in question bind to the receptor, and the hormone–receptor complex is taken into the cell where it exerts its effects. The crucial role of receptors in hormonal effects has led to the determination of these receptors in tumor tissue. In recent years, pathologists have been performing receptor determinations using immunohistochemical methods. The advantage of these methods is that they can localize positive immunoreactivity to specific sites in tissues.

The detection of receptors is predictive of higher response rates to hormonal therapy. Receptor determination is now performed routinely for breast cancers, in which both estrogen receptor (ER) and progesterone receptor (PR) status are determined. These determinations, and those of c-erbB2 (HER2/neu), epithelial growth

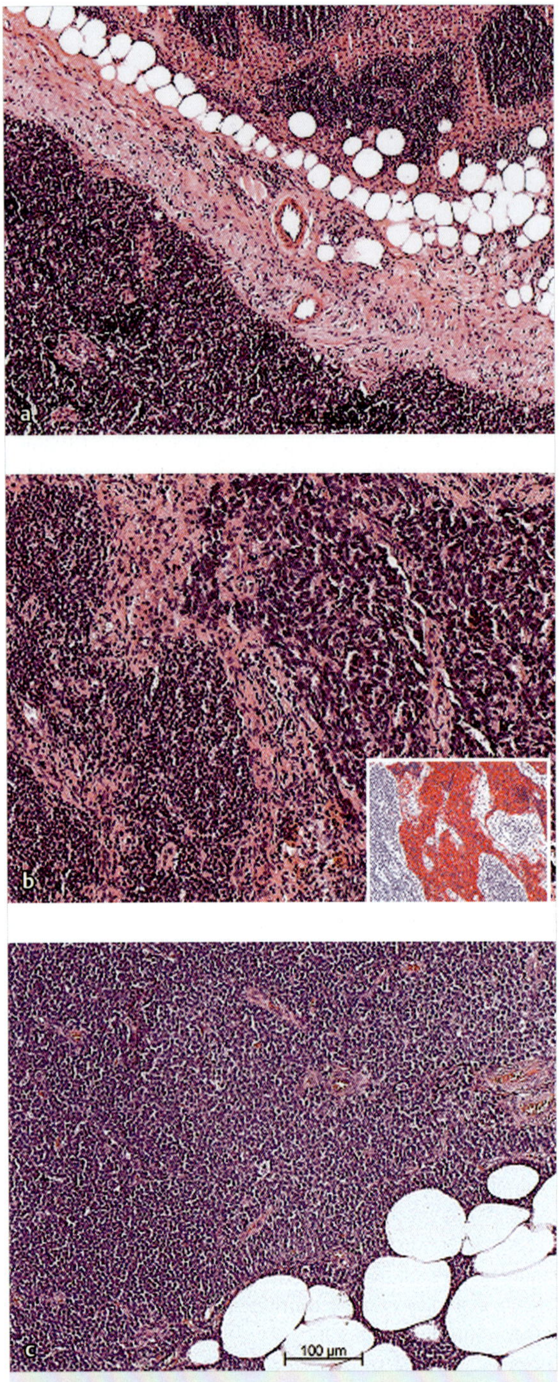

Fig. 5.5 Comparison of small-cell tumors.
a, b Lymph node metastasis from a small-cell carcinoma with CD56 expression (inset).
c NHL has infiltrated this lymph node and spread diffusely into perinodal fat. Lymph follicles can no longer be identified (H&E; original magnification × 20).

factor receptor (EGRF) or vascular endothelial growth factor (VEGF) and its receptors, can be performed on the primary tumor as well as metastases.

Receptor studies have prompted the development of agents that bind to receptors with high affinity but do not exert any effects. This pharmacological receptor blockade with agents such as tamoxifen (Nolvadex) has been found to increase 5-year survival rates in 75% of all women with a positive receptor status. Newer agents such as trastuzumab (Herceptin) produce an antiproliferative effect by binding to the c-erbB2 receptor.

References

[1] Caturelli E, Ghittoni G, Roselli P, De Palo M, Anti M. Fine needle biopsy of focal liver lesions: the hepatologist's point of view. Liver Transpl 2004; 10 suppl 1: S26–S29

[2] Stölzel U, Tannapfel A. Indications for liver biopsy in liver tumors [Article in German]. Zentralbl Chir 2000; 125: 606–609

[3] Tannapfel A, Dienes HP, Lohse AW. The indications for liver biopsy. Dtsch Arztebl Int 2012; 109: 477–483

[4] Wittekind C, Tannapfel A. Prinzipien der Pathologie in der Onkologie. In: Schmoll HJ, Hoeffken K, Possinger K, eds. Kompendium Internistische Onkologie. Berlin, Heidelberg, New York: Springer Verlag; 2002:307–337

[5] Friedman LS. Controversies in liver biopsy: who, where, when, how, why? Curr Gastroenterol Rep 2004; 6: 30–36

[6] Hamilton SR, Aaltonen LA, eds. World Health Organization Classification of Tumours. Pathology and Genetics of Tumours of the Digestive System. Lyon: IARC Press; 2000

[7] Wittekind C, Meyer HJ. TNM Klassifikation maligner Tumore. Weinheim: Wiley-Blackwell; 2010

[8] Dallenbach FE, Coupland SE, Stein H. Marginal zone lymphomas: extranodal MALT type, nodal and splenic [Article in German]. Pathologe 2000; 21: 162–177

6 Fine Needle Aspiration Cytology

C. Jenssen, T. Beyer

The fine needle aspiration cytology (FNAC) of tumors was first described in 1931 by the German pathologist Ernst Mannheim. He was the first to use small-gauge needles (1 mm in diameter) in the diagnosis of 43 patients with tumors of the breast and abdomen.[1] Lopes-Cardozo in the Netherlands and Söderström, Eneroth, Franzen, and Zjicek in Sweden published the first comprehensive case series in the 1950s and 1970s. It was not until ultrasound guidance became available for fine needle aspirations (US-FNA) that the barriers in traditional pathology were broken down, and the technique became widely practiced during the 1980s (for the history of FNAC, see reference [2] and review articles[3,4]). New impulses resulted from the introduction of endoscopic ultrasound-guided FNA (EUS-FNA) in 1982 and of endobronchial ultrasound-guided transbronchial needle aspiration (EBUS-TBNA) in 2004.[5,6]

Ideally, it is best to have one operator determine the need for the service, collect the specimens, and perform the cytologic evaluation (clinical cytology). At a few German centers the specimens are analyzed by the clinician who collects them, while in the United States, United Kingdom, Sweden, and Italy, specimen collection at some centers is performed by an interventional cytopathologist —but these are the exceptions. Most ultrasound diagnosticians work with a cytopathologist partner in their own facility or, increasingly, work contractually with an outside laboratory to which cytology samples are submitted for evaluation. In this setting, good communication and standardization are key factors in determining the quality of the cytologic diagnosis.

In this chapter, then, the collection, preparation, and processing of the cellular material obtained by US-FNA, EUS-FNA, and EBUS-TBNA will be described from the viewpoint of the ultrasound diagnostician and clinical cytologist. Rapid on-site evaluation (ROSE), common artifacts, sources of error, and limitations will also be explored.

6.1 Specimen Collection

6.1.1 Ultrasound-Guided Biopsy

The technique of ultrasound-guided biopsy is fully described in numerous monographs[2,7–10] and in video tutorials on the website of the Papanicolaou Society of Cytopathology (http://www.papsociety.org/fna.html). The technique of EUS-guided biopsy was recently described in detail.[11] Biopsy needles are used in sizes ranging from 27 to 22 gauge. Their length and design depend on the depth of the lesion and the specific sampling procedure (US-FNA, EUS-FNA, EBUS-TBNA).

6.1.2 Needle Movement and Aspiration

In the sampling of solid target lesions, the needle is introduced into the mass and moved quickly in and out in multiple, short excursions ("needling") to minimize the sampling error (http://www.papsociety.org/Needle%20Movement/index.html). In fine needle aspirations of the thyroid gland and lymph nodes and in EUS-guided fine needle aspirations, it has been shown that aspiration with suction and needling without suction (capillary method) are equally effective for sampling cellular material.[7,12–14] If aspiration yields a bloody aspirate, further sampling should be performed without suction. The aspiration of a solid lesion is concluded and the needle removed from the lesion as soon as cellular material or blood is seen in the transparent needle hub. Suction should be released before the needle is withdrawn from the lesion. Cystic lesions should be completely aspirated whenever possible.

6.2 Specimen Preparation

6.2.1 Fluid Aspirates

Mucinous or viscous aspirates can be smeared onto a slide using conventional technique. Hypocellular fluids collected from effusions or cystic lesions, on the other hand, are centrifuged to concentrate the cellular material. If swift transport and rapid processing in the cytopathology laboratory are ensured, fluid aspirates can be submitted directly. Otherwise the fluids should be stored in tightly sealed containers with a fixative solution (e.g., maximum of 50% alcohol in a 1:1 ratio, no formalin!) for submission according to the requirements of the cytology laboratory. With very bloody fluids, addition of 3.8% sodium citrate (2 mL per 20 mL aspirate) or heparin (e.g., 5000 IU standard heparin) is recommended to prevent clotting.

6.2.2 Centrifuging Effusions

Large volumes of aspirated effusion fluid are centrifuged using a clinical centrifuge at 2500 rpm for approximately 10 minutes. The supernatant liquid is carefully suctioned off, and smears are prepared from the upper layer of sediment. Bloody sediments require preliminary density gradient centrifugation. Clots or fibrin particles are fixed in formalin and embedded in paraffin for standard histologic processing. The question whether the examination of larger effusion volumes (> 50 mL) increases the diagnostic yield and sensitivity of effusion cytology has been investigated in one retrospective and two prospective studies, but the results were inconclusive.[15–17]

Cytocentrifugation (Cytospin)

Small amounts of fluid aspirate (e.g., from a cystic lesion) can be spun directly onto a special slide with a Cytospin centrifuge (▶ Fig. 6.1). The chamber of the cytocentrifuge can accommodate samples of 250 to 300 µL. The deposition area on the slide is rimmed by a filter card that absorbs residual fluid during centrifugation (750 rpm for 2 minutes). Higher spinning speeds should be avoided as they would cause mechanical destruction of the deposited cells. The resulting thin-layer preparations can be air-dried or wet-fixed, and various stains can be applied.

6.2.3 Aspirates from Solid Lesions

Material aspirated from solid lesions can be processed in various ways for cytologic evaluation. In many cases it is expedient to run multiple sample preparation techniques in parallel fashion. The selection of techniques will depend on the experience of the cytopathologist and clinician, the distance between the site of specimen collection and the cytopathology laboratory, the capabilities for on-site evaluation, the type of material, and the presumptive clinical diagnosis. Thus, the cytopathology partner should be consulted in selecting the technique. Several preparation options are available for materials aspirated from solid lesions[2,8,9]:

- Conventional smears (air-dried or wet-fixed)
- Liquid-based thin-layer techniques (e.g., thin preparations)
- Cell block

Additionally, residual aspirate can be flushed out with physiologic saline solution and submitted for cytomorphologic evaluation following micropore filtration or cytocentrifugation.

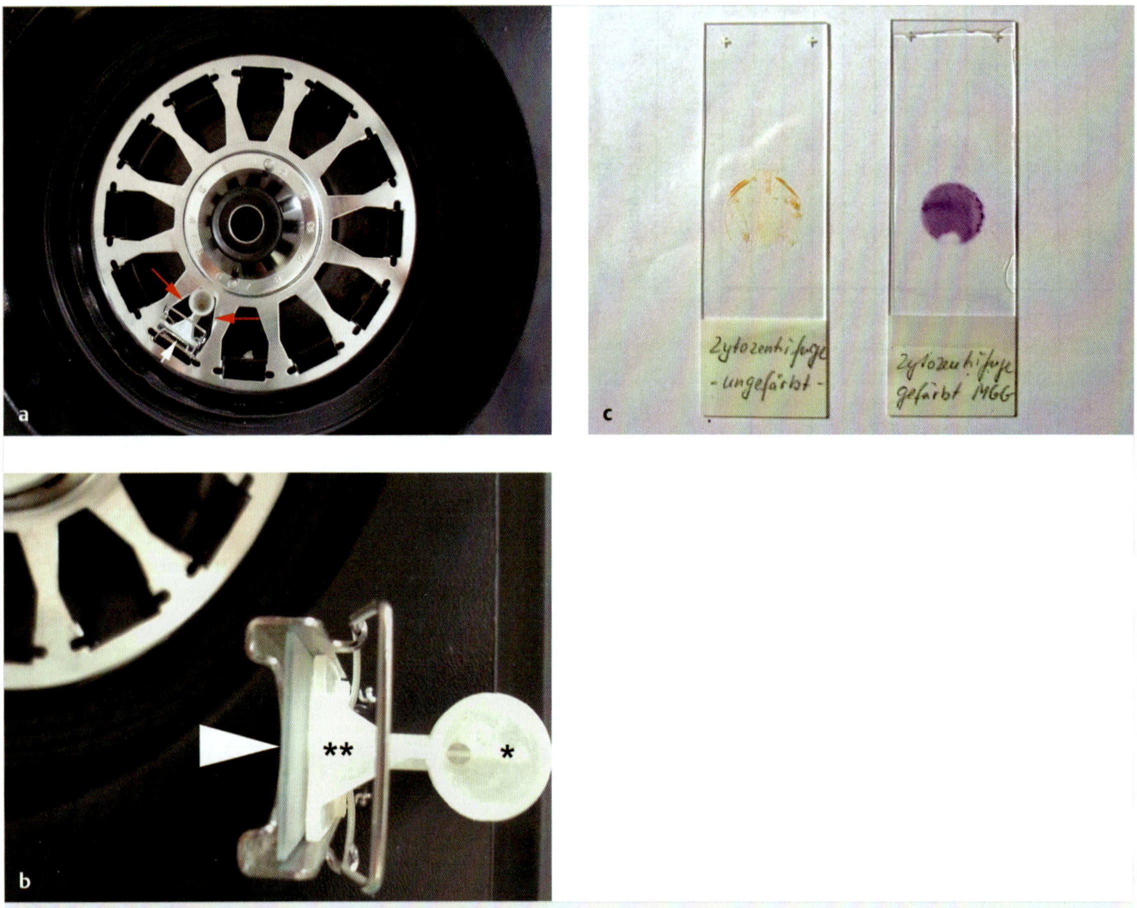

Fig. 6.1

a Overhead view of a cytocentrifuge with cytology funnel and sample chamber (red arrows) and a glass slide (white arrow).
b Close-up view of the cytology funnel (*), sample chamber (**) and glass slide (arrowhead), held in place with a metal clip.
c Cytospin slide with central deposition area. Left: unstained. Right: May–Grünwald–Giemsa (MGG)-stained.
Source: Images **a** and **b** reproduced with kind permission of B. Lucke, Wriezen, Germany. Image **c** with kind permission of B. Fiedler, Berlin, Germany.

Conventional Smears

Optimum smear preparation is essential for an accurate cytomorphologic evaluation. The goal is to produce uniform, artifact-free, thin-layer smears while avoiding the loss of material. Coherent cell clusters should be preserved whenever possible so that their specific aggregation patterns can be assessed during cytologic evaluation. The quality of a smear depends both on the smearing technique and on the nature and consistency of the sample. Admixture of blood or fluid is a very common source of artifacts. Various smear techniques have been described in the literature.[9,18] An instructional video on the website of the Papanicolaou Society of Cytopathology (http://www.papsociety.org/Basic%20Smearing%20Technique/index.html) demonstrates the optimum smearing technique and common errors.

Expelling the Material onto the Slide

To deposit the material sampled by FNA onto a slide, the needle tip is touched to an area of the slide near the frosted end while being held at an angle of approximately 45°, and a small amount of the harvested material is expelled onto the slide either with a stylet or by slowly depressing the plunger of an air-filled syringe (2–10 mL) (▶ Fig. 6.2a) (http://www.papsociety.org/Expulsion%20Onto%20Slide/index.html). The smaller the amount of material, the easier it is to prepare a thin smear. If there appears to be too much material on one slide for a thin-layer smear, the material can easily be divided by loosely applying a second slide to the original slide (http://www.papsociety.org/Dividing%20Material/index.html). The material should never be ejected onto the slide from a distance, as this may scatter tiny droplets over the slide that would dry before a smear can be prepared.

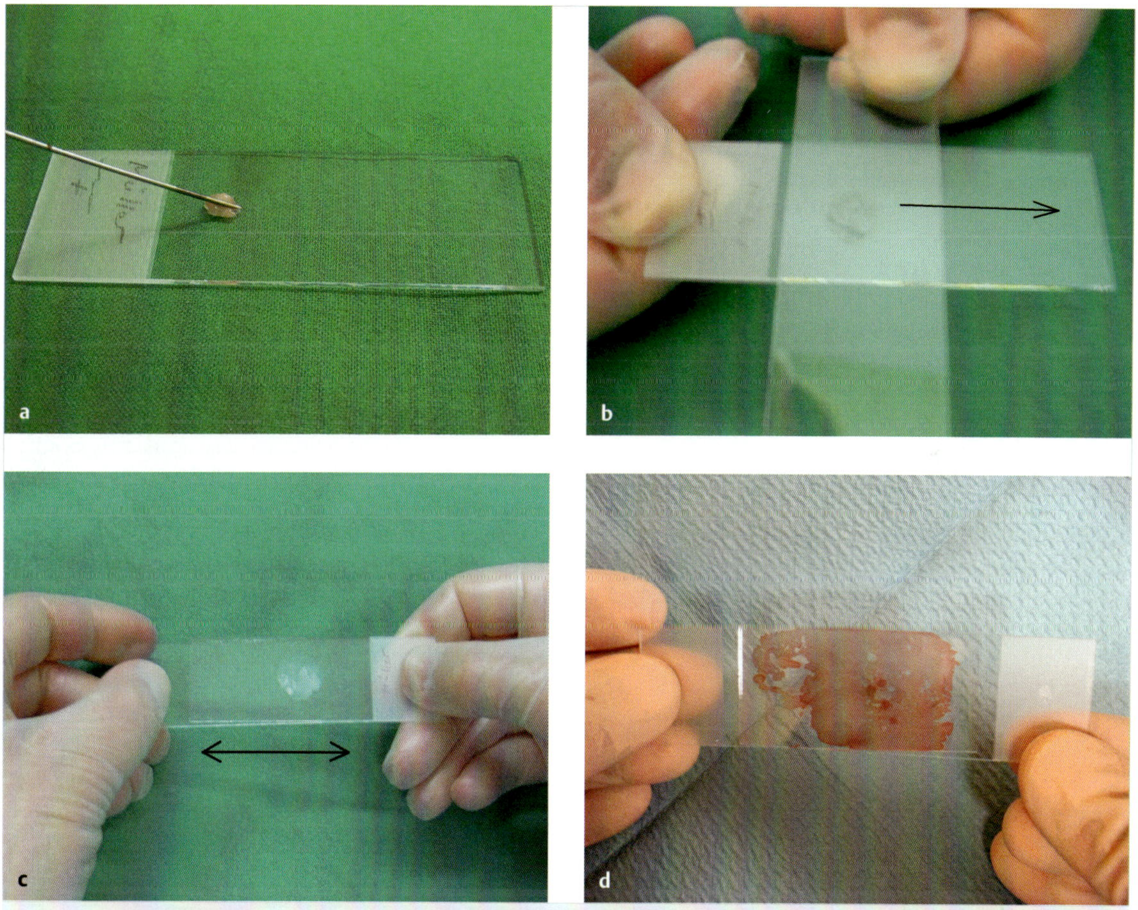

Fig. 6.2 Smearing technique.
a The needle, held at an angle, is touched to the glass slide near the frosted end, and a small amount of material is expelled onto the slide.
b, c The material is spread into a thin smear with a second slide, which is placed either across the bottom slide (**b**) or parallel to it (**c**) and slid along the bottom slide with light pressure.
d Another technique is to divide the material between two slides that are placed lightly together and then lifted apart without sliding.
Figures **a, b, c** from Beyer T. Tips and tricks for fine-needle puncture. In: Dietrich CF, ed. Endoscopic Ultrasound. An Introductory Manual and Atlas. Stuttgart, New York: Thieme; 2011:168–175.

Residual material is initially left in the needle, where it is protected from drying. Once a smear has been completed, additional material may be expelled from the needle onto a second slide. With some practice in smearing, material can be deposited on up to three slides in one run and then smeared in rapid succession. Material trapped in the needle hub can be deposited onto the slide using the "flip technique," i.e., fixing the needle barrel with two fingers and flicking the hub onto the slide repeatedly to eject the residual material (http://www.papsociety.org/Flip%20Technique/index.html).

Smearing Technique

The frosted end of the slide is held between the thumb and index finger of the left hand. The right hand then places the transparent side of a second, clean slide against the bottom slide containing the sample, positioning the top slide either across or parallel to the bottom slide. The top slide is initially tilted at an angle of 30° to 45° angle but is then rotated downward until it is parallel to the bottom slide. Gentle pressure is applied, depending on the consistency of the material, and the surface tension of the droplet should be sufficient to spread the material into a circular film between the slides. If the specimen is thin and uniform, it is unnecessary to smear the material any further. Both slides are lifted apart and fixed ("pull-apart" method, ▶ Fig. 6.2d).

If a thin, uniform specimen is not obtained, the top slide is slid along the bottom slide under light pressure, moving away from the frosted edge and keeping both slides parallel throughout the smearing process (▶ Fig. 6.2b, c). The top slide is removed, leaving a thin, oval-shaped smear on the bottom slide (▶ Fig. 6.3). Mostly isolated cells are found at the periphery of the smear, while cell clusters are found at the center. Some material is incidentally spread onto the top slide, but that smear is generally of poor quality.

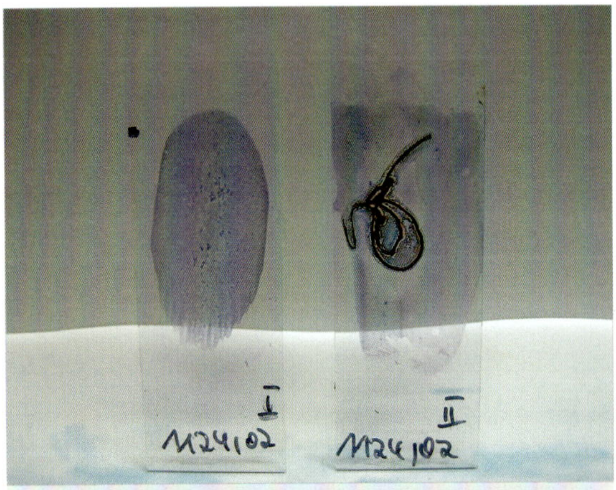

Fig. 6.3 May–Grünwald–Giemsa (MGG) stained smears: overhead view of two slides. Left: high-quality stain. Right: severe crush and air-drying artifacts. (Beyer T. Tips and tricks for fine-needle puncture. In: Dietrich CF, ed. Endoscopic Ultrasound. An Introductory Manual and Atlas. Stuttgart, New York: Thieme; 2011:168–175.)

If the harvested solid material is mixed with a significant amount of fluid, artifacts due to cellular swelling may occur. Before smearing, then, the slide can be tilted sideways, causing the fluid to collect along the bottom edge; then another slide can be used to scrape off some of the solid material, which is then smeared onto another slide. Another technique is to blot admixtures of body fluids and fresh blood from the edge of the tilted slide with filter paper or a gauze pad before the diagnostic material is smeared. If tiny tissue particles remain on the smear, they can be picked up with a needle and placed in fixative for paraffin block preparation (http://www.papsociety.org/Problem%20Material%201/index.html).

Caution

Aspirate should always be spread gently into a thin, uniform smear. This should be done swiftly to prevent air-drying of the specimen before smearing (smear: "less is more"). *Tissue particles or clots should not be crushed or discarded, but placed in fixative for later histologic examination (cell block).* (With tissue particles: "more is better.")

Possible Errors

Various technical errors may occur during the preparation of smears and may sometimes cause significant artifacts. In unfavorable cases this may prevent a correct diagnosis despite the collection of an adequate specimen.

The most common errors are as follows.

- Depositing too much material onto the slide (thick-layer artifacts, ▶ Fig. 6.3 and ▶ Fig. 6.4a, b)
- Leaving too much fluid on the slide (swelling artifacts)
- Smearing blood along with the diagnostic material (blood artifacts, ▶ Fig. 6.4c)
- Spraying the material onto the slide from a distance (air-drying artifacts)
- Working too slowly (air-drying artifacts)
- Applying too much pressure while smearing the material (crush artifacts)
- Failure to keep both slides parallel to each other throughout smearing (scratch artifacts)

Labeling

Materials from different sites must be carefully separated from each other and clearly labeled. The frosted end of the slide should be labeled either before or immediately after specimen collection. Generally a pencil should be used, because labeling done with other markers (e.g., fiber-tip pens, ballpoint pens) will be effaced by fixative and staining solutions.

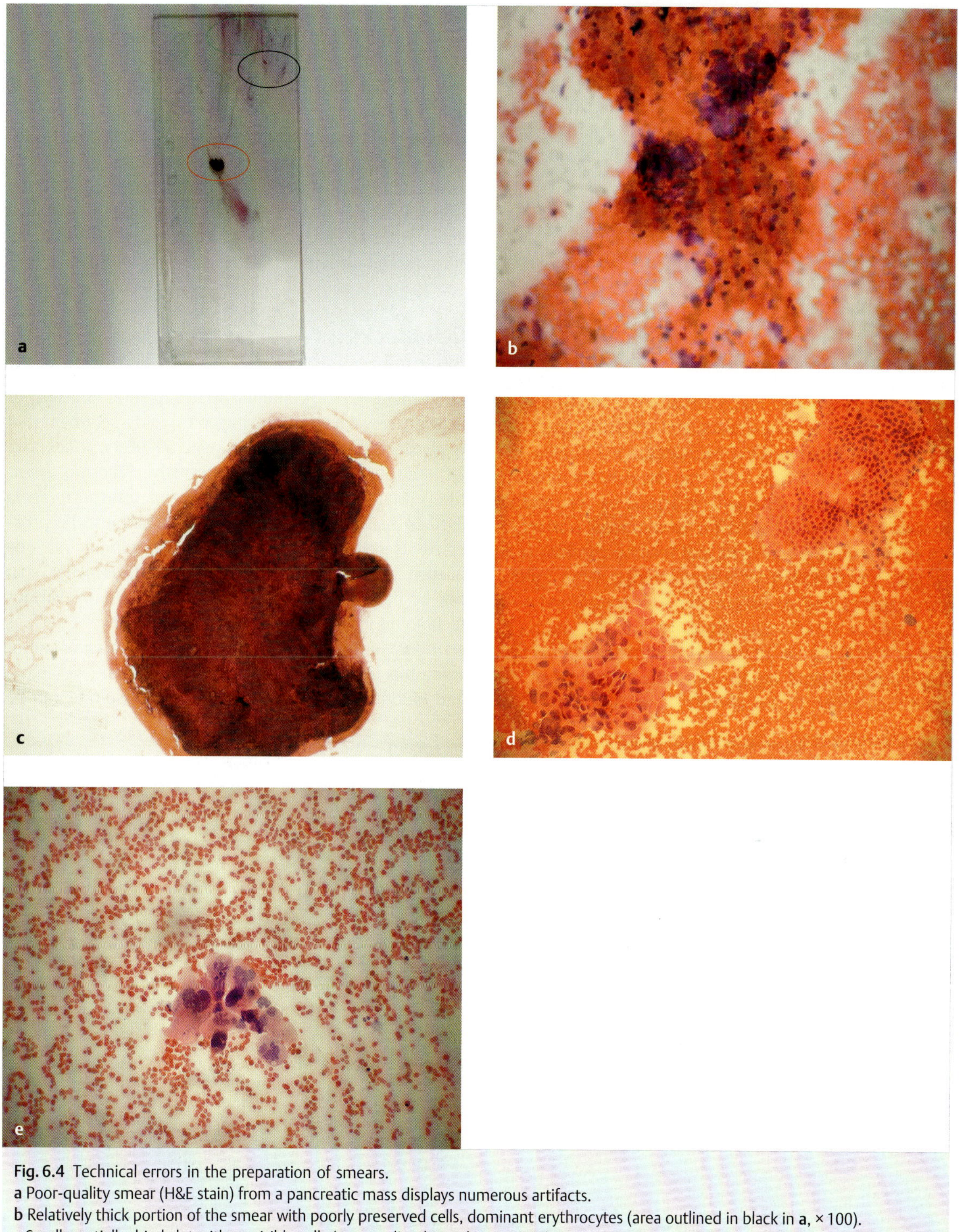

Fig. 6.4 Technical errors in the preparation of smears.
a Poor-quality smear (H&E stain) from a pancreatic mass displays numerous artifacts.
b Relatively thick portion of the smear with poorly preserved cells, dominant erythrocytes (area outlined in black in **a**, × 100).
c Small, partially dried clot with no visible cells (area outlined in red in **a**, × 200).
d Relatively thin portion of the smear (area outlined in green in **a**, × 200): dominant erythrocytes with normal glandular epithelium at upper right and tumor cells at lower left, consistent with adenocarcinoma.
e Detail from that portion of the smear shown in **d** (× 400). Cytologic diagnosis: poorly differentiated adenocarcinoma.
Source: All pictures courtesy of B. Fiedler, Berlin, Germany.

Cytocentrifugation (Cytospin)

When conventional smears have been prepared, residual material still trapped in the needle after it has been grossly emptied with a stylet and/or air-filled syringe can be rinsed into a transport container with approximately 1 mL of physiologic saline solution, Hank's balanced saline solution, or dilute Bouin fixative and then processed further by cytocentrifugation in the cytopathology laboratory.[2,8,9,19] If an expert in smearing technique is not available, the entire aspirated sample can simply be placed in transport solution and cytocentrifuged in the cytopathology laboratory.[20]

Thin-Layer Preparations

Liquid-based thin-layer preparations are an alternative or adjunct to conventional smears, and partially automated systems (e.g., PapSpin [Thermo Scientific]; ThinPrep and SurePath [Becton Dickinson]) can be used to produce them. The material obtained by aspiration, or residual material that was not used for conventional smears, is placed in a specific transport and fixation medium (e.g., CytoLyt solution [Cytyc Corporation]). After ultracentrifugation, the cellular material is transferred to a glass slide as a monolayer preparation in an automated process.[2,8,19] The main advantage of these methods is that they do not depend on the smearing technique of the clinical examiner. Other advantages are the removal of red cells, mucus, and protein precipitates, the concentration of diagnostically relevant material, an improved ability to evaluate individual cells, and an enhanced ability to perform ancillary tests (e.g., immunocytochemistry, molecular biology). As a result, screening and interpretation by the cytopathologist are faster and easier. Disadvantages of thin-layer techniques are the somewhat lower cellularity of the smears, the loss of diagnostically relevant extracellular background (e.g., mucin, necrosis), destruction of the architectural integrity of small cell clusters, and the significantly higher costs (▶ Table 6.1).[21]

Cell Blocks

Material for cell block preparations is obtained from aspirated fluids (cystic contents, ascites, pleural effusion) or needle rinse, which is centrifuged to yield a sediment that is placed in fixative solution (e.g., 50–96% alcohol, 10% formalin, or CytoRich Red preservative [Thermo Scientific]). Material from the fixation and transport media used to make thin-layer preparations can also be processed as cell blocks. Multiple centrifugations may be needed to obtain a consistent sediment, or pellet, that can be paraffin-embedded in a biopsy cassette. Various techniques for the aggregation of individual cells, such as artificial clot formation induced by adding plasma and/or thrombin, are used in preparing cell blocks.[2,8,9,19] Fibrin and blood clots forming in fine needle aspirate can be

Table 6.1 Advantages and disadvantages of different fixation methods for FNA material

Criterion	Air drying	Wet fixation	Thin-layer preparation
Immediate staining and on-site cytology	+++	+	–
Dependence on smearing technique	+++	++	–
Time loss	–	+	+
Cytochemistry, immunocytochemistry	++	+	++
Romanowsky staining (e.g., MGG)	+++	+	–
Papanicolaou staining	++	+++	+++
Artifacts	Enlarged cells and nuclei, increased pleomorphism, chromatin condensation	Shrinkage and rounding of cells	Optimum cell preservation, but significant changes in cellular architecture
Extracellular background	Distinct background with prominent extracellular substances	Faint	Clear background, almost complete disappearance of extracellular substances (mucin)
Cytoplasmic details	Well defined, good color gradation with MGG; keratinization visible	Poorly defined; transparent cytoplasm; keratinization visible	Preserved
Nuclear details and chromatin quality	Limited; good color gradation with MGG	Crisp visualization	Crisp nuclear details, prominent nucleoli
Stromal elements	Clearly defined	Poorly defined	Poorly defined
Partially necrotic tissue	Obscured cellular details	Good visualization of intact single cells	Good visualization of intact single cells

Source: Compiled from sources cited in the text.

placed in formalin and embedded in paraffin to produce "natural" cell blocks. There is no definition that uniquely distinguishes "natural" cell blocks from histologic preparations of small tissue cores like those obtained with 22-gauge needles.

Numerous paraffin sections can be produced from one aspiration sample and stored almost indefinitely for possible later tests. Essentially all histochemical and immunohistochemical techniques can be performed on cell blocks, just as on histologic preparations. This is particularly important in the evaluation of solid neoplasms, as in the differential diagnosis of malignant lymphadenopathy or of hepatic and pulmonary metastases from several possible primary tumors. For these reasons, cell blocks are prepared routinely as an adjunct to conventional smears at many institutions.[2,8,9,11,22]

6.3 Fixation and Staining

6.3.1 Basic Principles

Fixation is a crucial step for later cytologic assessment as it stabilizes the cellular architecture and produces permanent adhesion of the cells to the microscope slide. The dehydration and/or denaturing of structural and functional proteins terminates the autolysis that begins immediately after the specimen is collected.

A smear may be wet-fixed or air-dried. The selection of a particular fixation method determines the subsequent staining methods that can be used. The desired staining method in turn depends on the preference and experience of the cytopathology laboratory. May–Grünwald–Giemsa (MGG) is the standard stain used for air-dried smears, while Papanicolaou or hematoxylin and eosin (H&E) stain is preferred for wet-fixed smears. The advantages and disadvantages of the various fixation and staining methods are listed in ▶ Table 6.1.[2,8,9,19–21,23] Typical staining patterns are illustrated in ▶ Fig. 6.5 and ▶ Fig. 6.6.

6.3.2 Air Drying and Romanowsky Stains

The smears should be thin enough to appear visually dry within approximately 5 minutes. Smears should never be placed in closed transport containers before the drying process is complete. Drying artifacts such as indistinct cell borders, enlarged nuclei, and altered chromatin structure may lead to false-negative as well as false-positive diagnoses. Air-dried smears can be evaluated without delay by drying the smear with a small hand-held fan. This shortens the drying time by approximately two-thirds compared with ordinary air drying and does not degrade the quality of the smear.[24]

Air-dried smears are preferably stained with various Romanowsky stains (Diff-Quick [LT-SYS Diagnostika LABOR + TECHNIK], Hemacolor [Merck Millipore], May–Grünwald, Giemsa, May–Grünwald–Giemsa = Pappenheim; ▶ Fig. 6.3, ▶ Fig. 6.5a, ▶ Fig. 6.6a). Romanowsky stains contain methylene blue and eosin, which stain nuclear structures and cytoplasm differently depending on the pH (metachromasia). These stains are very good for (immuno) cytochemical testing because the slight protein denaturing gives excellent preservation of enzymes and antigen structures for immunocytochemistry. Papanicolaou (▶ Fig. 6.6c) and H&E stains (▶ Fig. 6.4, ▶ Fig. 6.5b, ▶ Fig. 6.6e) can also give excellent results on air-dried smears.[25–27]

While traditional MGG staining takes approximately 4 minutes, the commercial Diff-Quick and Hemacolor stains take less than 1 minute.

The MGG staining of air-dried smears, a method adopted from hematologic cytology, is preferred by most clinical cytologists, especially since it permits rapid on-site evaluation (ROSE) of specimens within about 2 minutes when fan drying and rapid staining are used. Air-dried smears have a virtually unlimited shelf life.

Note

Air-dried smears are compatible with nearly all staining methods as well as cytochemical and immunocytologic techniques.

6.3.3 Wet Fixation and Papanicolaou Staining

Wet fixation is advantageous because it can be done quickly and gives excellent preservation of cellular and nuclear morphology. Shrinkage artifacts aside, it provides pathologists less experienced in cytology with more familiar images that resemble histologic sections (▶ Fig. 6.5c, ▶ Fig. 6.6d). Immunocytochemistry is somewhat limited because wet fixation denatures structural proteins in the cell membrane, with the result that certain epitopes are no longer accessible to the monoclonal antibodies that are used. Cytoplasmic details are lost (▶ Table 6.1).

Wet fixations are prepared either by immersing the smear in special solutions (immersion fixation: absolute alcohol, mixed solutions of alcohol and ether or acetone, formalin, methanol, isopropanol) or by using a spray fixative (Cyto-Fix [BD Bio Sciences], CytoRAL [RAL Diagnostics], Merckofix [Merck Millipore]). Besides alcohol or acetone and occasionally isopropanol, most spray fixatives contain polyethylene glycol, which acts as a sealant. This protective film is removed from the slide before staining in the cytopathology laboratory by immersing it in 96% alcohol. Wet fixation must be done immediately (< 5 seconds) after the sample has been smeared on the slide. This is necessary to prevent air-drying artifacts that could seriously compromise morphologic evaluation. The thinner a smear is and the less moisture it contains, the

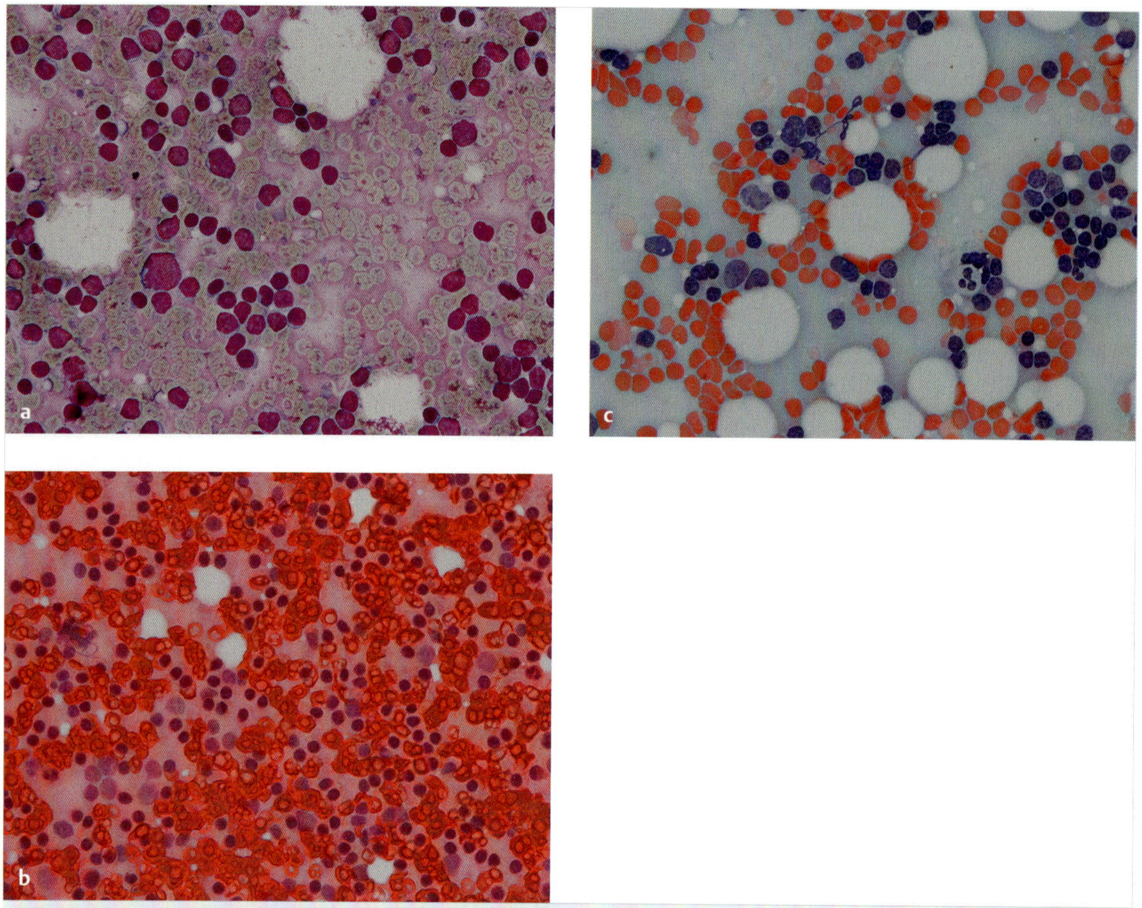

Fig. 6.5 Percutaneous FNA of a small inguinal lymph node in a woman with squamous cell carcinoma of the anal canal. Cytopathologic diagnosis: "benign" (only lymphocytes and macrophages, no tumor cells). The cells in the thin-layer smears at × 400 magnification are somewhat larger with MGG and H&E stain than with Papanicolaou. The nuclei and cytoplasm stain differently. The red-cell background is most troublesome with H&E stain.
a MGG stain.
b H&E stain.
c Papanicolaou stain.
With kind permission of S. Wagner, Königs Wusterhausen, Germany.

more rapidly it must be fixed.[2,9,19,21,23] If some drying has already occurred, the specimen can be wet-fixed after rehydrating it in physiologic saline solution (30 seconds) without loss of quality.[25]

Spray-fixed preparations are ready for submission in approximately 10 to 20 minutes. Immersion-fixed preparations should be submitted in screw-capped plastic containers filled with fixative solution whenever possible.

Wet fixation is most commonly used for cytology samples that will be submitted to an outside laboratory. Papanicolaou stain is generally used on wet-fixed preparations. A compelling feature of Papanicolaou-stained smears is the excellent depiction of nuclear chromatin structure. Cellular evaluation in thin smears is less compromised by extracellular mucin, mucus, or blood. Disadvantages of wet fixation are its relatively high time and labor costs and the photosensitivity of the preparations (▶ Table 6.1).[2,9,19,20,23]

Caution

Wet fixation must be done immediately after the smear is prepared.

6.3.4 Ancillary Tests

Ancillary tests that are well established in histology (cytochemistry, ▶ Fig. 6.7; immunocytochemistry [ICC]; molecular genetics) can generally be applied to cytologic preparations with certain slight modifications (especially regarding antibody concentrations and incubation techniques) and limitations (▶ Table 6.2, ▶ Table 6.3; details may be found in reference [8] and other cytopathology textbooks). This particularly applies to air-dried smears

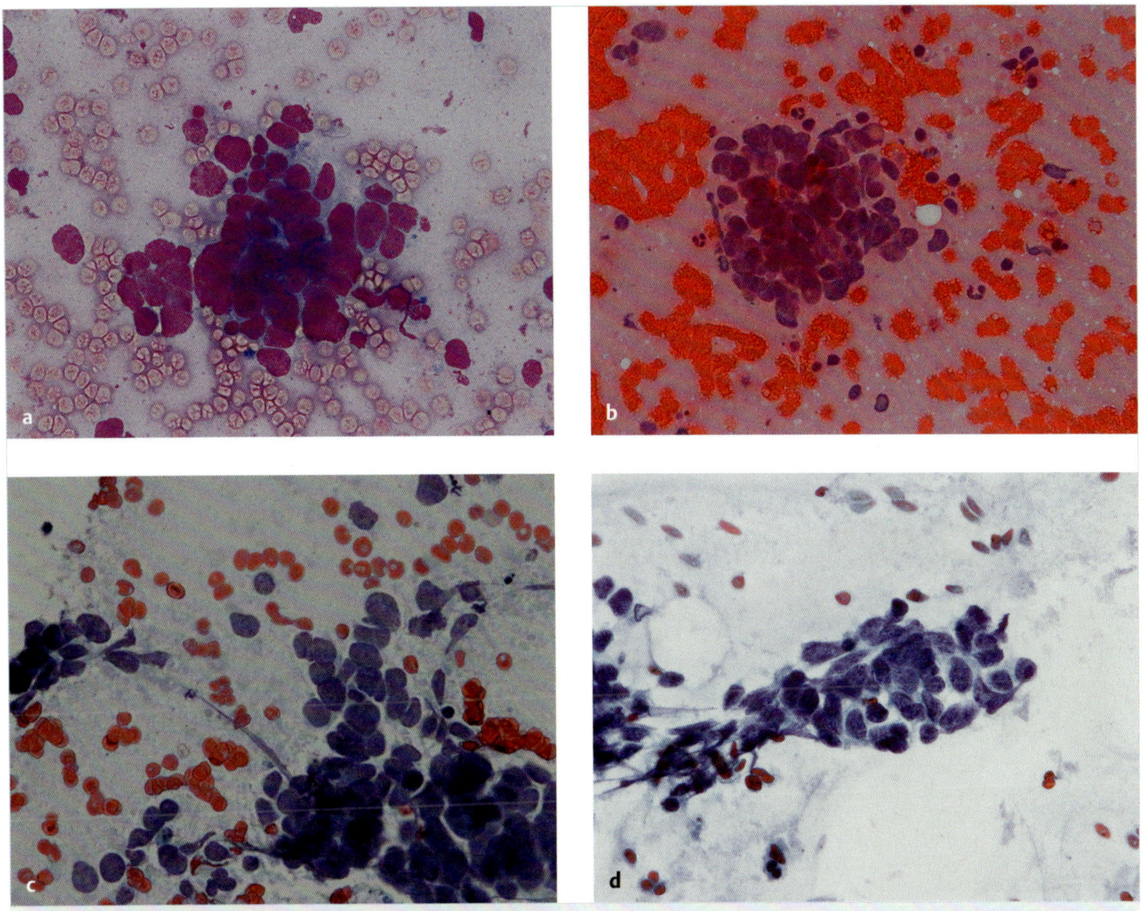

Fig. 6.6 Transesophageal EUS-FNA of an enlarged and morphologically abnormal infracarinal lymph node associated with an unknown primary tumor. Cytopathologic diagnosis: malignant small-cell neoplasm. Five different fixation and staining methods are shown (**a–e**). The diagnosis is evident in all five, but the different preparation methods cause marked differences with respect to apparent cell size (larger with air drying [**a–c**] than with wet fixation [**d**]), cytoplasmic and nuclear staining (metachronous with MGG [**a**] and H&E [**b, e**]), nuclear details and chromatin structure (better with Papanicolaou stain), and the architecture of the cell cluster (best in the cell block [**e**]). The marked differences are apparent even to a noncytologist. Immunocytochemistry on the cell blocks (**f–h**) reveals a lymph node metastasis from small cell lung cancer with high proliferative activity (all plates are × 400).
a MGG, air-dried.
b H&E, air-dried.
c Papanicolaou, air-dried.
d Papanicolaou, wet-fixed.
With kind permission of S. Wagner, Königs Wusterhausen, Germany.
(Continued on next page.)

and, within limits, to wet-fixed prestained smears. Cytospin and thin-layer preparations are excellent for ancillary studies owing to their low extracellular background and thin layer of cells. Spray-fixed smears that were subjected to temperature fluctuations during transport are unsuitable for ancillary testing. Generally speaking, smears that will undergo immunocytochemical staining should have a thin and uniform consistency.

Large, standardized immune panels generally cannot be used on smears because of the limited quantity of available representative smears. For this reason, a minimum of 10 to 12 smears should be prepared if possible whenever a malignant tumor is suspected. If only a few representative smears are available, a probability analysis should be done based on clinical information. Immunocytochemical markers selected on that basis can then be applied selectively and sequentially. If the number of smears is still insufficient, multiple reactions can be run on one slide. This is done by using a special slide marker (PAP pen) to outline two or at most four zones, which are then incubated with different antibodies. Cell blocks will generally provide an adequate number of sections for even complex multistep immunophenotypic tests. Immune panels suitable for immunocytochemistry are available for specific diagnostic situations (effusions, liver lesions, pancreatic lesions, mediastinal and lung lesions,

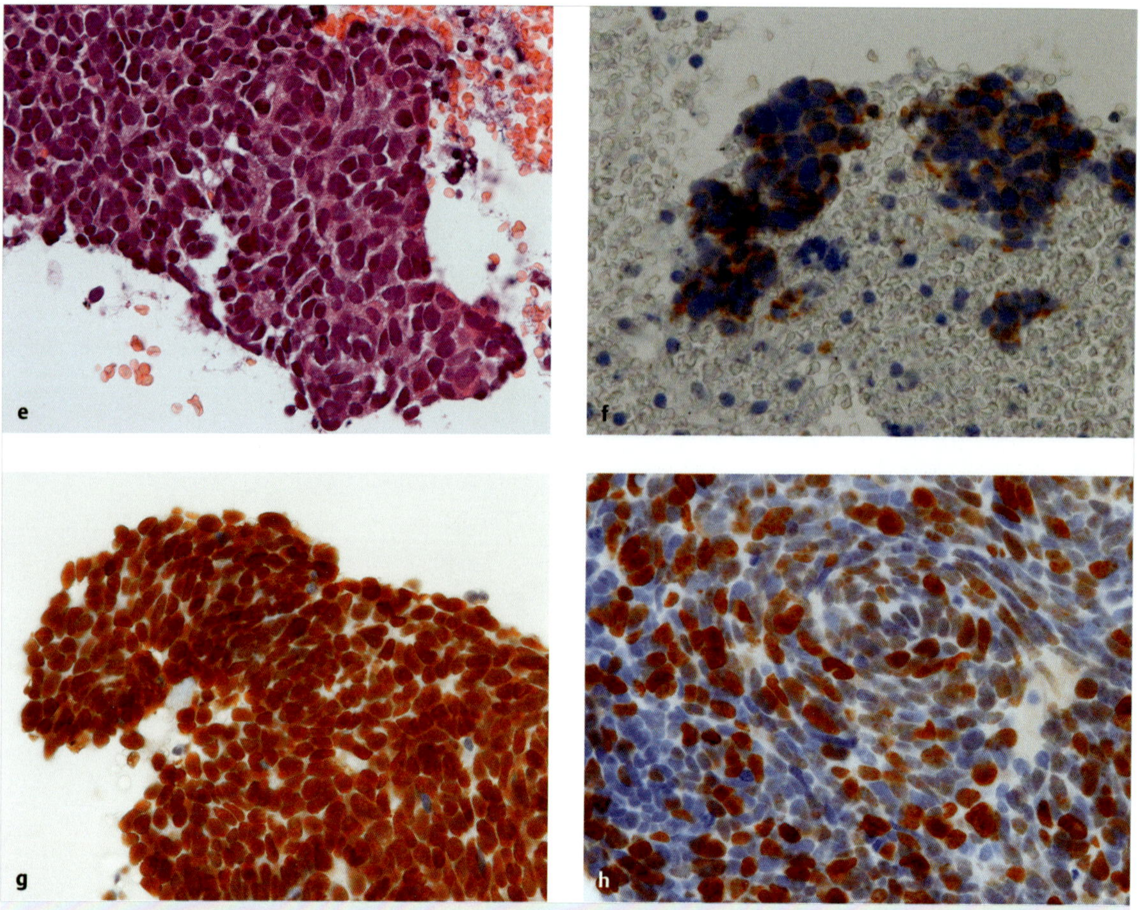

Fig. 6.6 (continued) Transesophageal EUS-FNA of an enlarged and morphologically abnormal infracarinal lymph node associated with an unknown primary tumor.
e H&E, "natural" cell block after formalin fixation.
f Positive cytoplasmic staining for AE1/AE3 = epithelial origin.
g TTF-1 positive = pulmonary origin. (LCA negative = excludes lymphatic origin; CK34β12 negative = differentiates from basaloid squamous cell carcinoma; LCA and CK34β12 not shown.)
h Ki-67 positive in approximately 70% of tumor cells = large proportion of mitotically active cells.
With kind permission of S. Wagner, Königs Wusterhausen, Germany.

lymph nodes, subepithelial tumors).[8,19,28–35] When a standardized technique is followed, some 85% of primary tumor sites can be identified immunocytochemically in effusion cytology, and approximately 90% can be identified in fine needle aspirations from the liver and lymph nodes[32–35] (▶ Fig. 6.6f–h, ▶ Fig. 6.8).

Note

For maximum diagnostic accuracy with FNAC, we recommend that additional material be harvested for special stains (especially cell block material).

Cytologic preparations are very receptive to molecular genetic tests (flow cytometry, fluorescence in situ hybridization [FISH], polymerase chain reaction [PCR], gene microarray analysis) owing to the intact condition of the cell nuclei.[8,19] With proper expertise, then, the diagnosis and classification of malignant lymphomas can be accomplished by the analysis of fine needle aspirate from lymph nodes using PCR (clonality), special stains for CD20 and CD3 epitopes (for typing cell lines) and MIB-1 (proliferative activity), and the molecular genetic detection of translocations by FISH (B-cell lymphoma-2, cycln D1).[36–38]

6.4 Cytomorphologic Evaluation

6.4.1 Rapid On-Site Evaluation

Contrasting with the situation in the United States, Rapid On-Site Evaluation ("ROSE") protocols have been instituted at only a few centers in Europe, due mainly to the growing numbers of decentralized cytopathology labora-

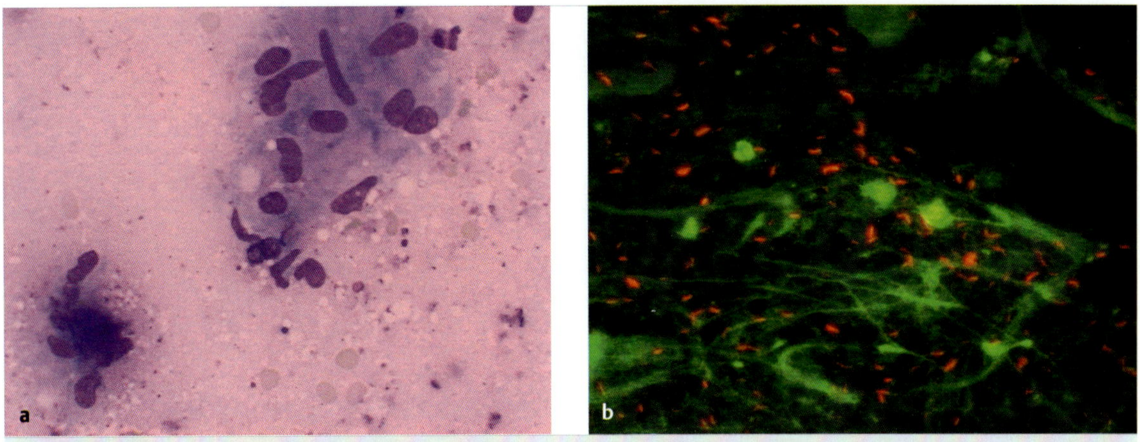

Fig. 6.7 Transesophageal FNA of a mediastinal lymph node.
a MGG-stained smear displays epithelioid cells and necrosis.
b Lymph node tuberculosis is diagnosed by fluorescent staining with acridine orange. Mycobacteria appear as bright reddish-orange rods against a dark-green background.
Source: Beyer T. Tips and tricks for fine-needle puncture. In: Dietrich CF, ed. Endoscopic Ultrasound. An Introductory Manual and Atlas. Stuttgart, New York: Thieme; 2011:168–175.

tories. ROSE is practiced routinely when specimen collection and cytomorphologic evaluation are performed by the same operator (clinical cytology).

Rapid Fixation and Staining

Various techniques have been described for performing the rapid fixation and staining that are necessary for immediate on-site evaluation. The most common technique is (fan-assisted) air drying followed by rapid staining (DiffQuick, Hemacolor), a method derived from hematologic cytology. Another option is to combine rapid alcohol fixation and modified ultrafast Papanicolaou staining. Rapid methylene blue and H&E staining are also possible. These techniques ensure that readable smears will be available for on-site evaluation within 2 to 3 minutes after aspiration. Immediate evaluation by telepathology provides an alternative to the on-site presence of a cytomorphologist[39,40] (▶ Fig. 6.9).

Table 6.2 Typical cytochemical reactions and special cytologic stains

Cytochemical reaction	Substance demonstrated
Periodic acid Schiff (PAS)	Glycogen
PAS diastase (PAS-d)	Mucin
Alcian blue	Mucin
Gram	Differentiation of bacteria
Ziehl–Neelsen	Acid-fast rods (tuberculosis)
Auramine–rhodamine	Acid-fast rods (tuberculosis)
Acridine orange	Nucleic acids, acid-fast rods (tuberculosis)
Feulgen	DNA
Prussian blue	Iron
Sudan red	Fat
Silver nitrate	Argyrophilic nuclear organizer regions (AgNOR)

Source: reference [8].

Goals

On-site cytology has several goals. They include increasing the diagnostic yield of FNAC, optimizing the number of fine needle passes required, optimizing the utilization of resources, and reducing risks. Moreover, an immediate preliminary diagnosis allows for rapid decision making on further actions.[41]

On-site cytopathology should answer the following questions:

- Is the sampled material representative of the aspirated lesion?
- Is the aspirate adequate for cytomorphologic evaluation?
- Is the finding benign or malignant? Can a preliminary diagnosis be made?
- Are additional aspirations necessary for special preparations (cell block, special stains)?
- Does the FNA need to be supplemented by core needle biopsy?

Importance

Numerous studies have been published on the importance of rapid on-site evaluation in FNA cytology. Analyses of the literature show that up to 32% (average of about 20%) of FNAs are nondiagnostic due to scant cellularity or poor preparation. In a large series of 5,688 percutaneous FNA cases at the University of Pennsylvania Medical Center over a 5-year period, the rate of nondiagnostic FNAs with on-site evaluation was only 0.98%. On-site cytology

Table 6.3 Important, frequently used immunocytochemical markers and their applications in (differential) diagnosis

Immunocytochemical stain	Application in (differential) diagnosis
Epithelial markers	
EMA	Epithelial membrane antigen (screening marker for epithelial neoplasms)
Pancytokeratin (AE1/AE3, MNF116)	Epithelial (positive) versus nonepithelial origin (negative)
CK5/6	Adenocarcinoma (negative) versus squamous cell carcinoma (positive) and mesothelioma (positive)
p63, CD56	Differentiation of lung cancers (adenocarcinoma: $p63^-$, $CD56^-$; squamous cell carcinoma: $p63^+$, $CD56^-$; small cell carcinoma: $p63^-$, $CD56^+$)
CK7/CK20	Differentiate adenocarcinomas of different origins, e.g., pulmonary adenocarcinoma ($CD20^-$, $CD7^+$) versus metastatic colorectal carcinoma ($CK20^+$, $CK7^-$)
Specific epithelial tumor markers	
CEA	Carcinoembryonic antigen, screening marker for adenocarcinoma
CA 125	Carbohydrate antigen 125, marker for ovarian carcinoma and pancreatic carcinoma
TTF-1	Thyroid transcription factor 1, highly sensitive and specific marker for the thyroid gland and relatively specific for adenocarcinoma of the lung
CDX2	Markers for an intestinal origin of adenocarcinoma
Hep Par 1	Hepatocyte paraffin 1, highly sensitive and specific marker for hepatocellular carcinoma
HMB-45	Highly sensitive and relatively specific marker for malignant melanoma
PSA	Prostate-specific antigen, specific marker for prostatic carcinoma
NSE (neuron-specific enolase), chromogranin, synaptophysin CD56	Markers for neuroendocrine differentiation
Mesenchymal tumor markers	
Vimentin	Screening marker for mesenchymal neoplasms and melanomas
CD34	Screening marker for mesenchymal and endothelial tumors
SMA (smooth muscle actin)	Marker for smooth muscle tumors (leiomyoma, leiomyosarcoma)
Desmin	Marker for smooth muscle tumors (leiomyoma, leiomyosarcoma)
CD117 (c-kit)	Marker for gastrointestinal stromal tumors (GIST)
Receptors	
Estrogen, progesterone	Markers for breast and endometrial cancers; used in selecting patients for receptor-blocking therapies
HER2-neu	Human epidermal growth receptor 2, used in selecting breast- and stomach-cancer patients for herceptin therapy
Markers for the diagnosis and differentiation of malignant lymphomas	
LCA (CD45)	Leukocyte common antigen, screening marker for neoplasms of the hematopoietic/lymphatic system; differentiation of small-cell neoplasms
CD3	T-cell marker
CD20	B-cell marker
CD5, CD10, CD15, CD30, cyclin D1, bcl-6, bcl-2, ...	Markers for specific types of malignant lymphoma
Proliferation marker	
Ki67 (MIB-1)	Correlates with the proliferative activity of malignant tumors, prognostic marker for mesenchymal and lymphatic neoplasms

Source: Compiled from sources cited in the text.

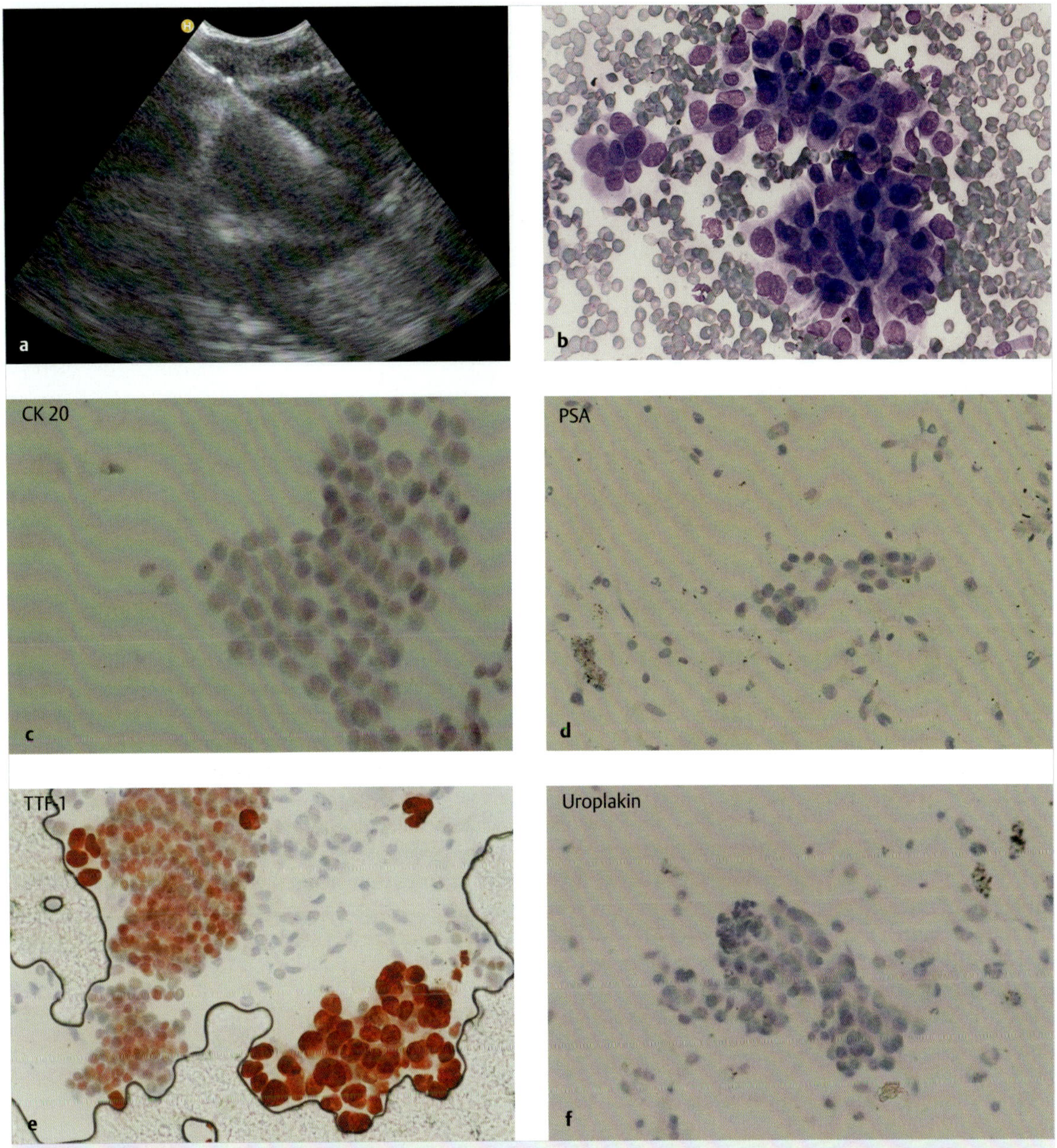

Fig. 6.8 Transbronchial FNA (**a**) from an enlarged mediastinal lymph node in a man with a prior history of three successfully treated cancers (colon cancer 9 years, bladder cancer 7 years, and prostate cancer 3 years before current presentation). Cytology (**b–h**) revealed a non-small cell tumor, most likely adenocarcinoma. Differentiation could not be made between bronchial carcinoma and a late metastasis from one of the three previous cancers. Immunocytochemistry identifies the lesion as a fourth malignancy: pulmonary adenocarcinoma.
a EBUS-TBNA.
b Hemacolor rapid stain.
c Immunocytochemistry: CD20 negative.
d Immunocytochemistry: PSA negative.
e Immunocytochemistry: TTF-1 positive (CD7 positive not shown).
f Immunocytochemistry: uroplakin negative.

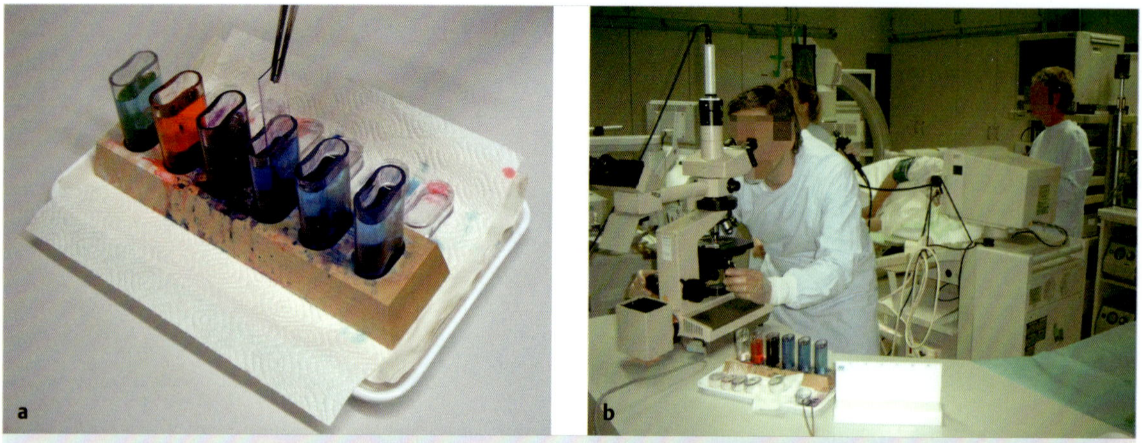

Fig. 6.9 ROSE (rapid on-site evaluation). Rapid staining is essential for an immediate on-site cytologic evaluation.
a Hemacolor rapid staining kit. (Source: from Beyer T. Tips and tricks for fine-needle puncture. In: Dietrich CF, ed. Endoscopic Ultrasound. An Introductory Manual and Atlas. Stuttgart, New York: Thieme; 2011:168–175.)
b Before the procedure (here EUS-FNA) is completed, the (clinical) cytologist performs a microscopic evaluation in the examination room and assesses the adequacy of the specimen.

increased the average cost per FNA (US$3,096) by approximately 7% ($231).

Assuming that a nondiagnostic FNA must be repeated, ROSE provided a definite cost benefit at the reporting center.[42] Another report from the same center showed that a correct on-site evaluation of air-dried and Diff-Quick-stained smears from thyroid FNA was achieved in 65% of histologically controlled cases, while subsequent interpretations of Papanicolaou-stained alcohol-fixed smears and of Millipore filter preparations were correct in 88% and 91% of cases, respectively.[43] In a comparative study of 883 thyroid FNAs at another U.S. center, it was found that the percentage of nondiagnostic FNAs was significantly lower with on-site evaluation than without it (5.9% versus 31.8%). Moreover, 8 malignant cases were missed by FNA in the group without on-site evaluation (13.8%), compared with zero misses in the group with on-site evaluation.[44]

Various studies have shown that on-site evaluation can significantly reduce the number of needle passes necessary for a diagnosis.[44–46]

Similar results on the diagnostic utility of ROSE have been documented for the FNA of liver masses,[47–49] renal masses,[50] retroperitoneal abdominal lesions,[48,51–53] nonpalpable breast tumors,[54,55] and head and neck masses.[56] Positive assessments of on-site cytology have also been published for EUS-FNA, especially in the aspiration of pancreatic lesions and lymph nodes,[57–63] and for (EBUS-) TBNA.[64–66] In one meta-analysis, the cumulative sensitivity of EUS-FNA for staging lung cancer was 80% in studies without ROSE but 88% in studies with ROSE.[67]

On the other hand, it should be noted that the evaluation of cost effectiveness is a controversial issue. One differentiated analysis came to the conclusion that on-site cytology under the conditions prevalent in the United States is cost-effective only when specimen collection and interpretation are performed by the same cytopathologist.[68] With the clinician or pathologist time averaging between 35 and 44 minutes, the presence of a cytopathologist during a sonographically or EUS-guided FNA performed by a clinician represents a time-consuming approach.[68,69] It should also be considered that the preliminary on-site diagnosis and the final cytologic interpretation differed from each other in 5.8%[70] to 8.4% of cases[71] in large series. The main reasons for the discrepant diagnoses were hypocellular smears with a dominant normal local cell population, contamination from the needle tract, and diagnostically challenging entities with overlapping cytomorphologic features.[70–72]

Note

With on-site cytology, the need for additional aspirations or a core needle biopsy can be assessed during the intervention.

Working without ROSE

If on-site cytology is not available, various authors recommend following a standard protocol with a predetermined number of needle passes (depending on the aspirated lesion, ▶ Table 6.4) and the parallel preparation of conventional smears (air-dried and/or wet-fixed), as well as concentrated preparations if needed for ancillary studies (cell block, Millipore filter, Thin-Prep).[58,61,73–76] It has been shown that combining cytological smears with cell block may enhance diagnostic performance of fine needle aspiration.[47,77–83]

Table 6.4 Number of fine needle passes needed to attain high sensitivity in the FNA of various target lesions

Target lesion	Collection method	Number of passes	Sources
Thyroid nodules	Percutaneous FNA	4	46,76
Renal tumors	Percutaneous FNA	3	50
Breast tumors	Percutaneous FNA	3 or 4	55,99
Liver tumors	Percutaneous FNA	1 or 2	49,100
Mediastinal lymph nodes	EUS-FNA	3	101
Mediastinal lymph node	EBUS-TBNA	2 or 3	74
Pancreatic tumors	EUS-FNA	5–7[a]	73,102

[a] Several studies limited to two passes still report approximately 80% sensitivity in the EUS-FNA of pancreatic lesions.

Note

When samples are sent to an outside cytopathology laboratory, details on material processing should always be precisely coordinated between the clinician and the laboratory.

As a general rule of thumb, approximately 10 to 12 smears should be prepared in settings where on-site cytology is not available.

6.4.2 Final Cytologic Diagnosis

Clinical Data

The final cytomorphologic diagnosis is based not only on the morphologic evaluation of smears and the results of ancillary tests (especially immunocytochemistry) but also on clinical data. For this reason, the requisition form should always include the following information:

1. Type of material
2. Preparation after collection (wet fixation or air drying, transport solution)
3. Site of specimen collection
4. Needle route (e.g., percutaneous, transbronchial, transgastric)
5. Patient history:
    - Previous tumor disease? (with histologic diagnosis)
    - Clinical diagnoses (especially diseases of the biopsied organ)
    - Relevant laboratory findings (e.g., tumor markers)
6. Indication

Cytopathology Reporting

The interpretation of FNA preparations is a multifaceted process that includes the evaluation of cellular morphology, intercellular interactions, cell cluster architecture, and the extracellular matrix along with the patient's history and clinical data, imaging results, and histologic material when available.[84,85] The criteria and principles of cytomorphologic interpretation, organ- and lesion-specific diagnostic algorithms, diagnostic pitfalls, and limitations of the method have been detailed in monographs and cytopathology atlases[2,7–9,13] and are beyond the scope of this chapter. Cytopathology reporting should include basic information (patient data, date and method of specimen collection, number and type of preparations) and should answer the following questions:

- Is the material representative and diagnostic?
- From what organ or tissue was the material sampled?
- Normal cellular findings, inflammation, or neoplasia?
- If neoplasia: benign or malignant?
- Can the neoplasia or inflammation be classified?
- Are there limitations on diagnostic certainty (possible differential diagnoses)?

Particularly with regard to benign/malignant differentiation, the clinician expects a clear, unambiguous report and a diagnosis that is as specific as possible. If a definitive diagnosis cannot be made, the report should include a differential diagnosis and recommendations for further investigation.[84] The degree of diagnostic (un)certainty must be reflected in the report.[86]

Clinicians and cytopathologists should agree on using one of the reporting nomenclatures that have been published in guidelines. Practitioners use cytology terminologies for FNAC of the thyroid gland[87,88] and breast[89] (Bethesda System), the consensus nomenclature for "Standardized Reporting in Extragenital Cytology" issued by the German Society for Pathology and the German Society for Cytology[90] (▶ Table 6.5), and the general nomenclature of the Papanicolaou Society of Cytopathology.[91] The guideline of the College of American Pathologists, drawing on histopathology practice, prefers a descriptive diagnosis and states that standard diagnostic categories should always be supplemented by a descriptive diagnosis.[84]

Caution

The categories "negative for malignancy" and "benign" do not exclude malignancy! There is always a potential for sampling error.

Diagnostic Certainty of FNAC

The rate of nondiagnostic and false-negative findings in FNAC varies greatly in published studies and depends on

Table 6.5 Grading the likelihood of malignancy in cytopathologic findings based on "Standard Reporting in Extragenital Cytology" issued by the German Societies for Pathology and of Cytology[90]

Diagnostic category	Interpretation
Negative	Malignant cells not detected
Equivocal	Malignant cells cannot be confidently excluded
Very suspicious	Malignant cells are probable
Positive	Malignant cells are detected
Inadequate	Inadequate specimen (only necrotic, autolytic or osmotically damaged cells or absence of cells from the aspirated mass in the specimen)

Source: Böcking A. Standardisierte Befunderstellung in der extragenitalen Zytologie. Pathologe 1998; 19(3):236–241, with kind permission from Springer Science + Business Media.

factors such as the target organ, the nature and size of the target lesion, the aspiration method (US-FNA, EUS-FNA, etc.), the number of needle passes, the presence of a cytopathologist during the aspiration, and the preparation methods that are used. The great majority of false-negative findings result from *sampling errors*, which are the responsibility of the clinical diagnostician. False-positive findings, on the other hand, are mostly *interpretive errors* caused by the overinterpretation of benign changes by the cytopathologist.[11,22,23,92,93]

False-positive FNAC is rare in most single-center retrospective studies, with a reported incidence of approximately zero to 1%. It is likely, however, that these figures underestimate true false-positive rates because the gold standard of surgical or postmortem histologic control was not available for all cases. A recently published analysis of a prospective database of 5,667 EUS-FNAs investigated the false-positive rates for EUS-FNA in 377 patients who underwent subsequent surgical resection (histology) without prior neoadjuvant therapy. EUS-FNA was false-positive for malignancy in 20 of the patients (5.3%). The false-positive rate increased to 27/377 (7.2%) when false-suspicious findings were included.

The risk of false-positive findings was significantly higher for nonpancreatic FNAs (15%) than for the EUS-FNA of pancreatic lesions (2.2%). Two-thirds of the nonpancreatic false-positive FNAs involved the sampling of periesophageal or perirectal lymph nodes in patients with Barrett esophagus or luminal neoplasms, suggesting that tumor-cell contamination of the needle was the most likely cause. However, a consensus re-review of the false-positive and false-suspicious cases by three pathologists found that half of the discordant findings (13 of 377 EUS-FNAs = 3.4% of all cases) were due to interpretive error by the cytopathologist.[94]

Data from the benchmarking program of the College of American Pathologists on the accuracy of interpretations in nongynecologic cytology indicated a substantially higher rate of incorrect benign/malignant determinations in benign fine needle aspirates from the kidney (60%), liver (37%), pancreas (10%), and salivary glands (6%).[95] Eleven percent of FNA specimens from granulomatous or specific inflammatory lung lesions[96] and 22% of FNA specimens from pulmonary hamartomas[97] were misdiagnosed as carcinomas or carcinoid tumors. The false-positive rate for FNA slides from salivary glands was 8%.[98] It should be noted, however, that the cytopathologists and cytotechnicians participating in this interlaboratory study received only one conventional smear per case. Ancillary tests were not possible, and no clinical information was provided. Even so, these data clearly indicate the potential for errors in cytomorphologic interpretation, especially when samples are submitted to an outside laboratory and interpreted by pathologists not specialized in cytology. The data also permit a concrete analysis of pitfalls.[95] Above all, though, we feel that these results underscore the key importance of the history and clinical information and of special stains and preparations in establishing an accurate cytologic diagnosis.

Caution

Without the history and clinical information, a reliable cytopathologic diagnosis cannot be made.

6.5 Conclusions

Sonographically and endosonographically guided fine needle aspiration cytology is an important, minimally invasive procedure for the tissue diagnosis of lesions and parenchymal changes in numerous organs. Each individual step—from patient selection to specimen collection, and from specimen preparation to interpretation—requires a sound knowledge of the overall process, good practical skills, and critical reflection. The cytomorphologic analysis plus the history and clinical data must converge to yield a precisely formulated diagnosis. Optimal results can be achieved when all the steps are handled by one operator (clinical cytology) and/or an immediate on-site evaluation of the aspirates can be made (ROSE).

References

[1] Mannheim E. Die Bedeutung der Tumorpunktion für die Tumordiagnose. Z Krebsforsch 1931; 34: 572–593

[2] Kocjan G. Fine Needle Aspiration Cytology. Diagnostic Principles and Dilemmas. Berlin, Heidelberg: Springer-Verlag; 2006

[3] Ansari NA, Derias NW. Fine needle aspiration cytology. J Clin Pathol 1997; 50: 541–543

[4] Diamantis A, Magiorkinis E, Koutselini H. Fine-needle aspiration (FNA) biopsy: historical aspects. Folia Histochem Cytobiol 2009; 47: 191–197

[5] Vilmann P, Jacobsen GK, Henriksen FW, Hancke S. Endoscopic ultrasonography with guided fine needle aspiration biopsy in pancreatic disease. Gastrointest Endosc 1992; 38: 172–173

[6] Yasufuku K, Chiyo M, Sekine Y et al. Real-time endobronchial ultrasound-guided transbronchial needle aspiration of mediastinal and hilar lymph nodes. Chest 2004; 126: 122–128

[7] Lopes Cardozo P. Atlas of Clinical Cytology. A Contribution to Precise Cytodiagnosis and Cytological Differential Diagnosis. Leiden: Paul Lopes Cardozo; 1976

[8] Bubendorf L, Feichter GE, Obermann EC, Dalquen P. Zytopathologie. Berlin, Heidelberg: Springer-Verlag; 2011

[9] Gherardi G. Fine-Needle Biopsy of Superficial and Deep Masses. Dordrecht, Heidelberg, London, Milan, New York: Springer Italia; 2009

[10] Pothier DD, Narula AA. Should we apply suction during fine needle cytology of thyroid lesions? A systematic review and meta-analysis. Ann R Coll Surg Engl 2006; 88: 643–645

[11] Jenssen C, Dietrich CF. Endoscopic ultrasound-guided fine-needle aspiration biopsy and trucut biopsy in gastroenterology – an overview. Best Pract Res Clin Gastroenterol 2009; 23: 743–759

[12] Sajeev S, Siddaraju N. A comparative analysis of fine-needle capillary cytology vs. fine-needle aspiration cytology in superficial lymph node lesions. Diagn Cytopathol 2009; 37: 787–791

[13] Sidawy MK, Ali SZ, eds. Fine Needle Aspiration Cytology. Philadelphia: Churchill Livingstone-Elsevier; 2007

[14] Storch IM, Sussman DA, Jorda M, Ribeiro A. Evaluation of fine needle aspiration vs. fine needle capillary sampling on specimen quality and diagnostic accuracy in endoscopic ultrasound-guided biopsy. Acta Cytol 2007; 51: 837–842

[15] Abouzgheib W, Bartter T, Dagher H, Pratter M, Klump W. A prospective study of the volume of pleural fluid required for accurate diagnosis of malignant pleural effusion. Chest 2009; 135: 999–1001

[16] Sallach SM, Sallach JA, Vasquez E, Schultz L, Kvale P. Volume of pleural fluid required for diagnosis of pleural malignancy. Chest 2002; 122: 1913–1917

[17] Swiderek J, Morcos S, Donthireddy V et al. Prospective study to determine the volume of pleural fluid required to diagnose malignancy. Chest 2010; 137: 68–73

[18] Abele JS, Miller TR, King EB, Lowhagen T. Smearing techniques for the concentration of particles from fine needle aspiration biopsy. Diagn Cytopathol 1985; 1: 59–65

[19] Bales CE. Laboratory techniques. In: Koss LG, Melamed MR, eds. Koss' Diagnostic Cytology and its Histopathologic Bases. 5th ed. Philadelphia, Baltimore: Lippincott, Williams & Wilkins, 2006:1569–1634

[20] Crystal BS, Wang HH, Ducatman BS. Comparison of different preparation techniques for fine needle aspiration specimens. A semi-quantitative and statistical analysis. Acta Cytol 1993; 37: 24–28

[21] Dey P, Luthra UK, George J, Zuhairy F, George SS, Haji BI. Comparison of ThinPrep and conventional preparations on fine needle aspiration cytology material. Acta Cytol 2000; 44: 46–50

[22] Jenssen C, Möller K, Sarbia M, Wagner S. EUS-guided biopsy – indications, problems, pitfalls, troubleshooting, and clinical impact. In: Dietrich CF, ed. Endoscopic Ultrasound. An Introductory Manual and Atlas. Stuttgart, New York: Thieme; 2011:91–167

[23] Beyer T. Tips and tricks for fine-needle puncture. In: Dietrich CF, ed. Endoscopic Ultrasound. An Introductory Manual and Atlas. Stuttgart, New York: Thieme; 2011:168–175

[24] Baig MA, Fathallah L, Feng J, Husain M, Grignon DG, Al-Abbadi MA. Fast drying of fine needle aspiration slides using a hand held fan: impact on turn around time and staining quality. Cytojournal 2006; 3: 12

[25] Chan JK, Kung IT. Rehydration of air-dried smears with normal saline. Application in fine-needle aspiration cytologic examination. Am J Clin Pathol 1988; 89: 30–34

[26] Yang GC. Ultrafast Papanicolaou stain is not limited to rapid assessments: application to permanent fine-needle aspiration smears. Diagn Cytopathol 1995; 13: 160–162

[27] Yang GC, Alvarez II. Ultrafast Papanicolaou stain. An alternative preparation for fine needle aspiration cytology. Acta Cytol 1995; 39: 55–60

[28] Fowler LJ, Lachar WA. Application of immunohistochemistry to cytology. Arch Pathol Lab Med 2008; 132: 373–383

[29] Kakar S, Gown AM, Goodman ZD, Ferrell LD. Best practices in diagnostic immunohistochemistry: hepatocellular carcinoma versus metastatic neoplasms. Arch Pathol Lab Med 2007; 131: 1648–1654

[30] Stelow EB, Murad FM, Debol SM et al. A limited immunocytochemical panel for the distinction of subepithelial gastrointestinal mesenchymal neoplasms sampled by endoscopic ultrasound-guided fine-needle aspiration. Am J Clin Pathol 2008; 129: 219–225

[31] Turner MS, Goldsmith JD. Best practices in diagnostic immunohistochemistry: spindle cell neoplasms of the gastrointestinal tract. Arch Pathol Lab Med 2009; 133: 1370–1374

[32] Böcking A, Pomjansky N, Buckstegge B, Onofre A. Immunocytochemical identification of carcinomas of unknown primaries on fine-needle-aspiration-biopsies [Article in German]. Pathologe 2009; 30 Suppl 2: 158–160

[33] Onofre AS, Pomjanski N, Buckstegge B, Böcking A. Immunocytochemical diagnosis of hepatocellular carcinoma and identification of carcinomas of unknown primary metastatic to the liver on fine-needle aspiration cytologies. Cancer 2007; 111: 259–268

[34] Pomjanski N, Grote HJ, Doganay P, Schmiemann V, Buckstegge B, Böcking A. Immunocytochemical identification of carcinomas of unknown primary in serous effusions. Diagn Cytopathol 2005; 33: 309–315

[35] Casimiro Onofre AS, Pomjanski N, Buckstegge B, Böcking A. Immunocytochemical typing of primary tumors on fine-needle aspiration cytologies of lymph nodes. Diagn Cytopathol 2008; 36: 207–215

[36] Garcia CF, Swerdlow SH. Best practices in contemporary diagnostic immunohistochemistry: panel approach to hematolymphoid proliferations. Arch Pathol Lab Med 2009; 133: 756–765

[37] Kaleem Z. Flow cytometric analysis of lymphomas: current status and usefulness. Arch Pathol Lab Med 2006; 130: 1850–1858

[38] Safley AM, Buckley PJ, Creager AJ et al. The value of fluorescence in situ hybridization and polymerase chain reaction in the diagnosis of B-cell non-Hodgkin lymphoma by fine-needle aspiration. Arch Pathol Lab Med 2004; 128: 1395–1403

[39] Alsharif M, Carlo-Demovich J, Massey C et al. Telecytopathology for immediate evaluation of fine-needle aspiration specimens. Cancer Cytopathol 2010; 118: 119–126

[40] Kim B, Chhieng DC, Crowe DR et al. Dynamic telecytopathology of on site rapid cytology diagnoses for pancreatic carcinoma. Cytojournal 2006, 3. 27

[41] Silverman JF, Finley JL, O'Brien KF et al. Diagnostic accuracy and role of immediate interpretation of fine needle aspiration biopsy specimens from various sites. Acta Cytol 1989; 33: 791–796

[42] Nasuti JF, Gupta PK, Baloch ZW. Diagnostic value and cost-effectiveness of on-site evaluation of fine-needle aspiration specimens: review of 5,688 cases. Diagn Cytopathol 2002; 27: 1–4

[43] Baloch ZW, Tam D, Langer J, Mandel S, LiVolsi VA, Gupta PK. Ultrasound-guided fine-needle aspiration biopsy of the thyroid: role of on-site assessment and multiple cytologic preparations. Diagn Cytopathol 2000; 23: 425–429

[44] Zhu W, Michael CW. How important is on-site adequacy assessment for thyroid FNA? An evaluation of 883 cases. Diagn Cytopathol 2007; 35: 183–186

[45] Lachman MF, Cellura K, Schofield K, Mitra A. On-site adequacy assessments for image-directed fine needle aspirations: a study of 341 cases. Conn Med 1995; 59: 657–660

[46] Redman R, Zalaznick H, Mazzaferri EL, Massoll NA. The impact of assessing specimen adequacy and number of needle passes for fine-needle aspiration biopsy of thyroid nodules. Thyroid 2006; 16: 55–60

[47] Ceyhan K, Kupana SA, Bektaş M et al. The diagnostic value of on-site cytopathological evaluation and cell block preparation in fine-needle aspiration cytology of liver masses. Cytopathology 2006; 17: 267–274

[48] Fornari F, Civardi G, Cavanna L et al. Ultrasonically guided fine-needle aspiration biopsy: a highly diagnostic procedure for hepatic tumors. Am J Gastroenterol 1990; 85: 1009–1013

[49] Pupulim LF, Felce-Dachez M, Paradis V et al. Algorithm for immediate cytologic diagnosis of hepatic tumors. AJR Am J Roentgenol 2008; 190: W208–W212

[50] Andonian S, Okeke Z, Okeke DA, Sugrue C, Wasserman PG, Lee BR. Number of needle passes does not correlate with the diagnostic yield of renal fine needle aspiration cytology. J Endourol 2008; 22: 2377–2380
[51] Azabdaftari G, Goldberg SN, Wang HH. Efficacy of on-site specimen adequacy evaluation of image-guided fine and core needle biopsies. Acta Cytol 2010; 54: 132–137
[52] Saleh HA, Masood S, Khatib G. Percutaneous and intraoperative aspiration biopsy cytology of pancreatic neuroendocrine tumors: cytomorphologic study with an immunocytochemical contribution. Acta Cytol 1996; 40: 182–190
[53] Stewart CJ, Coldewey J, Stewart IS. Comparison of fine needle aspiration cytology and needle core biopsy in the diagnosis of radiologically detected abdominal lesions. J Clin Pathol 2002; 55: 93–97
[54] Buchbinder SS, Gurell DS, Tarlow MM, Salvatore M, Suhrland MJ, Kader K. Role of US-guided fine-needle aspiration with on-site cytopathologic evaluation in management of nonpalpable breast lesions. Acad Radiol 2001; 8: 322–327
[55] Pennes DR, Naylor B, Rebner M. Fine needle aspiration biopsy of the breast. Influence of the number of passes and the sample size on the diagnostic yield. Acta Cytol 1990; 34: 673–676
[56] Eisele DW, Sherman ME, Koch WM, Richtsmeier WJ, Wu AY, Erozan YS. Utility of immediate on-site cytopathological procurement and evaluation in fine needle aspiration biopsy of head and neck masses. Laryngoscope 1992; 102: 1328–1330
[57] Cleveland P, Gill KR, Coe SG et al. An evaluation of risk factors for inadequate cytology in EUS-guided FNA of pancreatic tumors and lymph nodes. Gastrointest Endosc 2010; 71: 1194–1199
[58] Erickson RA, Sayage-Rabie L, Beissner RS. Factors predicting the number of EUS-guided fine-needle passes for diagnosis of pancreatic malignancies. Gastrointest Endosc 2000; 51: 184–190
[59] Jhala NC, Eltoum IA, Eloubeidi MA et al. Providing on-site diagnosis of malignancy on endoscopic-ultrasound-guided fine-needle aspirates: should it be done? Ann Diagn Pathol 2007; 11: 176–181
[60] Klapman JB, Logrono R, Dye CE, Waxman I. Clinical impact of on-site cytopathology interpretation on endoscopic ultrasound-guided fine needle aspiration. Am J Gastroenterol 2003; 98: 1289–1294
[61] LeBlanc JK, Emerson RE, Dewitt J et al. A prospective study comparing rapid assessment of smears and ThinPrep for endoscopic ultrasound-guided fine-needle aspirates. Endoscopy 2010; 42: 389–394
[62] Turner BG, Cizginer S, Agarwal D, Yang J, Pitman MB, Brugge WR. Diagnosis of pancreatic neoplasia with EUS and FNA: a report of accuracy. Gastrointest Endosc 2010; 71: 91–98
[63] Iglesias-Garcia J, Dominguez-Munoz JE, Abdulkader I et al. Influence of on-site cytopathology evaluation on the diagnostic accuracy of endoscopic ultrasound-guided fine needle aspiration (EUS-FNA) of solid pancreatic masses. Am J Gastroenterol 2011; 106: 1705–1710
[64] Baram D, Garcia RB, Richman PS. Impact of rapid on-site cytologic evaluation during transbronchial needle aspiration. Chest 2005; 128: 869–875
[65] Cameron SE, Andrade RS, Pambuccian SE. Endobronchial ultrasound-guided transbronchial needle aspiration cytology: a state of the art review. Cytopathology 2010; 21: 6–26
[66] Trisolini R, Cancellieri A, Tinelli C et al. Rapid on-site evaluation of transbronchial aspirates in the diagnosis of hilar and mediastinal adenopathy: a randomized trial. Chest 2011; 139: 395–401
[67] Micames CG, McCrory DC, Pavey DA, Jowell PS, Gress FG. Endoscopic ultrasound-guided fine-needle aspiration for non-small cell lung cancer staging: a systematic review and metaanalysis. Chest 2007; 131: 539–548
[68] Layfield LJ, Bentz JS, Gopez EV. Immediate on-site interpretation of fine-needle aspiration smears: a cost and compensation analysis. Cancer 2001; 93: 319–322
[69] Alsharif M, Andrade RS, Groth SS, Stelow EB, Pambuccian SE. Endobronchial ultrasound-guided transbronchial fine-needle aspiration: the University of Minnesota experience, with emphasis on usefulness, adequacy assessment, and diagnostic difficulties. Am J Clin Pathol 2008; 130: 434–443
[70] Woon C, Bardales RH, Stanley MW, Stelow EB. Rapid assessment of fine needle aspiration and the final diagnosis—how often and why the diagnoses are changed. Cytojournal 2006; 3: 25
[71] Eloubeidi MA, Tamhane A, Jhala N et al. Agreement between rapid onsite and final cytologic interpretations of EUS-guided FNA specimens: implications for the endosonographer and patient management. Am J Gastroenterol 2006; 101: 2841–2847
[72] Monaco SE, Schuchert MJ, Khalbuss WE. Diagnostic difficulties and pitfalls in rapid on-site evaluation of endobronchial ultrasound guided fine needle aspiration. Cytojournal 2010; 7: 9
[73] Jhala NC, Jhala D, Eltoum I et al. Endoscopic ultrasound-guided fine-needle aspiration biopsy: a powerful tool to obtain samples from small lesions. Cancer 2004; 102: 239–246
[74] Lee HS, Lee GK, Lee HS et al. Real-time endobronchial ultrasound-guided transbronchial needle aspiration in mediastinal staging of non-small cell lung cancer: how many aspirations per target lymph node station? Chest 2008; 134: 368–374
[75] Pellisé Urquiza M, Fernández-Esparrach G, Solé M et al. Endoscopic ultrasound-guided fine needle aspiration: predictive factors of accurate diagnosis and cost-minimization analysis of on-site pathologist. Gastroenterol Hepatol 2007; 30: 319–324
[76] Sidiropoulos N, Dumont LJ, Golding AC, Quinlisk FL, Gonzalez JL, Padmanabhan V. Quality improvement by standardization of procurement and processing of thyroid fine-needle aspirates in the absence of on-site cytological evaluation. Thyroid 2009; 19: 1049–1052
[77] Ardengh JC, Lopes CV, de Lima LF et al. Cell block technique and cytological smears for the differential diagnosis of pancreatic neoplasms after endosonography-guided fine-needle aspiration. Acta Gastroenterol Latinoam 2008; 38: 246–251
[78] Khurana U, Handa U, Mohan H, Sachdev A. Evaluation of aspiration cytology of the liver space occupying lesions by simultaneous examination of smears and cell blocks. Diagn Cytopathol 2009; 37: 557–563
[79] Kopelman Y, Marmor S, Ashkenazi I, Fireman Z. Value of EUS-FNA cytological preparations compared with cell block sections in the diagnosis of pancreatic solid tumours. Cytopathology 2011; 22: 174–178
[80] Liu K, Dodge R, Glasgow BJ, Layfield LJ. Fine-needle aspiration: comparison of smear, cytospin, and cell block preparations in diagnostic and cost effectiveness. Diagn Cytopathol 1998; 19: 70–74
[81] Nassar A, Cohen C, Siddiqui MT. Utility of millipore filter and cell block in thyroid needle aspirates: which method is superior? Diagn Cytopathol 2007; 35: 34–38
[82] Nathan NA, Narayan E, Smith MM, Horn MJ. Cell block cytology. Improved preparation and its efficacy in diagnostic cytology. Am J Clin Pathol 2000; 114: 599–606
[83] Noda Y, Fujita N, Kobayashi G et al. Diagnostic efficacy of the cell block method in comparison with smear cytology of tissue samples obtained by endoscopic ultrasound-guided fine-needle aspiration. J Gastroenterol 2010; 45: 868–875
[84] Crothers BA, Tench WD, Schwartz MR et al. Guidelines for the reporting of nongynecologic cytopathology specimens. Arch Pathol Lab Med 2009; 133: 1743–1756
[85] Kocjan G, Chandra A, Cross P et al. BSCC Code of Practice—fine needle aspiration cytology. Cytopathology 2009; 20: 283–296
[86] Skoumal SM, Florell SR, Bydalek MK, Hunter WJ. Malpractice protection: communication of diagnostic uncertainty. Diagn Cytopathol 1996; 14: 385–389
[87] Baloch ZW, LiVolsi VA, Asa SL et al. Diagnostic terminology and morphologic criteria for cytologic diagnosis of thyroid lesions: a synopsis of the National Cancer Institute Thyroid Fine-Needle Aspiration State of the Science Conference. Diagn Cytopathol 2008; 36: 425–437
[88] Cibas ES, Ali SZ. The Bethesda System for Reporting Thyroid Cytopathology. Thyroid 2009; 19: 1159–1165
[89] The uniform approach to breast fine needle aspiration biopsy. A synopsis. Acta Cytol 1996; 40: 1120–1126, discussion 1119
[90] Böcking A. Standardization of cytopathologic diagnosis [Article in German]. Pathologe 1998; 19: 236–241

[91] The Papanicolaou Society of Cytopathology Task Force on Standards of Practice. Guidelines of the Papanicolaou Society of Cytopathology for fine-needle aspiration procedure and reporting. Diagn Cytopathol 1997; 17: 239–247

[92] Jenssen C, Möller K, Wagner S, Sarbia M. Endoscopic ultrasound-guided biopsy: diagnostic yield, pitfalls, quality management part 1: optimizing specimen collection and diagnostic efficiency [Article in German]. Z Gastroenterol 2008; 46: 590–600

[93] Jenssen C, Möller K, Wagner S, Sarbia M. Endoscopic ultrasound-guided biopsy: diagnostic yield, pitfalls, quality management [Article in German]. Z Gastroenterol 2008; 46: 897–908

[94] Gleeson FC, Kipp BR, Caudill JL et al. False positive endoscopic ultrasound fine needle aspiration cytology: incidence and risk factors. Gut 2010; 59: 586–593

[95] Young NA, Mody DR, Davey DD. Misinterpretation of normal cellular elements in fine-needle aspiration biopsy specimens: observations from the College of American Pathologists Interlaboratory Comparison Program in Non-Gynecologic Cytopathology. Arch Pathol Lab Med 2002; 126: 670–675

[96] Auger M, Moriarty AT, Laucirica R et al. Granulomatous inflammation–an underestimated cause of false-positive diagnoses in lung fine-needle aspirates: observations from the College of American Pathologists Nongynecologic Cytopathology Interlaboratory Comparison Program. Arch Pathol Lab Med 2010; 134: 1793–1796

[97] Hughes JH, Young NA, Wilbur DC, Renshaw AA, Mody DR; Cytopathology Resource Committee, College of American Pathologists. Fine-needle aspiration of pulmonary hamartoma: a common source of false-positive diagnoses in the College of American Pathologists Interlaboratory Comparison Program in Nongynecologic Cytology. Arch Pathol Lab Med 2005; 129: 19–22

[98] Hughes JH, Volk EE, Wilbur DC; Cytopathology Resource Committee, College of American Pathologists. Pitfalls in salivary gland fine-needle aspiration cytology: lessons from the College of American Pathologists Interlaboratory Comparison Program in Nongynecologic Cytology. Arch Pathol Lab Med 2005; 129: 26–31

[99] Abati A, Simsir A. Breast fine needle aspiration biopsy: prevailing recommendations and contemporary practices. Clin Lab Med 2005; 25: 631–654, v

[100] Civardi G, Fornari F, Cavanna L, Di Stasi M, Sbolli G, Buscarini L. Value of rapid staining and assessment of ultrasound-guided fine needle aspiration biopsies. Acta Cytol 1988; 32: 552–554

[101] Wallace MB, Kennedy T, Durkalski V et al. Randomized controlled trial of EUS-guided fine needle aspiration techniques for the detection of malignant lymphadenopathy. Gastrointest Endosc 2001; 54: 441–447

[102] LeBlanc JK, Ciaccia D, Al-Assi MT et al. Optimal number of EUS-guided fine needle passes needed to obtain a correct diagnosis. Gastrointest Endosc 2004; 59: 475–481

7 Infections and Diagnostic Microbiology

T. Glueck, H. J. Linde, C. F. Dietrich

7.1 General Principles of Microbiological Testing

7.1.1 Microbiological Specimens

Specimens for microbiological testing can be collected from numerous organs and tissues by an experienced examiner using ultrasound-guided aspiration and biopsy:

- Ascites
- Cyst fluid
- Abscess contents
- Pleural effusion
- Pericardial effusion
- Synovial fluid
- Liver tissue
- Renal tissue
- Lymph node tissue

7.1.2 Prerequisites for Microbiological Testing

Skin Preparation

When a specimen is collected by percutaneous needle aspiration, rigorous precautions should be taken to avoid transferring pathogens from the skin surface to deeper tissues and to ensure that the sample is not contaminated by skin flora. Skin preparation is essential, therefore. The antiseptic solutions most commonly used for this purpose are 10% PVP-iodine and alcohols. Alcohol-based solutions appear to be more effective than aqueous iodine solutions and mixtures of alcohols and iodine or chlorhexidine.[1,2] Skin preparation should include mechanical cleansing of the site by scrubbing with a sterile gauze pad. Hair-bearing skin should not be shaved before the puncture, since shaving causes tiny skin abrasions that predispose to local infection. Any hairs at the puncture site may be carefully clipped with a scissors, however. Recommendations on necessary exposure times to antiseptic solutions must be observed. Most experts recommend an exposure time of 60 to 180 seconds. However, skin areas rich in sebaceous glands (e.g., the groin) may require a longer exposure (up to 10 minutes) to achieve an adequate reduction of microorganisms.

Specimen Collection and Volume

It is good practice to collect as much material as possible so that there will be enough for chemical, cytological, and microbiological tests. Scanty specimen volumes can reduce sensitivity and increase sampling errors. ▶ Table 7.1 lists recommendations on minimum specimen volumes required for different diagnostic tests. These figures may vary somewhat from laboratory to laboratory, depending on the specific methods used. Communication with the microbiologist is advised, especially with scanty specimens, so that the best culture method can be used.

If tissue for pathologic examination is collected in addition to material for microbiological testing, meticulous care should be taken that the sample for microbiological testing does not come into contact with formalin solution, as that would preclude any further microbiologic analysis.

Specimen Submission to the Microbiology Laboratory

Before a specimen is sent for microbiological testing, it needs to be placed in a transport container that is appropriate for the specimen and the desired tests. The type of container depends on the expected transport time and presumptive organisms. If transport conditions are unfavorable, the culture result may be tainted by the destruction of delicate microbes and the overgrowth of more robust organisms.

If the specimen can be transported to the microbiology laboratory in less than 2 hours, it is generally sufficient to submit a fresh specimen in a sterile tube (e.g., in the aspiration syringe itself).

If transport time will exceed 2 hours, even with immediate submittal, a suitable transport medium must be used. Blood culture media are excellent for liquid specimens. In this case, however, additional fresh material should *always* be submitted so that microscopic preparations, possible antigen tests, cultures for mycobacteria or

Table 7.1 Specimen volumes required for various microbiological detection methods (approximate volumes needed per test)

Test	Absolute minimum volume	Ideal volume
Gram stain	0.2 mL	0.5 mL
Aerobic culture	0.2 mL	2 mL
Anaerobic culture	0.2 mL	2 mL
Fungal culture	0.2 mL	2 mL
Mycobacteria culture	3 mL	10 mL
Blood cultures[a]	2–10 mL	10 mL
Borrelia burgdorferi –PCR	2 mL	5 mL
PCR testing	0.2 mL	1 mL
Serology (blood)	3 mL	10 mL

[a] It is important to follow manufacturer's recommendations.

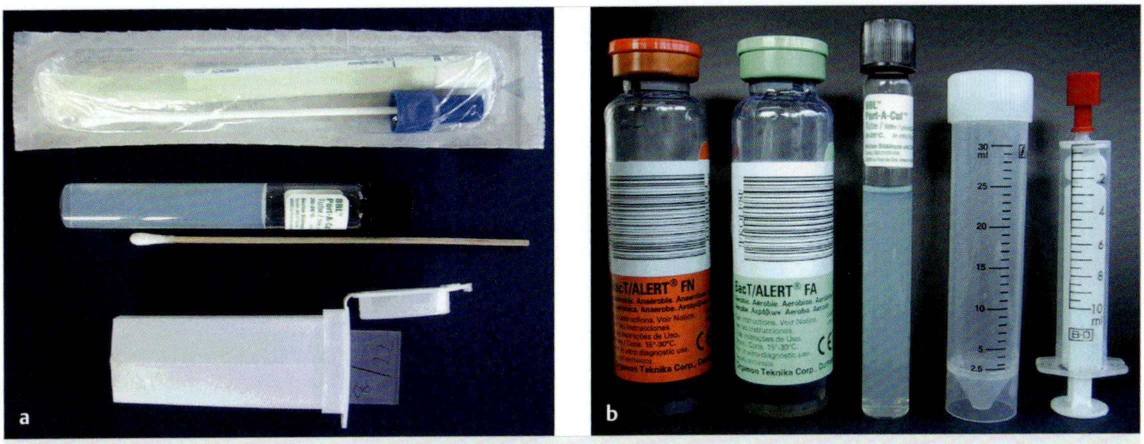

Fig. 7.1 Submission containers.
a Submission container for glass slides (bottom); transport container with semisolid prereduced transport medium (e.g., Port-A-Cul [Becton Dickinson]) (center); and swab kit with gel chamber (top).
b Containers for submitting liquid specimens (from left to right): two anaerobic/aerobic blood culture bottles, transport container with semisolid prereduced medium (e.g., Port-A-Cul), sterile tube, syringe with stopper.

fungi, and other special cultures can be grown. If the specimen were inoculated only into blood culture bottles, none of these tests could be performed; nor could a Gram stain be done to provide a plausibility check for culture results. Another option is to use a semisolid, prereduced transport medium (e.g., Port-A-Cul system, or similar). Microbiology laboratories will usually provide necessary submission supplies at no charge (▶ Fig. 7.1).

If there is clinical evidence that the lesion of interest has already given rise to a systemic infection, blood culture bottles (at least two pairs of aerobic and anaerobic) should also be submitted. With modern blood culture systems, care should be taken that the aerobic blood culture bottle is not "aerated" (risk of contamination). These systems provide optimum aerobic culture conditions with no need for additional measures. Transport to the microbiology laboratory should be as rapid as possible. If collected specimens cannot be submitted right away, blood cultures should be incubated at 35°C and all other materials stored at 4°C to prevent specimen contamination or overgrowth by fast-growing organisms.

Specimens must be labeled with the name of the patient, the sender, and specimen information and submitted to the laboratory with the proper request form. Information on the nature of the specimen along with clinical information and the presumed pathogen are essential so that the microbiologist can select the most appropriate culture techniques and detection methods.

Immediate Examination of Specimens

Macroscopic examination of the specimen should be done immediately after collection. If facilities are available, a portion of the specimen can be microscopically examined on-site by Gram staining a fresh sample. Gram staining (see below) can provide fast, valuable information on the causative organism(s), especially if the material cannot be sent to the microbiology laboratory right away.

7.2 Microbiological Techniques

7.2.1 Stains

Staining is the first step in microbiological testing. Stains can be performed in the microbiology laboratory immediately after specimen receipt or even on the ward and can provide an early source of valuable information. Stains supplement culture methods and often aid in their interpretation. This particularly applies to Gram staining. In addition, microscopic examination permits a semiquantitative assessment of the pathogen distribution in the specimen and an estimation of the degree of inflammatory response (WBC count in the specimen). Parasites (amebas, echinococci, etc.) can also be detected microscopically.

Gram Stain

The Gram stain is the most important stain in microbiology. It differentiates between gram-positive and gram-negative organisms owing to the fundamentally different cell wall structures of these two types of bacteria. Another advantage of the Gram stain is that it can be done quickly, even outside the microbiology laboratory.

The supplies necessary for Gram staining are illustrated in ▶ Fig. 7.2 and include the following:

- A microscope (× 10, × 40, × 100/oil)
- Glass slides
- Bunsen or gas burner
- Acetone or methyl alcohol
- Crystal violet 0.25%

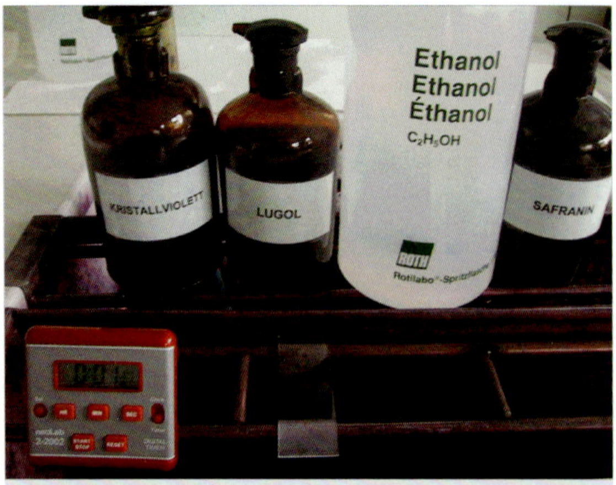

Fig. 7.2 Workstation with supplies for Gram staining.

- Lugol solution 1% (iodine and potassium iodide)
- 96% ethyl alcohol
- Safranin (fuchsin) 0.1%

For an outline of the Gram-staining procedure refer to ▶ Table 7.2 and ▶ Fig. 7.3. A Gram-stained preparation is illustrated in ▶ Fig. 7.4.

The most important gram-positive and gram-negative pathogens are listed in ▶ Table 7.3.

Table 7.2 Outline of the Gram staining procedure

Step in procedure	Action
1	Label the frosted end of the slide with a pencil.
2	Smear out the aspirated material (may dilute with sterile saline if necessary).
3	Air-dry the smear.
4	Fix: cover with acetone or concentrated methyl alcohol for 3 min or pass 3 times through the burner flame.
5	Cover with crystal violet for 1 min, pour off.
6	Cover with Lugol solution (iodine–potassium iodide), pour off.
7	Decolorize with 96% alcohol (until all blue is gone).
8	Rinse with water.
9	Cover with safranin.
10	Rinse off with water and dry.
Tips	Adequate decolorization is essential, so a thin smear is desired. Check: all body cells should stain red; blue staining means inadequate decolorization.
	The lower limit of detection is approximately 10^4 organisms/mL.

Ziehl–Neelsen Stain, Auramine Stain

Ziehl–Neelsen and auramine stains are used almost exclusively in microbiology laboratories for the detection of acid-fast rods (mycobacteria, *Nocardia* spp., *Actinomyces* spp.). Since bacterial counts in specimens are usually low, fluorescent stains (auramine stain, ▶ Fig. 7.5) are often used to increase the sensitivity of microbial detection (see the Box "Key Questions Relating to the Differential Diagnosis of Enlarged Lymph Nodes" (p. 73)).

Other fluorescent stains are available in the laboratory for the microscopic detection of microorganisms. These stains can reveal fungi or bacteria that are difficult to stain by other methods.

Detection of Parasites

Amebas and other parasites are on very rare occasions found in aspirates and are easily confused with leukocytes. It is important to inform the microbiologist of their suspected presence. On the other hand, serology is an

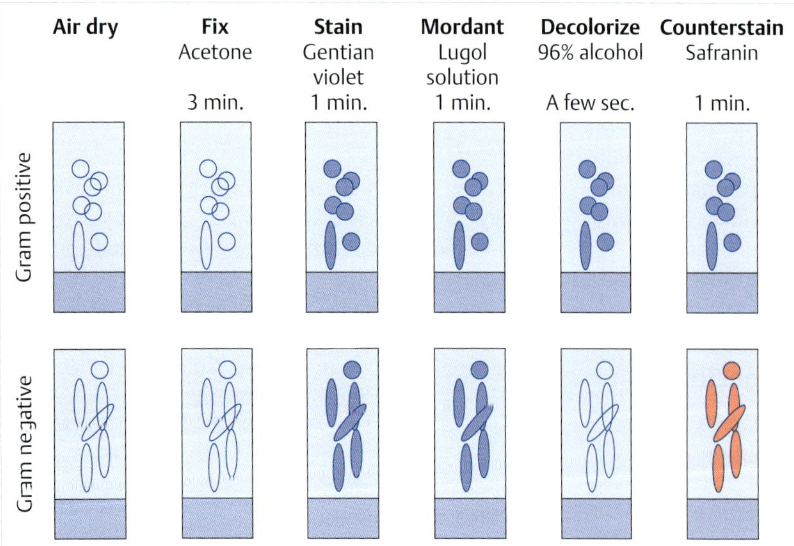

Fig. 7.3 Schematic representation of the Gram staining process.

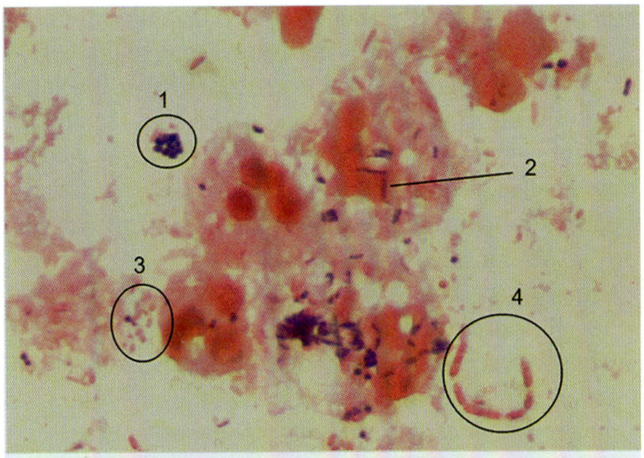

Fig. 7.4 Gram stain of abscess material with polymorphonuclear leukocytes in various stages of degeneration, gram-positive cocci (1), gram-positive rods (2), gram-negative cocci (3), and gram-negative rods (4) (× 1000 magnification).

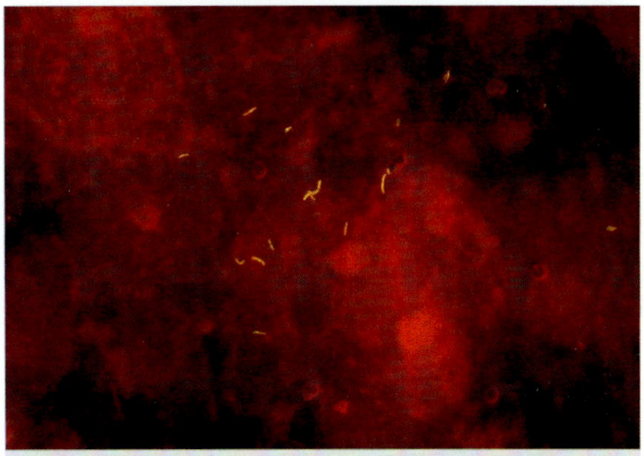

Fig. 7.5 Acid-fast rods in abscess material visualized by auramine staining.

important adjunct in patients with suspected parasitic diseases such as amebic liver abscess or hydatid liver disease, especially because needle aspiration of hydatid liver cysts should be avoided, as this could cause peritoneal seeding of worm larvae (protoscolices). Infections by *Echinococcus* spp. are detectable by serologic testing in almost all cases; only well-encapsulated cysts of *Echinococcus granulosus* (dog tapeworm) may be serologically negative in rare cases.

7.2.2 Culture Techniques

The isolation of microorganisms from invasively sampled materials is done under varying growth conditions on a combination of liquid and solid nutrient media. With fast-growing organisms, a preliminary differentiation can be made in just 24 hours. By 48 hours, it is generally possible to make a definitive identification and perform susceptibility testing in a bacterial isolate. In modern microbiology laboratories, this is usually done in fully automated incubators using standardized culture strips.

7.2.3 Nucleic Acid Amplification Techniques

Many specific and nonspecific nucleic acid amplification techniques are currently available to detect the DNA of microorganisms. Further differentiation is possible by sequencing of the amplification products. These techniques are particularly useful for detecting pathogens that are slow-growing or difficult to culture, such as viruses (DNA, RNA), and for the detection of pathogens in patients on antimicrobial therapy. Mycobacterial DNA is still detectable in tissue for years after the complete resolution of tuberculosis.

Specific assays are available for the *Mycobacterium tuberculosis* complex, for atypical mycobacteria, for *Aspergillus*, for *Rochalimaea*, for toxoplasmosis, and for many other pathogens, in specialized microbiology laboratories.

Bacterial 16S ribosomal DNA shows variable and highly conserved regions. Using primers that recognize the conserved regions, the variable sequences located beneath the highly conserved regions can be amplified, sequenced, compared with entries in gene banks, and then assigned to a particular species. The 16S rDNA assay is generally a highly sensitive procedure, but it may be compromised by nonspecifically inhibiting substances in the sample. The test is effective only for materials that are sterile under normal conditions but is still susceptible to contamination due to its high sensitivity. To date, nucleic acid amplification techniques for genotypic resistance analysis have been developed only for certain resistance mechanisms and only for a few organisms (e.g., MRSA). They have so far been unable to replace time-consuming culture methods.

Table 7.3 Most important gram-positive and gram-negative bacteria

Gram-positive cocci	Gram-positive rods	Gram-negative cocci	Gram-positive rods
Staphylococci	Clostridia	Neisseria spp.	Enterobacteriaceae
Enterococci	Cornybacteria	*Acinetobacter* spp.	*Pseudomonas* spp.
Streptococci	*Bacillus* spp.		*Bacteriodes* spp.

7.2.4 Serology

Serologic tests are of limited value for the detection of acute infections because a detectable antibody response appears only after a latent period of several days. Ordering serologic tests makes sense only if the result will have diagnostic or therapeutic implications. The confident serologic diagnosis of an infection generally requires drawing a second sample 1 to 2 weeks later that will show a significant rise in antibody titers. There are only a few serologies for which a single high IgG or IgM titer is diagnostic of an infection. Within the context of this book, these diseases include echinococcosis, amebiasis, schistosomiasis, hepatitis B/C, and HIV infection. Serologic analysis requires experience. Physicians should resist the indiscriminate ordering of serologic tests that are not appropriate for the disease in question. Another pitfall is the overinterpretation of positive IgM titers, especially if the titers are low. This is usually a nonspecific finding.

7.2.5 When Are Microbiological Test Results Available?

The turnaround time for issuing a final report on a microbiology sample is usually 48 hours for fast-growing organisms. Occasionally, however, even preliminary findings can help to optimize treatment and can be obtained simply by calling the laboratory. Average turnaround times are listed in ▸ Table 7.4. Exact times will vary depending on sample throughputs and laboratory organization.

7.2.6 Limitations of Microbiological Methods

The accuracy of microbiological testing depends directly on the desired scope of the tests before the sample is submitted. It should be emphasized that *Mycobacterium tuberculosis*, for example, would be missed in a sample submitted for testing for "pyogenic organisms" or the "presence of organisms" even if the sample contained massive numbers of the mycobacteria. It is essential, therefore, to *request tests that are consistent with clinical information*. A specific request is also helpful for limiting costs. In equivocal cases, it is advantageous to discuss the scope of the tests with the microbiologist or the infectious disease specialist. Moreover, the test results will depend in large measure on the quality of the material that is collected and submitted for analysis.

Table 7.4 Average turnaround times for microbiology requests

Result within:	Tests
1–3 hours	Gram stain, antigen detection, specific PCR (e.g., LightCycler [Roche Applied Science])
3–5 hours	Detection of acid-fast rods, other special stains
24 hours	Preliminary differentiation of fast-growing bacteria. Result of antimicrobial susceptibility testing done directly from patient samples (e.g., positive microscopic findings). Growth in blood cultures (yes/no, Gram stain)
48 hours	Differentiation and susceptibility testing of fast-growing aerobic organisms
>72 hours	Differentiation of anaerobes
Approximately 14 days	Mycobacteria in liquid culture, rapidly growing atypical mycobacteria (MOTT, NTM[a])
4–6 weeks	Mycobacteria in solid culture, slow-growing organisms

[a] *MOTT*, mycobacteria other than tuberculosis. *NTM*, nontuberculous mycobacteria.

Common reasons for unsatisfactory microbiological test results include the following.

- Sampling error due to an inadequate specimen volume
- Sampling error due to low bacterial counts
- Slow or delayed transport, improper transport container, failure to culture fastidious pathogens (e.g., anaerobes) due to overgrowth of other organisms
- Detection of ubiquitous organisms, typical (skin) commensals or contamination (e.g., coagulase-negative staphylococci, corynebacteria, etc.), especially when determined in liquid culture media, blood cultures or PCR assays, since only a few organisms are sufficient to produce a positive result in these procedures. The significance of detecting these organisms must be questioned, especially when they do not match the clinical information and/or the Gram stain result. A Gram stain that matches the isolated organism, or the repeated detection of one of these organisms, is less suggestive of contamination and is more consistent with an infecting organism.
- Previous antimicrobial therapy
- In purulent materials (i.e., materials containing large numbers of white cells), the antimicrobial substances released from degenerating granulocytes may produce false-negative culture results. Consequently, purulent materials should always be diluted in transport media (e.g. in blood culture bottles) when submitted for testing.
- Inadequate request or unreasonable expectation for microbiological testing, such as the growth of mycobacteria in ordinary blood culture bottles, the growth of parasites in a bacterial culture, and so on
- Expecting culture results within a few hours
- Nonculturable organisms (e.g., parasites)

7.2.7 Specimen Receipt during Off-hours (Nights, Weekends, Holidays)

Not infrequently, material for microbiological testing is received outside of normal working hours. In this case the sample should be stored under the most favorable conditions available to ensure that optimal microbiological testing can be performed at a later time. It should be noted that the overgrowth of one or more organisms may occur over time in a specimen with polymicrobial flora, with the result that the actual pathogen is no longer detectable. This can be avoided by refrigerating the sample, although this will limit the detection of very cold-sensitive organisms such as pneumococci. Liquid materials should therefore be divided into separate portions if a sufficient volume of material is available. A portion of the material can then be refrigerated for Gram staining, classic cultures, and possible examination for parasites, viruses, or mycobacteria. Another portion of the sample should be inoculated into blood culture bottles (aerobic and anaerobic) and immediately incubated at 35°C. The preincubation should be reported to the microbiology laboratory that will be performing the tests.

7.3 Specific Guidelines for Microbiological Testing and Differential Diagnosis by Organ Systems and Syndromes

Detailed microbiological testing is an important basis for providing rational antimicrobial therapy. With an acute or life-threatening infection, it is mandatory to initiate antibiotic therapy with a reasonably broad spectrum on an empirical basis instead of waiting 24 to 48 hours for microbiological results. When the results are reported, it will often be possible to change from the initial empirical broad-spectrum therapy to an agent with a narrower antimicrobial spectrum that will be more effective and will usually reduce costs. Thus, the therapeutic recommendations given in this chapter for some selected situations are intended only as guidelines for initiating empirical therapy. They should always be checked and modified on the basis of the results of microbiological testing.

7.3.1 Investigation of Enlarged Lymph Nodes

The investigation of lymph node enlargement is aimed at determining whether the enlargement is due to reactive inflammatory changes or neoplasia, i.e., primary lymph node neoplasms (non-Hodgkin or Hodgkin lymphoma) or metastases from solid tumors. The differential diagnosis is based on a combined assessment of clinical, microbiological, and histological findings.

In the investigation of lymphadenopathy, the key questions listed in the Key Questions box should be answered before any invasive tests are performed. As a general rule, any lymph node enlargement that persists longer than 3 weeks, even with antibiotic therapy, and has no other apparent explanation requires further investigation, which may include histology.

The differential diagnosis of infectious causes (see the box below) should also include less common pathogens such as HIV, *Toxoplasma*, *Brucella* and mycobacteria, particularly in children, migrants, and groups with special exposure (farmers, hunters).

Key Questions Relating to the Differential Diagnosis of Enlarged Lymph Nodes

- Age of the patient (significant differences between children and adults)
- Is the enlargement definitely abnormal? (depends on age, site)
- Watch for "age-typical" lymph nodes: size < 1 cm (< 1.5–2 cm at the mandibular angle); lymph nodes usually soft, movable; usually not tender or painful, no inflammatory reaction; typical sites (cervical), preschool and school-age children
- Is the lymph node swelling progressive over time? Any significant lymph node enlargement lasting more than 2 to 6 weeks requires a histologic diagnosis.
- Where are the enlarged lymph nodes located? Inguinal and cervical lymphadenopathy are often reactive. Clavicular, para-aortic, and iliac lymphadenopathy are suspicious for malignancy.
- Is there evidence of an infectious cause? Cardinal feature: painful lymph node enlargement, especially in children with "age-typical" (postinfectious) lymphadenopathy.
- Is there reason to suspect a malignant cause? Cardinal features: painless lymphadenopathy, weight loss, malignancy elsewhere in the body.
- Are there any associated suggestive clinical findings (splenomegaly, etc.)?
- Iatrogenic conditions: immunosuppression (e.g. post-transplant lymphopoliferative disease [PTLD]) or other significant immunosuppression, medications (e.g., phenytoin, allopurinol, hydralazine, procainamide, isoniazid, dapsone)?

Differential Diagnosis of Infectious Causes of Lymph Node Enlargement

- Look for local portals of entry (nasopharynx, tonsils, any type of skin lesion).
- Systemic disease (e.g., mononucleosis, cytomegalovirus infection, all childhood diseases such as mumps and rubella)?
- Is there any process involving an organ in the region drained by the affected node?
- Travel history?
- Food history: unpasteurized milk? foreign "specialities"? "raw" foods?
- Animal contact: bites? scratched skin? contact with animal saliva?

Further diagnostic actions are directed by noting "age-typical" lymph nodes, associated clinical findings, and necessary laboratory tests (▶ Table 7.5, ▶ Table 7.6, ▶ Table 7.7).

Table 7.5 Suggestive clinical findings and typical circumstances associated with enlarged lymph nodes

Associated clinical finding: Lymphadenopathy and...	Suggestive of:
Pustule or erythema in region drained by enlarged lymph node	Bacterial lymphangitis Cat-scratch disease (contact with cat saliva?)
Cutaneous manifestations	Many bacterial and viral infections Also: fungal infections, systemic lupus erythematosus (SLE), dermatomyositis
Recurrent skin infections	Immunodeficiency, hyper-IgE syndrome Colonization with Panton–Valentine leukocidin-producing *Staphylococcus aureus* strains
Skin rash, lip rhagades, fever in children	Kawasaki syndrome
History and possible associated atopic dermatitis	Allergies
History of tick bite, erythema migrans	Lyme disease
Joint swelling, bone and soft-tissue pain	Rheumatic diseases, reactive arthritis, septic arthritis Leukemia
Enteritis and joint swelling	Infection by *Yersinia*, *Campylobacter* (reactive arthritis)
Enlarged inguinal lymph nodes	Sexually transmitted diseases (gonorrhea, chlamydia, *Haemophilus ducreyi*) Look for associated symptoms with joint pain, conjunctivitis, arthropathy (Reiter syndrome)! Infections involving the lower limb or perineum
Very pronounced lymph node swelling	Lymphoproliferative diseases Rosai–Dorfman disease (= sinus histiocytosis with massive lymphadenopathy)
Splenomegaly and neurologic symptoms	Storage diseases
Enlarged, grayish-yellow tonsils, with or without lymph node enlargement	Tangier disease

Table 7.6 Recommended diagnostic studies

Type of lymphadenopathy	Primary tests, serology	Comments
Solitary or circumscribed lymphadenopathy	Microscopy, differential blood count, ESR, CRP, LDH Optional: uric acid, creatinine, urea Toxoplasmosis serology Abdominal ultrasound Head and neck ultrasound Axillary and inguinal ultrasound Chest radiograph With history or clinical indicators: • Serology for HIV, hepatitis B/C, *Borrelia burgdorferi* • If indicated: TB testing, TB interferon release assay and/or organ-specific TB tests	Lymph node biopsy or lymphadenectomy indicated after exclusion of inflammatory cause or with high likelihood of metastasis from a known (or presumed) primary tumor Lymphoma diagnosis requires complete excision of a suspicious lymph node
Cervical lymphadenopathy	Toxoplasmosis serology is mandatory	Look for infectious foci in the head and neck region, teeth, and paranasal sinuses In children: atypical mycobacteria; consider sarcoidosis or lymphoma
Mediastinal lymphadenopathy	TB testing is mandatory! Transesophageal and transbronchial endosonography! Sarcoidosis parameters, evaluation for lymphoma (differential blood smear)	Look for bacterial infections. TB is a particularly common cause of mediastinal lymphadenopathy
Axillary lymphadenopathy		Look for infectious foci in the upper limb and breast Differential diagnosis: breast malignancy

Table 7.6 (continued) Recommended diagnostic studies

Type of lymphadenopathy	Primary tests, serology	Comments
Abdominal lymphadenopathy	Serology for HBV, HCV in patients with enlarged portal lymph nodes *Yersinia* testing (culture and serology) in patients with enlarged mesenteric nodes and Peyer plaques in terminal ileum	Consider abdominal TB and/or atypical mycobacteria (in migrants may coexist with HIV)
Inguinal lymphadenopathy	TPHA, VDRL serology *Chlamydia trachomatis* Genital smear if indicated (*Chlamydia* PCR, culture or PCR for gonococci)	Look for infectious foci in the lower limb and perineum Sexually transmitted diseases
Multifocal lymphadenopathy, with possible associated splenomegaly	EBV, CMV and HIV serology Test for lymphoma! Consider Rosai–Dorfmann disease	

Abbreviations: CMV, cytomegalovirus; CRP, C-reactive protein; EBV, Epstein–Barr virus; HIV human immunodeficiency virus; LDH, lactate dehydrogenase; TB, tuberculosis; TPHA, Treponema pallidum hemagglutination; VDRL, Venereal Disease Research Laboratory (test for syphilis).

Table 7.7 Value of serology and other microbiological tests in the investigation of lymphadenopathy (taking into account the history, clinical findings, and possible splenomegaly)

Test	Comments
HIV test	Mandatory for unexplained multifocal lymphadenopathy
Toxoplasmosis serology	Unexplained lymphadenopathy with isolated cervical involvement
EBV serology	Unexplained lymphadenopathy with severe malaise, tonsillitis, and splenomegaly The mononucleosis rapid test (Paul–Bunnel test) is nonspecific and not very sensitive; better to perform complete EBV serology Positive anti-EBV IgM indicates an acute infection. Reactivation may produce low IgM titers Positive anti-EBV-EBNA-1 indicates a past infection and immunity and is not an adequate explanation for lymph node enlargement Frequently coexisting hepatitis
CMV serology	Acute, severe malaise and splenomegaly
Serologies for HAV, HBV, HCV, HEV, and possibly HDV	Patients with portal lymphadenopathy Quantitative assay of viral concentrations in the blood Check for multiple extrahepatic manifestations of hepatitis C and B infection
Bartonella henselae serology	Cat exposure (scratching or licking → history?) Bartonellosis takes a severe, atypical course in immunosuppressed patients (cutaneous manifestations!) Bartonella DNA in lymph nodes detectable by PCR. Pathogen demonstrable by Warthin–Starry stain
Rubella serology	Typical skin rash with small pink spots in children; typical retroauricular lymphadenitis Caution: infection during pregnancy
Measles serology	Look for coexisting, confluent exanthema and enanthema(!)
Parvovirus B19 serology	Characteristic “slapped cheek” rash Possible diffuse lymphadenopathy
Anti-streptolysin titers	In patients with (past/recurrent) tonsillitis to detect immune reaction to group A β-hemolytic streptococci. May be important in the differential diagnosis of cervical lymphadenopathy when antibiotic therapy has already been initiated For other lymph node sites in patients with (recurrent) erysipelas
Brucellosis serology	Patients suffering from brucellosis may have varying degrees of lymph node enlargement and splenomegaly With suspected brucellosis, a detailed travel and food history should be taken (unpasteurized milk products?)

(Continued on next page.)

Table 7.7 (continued) Value of serology and other microbiological tests in the investigation of lymphadenopathy

Test	Comments
Borrelia serology	Check for erythema migrans with possible associated lymphadenopathy
Tularemia (rabbit fever) serology	Suppurative lymphadenopathy (differential diagnosis: bartonellosis!), patients usually severely ill. Very rare disease, largely limited to groups at risk (hunters, farmers, butchers)
Chlamydia serology (*Chlamydia trachomatis*)	Inguinal lymphadenopathy. Genital symptoms are often absent. Possible cross reactivity with respiratory chlamydia, depending on test Smear for PCR testing is preferred
Gonococcal serology (*Neisseria gonorrhoeae*)	Inguinal lymphadenopathy. Patients may have no genital symptoms. Smear for PCR testing (combined with chlamydia PCR)
Syphilis serology (*Treponema pallidum*)	TPHA screening test FTA-ABS IgM and VDRL tests for active infection
Yersinia serology	Included in tests for intestinal pathogens in patients with GI infections. Serology positive only about 2 weeks after symptom onset, by which time stool cultures are usually negative
Tests for tuberculosis	Mendel–Mantoux skin test with 2–5 IU of PPD, very nonspecific Interferon release TB tests (QuantiFERON-TB Gold test, ELISPOT test) are more specific but do not differentiate between latent and active TB (see text for details)
Atypical mycobacteria	Cause lymph node swelling/lymphadenitis only in children or immunosuppressed patients Diagnosed by PCR in biopsy/abscess material, culture may be tried. Serology not available
Actinomycosis	Serology not available. May try culture or PCR after consulting with microbiologist (specific request!)
Fungi: • Histoplasmosis • Blastomycosis • Coccidioidomycosis	Specific serologies are available. Obtain travel history!
Parasites: • *Leishmania* • Trypanosomes • Microfilariae	Specific serologies are available. Obtain travel history!
Bacterial smears from lymph nodes or skin lesions, possible blood cultures	Suspected bacterial infection

Abbreviations: HAV, HBV, HCV, HDV, HEV, hepatitis A,B, C, D, E virus; PPD, purified protein derivative (of tuberculin); and see ▸ Table 7.6.

Circumscribed lymph node enlargement in one region should also prompt ultrasound imaging of the abdomen, head and neck region, axillae, and groin.

Further work-up should include a differential blood count, LDH, CRP, and ESR with optional testing of uric acid, creatinine, and urea. Serologies for *Borrelia burgdorferi*, toxoplasmosis, HIV, hepatitis B/C, etc. may be appropriate, depending on clinical findings. Suspected mycobacterial infection should be investigated by obtaining a chest radiograph, sputum culture, and interferon release assay for detection of tuberculosis (e.g., QuantiFERON-TB Gold blood test [Cellestis Ltd]).

If these tests are not diagnostic, other entities should be considered: lymphoma, sarcoidosis, infection with an atypical presentation, and infections by rare pathogens.

If lymph node enlargement is progressive over time, a suspicious node should be extirpated *in toto* for histologic, immunohistologic, and microbiological testing (culture, PCR) to establish a definitive diagnosis.

7.3.2 Microbiological Testing and Antimicrobial Therapy for Suspected Tuberculosis

Tuberculosis (TB) is one of the most common infectious diseases in the world. It has become more prevalent also in industrialized countries in recent years as a result of growing immigration. A special problem is posed by the rising incidence of drug-resistant mycobacteria, with geographically variable resistance rates. Because TB often presents with nonspecific symptoms but may take a severe course, it should always be considered in the investigation of enlarged lymph nodes, intra-abdominal masses, and abscesses. In addition to the specific examination of lymph node biopsies and aspirated abscess contents by staining, PCR for *Mycobacterium tuberculosis* complex, and mycobacterial culture, every such patient should also be tested for pulmonary TB.

With the recent availability of the tuberculosis PCR assay, the diagnosis of TB can be established within 24 hours. The sensitivity of PCR is higher than that of microscopy and ranges from 60 to 90% even in microscopically negative cases.[3] Specific PCR tests can also be used to investigate a suspected infection with nontuberculous mycobacteria (NTM, MOTT). The clinical suspicion of these "atypical mycobacteria" must be explicitly reported to the microbiologist, however, because the *M. tuberculosis*-complex-specific primers used for a generic request of "TB PCR" would not be able to detect atypical mycobacteria.

The culture detection of mycobacteria requires parallel cultures on solid nutrient media and in liquid media. A positive culture requires bacterial counts of 10^2 to 10^3 per mL on solid media and 10^1 to 10^2 per mL in liquid media.[4] If culture detection is unsuccessful because there are too few bacteria in the sample, the histopathologic examination of caseating granulomas combined with a positive interferon gamma release test can rule in TB.

The interferon gamma release test has largely replaced the classic Mendel–Mantoux skin test in recent years. It is an in-vitro assay that measures the production of TB-antigen-specific interferon gamma by peripheral blood mononuclear cells within 24 hours after antigen contact. This is done in either an ELISA (QuantiFERON-TB Gold test) or ELISPOT assay (T-SPOT-TB [Oxford Immunotec]). The interferon gamma test has a sensitivity of 76 to 100% for the diagnosis of tuberculosis. It has a higher specificity than the Mendel–Mantoux test. Active TB is diagnosed in most cases by a combination of history, radiologic findings, interferon gamma release test, and microbiological results (microscopy/culture, also PCR from sputum or other materials, possibly including samples acquired by invasive techniques).

Recommended Treatment

After an adequate number of specimens have been collected for TB cultures (3 × sputum, urine, possible aspirate), a four-drug regimen is currently used for the initial treatment of tuberculosis. This regimen generally consists of rifampin at a dose of 10 mg/kg (typically 600 mg, once daily oral or IV), isoniazid at 5 mg/kg (typically 300 mg, once daily oral or IV) combined with vitamin B_6 (50–100 mg once daily oral or IV), ethambutol at 20 mg/kg (typically 1200 mg, once daily oral or IV), and pyrazinamide at 30 mg/kg (typically 1500–2000 mg, once daily oral). The treatment regimen may have to be modified based on culture sensitivity testing.

7.3.3 Liver Mass Suspicious for an Abscess (Including Amebic Abscess)

Cystic liver masses in febrile patients are always suspicious for an abscess. Liver abscesses are caused by hematogenous spread via the portal vein, and the spectrum of causative organisms includes aerobic/anaerobic and gram-positive/gram-negative intestinal flora. Mixed infections are common.

Amebic liver abscess also results ultimately from the hematogenous spread of an intestinal amoebic infection that may produce few symptoms and may have been acquired months earlier. By the time the amoebic liver abscess is manifested, the intestinal symptoms of amebiasis are generally long past. For this reason, a detailed travel history should be taken to determine the possible cause of a liver abscess. The differential diagnosis of cystic liver masses should also include echinococcal cysts, but these lesions cause fewer acute complaints than a bacterial or amoebic liver abscess. Echinococcosis of the liver is discussed in Chapter 17.

Bacterial Liver Abscess

Diagnosis

The contents of a bacterial abscess usually have a liquid to creamy consistency and are often foul-smelling when the flora includes anaerobes. Material collected by needle aspiration should be sent for Gram staining and culturing for pyogenic organisms and anaerobes. Suitable transport media are aerobic/anaerobic blood culture bottles or special transport tubes that are favorable for anaerobes.

Treatment

The empirical antibiotic treatment of a bacterial liver abscess should cover the main intestinal organisms and should also have anaerobic efficacy. Empirical agents may consist of an aminopenicillin/β-lactamase inhibitor combination (ampicillin/sulbactam, 3 g IV three times a day or ampicillin/clavulanic acid, 2.2 g IV three times a day), for example, or a fluoroquinolone such as ciprofloxacin (400 mg IV twice a day or 500 mg oral twice a day) plus metronidazole (400–500 mg oral three times a day or 500 mg IV three times a day). Severe cases can be treated with an ureidopenicillin/β-lactamase inhibitor combination (piperacillin/tazobactam, 4.5 g IV three times a day), for example. An important element of treatment is drainage of the abscess, which will usually lead to prompt clinical improvement.

Amebic Liver Abscess

Diagnosis

Amebic abscesses typically contain a chocolate-colored material with a somewhat viscous consistency. The microscopic detection of amebas in aspirate is successful in less than 20% of cases because these organisms are found almost exclusively in the peripheral part of the abscess. The diagnosis of amebic abscess is aided greatly by the macroscopic appearance of the aspirated fluid and the patient's travel history, which should be sufficient to make a presumptive diagnosis and start empirical therapy. Chemical laboratory tests usually show a nonspecific inflammatory response with leukocytosis, elevated ESR and CRP, and frequent elevation of alkaline phosphatase (AP) or transaminases. Eosinophilia is usually not present.

The definitive diagnosis of an amebic causation is typically based on the detection of amebas in the stool. The **stool antigen test** has proven superior to microscopic identification, with a sensitivity of 94% versus 37% and specificity of 94% versus 99%. The diagnosis can also be made serologically. Positive titers can be demonstrated in 92 to 97% of patients but do not necessarily signify acute disease.

Treatment

The agent of choice for the treatment of amebic liver abscess is metronidazole (400–500 mg three times a day; children 35–50 mg/kg BW) administered IV or orally for 10 days. An alternative to metronidazole is tetracycline 250 mg four times a day orally for 10 days). Dehydroemetine (1.5 mg/kg BW [maximum of 90 mg]) or emetine (1 mg/kg BW [maximum of 60 mg] daily) and chloroquine phosphate (500 mg [= 600 mg base] twice a day orally for 2 days, followed by 250 mg twice a day orally for 2 weeks) may also be used but are less well tolerated.

Because the above therapeutic agents will not definitely eradicate the luminal forms of amebas in the bowel, the treatment regimen should conclude with an intraluminal agent that can kill cysts still present in the bowel and prevent a recurrence. This can be accomplished with either nonabsorbable paromomycin (500 mg three times a day orally for 10 days) or diloxanide furoate (500 mg three times a day, or 20 mg/kg BW in children) taken for 10 days.

Unlike pyogenic liver abscesses, amebic abscesses will generally show excellent response to pharmacologic therapy alone without drainage, although the amebic abscess will usually not resolve completely by the end of medical therapy. This is no reason to prolong treatment, and residual abscess will generally be reabsorbed within a few weeks. Therapeutic response is assessed clinically and sonographically. Only large amebic liver abscesses require puncture and drainage of the "anchovy-like" fluid contents to reduce the size of the abscess and expedite healing. Surgical treatment is indicated only in exceptional cases.

Pleural Effusion

Pleural effusion may be caused by a primary infectious process or by infection spreading from the lung. The most common pathogens isolated from pleural effusion are gram-positive organisms such as pneumococci, streptococci, and staphylococci, although virtually any bacterial lung infection including legionnaires' disease may incite a pleural inflammation.

Tuberculous pleurisy is a characteristic manifestation of TB, and any pleural effusion that is not otherwise explained should be considered suspicious for TB. Not infrequently, however, the causative organism can be identified in a fresh specimen. The failure to detect pathogens in stains or bacterial cultures is in itself suspicious for a mycobacterial infection when exudate is present.

The differential diagnosis should include rare pathogens such as *Nocardia* and *Actinomyces* as well as noninfectious diseases that are associated with pleural exudate such as tumors and severe congestive heart failure.

Diagnosis

An infectious cause is suggested by a white blood count > 5×10^9/L (5000/µL) and a protein content > 25 g/L (2.5 g/dL) in aspirated fluid. A bacterial infection is typically associated with a very purulent exudate (pleural empyema), which consists on cytologic examination almost entirely of neutrophils. Before antibiotic therapy is initiated, pleural fluid should always be submitted for microbiological testing (Gram stain, culture for pyogenic organisms; anaerobic cultures may generally be omitted). The very specific determination of *Legionella* antigen in the urine may be helpful depending on the lung findings, "season," and travel history.

The pleural exudate in tuberculous pleurisy displays a high protein content and moderately high cellularity. Mononuclear cells are abundant in addition to granulocytes. The Ziehl–Neelsen stain for mycobacteria from pleural aspirate has low sensitivity for pathogen identification. PCR from pleural aspirate has better sensitivity for diagnosing tuberculous pleurisy, generally providing > 80% sensitivity and specificity. An interferon gamma assay in pleural aspirate is also considered sensitive and specific for TB and has proved useful, although the test is not approved for this application.

It should be added that it is unnecessary to perform microbiological tests on every pleural aspirate if there is no clinical or other evidence of an infectious or inflammatory process (e.g., pleural effusion in patients with congestive heart failure). The diagnostic value of microbiological testing in these cases is extremely low.[8]

Treatment

If there is clinical evidence of a pleural infection arising from a pulmonary process, cephalosporins (cefazolin,

2 g IV three times a day or cefuroxime, 1.5 g IV three times a day, for example) can be used in conjunction with a macrolide (clarithromycin, 500 mg IV or orally twice a day), unless the infection is a nosocomial process or there is known colonization by a multidrug-resistant organism such as MRSA. This should be considered when selecting the antibiotic regimen.

Pericardial Effusion

Infections of the pericardium and/or myocardium present with nonspecific symptoms in the early stage. Echocardiography is important in its ability to detect small amounts of pericardial effusion and even mild systolic dysfunction that may indicate myocarditis. The etiologic differential diagnosis is broad and should include viruses (e.g., coxsackievirus or other enteroviruses), Lyme disease (which typically causes conduction disorders, e.g., heart blocks) or mycobacterial or classic bacterial pathogens similar to those found in pleurisy. Tuberculous pericarditis was once considered a common manifestation of TB but has rarely been diagnosed in Central Europe and North America during recent years (most commonly in migrants).

Infectious pericarditis or myocarditis with pericardial effusion always requires differentiation from malignant and autoimmune processes. Pericarditis with effusion may be an isolated manifestation or may occur in the setting of polyserositis, in connective tissue diseases, vasculitis, or sarcoidosis (rarely in rheumatoid arthritis).

Diagnosis

In many cases, large pericardial effusions are managed not only by needle aspiration but also by the temporary placement of a pericardial drain. Cell counts and cell differentiation are determined in the pericardial aspirate, which should also be evaluated by clinical chemistry for LDH, cholesterol, and total protein. A cytologic examination is advisable in most cases. Purulent pericardial aspirate should be submitted for microbiological testing, similarly to pleural effusions, and blood culture bottles are highly suitable for this purpose. A tube of fresh aspirate should also be submitted for Gram staining. Microbiological testing for mycobacteria (stain, PCR, and culture) should also be considered. Specific PCRs and serologies are available for diagnosis of viruses and Lyme disease (very rare causes of pericardial effusion!). High IgM titers in the serologic tests for these pathogens are suggestive for a role in the pathogenesis of pericarditis. A marked rise in titers in follow-up serologic tests will confirm the diagnosis.

Treatment

Causal treatment is not available for viral pericarditis and myocarditis; physical rest and supportive measures are recommended.

The empirical treatment for a purulent pericardial effusion should employ broad-spectrum antibiotics with staphylococcal activity, such as cephalosporins (cefuroxime, 1.5 g IV three times a day or ceftriaxone, 2 g IV once a day) or a ureidopenicillin/β-lactamase inhibitor combination such as piperacillin/tazobactam (4.5 g IV three times a day). Any therapy that has been initiated empirically should be adjusted based on culture results. It is recommended that treatment be continued for at least 2 to 3 weeks.

Ceftriaxone would be the agent of choice for the treatment of very rare Lyme pericarditis or myocarditis with pericardial effusion.

The treatment of tuberculosis follows the principles of antituberculous combination therapy outlined above.

Ascites, Peritonitis

The etiology of ascites has a broad differential diagnosis. Bacterial, mycobacterial, or fungal infections of the abdominal cavity with ascites formation are classified as follows:

- **Primary peritonitis** (without a hollow viscus perforation):
  - Spontaneous bacterial peritonitis in patients with liver cirrhosis
  - Tuberculous peritonitis
  - Peritoneal dialysis-related infections
  - Ascending genital infections in females
- Secondary peritonitis
  - Peritonitis due to a hollow viscus perforation in the abdomen
  - Peritonitis from an infectious process in an abdominal organ
- Tertiary peritonitis
  - Sequel to secondary peritonitis, e.g., due to anastomosis leakage, generally with accompanying sepsis

Additionally, there are a number of noninfectious abdominal processes with associated ascites formation, most notably hepatic cirrhosis or other causes of portal hypertension (e.g., portal vein thrombosis), severe congestive heart failure, peritoneal carcinomatosis due to an intraperitoneal malignancy, and finally rare causes such as autoinflammatory diseases with polyserositis or familial Mediterranean fever.

Diagnosis

Cell counts are important in the evaluation of ascites. The presence of $> 0.25 \times 10^9$ neutrophilic granulocytes per liter of ascites (250/µL) (helpful but less precise: $> 0.5 \times 10^9$ WBC/L [500/µL]) indicates an ascitic fluid infection. Measurement of the protein content, on the other hand, is less important in distinguishing between sterile and infected ascites. Glucose and LDH are helpful in distinguishing spontaneous bacterial peritonitis from secondary peritonitis. In secondary peritonitis, glucose is usually well below 2.77 mmol/L (50 mg/dL) and LDH is usually elevated to well above 3.76 µkat/L (225 U/L). Cholesterol values > 1.17 mmol/L (45 mg/dL) increase the likelihood that the ascites has a malignant cause. This is determined by cytologic examination of the ascites for malignant cells and by measuring carcinoembryonic antigen (CEA).

For microbiological testing of a suspected ascitic fluid infection, aspirated fluid should be transferred immediately after collection (at bedside) to paired aerobic/anaerobic blood culture bottles. Additionally, a fresh sample should be submitted in a sterile tube for Gram staining and optional special tests (e.g., PCRs). The pathogen density in spontaneous bacterial peritonitis is only about 1 organism/mL: that is why Gram stain results are generally negative. Moreover, 90% of spontaneous bacterial peritonitis cases involve an infection with only one organism. A positive Gram stain and the detection of more than one bacterial species are suspicious for secondary peritonitis.

Treatment

Spontaneous bacterial peritonitis is most commonly treated with a group 3a cephalosporin such as cefotaxime (2 g IV three times a day) or ceftriaxone (2 g IV once a day). Enterobacteriaceae (e.g., *Escherichia coli*) are the most common pathogens in this situation and current resistance rates of these pathogens to ciprofloxacin and aminopenicillin/β-lactamase inhibitor combinations are significantly higher than to group 3a cephalosporins. The former drugs can therefore no longer be recommended as an initial first-line therapy. When spontaneous bacterial peritonitis occurs as a nosocomial infection, a more resistant spectrum of pathogens can be assumed including vancomycin-resistant enterococci (VRE), MRSA, or resistant gram-negative isolates (e.g., ESBL-producing *E. coli*). In such cases antibiotic therapy should be individually tailored to the specific clinical situation.

The choice of antibiotic therapy for secondary peritonitis (due to hollow viscus perforation) should be preceded by risk stratification to assess the overall level of risk:

- **Low risk:** a localized recent infection arising from an abdominal process that is easily curable by surgical treatment. Low-risk cases should respond well to a classic combination such as a group 2 cephalosporin (e.g., cefuroxim 1.5 g IV three times a day) or group 3a cephalosporin (ceftriaxone 2 g IV once a day) plus metronidazole (400–500 mg three times a day) or an aminopenicillin/β-lactamase inhibitor combination (e.g., ampicillin 2 g/sulbactam 1 g IV three times a day).
- **Higher risk:** a longer standing process, preceding antibiotic therapy, including delayed diagnosis, four-quadrant peritonitis, sepsis, and/or a nosocomial situation such as anastomosis leakage. This higher-risk constellation calls for therapy with a broader spectrum, e.g., with an ureidopenicillin/β-lactamase inhibitor combination such as piperacillin/tazobactam (4.5 g IV three time a day) or a carbapenem (e.g., meropenem 1 g IV three time a day).
- Yeast infections are relatively common in such situations, and empirical treatment with an antifungal agent (e.g. fluconazole 400 mg once a day) should also be considered.

Abscesses

Abscesses in the skin and limbs are often caused by gram-positive organisms, mainly by staphylococci and occasionally by streptococci, which typically enter the tissue through a break in the skin.

Intra-abdominal abscesses result from spontaneous (e.g., diverticulitis) or iatrogenic perforation (e.g., anastomosis leakage) of a hollow viscus. As a result, the causative organisms are a mixed population of gram-positive/gram-negative and aerobic/anaerobic pathogens that may even include fungi. Together with enterococci, the latter may play a significant role, especially in patients with perforations after previous antibiotic therapy.

A perinephritic abscess arising from pyelonephritis may develop in patients with complicated urinary tract infections. The causative organisms are the same as in urinary tract infections, i.e., predominantly Enterobacteriaceae (e.g., *E. coli*).

Diagnosis

The material collected by needle aspiration or drainage should be submitted for microbiological testing without delay. The submission of fresh specimens (e.g., a whole syringe with aspirated pus packed in a plastic bag) is adequate in many cases. A transport medium should be used if the transport time to the laboratory is expected to exceed 2 to 4 hours.

Treatment

The choice of antibiotic therapy is dictated by the location, clinical situation, and presumed pathogen.

For suspected gram-positive organisms (e.g., in skin abscesses), basic cephalosporins (cefazolin, 2 g IV three times a day, or cefuroxime, 1.5 g IV three times a day) or a penicillinase-fast penicillin (flucloxacillin, 2 g IV four times a day) would be recommended provided that there is a low local prevalence of (community-acquired) MRSA. For countries with a high prevalence of such pathogens, empirical treatment of abscesses often includes vancomycin.

In the treatment of primary intra-abdominal abscesses without prior antibiotic therapy, suitable agents would include aminopenicillin/β-lactamase inhibitor combinations (e.g., ampicillin/clavulanic acid, 2.2 g IV three times a day, or amoxicillin/sulbactam 3 g IV three times a day). In severe cases with prior antibiotic therapy, severe sepsis, or an immunosuppressed patient, a broader spectrum is preferred (e.g., piperacillin/tazobactam, 4.5 g IV three times a day). Empirical antifungal treatment with fluconazole (400 mg once a day) would also be appropriate in these situations.

Joint Effusion

Joint inflammation may result from a bacterial infection or may be an aseptic inflammation in the setting of rheumatic disease, reactive arthritis, gouty arthropathy, or activated osteoarthritis. Differential diagnosis is not easily made on clinical findings. The diagnostic problem is compounded by the fact that bacterial ("septic") arthritis may supervene upon severe degenerative or arthritic joint changes.

The WBC count in aspirated joint effusion is important in establishing the cause of arthritis. WBC counts < 5×10^9/L (5000/µL) signify a reactive process as in activated osteoarthritis, while counts from 5×10^9 to 40×10^9/L (5000–40,000/µL) would indicate a rheumatic disorder or Lyme disease. Septic arthritis, on the other hand, has white cell counts typically well above 5×10^9/L (> 50,000/µL) and the aspirate usually has a purulent or "chocolate sauce" appearance.

Differentiation of the various etiologies of arthritis is of key clinical importance because of the significantly different treatment. Furthermore, septic arthritis is always an indication for early surgical treatment, including joint lavage, to eradicate the infectious focus and prevent systemic spreading.

Diagnosis

Percutaneous aspiration of a joint effusion should follow the standard access route for the affected joint (see Musculoskeletal Interventions, Chapter 28) using strict aseptic technique, a fenestrated drape, and strict adherence to the exposure times recommended for skin antiseptics. The aspirated fluid has to be sent immediately for microbiological analysis in a sterile tube. If transport times longer than 2 to 4 hours are anticipated, a portion of the aspirate should be submitted in a transport tube or an aerobic blood culture bottle. In all cases, part of the aspirate should also be submitted to the laboratory in a tube (ideally containing EDTA as anticoagulant) for the determination of cell counts. Blood cultures should be taken as well. Clinical suspicion of arthritis due to Lyme disease, which is characterized by large and relatively painless effusions and typical involvement of the knees, can be confirmed by positive *Borrelia* serology (ELISA + western blot) and optionally by *Borrelia*-PCR from effusion aspirate.

Treatment

- The empirical treatment of a purulent joint effusion should employ antibiotics with staphylococcal activity, such as a group 2 cephalosporin (cefuroxime, 1.5 g IV three times a day) or a penicillinase-fast penicillin (flucloxacillin 2 g IV four times a day) or a group 3a cephalosporin (ceftriaxone, 2 g IV once a day) or a ureidopenicillin/β-lactamase inhibitor combination such as piperacillin/tazobactam (4.5 g IV three times a day). All therapies that have been initiated empirically should be adjusted according to culture results. It is recommended that treatment be continued for at least 3 weeks. Treatment should be prolonged in patients with a foreign-body infection (metal implants, prosthetic joint replacement) and should generally be accompanied by surgical intervention.
- For Lyme disease (positive serology, positive history of tick bite, typical joint aspirate, knees generally affected, optionally positive *Borrelia*-PCR): initiate doxycycline therapy (100 mg orally twice a day for 2 to 3 weeks).
- For gouty arthritis: nonsteroidal anti-inflammatory drugs (NSAIDs) (caution: no NSAID if kidney function is impaired!) or corticosteroids

References

[1] Mimoz O, Pieroni L, Lawrence C et al. Prospective, randomized trial of two antiseptic solutions for prevention of central venous or arterial catheter colonization and infection in intensive care unit patients. Crit Care Med 1996; 24: 1818–1823

[2] Caldeira D, David C, Sampaio C. Skin antiseptics in venous puncture site disinfection for prevention of blood culture contamination: systematic review with meta-analysis. J Hosp Infect 2011; 77: 223–232

[3] Roth A, Schaberg T, Mauch H. Molecular diagnosis of tuberculosis: current clinical validity and future perspectives. Eur Respir J 1997; 10: 1877–1891

[4] Lange C, Schaberg T, Diel R, Greinert U. [Current position regarding the diagnosis of tuberculosis] Dtsch Med Wochenschr 2006; 131: 341–347

[5] Lima DM, Colares JK, da Fonseca BA. Combined use of the polymerase chain reaction and detection of adenosine deaminase activity on pleural fluid improves the rate of diagnosis of pleural tuberculosis. Chest 2003; 124: 909–914

[6] Bandyopadhyay D, Gupta S, Banerjee S et al. Adenosine deaminase estimation and multiplex polymerase chain reaction in diagnosis of extra-pulmonary tuberculosis. Int J Tuberc Lung Dis 2008; 12: 1203–1208

[7] Dheda K, van Zyl-Smit RN, Sechi LA et al. Utility of quantitative T-cell responses versus unstimulated interferon-gamma for the diagnosis of pleural tuberculosis. Eur Respir J 2009; 34: 1118–1126

[8] Barnes TW, Olson EJ, Morgenthaler TI, Edson RS, Decker PA, Ryu JH. Low yield of microbiologic studies on pleural fluid specimens. Chest 2005; 127: 916–921

8 Hygiene Management

H. Martiny, D. Nuernberg

Image-guided interventional procedures are increasingly used for a variety of therapeutic and diagnostic applications. To date, however, the procedures themselves and the hygienic requirements for medical products used in these procedures have not been consistently or adequately regulated due to a lack of guidelines. Besides the proper manufacture and preparation of the medical products themselves, a practical and effective approach to hygiene must involve a comprehensive process in which the individual steps are identified and described in detail.

8.1 General Hygienic Requirements

Hygienic requirements must be tailored to the specific diagnostic procedure that is to be performed. The scope of necessary measures should be described within the framework of the risk management program of the office or department of a medical facility.

8.1.1 Personal Protective Equipment and Coverings

Personal protective equipment includes gowns, gloves, masks, hair coverings (caps), and protective eyewear. Not all of these items will be needed in every case. Surgical gowns, gloves, masks, and hair coverings are also classified as medical products. Since personal protective equipment involves various regulatory areas relating to infection prevention and occupational safety, it should be of interest to hygienists as well as occupational physicians. The information in this chapter is intended as a guide to be considered in the formulation of standard operating procedures.

Recommendations issued by the Commission on Hospital Hygiene and Infection Prevention at the Robert Koch Institute address the hygienic aspects of surgical operations and minor invasive procedures with or without an increased risk of infection. For minor invasive procedures that are not associated with an increased risk of infection, it is sufficient to carry out a hygienic handwash or handrub and don a protective gown and (generally sterile) gloves. Operations or minor invasive procedures that are associated with an increased risk of infection require a cap, mask, sterile protective gown (surgical gown), and sterile gloves.[1]

Protective gowns should be changed for each new patient, or replaced after every procedure. Sterile gowns should have long sleeves, while short sleeves are preferred for nonsterile gowns. If disposable gowns are not used, a validated decontamination process should be used, even at the office level, to ensure proper cleaning and disinfection.[2,3]

Sterile gloves are changed for each new patient and are donned over the air-dried hands following surgical hand antisepsis (surgical scrub). In selecting a glove, the properties of the material should be considered in addition to worker safety laws.[4] Polyethylene is a recommended glove material for light-duty situations and for double gloving in patients with a possible latex intolerance, for example. Powder-free Biogel gloves containing natural latex rubber have also proven effective with their good tactile sensitivity and inner coating for easier donning. A double glove configuration with a puncture indicator system is also available if needed. Latex (or appropriate latex-free) gloves should be used in heavy-duty situations such as surgical operations and catheter insertions.[2]

A multi-layer **surgical mask** may be necessary for the protection of staff or patients.[1] Masks can prevent contamination of medical personnel and can also protect patients, especially ones who are immunocompromised. An effective mask should completely cover the mouth, nose, and beard if present. The level of protection afforded by the mask should conform to the hygiene program of the institution. It may be necessary, for example, to use masks with an FFP1 rating that are impermeable to fluids. The quality rating of a mask also indicates its filtration efficiency.[5,6] Filter efficiencies for various masks are listed in ▶ Table 8.1. Masks are changed for each new patient and must also be changed if contaminated or wetted through. Masks should not be reused after removal from the mouth and/or nose (pulled below the chin). It has been shown that just one well-fitting face mask can prevent the inhalation of microorganisms.[5,6]

Table 8.1 Filtering efficiency of respiratory protection masks according to DIN EN 149 (2001) and of surgical masks according to DIN EN 14683 (2005)

Type of mask		BFE	Total leakage (particle size ≤ 0.6 μm)
Surgical mask	Type I	> 95%	
		Type II	> 98%
Respiratory protection	FFP 1 (R or NR)		> 22%
	FFP 2 (R or NR)		> 8%
	FFP 3 (R or NR)		> 2%

Abbreviations: BFE, bacteriological filtering efficiency; FFP, filtering face piece; NR, not reusable; R, reusable.

The wearing of a **cap** and/or **protective eyewear** that is changed for each new patient may also be necessary for reasons of staff and patient safety.[1] In selecting protective eyewear, it should be determined whether blood or secretions are likely to be spattered, as this would require protective eyewear with side shields. It should also be determined whether the protective eyewear material is compatible with the disinfectants used in the facility and whether corrective eyeglasses should be covered.

8.1.2 Disposable Probe Covers

In the procurement of **disposable ultrasound probe covers**, it should be noted that both sterile and nonsterile products are available. Sterile products should be individually packaged in pouches that have been tested for their integrity. As a general rule, only sterile, disposable probe covers should be used in interventional procedures. According to Schrader, tests for package integrity are not regulated, and random testing may be done at the facility without testing an entire batch.[7] It should be determined whether covers made of latex-free material are available. Even the use of disposable probe covers does not eliminate the need for probe decontamination as described in the next subsection, since studies have detected microorganisms on used ultrasound probes even when disposable covers were used.[8–12] Probe contamination rates of 2 to 5% have been described with latex condom sheaths.[10,12] As a result, the ultrasound probe should be cleaned and disinfected after every examination even when a disposable probe cover has been used[13,14] and the probe will be sterilized.

8.1.3 Ultrasound Gel

The **ultrasound gel** used in interventional ultrasound procedures should be sterile. Package sizes should match the gel requirement for one examination to ensure that residual product will not be used on additional patients. Ultrasound gel comes packaged in syringes or foil pouches. A hygienically safer and more user-friendly option is to purchase sterile, disposable probe covers that are prefilled with sterile gel. Disposable probe covers can be applied under aseptic conditions when manufacturers' instructions are followed. Ultrasound gels have been identified as a potential vehicle for nosocomial infections.[14–21]

8.2 Hand Antisepsis and Skin Preparation

► **Hand antisepsis.** Hand antisepsis is the most important measure for protecting both staff and patients in the everyday practice of medicine. Fingernails should be trimmed short and round because most hand flora occur around and under the nails.[4] Nail polish should not be used, as it can shield microorganisms from the effects of hand antiseptics, and artificial nails should not be worn.[22] The hands should be free of injuries, especially in the nail bed, and free of inflammatory processes. Watches, jewelry, and rings (including wedding rings) should not be worn on the hands or forearms.[4]

► **Hygienic hand antisepsis.** Hygienic hand antisepsis is always performed before or after patient contact, regardless of whether protective gloves will be or have been worn. To protect the skin, the hands should not be washed immediately before hygienic antisepsis, but the hands should definitely be dry. The alcohol-based handrub that is used should be on the list approved by the VAH (Association for Applied Hygiene).[23] Only a small percentage of these products require an application time of 1 minute, and most products are listed for a shorter contact time. In this case a sufficient amount of the antiseptic agent (at least 3 mL) should be rubbed over all surfaces of the hands for at least 30 seconds. The hands should be moist throughout the contact period. It should be noted that most antiseptic dispensers are set to deliver only 1.5 mL of the agent at one time. It has proven helpful to follow a fixed routine for hand antisepsis, and most manufacturers supply a recommended routine with their product.

► **Surgical hand antisepsis.** Surgical hand antisepsis (surgical hand scrub) should be performed before all surgical operations and minor invasive procedures that are associated with an increased risk of infection.[1] The hygiene program at the institution should stipulate whether and for how long surgical hand antisepsis is preceded by handwashing. The recommendations of the KRINKO Commission are helpful in this regard. In interventional ultrasound procedures such as percutaneous liver biopsy or the percutaneous aspiration of ascites, which can be performed quickly and do not place high mechanical stresses on surgical gloves, hygienic hand antisepsis is considered sufficient. In other procedures such as percutaneous transhepatic cholangiography and drainage (PTCD), nephrostomy, or tumor therapies that are classified as operative or minor invasive procedures with an increased risk of infection, aseptic technique is essential, and the interventionalist should perform surgical hand antisepsis (surgical hand scrub) before donning a sterile gown and sterile gloves.

As in hygienic antisepsis, an alcohol-based product should be used for surgical hand antisepsis. Only certified products should be used.[23] A small number of these products require an application time of 5 minutes, but most are listed for shorter contact times. The necessary contact time may be 1 minute or longer, depending on the product. It should be noted, however, that the contact times recommended by manufacturers do not start until the hand has been completely wetted and the product is rubbed onto the hand areas that are to be scrubbed. Wetting of the forearms is not included in the actual contact time.[23]

▸ **Patient skin preparation.** Patient skin preparation ("skin prep") should follow recommendations of the Robert Koch Institute[24] on the "Prevention of Surgical Site Infections." In skin preparation with a listed (alcohol-based) antiseptic, it is important to follow the recommended contact times, which depend on the specific product, on the hygiene program of the institution, and on whether the skin area to be prepped is rich or poor in sebaceous glands. For skin with few sebaceous glands, the VAH listing distinguishes prepping for hypodermic injections and needle punctures (listed effective contact times are ¼ minute and 1 minute) from prepping for needle aspirations of joints, body cavities, and hollow organs and for surgical operations (listed effective contact time ≥ 1 minute). For skin areas rich in sebaceous glands, the listed contact times are ≥ 1 minute to ≥ 5 minutes or ≥ 10 minutes.[23]

When hair removal is necessary, it is done immediately before the surgical procedure, preferably by trimming the hair or by chemical epilation. The skin prep begins with thorough cleansing of the skin.[1] Then the area is scrubbed with sterile sponges on (Kocher) forceps, all of which should be packaged in sterile packaging with an adequate number of sponges available. The boundaries of the skin prep should be wide enough to allow for possible adjustment of the entry site, and therefore of the sterile drapes, without contaminating the puncture needle. Fluid-impermeable drapes should be used in settings where fluid might soak through the drape material.[1]

8.3 Ultrasound Probe and Accessories

8.3.1 Decontamination of the Ultrasound Probe

Ultrasound probes can be classified as noncritical, semicritical, or critical medical products depending on their intended use and the associated risk.[24] Semicritical medical products are defined as objects that come into contact with mucous membranes or skin that is not intact. Critical medical products, which include ultrasound probes that are used intraoperatively, may come into contact with blood, internal tissues, or organs. Semicritical medical products are always cleaned and disinfected with a virucidal agent before use.[1] Critical medical products are always cleaned, disinfected, and sterilized before use (see below). If the ultrasound probe itself cannot be sterilized, it should always be cleaned and disinfected with a virucidal agent before the sterile, disposable probe cover is applied.

The ultrasound probes used in image-guided interventional procedures are generally classified as semicritical objects, although they may come into contact with critical medical products such as needles and catheters. For this reason, direct contact with critical medical products should be avoided during the procedure despite the use of sterile, disposable probe covers. When a sterile ultrasound probe is used, there is no need to use a sterile disposable cover.

The manufacturers of ultrasound probes are providing users with increasingly detailed recommendations on decontamination that are highly effective when followed. Moreover, the ultrasound probes themselves are sterilizable in many cases. Manufacturers provide comprehensive lists of compatible cleansers and disinfectants and also furnish sterilization instructions for probes that can be sterilized.

The ultrasound probe should be cleaned and disinfected after every examination, even when a disposable probe cover has been used[13,14] and the probe itself can subsequently be sterilized.

The cleaning of an ultrasound probe should follow the manufacturer's recommendations on the type of cleanser (material compatibility) that should be used. After every examination, residual ultrasound gel should be carefully removed with a disposable towel. Next the ultrasound probe and cord are wiped off with a towel moistened with cleanser to remove gross contaminants and body fluids. The next cleaning step may involve immersion or wiping. If the probe is immersed, the manufacturer's instructions on immersion depth should be closely followed. Next the probe is thoroughly rinsed and dried with a towel.

Cleaning is followed by disinfection. Manufacturer's recommendations should always be noted in selecting a disinfectant. Additionally, the recommendations of the Robert Koch Institute state that medical products that are not subsequently sterilized, or cannot be sterilized, should be disinfected with a virucidal agent that is active against both enveloped and nonenveloped viruses.[25]

Before further decontamination or prior to use, the ultrasound probe should be carefully examined for possible damage such as cracks, chips, or sharp corners or edges.

If subsequent sterilization is not done or cannot be done, disinfection is followed by a final rinse with water of at least drinking-water quality. If this is uncertain, sterilely filtered (or sterile) water should be used. The probe is dried with a disinfected or sterile towel.

In procedures such as liver biopsy where the needle is inserted in close proximity to the ultrasound probe, there is a possibility that the probe will come into contact with the needle. In this case the probe is classified as a semicritical medical product, which should be disinfected with a virucidal agent and used with a sterile, disposable probe cover. A sterile ultrasound probe is necessary whenever a needle will be introduced through the probe for abscess drainage or PTCD, for example.

Various manufacturers recommend that ultrasound probes be sterilized by steam sterilization, ethylene oxide sterilization, or plasma sterilization. The sterilization process should always conform to standard operating procedures and validated methods. The sterilization of medical products in an unpackaged condition is not recognized in Germany as a valid sterilization process, though it is widely practiced in other countries.

8.3.2 Decontamination of Ultrasound Accessories

Whenever available, biopsy instruments, cannulas, hollow needles (see Chapter 2), etc. should be used in the form of disposable, single-use items. But if these types of medical devices require decontamination, the method of choice is machine decontamination (cleaning and disinfection) in a tested cleaning and disinfection device, which is then followed by sterilization. All steps, regardless of whether they involve a machine or manual process, require detailed standard operating instructions so that a validated procedure can be followed.

References

[1] Kommission für Krankenhaushygiene und Infektionsprävention am Robert Koch-Institut (RKI). Anforderungen der Hygiene bei Operationen und anderen invasiven Eingriffen. Bundesgesundheitsblatt Gesundheitsforschung Gesundheitsschutz 2000; 43: 644–648

[2] DGKH-Sektion "Hygiene in der ambulanten und stationären Kranken- und Altenpflege/Rehabilitation". Kleidung und Schutzausrüstung für Pflegeberufe aus hygienischer Sicht. HygMed 2009; 34: 102–107

[3] Kommission für Krankenhaushygiene und Infektionsprävention am Robert Koch-Institut. Anforderungen der Krankenhaushygiene und des Arbeitsschutzes an die Hygienebekleidung und persönliche Schutzausrüstung. Epidemiologisches Bulletin 2007 2007; 1. Available from: http://www.rki.de/DE/Content/Infekt/Krankenhaushygiene/Kommission/Downloads/Arbeitsschutz_pdf.html

[4] Biologische Arbeitsstoffe im Gesundheitswesen und in der Wohlfahrtspflege (TRBA 250), Release March 2014. GMBL. 2014 (March); No. 10/11: 206. Available from: http://www.baua.de/de/Themen-von-A-Z/Biologische-Arbeitsstoffe/TRBA/TRBA-250.html

[5] Checchi L, Montevecchi M, Moreschi A, Graziosi F, Taddei P, Violante FS. Efficacy of three face masks in preventing inhalation of airborne contaminants in dental practice. J Am Dent Assoc 2005; 136: 877–882

[6] Oberg T, Brosseau LM. Surgical mask filter and fit performance. Am J Infect Control 2008; 36: 276–282

[7] Schrader G. Vaginalsonden - Einsatz und Aufbereitung. HygMed 2005; 30: 437–439

[8] Amis S, Ruddy M, Kibbler CC, Economides DL, MacLean AB. Assessment of condoms as probe covers for transvaginal sonography. J Clin Ultrasound 2000; 28: 295–298

[9] Kac G, Podglajen I, Si-Mohamed A, Rodi A, Grataloup C, Meyer G. Evaluation of ultraviolet C for disinfection of endocavitary ultrasound transducers persistently contaminated despite probe covers. Infect Control Hosp Epidemiol 2010; 31: 165–170

[10] Milki AA, Fisch JD. Vaginal ultrasound probe cover leakage: implications for patient care. Fertil Steril 1998; 69: 409–411

[11] Rutala WA, Gergen MF, Weber DJ. Disinfection of a probe used in ultrasound-guided prostate biopsy. Infect Control Hosp Epidemiol 2007; 28: 916–919

[12] Storment JM, Monga M, Blanco JD. Ineffectiveness of latex condoms in preventing contamination of the transvaginal ultrasound transducer head. South Med J 1997; 90: 206–208

[13] Empfehlungen des BfArM. Aufbereitung von Ultraschallsonden mit Schleimhautkontakt. Reference no. 4306/05. Available from http://www.bfarm.de/SharedDocs/Risikoinformationen/Medizinprodukte/DE/ultraschallsonden-2.html

[14] Merz E. Schallkopfhygiene - ein unterschätztes Thema? [Transducer hygiene - an underrated topic?]. Ultraschall Med 2005; 26(1): 7-8. DOI: 10.1055/s-2004-813948

[15] Gaillot O, Maruéjouls C, Abachin E et al. Nosocomial outbreak of Klebsiella pneumoniae producing SHV-5 extended-spectrum beta-lactamase, originating from a contaminated ultrasonography coupling gel. J Clin Microbiol 1998; 36: 1357–1360

[16] Hutchinson J, Runge W, Mulvey M et al. Burkholderia cepacia infections associated with intrinsically contaminated ultrasound gel: the role of microbial degradation of parabens. Infect Control Hosp Epidemiol 2004; 25: 291–296

[17] Jacobson M, Wray R, Kovach D, Henry D, Speert D, Matlow A. Sustained endemicity of Burkholderia cepacia complex in a pediatric institution, associated with contaminated ultrasound gel. Infect Control Hosp Epidemiol 2006; 27: 362–366

[18] Schabrun S, Chipchase L, Rickard H. Are therapeutic ultrasound units a potential vector for nosocomial infection? Physiother Res Int 2006; 11: 61–71

[19] Weist K, Wendt C, Petersen LR, Versmold H, Rüden H. An outbreak of pyodermas among neonates caused by ultrasound gel contaminated with methicillin-susceptible Staphylococcus aureus. Infect Control Hosp Epidemiol 2000; 21: 761–764

[20] Marigliano A, D'Errico MM, Pellegrini I, Savini S, Prospero E, Barbadoro P. Ultrasound echocardiographic gel contamination by Burkholderia cepacia in an Italian hospital. J Hosp Infect 2010; 76: 360–361

[21] Olshtain-Pops K, Block C, Temper V et al. An outbreak of achromobacter xylosoxidans associated with ultrasound gel used during transrectal ultrasound guided prostate biopsy. J Urol 2011; 185: 144–147

[22] Deutsche Gesellschaft für Krankenhaushygiene e.V. Schmuck, Piercing und künstliche Fingernägel in Arztpraxen und anderen Einrichtungen des Gesundheitswesen. Release October 2010. http://www.krankenhaushygiene.de/informationen/fachinformationen/empfehlungen-der-dgkh/279

[23] Desinfektionsmittel-Kommission im VAH. Flächendesinfektion/Surface disinfection. In Desinfektionsmittel-Liste des VAH. Wiesbaden: mhp-Verlag; 2008: 52–87

[24] Kommission für Krankenhaushygiene und Infektionsprävention beim Robert Koch - Institut (RKI) und Bundesinstitut für Arzneimittel und Medizinprodukte (BfArM).. Anforderungen an die Hygiene bei der Aufbereitung von Medizinprodukten. Bundesgesundheitsblatt Gesundheitsforschung Gesundheitsschutz 2001; 44: 1115–1126

[25] Robert Koch-Institut. Deutschen Gesellschaft zur Bekämpfung der Viruskrankheiten. Disinfektionsmittelkommission der Deutschen Gesellschaft für Hygiene und Mikrobiologie. Evaluation and declaration of effectiveness of disinfectants against viruses. Position of the Virucide Study Group of the Robert Koch Institute (RKI) and the "Virus Disinfection" Professional Committee of the German Society for Control of "Virus Infections" and the Disinfectant Committee of the German Society of Public Health and Microbiology [Article in German]. Bundesgesundheitsblatt Gesundheitsforschung Gesundheitsschutz 2004; 47: 62–66

9 Contraindications, Complications, and Complication Management

C. Jenssen, C. F. Dietrich

The efficacy and safety of ultrasound-guided interventions depend on the type of intervention, the access route, patient-specific risk factors, the experience and expertise of the interventionalist and assistants, respect for contraindications, and the prompt recognition and treatment of complications.

9.1 Interventional Risk

9.1.1 Complication Rates and Mortality

Large retrospective surveys indicate that ultrasound-guided fine needle biopsy (needle diameter up to 1.0 mm) has complication rates in the range of 0.51%[1] to 0.81%,[2] including a 0.06 to 0.095% incidence of major complications. The mortality rates in these studies range from 0.0011%[2] to 0.018%.[3] While it should be noted that these studies significantly underestimate complication rates due to their methodologies, they still provide valuable clues to the frequency distribution of biopsy-related complications.

Besides pain, which was not assessed in all the surveys, bleeding is the most common major complication of ultrasound-guided biopsies, followed by infections and malignant seeding along the needle tract. The relative frequency of organ-specific complications (pancreatitis, pneumothorax, bile leakage, abortion) relates to the inclusion of various targeted sites in the statistical data. Deaths were caused mainly by severe hemorrhage, pancreatitis, and sepsis[1,2,4,5] as well as needle tract seeding.[6] Retrospective and prospective single-center studies with high case numbers that reported on biopsies of the liver and other abdominal organs with needle diameters > 1.0 mm have shown markedly higher complication rates from 0.4%[7,8] to 2.5%.[9,10]

9.1.2 Factors that Influence Interventional Risk

Needle Diameter, Needle Type

Data from surveys with high case numbers have yielded controversial results on the diameters and types of biopsy needle used.[2,11] Retrospective analyses of parenchymal liver biopsies[7,12] and biopsies of focal liver lesions[12] have consistently shown higher complication rates associated with the use of cutting biopsy needles compared with aspiration needles. On the other hand, comparative studies do not support the thesis that needle diameters between 18 gauge and 14 gauge (1.2–1.6 mm) are associated with a higher biopsy risk than fine needles.[13–18]

Number of Biopsies

There is evidence from various studies that the risk of complications depends on the number of biopsies performed.

Target Site

The risk of biopsy depends on the targeted site (see Section 9.6, Specific Biopsy Sites, p. 95). Higher complication rates have been reported for the ultrasound-guided biopsy of liver tumors than for parenchymal liver biopsies.[8,19]

Diagnostic and Therapeutic Interventions

The complication rates associated with ultrasound-guided therapeutic interventions are significantly higher than those in purely diagnostic procedures.[8,20,21]

Examiner Experience

Data on the relation of complication rates to operator experience are based almost entirely on percutaneous liver biopsies. In a Swiss survey that evaluated 3,501 liver biopsies (only 32.3% of which were ultrasound-guided), the complication rate among internists who performed fewer than 12 biopsies per year (1.68%) was higher than that of physicians who performed at least 50 liver biopsies per year (0%). Gastroenterologists had lower complication rates (0.11%) than internists (0.55%).[11] Similar results were reported in a British survey[22] and in a retrospective analysis of percutaneous liver and renal biopsies from two U.S. centers.[23] A more recent French study that analyzed 600 ultrasound-guided liver biopsies found no significant difference in complication rates between experienced operators (> 150 liver biopsies) and inexperienced operators (< 15 liver biopsies performed alone). This series included only one major complication, however, and inexperienced operators performed only 25% of the biopsies.[24]

9.2 Frequent Complications and Their Risk Factors

9.2.1 Pain and Vasovagal Reactions

Pain and vasovagal reactions are frequent complications of ultrasound-guided interventions and occur after 10 to

50% of percutaneous liver biopsies,[25] approximately 7% of renal biopsies,[26] and approximately 5% of pancreatic biopsies.[27] Severe vasovagal reactions were observed in up to 2.8% of patients who underwent prostatic biopsy.[28] The pain following liver and splenic biopsies is usually caused by minor bleeding or bile leakage and typically radiates to the shoulders.

9.2.2 Bleeding Complications

Incidence

The largest single-center study published to date was a retrospective review of 15,181 image-guided percutaneous core biopsies (needle diameter at least 20 gauge; kidney, liver, lung, pancreas, others) performed at a British center over a 6-year period.[29] Severe bleeding occurred in 0.5% of all cases. The incidence of bleeding was 0.7% after renal biopsy, 0.5% after liver biopsy, 0.2% after lung biopsy, 1.0% after pancreatic biopsy (mostly allografts), and 0.2% after biopsies of other organs (adrenal glands, retroperitoneum, bone, soft tissues, mesentery). This is in good agreement with other data.[8,30]

Predictors of Bleeding Risk

Several studies have shown that both the platelet count and the prothrombin time (or international normalized ratio, INR) are significant predictors of bleeding risk after percutaneous renal biopsy.[8,17,29–31] In the study by Atwell et al, the mean INR was 1.2 ± 0.9 in the small group of patients with severe bleeding but was only 1.0 ± 0.2 in the group without severe bleeding ($n = 15,116$). The platelet count in the group with major bleeding was 194 ± 88 × 10⁹/L (194 ± 88 × 10³/mm³), and thus significantly lower than in the group without bleeding complications (257 ± 111 × 10⁹/L).[29] In a multicenter study that investigated the complications of 2,740 percutaneous liver biopsies in patients with hepatitis C and advanced cirrhosis of the liver (HALT-C Trial), bleeding complications (16 cases; 0.6%) were more common in patients with an INR ≥ 1.3, and the rate increased significantly in patients with a platelet count of 60 × 10⁹/L or less (0.6% versus 5.2%). Withholding percutaneous liver biopsy from patients with a platelet count < 60 × 10⁹/L would have prevented bleeding in 25% (4 of 16) cases.[30] Similar results were found for renal biopsies in an HIV-infected population, where a reduction of platelet count by 10 × 10⁹/L was associated with a 1.05 times higher risk of bleeding.[31]

In a prospective single-center German study, 8 of 1,923 patients (0.4%) who underwent a diagnostic ($n = 1,696$) or therapeutic ($n = 227$) ultrasound-guided intervention of the liver or pancreas suffered bleeding severe enough to require a transfusion. Another 52 patients had a significant fall in Hb (> 1.24 mmol/L [2 g/dl]). The bleeding rate was higher in therapeutic interventions (2%) than in diagnostic interventions (liver: 0.12%; pancreas: 1.1%). Severe bleeding did not occur after parenchymal liver biopsy, but the bleeding rate after the biopsy of liver masses was 0.5%. The principal risk factor for bleeding and a fall in Hb in this study[8] was hepatic cirrhosis with a Quick value (prothrombin time ratio) < 50%, even though fresh plasma infusion was performed in patients with a Quick value in that range (T. Bernatik, personal communication, 2010).

A retrospective analysis of 629 percutaneous liver biopsies at a German center found that 58% of all biopsy-related bleeding occurred in patients with risk factors. In this cohort of patients with a high percentage of patients at risk, the following diseases and factors increased the risk of bleeding events[32]:

- Mycobacteriosis
- Need for prophylactic platelet transfusion
- Acute liver failure
- Heparin administration on the day of the biopsy
- Advanced hepatic cirrhosis
- Treatment with corticosteroids or metamizole
- Hematologic systemic disease

Most reports of fatal bleeding after ultrasound-guided liver biopsies recorded in large surveys involve the biopsy of liver masses (especially hepatocellular carcinoma [HCC] and hemangioma),[5,33] although sporadic deaths have also been described in large series of parenchymal liver biopsies. These deaths occurred exclusively in patients with special risk factors (coagulopathy, systemic disease, age).[11,22,17,32,34]

The biopsy of liver masses not covered by liver parenchyma is often thought to be associated with an increased bleeding risk. While plausible, this hypothesis has not been substantiated by published data.

The following parameters/diseases have been identified as risk factors for bleeding in patients undergoing percutaneous renal biopsy[26,35–40]:

- Arterial hypertension
- Acute renal failure
- Severe, chronic renal function impairment
- Number of needle passes
- Female sex
- Steroid medication
- Increased INR
- Hepatitis C infection
- Coinfection with HIV and hepatitis C
- Amyloidosis

The increased bleeding risk in patients with severe renal function impairment is due mainly to impaired platelet function.[41] Data on the role of platelet function tests (traditional bleeding time, PFA-100) for evaluating bleeding risk in renal and liver biopsies are controversial, however.[37,42–47]

Clinical Significance

The clinical significance of postinterventional bleeding is variable and ranges from asymptomatic hematomas or arteriovenous fistulas detectable by imaging and an asymptomatic drop in serum hemoglobin to symptomatic intraparenchymal, subcapsular, retroperitoneal, pleural, and free intraperitoneal hemorrhages. Rare manifestations are visceral pseudoaneurysms and bleeding into the biliary tract (hemobilia) or urinary tract (hematuria) and bleeding into the pancreatic duct (hemosuccus pancreaticus). There have been isolated case reports of acute cholecystitis, cholangitis, and biliary pancreatitis as a sequel to liver biopsy with bleeding into the biliary system (portobiliary fistula). Severe postinterventional splenic or renal hemorrhage may lead to organ failure.

Infectious Complications and Peritonitis

Antiseptic preparation of the skin site and the use of sterile equipment ensure low rates of infectious complications. On the other hand, abscesses, abdominal or chest wall infections, sepsis, or peritonitis may result from passing a needle or drain through bacterially contaminated spaces (e.g., abscesses, renal pelvis and parenchyma in pyelonephritis, intestinal structures). In a very large, single-center series of various ultrasound-guided procedures ($n = 13{,}534$), the rate of postinterventional infectious complications was very low at 0.1%. While no infections were observed after ultrasound-guided thoracentesis or fine needle aspiration, the incidence of infections after ultrasound-guided diagnostic biopsy was 0.2%. Biopsy of a liver transplant had the highest incidence (1%).[48] Biliary peritonitis was observed in 0.03 to 0.22% of liver biopsies and resulted from accidental puncture of the gallbladder or passing a needle or drain through bile ducts with obstructed drainage.[7,49] Ten septic complications (urosepsis, perirenal abscess; 1%) were found in a retrospective analysis of 1,005 parenchymal renal biopsies, only some of which were ultrasound-guided.[35] In another series of 1,090 ultrasound-guided parenchymal renal biopsies, no instances of infectious complications were reported.[50]

Of course, the risk of infectious complications is particularly high in ultrasound-guided transrectal prostatic biopsies. Uncomplicated urinary tract infections are likely to develop in approximately 11% of cases, fever in 2 to 3.5%, acute prostatitis in 1 to 2%, and urosepsis in only about 0.1 to 0.2%.[28,51,52] Risk factors for sepsis after prostatic biopsy are an indwelling transurethral catheter, the presence of diabetes mellitus, and the number of repeat biopsies.[53] Isolated cases of fatal septic complications have been reported in the literature. In the event of infectious complications after prostatic biopsy, the causative organisms are likely to be resistant to the antibiotic used for infection prophylaxis (usually a gyrase inhibitor).[54] A population-based study in Ontario, Canada, showed that hospital admission rates for urologic complications of transrectal prostate biopsy increased during the years 1996 to 2005, rising from 1 to 4.1%. Most of the hospital admissions (72%) were for infectious complications.[55]

9.2.3 Needle Tract Seeding

Incidence

Older surveys with large case numbers reported an incidence of 0.003%[1] to 0.009%[3] for seeding of malignant cells along the needle tract in ultrasound-guided fine needle biopsies of abdominal and retroperitoneal malignancies. One survey reported an incidence of 0.012% after transthoracic needle biopsy.[56] It is reasonable to assume, however, that these data understate the true incidence because tumor seeding generally appears with a latency of several months to as much as 25 months after needle biopsy.[2,5,57,58] In percutaneous biopsies of hepatocellular carcinomas, needle tract seeding was detected by imaging an average of 267 days (116–619 days) after the procedure.[57] There is another factor that contributes to the significant underestimation of needle tract seeding risk in large survey studies: the number of inoculation metastases was related statistically not only to the number of biopsies of malignant masses but to the total number of all ultrasound-guided biopsies.

More recent studies indicate a higher risk of malignant needle tract seeding after both diagnostic and therapeutic ultrasound-guided interventions for malignant tumors.

Liver Metastases

Individual single-center case series showed that tumor seeding after the percutaneous (fine needle) biopsy of colorectal liver metastases occurred with incidences of 10%,[6] 16%,[59] or 19%[60] respectively in different series.

Hepatocellular Carcinoma

A literature search published in 2007 yielded 179 cases of tumor seeding after percutaneous biopsy, percutaneous ethanol injection (PEI), or thermal ablation (radiofrequency ablation [RFA] or microwave ablation) of hepatocellular carcinoma (HCC). The median frequency of tumor seeding in the 41 papers reviewed was calculated to be 2.29% after biopsy, 1.4% after biopsy and PEI, 0.61% for RFA, and 0.72% for RFA for biopsy and ablation.[61] In another meta-analysis of a total of 8 studies, the incidence of metastatic implants in the needle tract after percutaneous biopsy of HCC was 2.7% (0.9% per year).[62] Only one study investigated the possibility of hematogenous tumor cell dissemination but did not demonstrate an increase in circulating tumor cells after the percutaneous biopsy of HCC.[63]

Lung Cancer and Pleural Mesothelioma

In a series of operatively treated stage I lung cancers, a higher incidence of needle tract seeding and pleural recurrence was found in the subset of tumors that had been confirmed by preoperative percutaneous or intraoperative needle biopsy with an 18-gauge cutting biopsy needle (8.6% versus 0.9%).[64] A relatively high risk of needle and drain tract seeding also exists after percutaneous biopsies and interventions for pleural mesothelioma, although the reported incidences vary over a wide range (all interventions: 0–48%; needle biopsy: 0–22%).[65] The study with the largest case numbers to date found a 4% incidence of needle tract seeding, which was significantly less than the incidence of tumor seeding after surgical biopsy (thoracoscopy or thoracotomy: 22%).[66]

Breast Cancer

In a systematic review of a total of 15 studies, epithelial tumor cell seeding after the core needle biopsy of breast cancers was found in an average of 22% of surgical specimens. Preoperative core needle biopsy was not associated with a decrease in survival, however.[67]

Other Malignant Tumors

Needle tract seeding has also been reported after the ultrasound- or CT-guided biopsy of pancreatic cancers and other malignancies, although no reliable incidence rates are available. There have been individual case reports of pleural, peritoneal, and cutaneous seeding from pancreatic, biliary, and renal cell carcinomas occurring after percutaneous biliary tract drainage and nephrostomy. Weiss et al compiled case data from their own files and from published reports on 29 cases of malignant seeding after ultrasound guided needle biopsy of dominant pancreatic carcinoma ($n = 11$) as the targeted site.[2] Very few data have been published from single-center studies on the incidence of malignant seeding after the percutaneous biopsy of pancreatic carcinoma. One Japanese group reported an incidence of 1.4% (1 in 73 cases).[58]

Clinical Significance

In one retrospective comparison, the 4-year survival rates of 90 patients who underwent preoperative biopsy were significantly lower due to a high incidence of needle tract seeding (19%) than in 509 patients who were not biopsied prior to the resection of colorectal hepatic metastases.[60] A Spanish study found that the percutaneous biopsy of HCC done before liver transplantation significantly increased the recurrence rate from 5.9% in the group without preoperative biopsy to 31.8% in the biopsy group. The number of hepatic recurrences was roughly the same in both groups (3.9% versus 4.5%). Extrahepatic recurrences (lung, needle tract) developed in 27.3% of the preoperative biopsy group but were rare (2%) in the nonbiopsy group.[68,69] Another study in 85 patients with large hepatocellular carcinomas found that preoperative biopsy significantly increased the incidence of postoperative intraperitoneal recurrence (12.5% versus 1.6%) while significantly reducing 5-year disease-free survival (24% versus 52%).[70]

9.2.4 Specific Complications

Some complications are specific for ultrasound-guided biopsies or interventions in particular organs or lesions, such as pneumothorax and hemothorax after percutaneous chest biopsy, pancreatitis after pancreatic biopsy, hematuria after renal biopsy, hypertensive crisis after biopsy of pheochromocytoma, anaphylactic shock after hydatid cyst biopsy, and injuries to cervical vessels and other structures after biopsies of the thyroid gland, cervical lymph nodes, and salivary glands.

9.3 Prevention of Complications

9.3.1 Risk Assessment and Patient Selection

Selecting patients for ultrasound-guided biopsies and interventions should always be done responsibly while giving due consideration to the expected clinical benefit, the individual procedural risk, the experience of the interventionalist, and alternative techniques. In particular, it should be determined whether the result of a biopsy is likely to influence patient management and whether noninvasive studies (especially contrast-enhanced ultrasonography [CEUS] and other imaging procedures) could provide diagnostic information adequate for treatment planning.

The decision on ultrasound-guided interventions in patients treated with anticoagulants or antiplatelet drugs should be based on a conscientious assessment of procedure-related and thromboembolic risks (▶ Table 9.1, ▶ Table 9.2). The urgency of the intervention should also be considered.

In patients with advanced liver or kidney disease, it should be noted that the increased risk of bleeding complications after percutaneous interventions is based on complex mechanisms and is not fully reflected in global markers such as platelet count, PT (or Quick value), INR, PTT, and bleeding time. The clinical bleeding history is of much greater importance in this regard.[71–73] Nevertheless, we still recommend the routine determination of PT or thromboplastin time (Quick value), INR, PTT, and platelet count before any elective intervention, both for

Table 9.1 Risk stratification for the interruption of treatment with clopidogrel and other thienopyridine-class antiplatelet drugs

High risk	Low risk
< 12 months after implantation of a coronary drug-eluting stent	Coronary heart disease without a coronary stent
< 1 month after implantation of a coronary bare metal stent	Cerebrovascular disease
< 1 month after implantation of a peripheral vascular stent	Peripheral arterial occlusive disease

Table 9.2 Risk stratification for the interruption of oral anticoagulant therapy

Condition or disease	High risk	Moderate risk	Low risk
Mechanical heart valve prosthesis	Mitral valve prosthesis	Bileaflet aortic valve prosthesis plus one of the following criteria: • Atrial fibrillation • Prior stroke or TIA • Arterial hypertension • Diabetes mellitus • Congestive heart failure • Age > 75 years	Bileaflet aortic valve prosthesis without other risk factors
	Older aortic valve prosthesis		Biological valve replacement
	Valve replacement and myocardial infarction or TIA ≤ 6 months		
Atrial fibrillation	Atrial fibrillation and mitral stenosis	$CHADS_2$ score of 3 or 4	$CHADS_2$ score of 0–2 (and no prior stroke or TIA)
Venous thromboembolism	< 3 months after VTE	3–12 months after VTE	> 12 months after VTE without other risk factors
	Severe thrombophilia	Mild thrombophilia (heterozygous factor V Leiden or factor II mutation)	
		Active cancer	
	Vena cava filter	Recurrent VTE	

Abbreviations: TIA, transient ischemic attack; VTE, venous thromboembolism.
Source: reference[76].

legal reasons and for best practice. The determination of bleeding time or a platelet function test with PFA-100 are advised in patients with advanced renal failure or advanced liver damage, and in patients who have a positive bleeding history with normal global coagulation tests.

Caution

The assessment of risks before a percutaneous ultrasound-guided procedure is based mainly on the patient's history and clinical data.

Global coagulation tests in themselves are inadequate for the assessment of bleeding risk.

9.3.2 Modification of Risk Factors

Interruption of Dual Antiplatelet Therapy

Drawing on current recommendations for endoscopic procedures, aspirin should be stopped 5 to 7 days before an ultrasound-guided intervention and clopidogrel and the new ADP-receptor antagonists should be stopped 7 to 10 days before, if this is considered to be necessary and reasonable (▶ Table 9.1). In patients with a high cardiovascular risk and especially in patients with coronary drug-eluting stents (DES), the procedure and the timing of the intervention should be coordinated with the cardiologist. Ordinarily, clopidogrel and other ADP-receptor antagonists can be discontinued at least 1 month after implantation of a bare metal stent and 12 months after implantation of a DES while aspirin is continued. If an intervention cannot be postponed, only the therapy with clopidogrel and other ADP-receptor antagonists should be interrupted while aspirin is continued.[74,75] Aspirin monotherapy does not necessarily have to be stopped.

Interruption or Reversal of Anticoagulant Therapy

In patients with a low thromboembolism risk (▶ Table 9.2), treatment with traditional oral anticoagulants (vitamin K antagonists, VKAs) can be stopped for approximately 5 to 7 days before the scheduled intervention, and the ultrasound-guided intervention may proceed when the INR is 1.5 or less.[76] It should be noted that the anticoagulant effect will subside at varying rates in difference individuals, and this process may take more than one week in patients with an initially high therapeutic INR, impaired liver function, or a low maintenance dose. Novel oral anticoagulants (NOACs, e.g., dabitragan, apixaban, rivaroxaban) in patients with normal renal function should be stopped just 24 hours before a scheduled ultrasound-guided intervention, whereas treatment in patients with renal insufficiency should be interrupted for a longer period depending on the glomerular filtration rate.

In cases where there is an acute or emergent need for an ultrasound-guided intervention, the effects of VKAs can be reversed with PPSB (a prothrombin concentrate: prothrombin = F II, proconvertin = F VII, Stuart-Power factor = F X, antihemophilic factor B = F IX, e.g., Beriplast) or FFP (fresh frozen plasma) or can be antagonized by the oral or intravenous administration of vitamin K. A 5- to 10-mg dose of vitamin K is necessary for the complete reversal of anticoagulation.[77] An adequate response to vitamin K use depends on the dose, mode of administration, baseline INR, and liver function and is usually obtained in approximately 24 to 48 hours. The decrease in INR observed only a few hours after the intravenous administration of vitamin K is initially due only to the rise in factor VII concentration; a sufficient rise in factor II concentration takes approximately 24 hours.[77] By contrast, PPSB and FFP are active immediately after intravenous administration. PPSB is faster and more effective than FPP for the reversal of anticoagulation and should be preferred for that reason and for its lower volume load and infection risk. One IU of PPSB per kg body weight increases the Quick value by approximately 1%. With a baseline INR of 2 to 3, a PPSB dose of 20 IU/kg BW is usually sufficient to achieve an INR < 1.5. Another option is to administer 20 mL of FFP per kg BW.[77] The intervention should be performed without delay because the half-life of the administered factors is only 5 to 8 hours and their efficacy will diminish over time. Importantly, the anticoagulant effect of NOACs is not reversible by PPSB or FFP.

Bridging

Bridging with low-molecular weight heparin (LMWH) is indicated in patients with a high or moderately high risk of arterial or venous thromboembolism in cases where VKA therapy will be interrupted or reversed.[76] Heparin can be given at a therapeutic dose in patients with a high thromboembolic risk. The therapeutic dose per kg body weight should be reduced in patients with impaired renal function. Registry studies have shown that bridging with a half-therapeutic dose provides adequate protection from thromboembolic events in patients with a moderately high thromboembolic risk.[78,79] Prophylactic dosing is adequate in patients with a low thromboembolic risk. The procedure may be scheduled for approximately 6 hours after the last dose of standard heparin or approximately 8 hours after the last dose of a LMWH. In patients with severe renal failure (KDOQI stage 3 or higher), the interval from the last dose of LMWH to the procedure should be lengthened to at least 12 hours. Ordinarily, the last heparin dose before the intervention will be administered on the eve of the procedure.

The continuation of heparin bridging and/or the resumption of oral anticoagulant therapy depends on the course of the intervention. After an uncomplicated biopsy and in the absence of other risk factors for delayed bleeding complications, heparin therapy can be continued the evening after the intervention and oral anticoagulant therapy can be resumed the next day. A longer interval (up to 4 weeks) is recommended after renal biopsy. Decisions should be made on a case-by-case basis following therapeutic interventions and in patients with specific risk factors.

The pharmacologic characteristics of NOACs (short half-life of 8–15 hours) obviate the need for bridging in patients on these drugs.

Caution

Weighing the bleeding risk, cardiovascular risk, and risk of thromboembolism should always be an interdisciplinary, case-by-case decision.

Prevention of Bleeding in Patients with Acquired Hemostatic Disorders

Patients with a low platelet count ($< 50 \times 10^9$/L) or impaired plasmatic coagulation due to liver disease (INR > 1.5; PTT > 50 s) may require the administration of platelet concentrates or FFP, depending on the planned interventional procedure, the target and access route, and the needle diameter. Each unit of platelet concentrate contains approximately 3 to 4×10^{11} platelets and raises the platelet count by approximately 30×10^9/L, although platelet concentrates may be less effective in patients with platelet antibodies, splenomegaly, or sepsis. The necessary dose can be calculated as follows:

$$\begin{aligned}&\text{Need for replacement (platelet count)}\\&= \text{desired increase in platelet count}\left(\frac{n \times 10^9}{L}\right)\\&\times \text{blood volume (approximately 70mL/kg)} \times 1.5\end{aligned} \tag{9.1}$$

Guidelines on the correction of plasmatic coagulation defects or deficits recommend the transfusion of 10 to 20 mL FFP per kg BW. It should be noted, however, that the effect of PPSB and FFP depends on the pretransfusion INR. For example, in the case of a basic value of INR of 3.0, 2,000 mL of FFP is needed to correct the INR to 1.5. If INR is 5.0, 3,000 mL FFP is necessary.[80] Correcting plasmatic coagulation and bleeding risk in patients with mild plasmatic coagulation disorders (INR = 1.1–1.85) is of questionable benefit.[80–83] As a rule, the use of FFP is preferred over PPSB in patients with coagulopathy due to liver disease. An (expensive) alternative is recombinant coagulation factor VIIa (NovoSeven, 90–150 µg/kg BW), which can also be used to correct platelet dysfunction.[84]

A prolonged bleeding time (> 10 minutes) in patients with severe renal and liver dysfunction, other types of acquired and congenital platelet dysfunction, von

Willebrand disease, mild hemophilia A, or antiplatelet drug therapy can be corrected by the intravenous administration of 1-deamino-8-D-arginine vasopressin (DDAVP, desmopressin). Desmopressin improves primary hemostasis (endothelial platelet adhesion and aggregation) by inducing the endothelial release of large multimers of von Willebrand factor.[85–88] It can be administered parenterally (brief intravenous infusion, subcutaneous injection: 0.3 µg/kg BW) or intranasally (≥ 50 kg BW: 300 µg). A meta-analysis has shown that the prophylactic use of desmopressin in surgical patients can reduce blood loss and lessen the need for transfusion to a slight degree.[89] The use of desmopressin to correct a significantly prolonged bleeding time before percutaneous renal biopsy is recommended in several reviews, although there are no hard data to support this practice.[47,45,90] Oral conjugated estrogens and dialysis therapy also reduce bleeding time and clinical bleeding events in uremic patients.[91]

Caution

Preinterventional corrective measures cannot entirely eliminate the increased bleeding risk in patients with acquired hemostatic disorders.

Prevention of Bleeding in Patients with Congenital Hemostatic Disorders

The factor level should be increased to at least 70% in hemophilia patients scheduled for liver biopsy. Recommendations on the duration of the correction range from 1 to 7 days.[92] A target level of 50% is considered adequate at some centers (T. Bernatik, personal communication, 2010). An IU factor concentrate will raise the factor level by approximately 2% (factor VIII, hemophilia A) or 1% (factor IX, hemophilia B). A consultation with a hemostasis expert is strongly advised before any intervention.

9.3.3 Risk Reduction Techniques

Prevention of Bleeding

Many methods have been described for making percutaneous biopsies safer in patients with an increased bleeding risk. All employ coaxial techniques to plug the needle tract with a hemostatic agent (Floseal, Gelfoam, Fclaspon)[93–97] or seal it by radiofrequency cauterization.[94,98,99]

Prevention of Pneumothorax

The risk of pneumothorax after percutaneous lung biopsy could be reduced in animal experiments and in a small comparative study by plugging the needle tract with fibrin glue.[100,101] The use of a coaxial needle with continuous suction also reduced the risk of pneumothorax during CT-guided lung biopsies in experimental animals.[102]

Prevention of Needle Tract Seeding

Prophylactic radiotherapy to the needle tract is often practiced after the transthoracic biopsy of pleural mesothelioma, although two of three randomized controlled studies showed no benefit from this procedure.[65]

Further studies are needed to determine whether different methodologies such as the coaxial biopsy technique,[103] specific biopsy needles,[57] or ablation of the needle tract[99] after percutaneous biopsy or other interventions for malignancies can reduce the risk of tumor seeding.

Prevention of Damage to Adjacent Organs during Thermoablation

A thermal protection technique such as the local injection of saline solution (hydrodissection) is an important precaution in cases where the target lesion for thermoablation (radiofrequency ablation [RFA] or microwave ablation [MWA]) is located close to nearby organs (gallbladder, colon) or duct systems (bile duct, urinary tract). The ureter can be splinted in retrograde fashion (see local tumor therapies in Chapter 19).

9.3.4 Local Anesthesia and Intravenous Sedation

Thorough local anesthesia with a moderately long-acting agent (e.g., lidocaine 1%, prilocaine 1%) is a fundamental requirement for preventing pain, uncontrolled movements, and associated complications during percutaneous interventions. After a skin wheal is raised, the proposed needle tract and especially the peritoneum in the needle path should be adequately anesthetized using a very thin needle (25–22 gauge) under ultrasound guidance. All air should be expelled from the needle and syringe before the injection; otherwise tiny air bubbles would enter the needle track, causing troublesome artifacts that could hamper the biopsy or intervention. A periprostatic nerve block with 1 to 2% lidocaine is effective prior to ultrasound-guided transrectal prostatic biopsy.

Intravenous sedation (midazolam, possibly combined with pethidine, fentanyl, or piritramide) limits the ability of the patient to cooperate with the intervention (respiratory maneuvers) but may be advisable before diagnostic biopsies in very anxious and restless patients. Intravenous sedation is generally necessary for prolonged and painful therapeutic interventions such as percutaneous transhepatic cholangiodrainage (PTCD) and tumor ablation.

> **Note**
>
> Preinterventional patient education and trust are the best remedies in anxious or uncooperative patients.

9.3.5 Prevention of Infection

It is widely agreed that the ultrasound probe used in a percutaneous biopsy should be disinfected, sterilized, or preferably covered with a sterile sheath, especially in therapeutic interventions and in immunocompromised patients. The disinfection and sterilization of ultrasound probes should follow manufacturers' recommendations, which often prohibit the use of alcohol-based disinfectants (see Chapter 8). Sterilization is feasible only for biopsy transducers. Alcohol-free wipes (e.g., Mikrobac Tissues from BODE) are excellent for probe disinfection. Following antiseptic skin preparation at the puncture site (e.g., with an isopropyl alcohol–based disinfectant) and sterile draping of the field, a sterile ultrasound gel or disinfectant spray is applied to the skin for acoustic coupling. The operator and any assistants should clean their hands with a hygienic handrub and don sterile gloves. In therapeutic interventions, the intervention team should also wear a sterile gown, mask, and cap, and a sterile instrument table should be prepared[104–106] (see Chapter 8).

Antibiotic prophylaxis (especially with ciprofloxacin and other gyrase inhibitors) is standard practice for ultrasound-guided transrectal prostate biopsy.[107–109] One preinterventional dose is sufficient.[110,111] Rectal preparation has proven beneficial before ultrasound-guided prostate biopsy.[112] Several studies have also shown that a povidone-iodine enema or suppository before transrectal ultrasound-guided biopsy can lower the rate of infectious complications.[113–115]

9.3.6 Optimal Approach and Alternatives

Numerous studies have shown that liver and renal biopsies performed with ultrasound guidance have lower complication rates than when the biopsy site is selected based on clinical criteria. Thus, imaging guidance (generally by ultrasound) should be used not only for biopsies of focal lesions and therapeutic interventions but also for parenchymal biopsies of the liver and kidney.[116–118] One study found that in 15.1% of cases, ultrasound biopsy guidance prompted a change in the biopsy site that had been chosen based only on clinical criteria. Ultrasound guidance facilitated avoidance of intervening blood vessels and other organs.[119] Before the needle is introduced, time should be taken to check various patient positions and depths of respiration to find the safest access route to the lesion. Proper selection of the ultrasound probe is also important for a safe and successful intervention. In the case of patients and/or needle paths with a high risk of complications, alternatives to the ultrasound-guided intervention should be considered. In some situations, computed tomography or endosonography will provide safer and easier guidance for lesions that are difficult to visualize with ultrasound or are located in the mediastinum, posterior retroperitoneum, or lesser pelvis. Endosonographic guidance should particularly be considered for the diagnostic biopsy or drainage of lesions located in the posterior mediastinum or close to the gastrointestinal tract, in the left suprarenal area, or in the pancreas. Even very small lesions of the liver and spleen can be biopsied endosonographically with high accuracy and very low risk (see Chapter 22).[120] Other alternatives are a transjugular parenchymal biopsy of the liver or kidney, especially in patients with a high bleeding risk, morbid obesity, or significant ascites[121–124]; laparoscopic biopsy; and open biopsy.

> **Note**
>
> Invest time and patience in selecting the optimum position and biopsy route ("measure twice and cut once").

9.4 Contraindications

For the most part, contraindications to ultrasound-guided interventions have not been validated by clinical studies but are based on traditional experience and "good clinical practice." Of course, an invasive procedure should not be performed if the patient (or guardian) is inadequately informed or has not consented to the procedure (▶ Table 9.3). This principle may be violated only in life-threatening situations and emergent procedures to which the patient cannot give informed consent. Inability of the patient to cooperate with the procedure or inadequate sonographic needle guidance may create a situation in which an ultrasound-guided procedure cannot be performed with reasonable risk or must be terminated.

Before every biopsy, it should be determined by interdisciplinary consultation whether the result is likely to have a significant impact on further diagnosis and management. Since there is a relative risk of seeding tumor cells along the needle tract, adversely affecting the prognosis, preoperative biopsy confirmation should generally be withheld in patients with presumed liver malignancies that are considered resectable.[125]

9.4.1 Coagulopathies

The limits stated in textbooks and reviews for parameters such as platelet counts and plasmatic coagulation factors differ slightly from one another, due mainly to a lack of

Table 9.3 Contraindications to ultrasound-guided interventions

Type (absolute or relative contraindication)	Contraindication
Absolute contraindications	Lack of patient education and informed consent
	Lack of patient cooperation
	Biopsy result is unlikely to influence further diagnostic and therapeutic actions
	Poor ultrasound needle guidance
	Treatment with oral anticoagulants or severe plasmatic coagulation disorder: INR > 1.5, PTT > 50 s, platelets < 50×10^9/L, therapeutic heparinization, treatment with thrombin inhibitors (e.g., hirudin, dagibatran) or factor Xa antagonists (e.g., fondaparinux, rivaroxaban, apixaban, edoxaban)
	Treatment with antiplatelet drugs of the thienopyridine class or ADP-receptor antagonists (clopidogrel, ticlopidine, prasugrel, ticagrelor) or glycoprotein IIb/IIIa receptor antagonists (abciximab, eptifabatide, tirofiban)
Relative contraindications	Preoperative biopsy of resectable liver malignancies
	High-risk access route (blood vessels, bowel)
	Target lesion assumed to have a high bleeding risk (e.g., suspected hepatic adenoma or subcapsular hemangioma)
	Superficial lesions in parenchymal organs (scant parenchymal coverage)
	Close proximity of the target lesion for ultrasound-guided ablation to major vessels, the gallbladder, or tubular structures (bile duct, renal pelvis, ureter)
	Adrenal masses whose differential diagnosis includes pheochromocytoma
	Suspected hydatid cyst

confirmation by controlled studies. The figures stated in ▶ Table 9.3 should be considered as guidelines only. They may have to be modified in selected cases depending on the urgency of the indication, the risk of the proposed intervention, and individual risk factors for bleeding complications. In one series of 47 patients with focal liver lesions and severe coagulopathy (platelet count < 50×10^9/L and/or prothrombin time ratio < 50%) who underwent fine needle liver biopsy guided by color Doppler ultrasound, there were no instances of severe bleeding, and minor complications occurred in only 3 patients (8.5%).[126] Embolization of the needle tract with procoagulant agents after biopsy was found to be a safe technique in similar populations.[96,127,128] Any departures from the above contraindications should be noted during the informed consent process and should be documented along with the reason for deviating from standard recommendations.

9.4.2 Procoagulant Therapy and Antiplatelet Drugs

Regarding treatment with procoagulant agents and antiplatelet drugs, it is important to weigh the benefits and risks of an ultrasound-guided intervention on the one hand and the discontinuation or reversal of this therapy on the other hand, as well as the urgency of the proposed intervention. In making this decision, the indication for anticoagulant or antiplatelet therapy must be known. In some cases the risks should be assessed in consultation with the prescribing physician (cardiologist, angiologist, vascular surgeon, neurologist). The risk assessment should be expressly noted during informed consent and should be documented. Pharmacologic parameters should be considered in timing the intervention and in reversing anticoagulant or antiplatelet therapy.

9.4.3 “Risky” Lesions and Access Routes

Hemangiomas, among others, have been cited in the literature as “risky lesions” for ultrasound-guided biopsy. Nevertheless, small case series have been published that report the uncomplicated ultrasound-guided biopsy of liver hemangiomas.[129,130] There is even more evidence to document the safety of ultrasound-guided biopsies of splenic parenchyma and focal splenic lesions.[13,131–136]

The access route for a needle biopsy is considered a relative risk that depends on the experience of the interventionalist. The ultrasound-guided percutaneous biopsy of deep retroperitoneal lymph nodes as well as mesenteric, gastrointestinal, perivascular, and splenic masses was long considered to be a risky procedure. But ultrasound guidance, with its capability for real-time visualization of target lesions in various planes and for graded compression, is useful for optimizing the access route. Indeed, studies in recent years have shown that even the lesions mentioned above as involving "risky access" can be biopsied under ultrasound guidance with little risk[106,137–147] (see Section 9.6, Specific Biopsy Sites).

Caution

When relative contraindications are present, it is important to weigh the risks carefully and also to make a critical appraisal of one's own expertise.

9.5 Management of Complications

9.5.1 Postinterventional Care and Detection of Complications

Ultrasound imaging is performed immediately after the intervention to check for new fluid collections, free air, pneumothorax, catheter malposition, or other evidence of a complication. A sign suggestive of clinically significant bleeding is the persistence of a "patent track," or flow along the needle tract detectable by color duplex scanning (▶ Fig. 9.1).

In a study of 352 patients who underwent ultrasound-guided liver biopsy, postbiopsy Doppler ultrasound detected flow along the needle tract in 43 cases (12%). In 39 patients the flow disappeared in less than 5 minutes. Clinically significant bleeding occurred in 5 patients. Four of these patients had a patent track that was demonstrable more than 5 minutes post biopsy in three cases.[148] A perirenal hematoma detectable after percutaneous renal biopsy is a predictor of clinically significant bleeding complications (positive predictive value [PPV] 43%, negative predictive value [NPV] 95%) (▶ Fig. 9.2).[36,149]

Every ultrasound-guided biopsy or therapeutic intervention should be followed by appropriate postinterventional care. We suggest that a percutaneous ultrasound-guided biopsy be followed by bed rest for 2 hours with vital signs checked every 30 minutes (general status, pain or other symptoms, blood pressure, pulse). If there are clinical signs suggestive of a complication, the first measure is a repeat ultrasound, which may be supplemented if needed by other imaging studies (CT, angiography). Contrast-enhanced ultrasound (CEUS) is an excellent and repeatable study for detecting persistent active bleeding (▶ Fig. 9.3)[150] or catheter malposition.[151]

The great majority of complications occur immediately or within 4 hours after the intervention. More than 80% occur within 24 hours.[7,8,29,40,152] In one study distinguished by a large percentage of patients with a high bleeding risk (40%), 70% of the complications occurred more than 24 hours after liver biopsy.[32] But in cooperative and mobile patients with no apparent risk factors, an observation period of several hours to 24 hours should be adequate after an ultrasound-guided biopsy. A postinterventional ultrasound examination is recommended before the patient is discharged. The discharge interview with the patient should note the possibility of late complications and describe their symptoms, and this information should be documented. Any complications that arise in association with ultrasound-guided interventions should be documented in a standardized, prospective format at every center.

Note

Standardized postinterventional care and the documentation of complications are mandatory.

9.5.2 Treatment of Complications

In the event of complications, immediate treatment should be instituted that includes basic stabilizing measures plus any complication-specific interventions that are required. Pain without a clinically or radiologically apparent cause is managed with standard analgesics (e.g., novaminsulfon and/or pethidine, fentanyl, or piritramide). Infectious complications require appropriate antibiotic therapy, which should take into account any preinterventional antibiotic prophylaxis.

If significant bleeding occurs, coagulation tests should be performed. Depending on the test results and known risk factors, replacement therapy or the intravenous administration of desmopressin may be indicated. Hemostasis can usually be obtained with conservative measures (▶ Fig. 9.2). The possibility of an ultrasound-guided intervention should always be considered, such as the CEUS- or color-Doppler-guided injection of human thrombin solution, fibrin glue, cyanoacrylate, or hemocoagulase into a pseudoaneurysm or intraparenchymal bleeding site (▶ Fig. 9.1e, f).[153,154] The angiographically or EUS-guided obliteration of a bleeding artery or pseudoaneurysm is a less invasive alternative to an operative procedure (see Chapter 22).

9.6 Specific Biopsy Sites

9.6.1 Liver Biopsy

Data Source

Several survey studies and numerous retrospective single-center and multicenter studies.

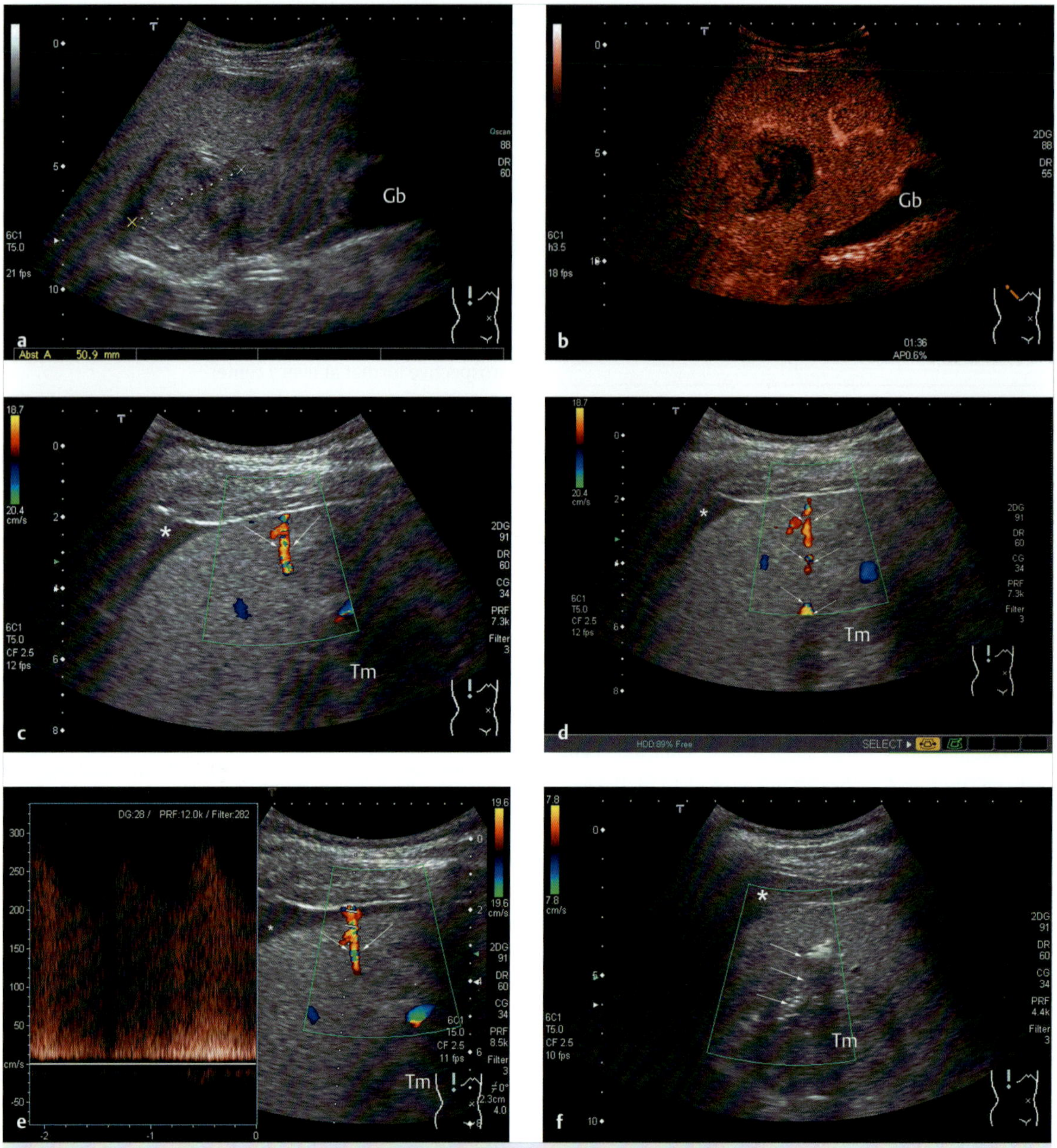

Fig. 9.1 "Patent track sign" and intra-abdominal bleeding after biopsy (18-gauge BioPince, Pflugbeil) of a liver mass in a cirrhosis patient (male, 60 years old; histology: hepatocellular carcinoma in a setting of hemochromatosis).

a Heterogeneous mass approximately 5 cm in diameter with an echogenic pseudocapsule (Gb: gallbladder).

b On contrast-enhanced ultrasound (1.5 mL SonoVue, Bracco) the mass shows arterial-phase hypervascularity with partial washout in the late phase.

c, d Image at 1 min post biopsy (18-gauge BioPince) shows a hypoechoic stripe between the liver and peritoneum (asterisk) and a high-frequency flow signal (arrows) between the tumor mass (Tm) and liver capsule. Blood flow past the liver capsule is also well defined by PW Doppler.

e, f When bleeding persisted for more than 5 min and the patient developed pain and hypotension, thrombin solution was injected into the biopsy tract with a 22-gauge needle under sonographic guidance. Bleeding ceased immediately after the injection (arrows: high-level echoes after thrombin injection). The initially hypoechoic subphrenic hematoma appears markedly more echogenic 25 minutes after the onset of bleeding (asterisk). It was no longer detectable the following day.

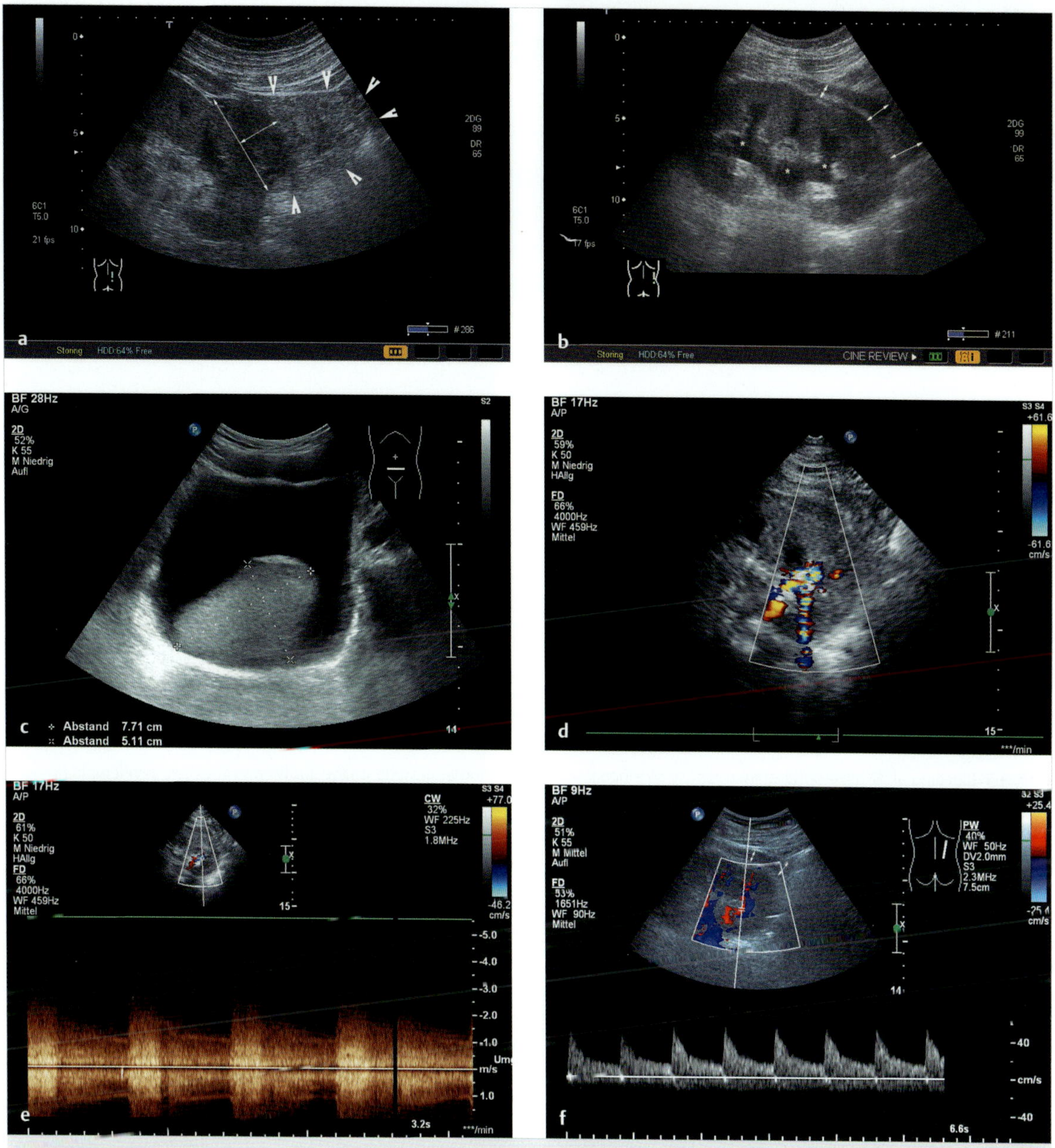

Fig. 9.2 Clinically significant bleeding and small arteriovenous fistula after parenchymal renal biopsy (18-gauge BioPince) in a patient with nephrotic syndrome.

a Immediate postbiopsy image in complaint-free patient shows a hypoechoic subcapsular hematoma (between the markers) and an echogenic pararenal hematoma (arrowheads) at the biopsy site (lower third of kidney).

b At 7 hours post biopsy the patient has flank pain, hematuria, incomplete bladder emptying and strangury, hydronephrosis (asterisks), and a slightly progressive hematoma (arrows).

c Another image at 7 hours post biopsy demonstrates a large echogenic clot (between markers) in the distended bladder.

d The cause of bleeding into the renal collecting system is an arteriovenous fistula in the lower third of the kidney (color Doppler).

e Fistula flow sampled by CW Doppler: peak systolic velocity (PSV) 3 m/s, end diastolic velocity (EDV) 1.3 m/s.

f The patient was reexamined after treatment (bed rest, bladder irrigation, transfusion of two units of packed red cells). The bleeding stopped in 3 days. At discharge the patient had normal urination and no complaints. Ultrasound scan before discharge shows a small residual hematoma (arrows). A normal Doppler waveform is sampled from the segmental artery in the lower third of the kidney.

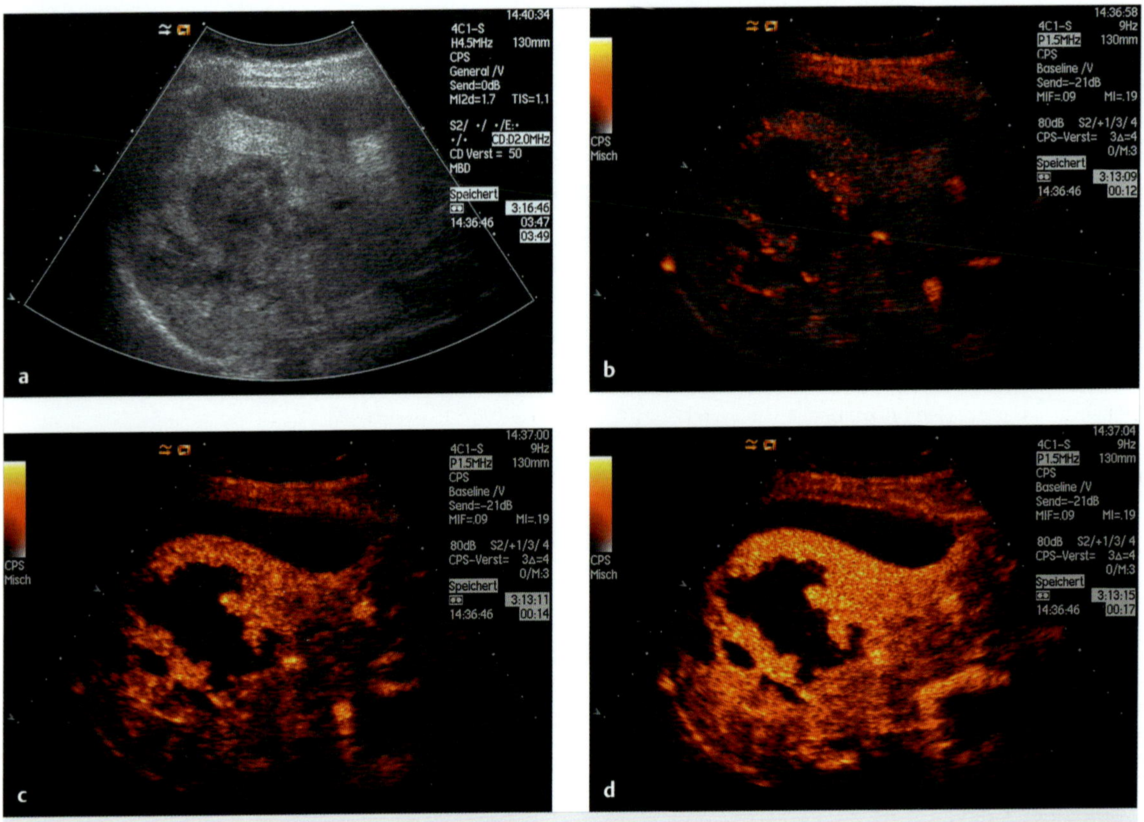

Fig. 9.3 Bleeding after ultrasound-guided biopsy of a hepatocellular adenoma. B-mode image shows a hypoechoic perihepatic fluid collection (**a**). Contrast-enhanced ultrasound images (**b–d**) display the true extent of the hemorrhage.

Complication Rates

More comprehensive data are available on ultrasound-guided parenchymal liver biopsies than on biopsies of focal liver lesions. An Italian study reported no serious complications or deaths in a total of 16,648 ultrasound-guided biopsies of focal liver lesions performed over a 22-year period.[20] Other groups of authors have reported major complications in up to 3.5% of cases, most consisting of intraperitoneal hemorrhage (▶ Fig. 9.1, ▶ Table 9.4).

Specific Complications

Hemobilia (0.059–0.2%); biliary peritonitis (0.03–0.22%); pneumothorax or pleural effusion (0.08–0.28%); arteriovenous or arterioportal fistula (5.4%); obstructive cholestasis, cholecystitis, cholangitis and/or biliary pancreatitis due to hemobilia (sporadic cases); sepsis (sporadic cases); and accidental puncture or perforation of nearby organs (sporadic cases). (Incidence data are drawn from sources cited in ▶ Table 9.4 and from statistical data in reference [49].)

Table 9.4 Complication rates of ultrasound-guided liver biopsy

	Mortality	Major complications	Minor complications	Bleeding	Needle tract seeding
Parenchymal biopsy	0–0.25% (0.48%)[a]	0.09–2.3%	Up to 13.6%[b]	Major, ca. 0.5% (up to 1.6%)[a] Minor, up to 9.9%[a]	–
Biopsy of liver masses	0–0.8%[c]	0.5–3.5%[d]	0–8.5%[e]	Up to 1.3%[d]	Hepatocellular carcinoma: 2.7%[f] Metastases: up to 19%[g]

[a] Data from a prospective single-center study with a large percentage (40%) of high-risk patients.[32]
[b] Data from a 20-year review of parenchymal liver biopsies at an Australian center ($n = 1398$).[17]
[c] One death in 129 fine needle biopsies of focal liver lesions due to fatal hemorrhage.[207]
[d] Fourteen major complications (tumor seeding in 9 patients, bleeding in 5) in 391 biopsies for suspected hepatocellular carcinoma.[208]
[e] Three minor complications in 47 biopsies of focal liver lesions in patients with severe coagulopathy.[126]
[f] Meta-analysis of 8 studies.[62]
[g] Percutaneous and intraoperative biopsy of liver metastases from colorectal cancer.

Table 9.5 Complication rates of ultrasound-guided renal biopsy

	Mortality	Major complications	Minor complications	Bleeding	Needle tract seeding
Parenchymal biopsy	0–0.2%	0–6.4%	3–13%	Minor, up to 35% Major, 0–3.7%	–
Biopsy of renal masses	None	0–0.9%[a]	0–5.3%		7 cases in the literature[b]

[a] Two major complications in 235 percutaneous renal biopsies of small, incidental renal tumors.[209]
[b] Survey in reference [90].

Specific Contraindications

Specific (relative) contraindications to percutaneous liver biopsy are an untreated biliary obstruction (risk of biliary peritonitis), lack of parenchymal coverage of focal target lesions, and a risky access route (major blood vessels, gallbladder, interposed colon). Moreover, all noninvasive diagnostic options (CEUS) should be exhausted in an effort to avoid the biopsy of lesions with a very high bleeding risk (adenomas, focal nodular hyperplasia, hemangioma). It is also better to avoid the biopsy of a probable HCC and instead rely on noninvasive studies meeting the criteria of the American Association for the Study of Liver Diseases (AASLD) or the European Association for the Study of the Liver (EASL)—especially before a planned liver transplantation. We also feel that the biopsy of imaging-confirmed hepatic metastases from colorectal cancer is contraindicated if, for example, neoadjuvant chemotherapy might allow for a resection with curative intent.

Alternatives

Recommended alternatives are

- Endosonographically guided fine needle aspiration (EUS-FNA) and EUS-guided Trucut biopsy (EUS-TCB) (especially with very small masses in the hepatic left lobe that are difficult to demonstrate and reach percutaneously; parenchymal liver biopsy in a patient with coagulopathy[155–158]
- Transjugular liver biopsy (especially in patients with a high bleeding risk, significant ascites, or morbid obesity)[124]
- Laparoscopic biopsy

9.6.2 Renal Biopsy

Data Source

Numerous retrospective single- and multicenter studies.

Complication Rates

Renal biopsies have a somewhat higher complication rate than liver biopsies (▶ Table 9.5). The risk of organ loss due to complications is less than 0.1%, however, and was 0.4% in only one study.[159] The complication rates of biopsies are lower in renal allografts than in native kidneys.[159]

Specific Complications

Subcapsular or perirenal hematoma (up to 91%; ▶ Fig. 9.2a); hematuria (7.4–35%; ▶ Fig. 9.2c); arteriovenous fistula (0.4–9%; ▶ Fig. 9.2d, e); urinary tract infection (up to 1%); urosepsis (up to 0.7%); hydronephrosis/bladder tamponade (no data available, ▶ Fig. 9.2b, c); renal function impairment (> 0.2 mg/dL; 2.2%); pneumothorax. (Incidence data from sources and reviews cited in ▶ Table 9.5.[47,90,160–163])

Specific Contraindications

Specific contraindications to percutaneous renal biopsy are uncontrolled arterial hypertension (> 140/90 mmHg), ureteral obstruction with insufficient drainage (risk of urinoma and abscess), acute pyelonephritis, a suspected vascular malformation or vascular tumor, and a solitary native kidney.[47] The percutaneous biopsy of suspected urothelial cell carcinoma is not recommended due to its very high metastatic potential.[161,162]

Alternatives

- Transjugular biopsy, especially in patients with coagulopathy or severe obesity[47,122]
- CT-guided biopsy in obese patients
- Laparoscopic and open surgical biopsy
- Left kidney: EUS-guided FNA[164]

9.6.3 Pancreatic Biopsy

Data Source

Several retrospective single- and multicenter studies in a total population of more than 3,500 patients.

Complication Rates

The overall complication rate ranges from 1.5 to 20% (review of the literature in Zamboni[165]). A multicenter Italian survey study ($n = 510$) found an overall complication rate of 4.9%.[27] A large single-center retrospective study in Italy ($n = 545$) reports an overall complication rate of 1.5% including minor complications such as pain, vasovagal reactions, or free fluid.[165] The biopsy of pancreatic allografts does not have a higher risk than biopsies of the native pancreas.[106]

Comparison with the complication rates of EUS-FNA determined in prospective studies, some carefully designed, is difficult due to the differences in study design. In one prospective single-center study of 355 cases, the 30-day rate of major complications in the EUS-FNA of pancreatic masses was 2.5%.[166]

Specific Complications

Acute pancreatitis; pancreatic pseudocyst.

Specific Contraindications

Due to the risk of peritoneal tumor seeding, the percutaneous biopsy of a solid pancreatic tumor should be avoided if operative treatment is planned. Even with EUS guidance, a pancreatic mass should be biopsied only if necessary for differential diagnostic reasons or to provide definitive histology in a palliative setting.[120]

Alternatives

- EUS-FNA

9.6.4 Splenic Biopsy

Data Source

Retrospective multicenter survey study ($n = 398$)[132] and several retrospective single- and multicenter studies totaling more than 2000 cases.

Complication Rates

The complications of splenic biopsy consist almost entirely of bleeding and associated organ rupture. The risk of complication-related organ loss is as high as 1.6%.[133] Two retrospective studies of ultrasound-guided percutaneous fine needle biopsies of the spleen—one Italian (160 cases) and one Indian (95 cases)—reported zero complications.[131,134] The overall complication rate in a multicenter Italian study was 5.2%, with a < 1% rate of major complications and no reported deaths.[132]

Overall complication rate: 0 to 16.7%; major complications: 0 to 3.2%.[131–134]

Specific Complications

None.

9.6.5 Biopsy of Gastrointestinal Hollow Organs and Mesenteric Masses

Data Source

Several retrospective case series with small numbers of patients (total $n = 190$).

Complication Rates

The seven case series to date have reported a total of 9 minor complications (pain, hematoma, abdominal wall infection) and one major complication (biliary peritonitis).[137,139–143,145]

Specific Complications

Peritonitis.

Specific Contraindications

Immune deficiency.

Alternatives

- EUS-FNA and EUS-TCB (wall lesions of the rectum and upper digestive tract)

9.6.6 Adrenal Biopsy

Data Source

Small case series, mostly involving CT- and ultrasound-guided interventions.

Complication Rates

The complication rates reported for image-guided adrenal biopsies range from 0 to 8.4%.[167–172] The largest series consisted of 277 adrenal biopsies, some with ultrasound guidance, and reported a complication rate of 2.8%.[172] Surgical authors have described small, selected case series of patients with very high complication rates after adrenal biopsy.[173,174]

To date, only one case of a procedure-related complication has been reported after the EUS-FNA of adrenal masses.[175]

Specific Complications

Hypertensive crisis due to pheochromocytoma biopsy; pneumothorax; bleeding.

Specific Contraindications

Suspected pheochromocytoma. Urinary or plasma metanephrines should be determined before adrenal biopsy is performed in patients with no prior history of a malignant tumor.

Alternatives

- EUS-FNA (suspected left adrenal mass),[176] laparoscopic biopsy or adrenalectomy.

9.6.7 Lungs, Pleura, and Mediastinum

Data Source

Numerous retrospective case series and one large, prospective single-center series.[177]

Complication Rates

Pleural biopsy: major complications in < 1%[178]; biopsy of peripheral lung nodules: approximately 10%.[179]

Specific Complications

Pneumothorax (in a collective statistical analysis of 1,760 ultrasound-guided transthoracic biopsies: 2.8%, with 1% requiring a chest tube; in a prospective series of 307 patients: 2.9%).[180] Hemoptysis (0–2%); bronchopleural fistula; pleural empyema; hemothorax; hemopericardium (very rare); air embolism; chest wall infection (sporadic cases). Risk factors for the development of pneumothorax are COPD/emphysema, cough, age, number of needle passes, depth of lesion, and use of aspiration needles.[179,181]

The risk of needle tract seeding in the percutaneous biopsy of a pleural mesothelioma is between 0% and 22%.[65]

Specific Contraindications

Pulmonary arterial hypertension contraindicates the transthoracic biopsy of peripheral lung nodules and pleural lesions due to the significantly increased risk of bleeding. Decompensated COPD or severe pulmonary emphysema are also contraindications due to the markedly increased risk of pneumothorax and air embolism. Additionally, an ultrasound-guided lung or pleural biopsy would be contraindicated if the development of a procedure-related pneumothorax or hemothorax would be acutely life-threatening due to severe ventilatory impairment or status post contralateral pneumonectomy.[179,181]

Alternatives

- CT-guided biopsy (masses distant from the pleura)
- EUS-FNA (endoscopic ultrasound-guided fine needle aspiration)
- EBUS-TBNA (endobronchial ultrasound-guided transbronchial needle aspiration)
- Bronchoscopic biopsy
- Transbronchial needle aspiration (depending on location)
- Mediastinoscopic biopsy
- Thoracoscopic biopsy

9.7 Specific Interventions

9.7.1 EUS-FNA, EUS-TCB, EBUS-TBNA

- EUS-FNA (endoscopic ultrasound-guided fine needle aspiration)
- EUS-TCB (endoscopic ultrasound-guided Trucut biopsy)
- EBUS-TBNA (endobronchial ultrasound-guided transbronchial needle aspiration)

Data Source

Numerous prospective and retrospective single-center and multicenter studies, some with specific indications and target organs, registry studies, and retrospective multicenter surveys.

Complication Rates

Overall complication rates

- EUS-FNA: 0.3–2.2%[120]; in a current meta-analysis of 51 studies with 10,941 cases: 0.98% (mortality 0.02%)[182,183]
- EUS-TCB: up to 2.4%[184]
- EBUS-TBNA: 0%[185]

Specific Complications

Bleeding (intraluminal: 4%; extraluminal: 1.3%); site-dependent septic complications (especially in EUS-FNA of cystic lesions in the mediastinum and pancreas); acute pancreatitis (0.29–2.0%); tumor seeding (7 documented sporadic cases).[120,182,183]

Specific Contraindications

EUS-FNA of cystic mediastinal lesions and liver lesions associated with insufficient drainage of obstructed bile ducts.

Alternatives

- Percutaneous biopsy
- Endoscopic biopsy
- Ductal brush cytology
- Bronchoscopic biopsy
- TBNA (transbronchial needle aspiration)
- Laparoscopy
- Mediastinoscopy
- Thoracoscopy

9.7.2 EUS-Guided Therapeutic Interventions

Data Source

Numerous retrospective studies.

Complication Rates

Overall complication rates[186]

- EUS-guided pseudocyst drainage: 0 to 18%
- EUS-guided drainage of pancreatic necrosis and abscesses: 0 to 31%
- EUS-guided celiac plexus block (EUS-CPB) or celiac plexus neurolysis (EUS-CPN): 1.6 to 8.2%; major complications: 0.5 to 0.6%
- EUS-guided cholangiodrainage (EUS-CD): 0 to 20%; mortality up to 4%
- EUS-guided pancreatic duct drainage (EUS-PD): 14 to 25%

Specific Complications

Procedure-specific complications

- EUS-guided drainage of pseudocysts, necrosis, abscesses: bleeding (intraluminal, intraperitoneal, intracystic), stent migration or occlusion, secondary pseudocyst infection, pneumoperitoneum, perforation/peritonitis, gallbladder perforation, air embolism
- EUS-CPB, EUS-CPN: self-limiting hypotension, self-limiting diarrhea, self-limiting pain, retroperitoneal infection, retroperitoneal bleeding, end-organ ischemia of the celiac trunk (spleen, stomach: sporadic cases)
- EUS-CD: stent migration or occlusion, cholangitis, cholecystitis, pneumoperitoneum, bilioma, biliary peritonitis, intraluminal bleeding, hemobilia, pancreatitis
- EUS-PD: pancreatitis, pseudocyst development, bleeding, infection, pneumoperitoneum, perforation
- EUS-guided tumor ablation (neuroendocrine pancreatic tumors, pancreatic cysts): pancreatitis

Specific Contraindications

Portal hypertension with interposition of collateral vessels in the needle tract, hemorrhagic pseudocysts.

Alternatives

Alternatives to specific procedures

- EUS-guided drainage of pseudocysts, necrosis, abscesses: percutaneous drainage, open drainage
- EUS-CPB/CPN: percutaneous approach (largely abandoned)
- EUS-CD: retrograde drainage (ERC), PTCD, biliary-enteric anastomosis
- EUS-PD: drainage operations

9.7.3 Transrectal Prostatic Biopsy

Data Source

Numerous prospective and retrospective single- and multicenter studies.

Complication Rates

The incidence of hospital admissions for urologic (mainly infectious) complications of ambulatory transrectal prostate biopsy increased dramatically in Ontario, Canada, rising from 1.0% in 1996 to 4.1% by 2005. The 30-day mortality rate remained unchanged at 0.09%.[55] Increasing numbers of biopsies may play a role, accompanied by a rise of bacterial resistance to peri-interventional gyrase inhibitors.[53,54] Bleeding is a frequent occurrence (hematuria in approximately 80%, hematospermia up to 50%, rectal bleeding up to 14%) but is rarely severe (up to 2.5%).

Specific Complications

Urinary tract infection (up to 11%[28]; caution: infections with extended spectrum beta-lactamase-producing bacteria); prostatitis (up to 2%[187]); bacteremia, sepsis (up to 3.1%[53]); meningitis (sporadic cases); bladder dysfunction and/or urinary retention (up to 0.4%[51]).

Specific Contraindications

None.

Alternatives

- Perineal biopsy
- Transurethral biopsy

9.7.4 Ultrasound-Guided Drainage (of Cysts, Pseudocysts, Abscesses, Cholecystitis)

Data Source

Numerous studies, mostly single-center, that are very heterogeneous and difficult to compare with one another.

Complication Rates

There is a lack of prospective data comparing, say, percutaneous needle drainage and catheter drainage as well as different drainage techniques. It is difficult to differentiate between abscess-related and procedure-related mortality and morbidity. The risks depend on patient-specific factors, the anatomical location and size of the fluid collection, and the technique that is used, to name but a few factors. Bacteremia immediately after the percutaneous drainage of intra-abdominal abscesses is common and was observed in 7 of 27 patients (26%) in one series.[188] Also common are technical drainage complications (dislodgment, occlusion), which occurred in 11.2% of cases in a series of 107 image-guided drainage procedures for abdominopelvic fluid collections.[189] Larger published case series report overall procedure-related complication rates ranging from 0 to approximately 30% and a procedure-related mortality of 4.2%.[189–196]

Specific Complications

Bacteremia and sepsis; intraperitoneal bleeding; bleeding into parenchyma or abscesses; perforation of an abscess or pseudocyst; hollow viscus injury with peritonitis; secondary abscess formation; pleural empyema; drain occlusion or dislodgment with secondary infection; fistula formation.

Specific Contraindications

Transpleural or transintestinal catheter drainage should be avoided.

Alternatives

- EUS-guided transesophageal, transgastric, transduodenal or transrectal drainage of an abscess or pseudocyst (see Chapter 22)[186]

9.7.5 Ultrasound-Guided PTCD and Cholecystotomy

Data Source

Several studies, mostly single-center.

Complication Rates

- **PTCD (percutaneous transhepatic cholangiodrainage):** mortality 0 to 2%; overall complication rate 0 to 22%[197,198]
- **Percutaneous gallbladder drainage:** mortality 0.36%, overall complication rate 6.24% (based on meta-analysis of 53 studies with 1,198 patients, including cases with image-guided percutaneous cholecystotomy[199])

Specific Complications

Hemobilia, portobiliary fistula; complications of hemobilia (drain occlusion, cholangitis, cholecystitis, biliary peritonitis); sepsis; pleural empyema; hemothorax; peritonitis.

Specific Contraindications

Transpleural catheter drainage should be avoided.

Alternatives

- Endoscopic retrograde cholangiopancreatography (ERCP) with retrograde bile duct drainage
- EUS-guided bile duct and gallbladder drainage
- Percutaneous-endoscopic and endosonographic-endoscopic rendezvous techniques
- Operative biliary-enteric anastomosis

9.7.6 Ultrasound-guided Tumor Ablation Therapy

Data Source

Numerous studies, mostly single-center, that are heterogeneous and difficult to compare with one another (patients, indications, interventional technique).

Complication Rates

Procedure-specific complication rates

- **Percutaneous ethanol injection (PEI) and percutaneous acetic acid injection (PAI) for liver tumors:** major complications 2.7%; all complications 10.5% (based on meta-analysis of 5 studies comparing PEI and RFA[200])
- **Radiofrequency ablation (RFA) of liver tumors:** mortality 0.3%; major complications 2.4%; minor complications 4.7% (data from Italian multicenter study, $n = 3{,}554$[201]), A meta-analysis of 5 studies comparing PEI and RFA: major complications 4.1%, all complications 19.2%[200,202]
- **RFA of renal tumors:** a survey of 6 case series with image-guided RFA of renal tumors ($n = 401$) that includes CT-guided RFA: mortality 0.25%, major complications 8.2%[178]

Specific Complications

Procedure-specific complications

- **PEI of liver tumors:** needle tract seeding (PEI with biopsy: 1.4%[61])
- **PEI of hydatid cysts:** mortality 0.7%; major complications (anaphylaxis, abscess formation, bleeding, fistulation) 3.5%; minor complications 2.1% (pain) (data from a prospective study with 143 patients[203])
- **PAI of HCC:** fever in 9.2%; bacteremia in 1%; abscess formation in 0.25% of cases after PAI of HCC[204]
- **RFA/microwave ablation (MWA) of liver tumors:** deterioration of liver function; liver infarction; bleeding; infection (abscess formation, sepsis); pleural effusion; hemothorax; pneumothorax; perforation of nearby organs (gallbladder, bowel); cholecystitis; biliary tract lesion/bilioma; portal vein thrombosis; skin burn[205,206]; needle tract seeding (RFA: 0.61%; RFA with biopsy: 0.95%[61])
- **RFA of renal tumors:** retroperitoneal bleeding; hematuria; urinary tract damage; pneumothorax; damage to the genitofemoral nerve (chronic pain syndrome)[202]

Specific Contraindications

None. Tumors near the capsule are treatable by RFA when precautionary measures are taken.

Alternatives

- Cryoablation
- Open resection
- Liver transplantation
- Transarterial chemoembolization (TACE)
- Selective internal radiotherapy (SIRT)

References

[1] Weiss H, Düntsch U, Weiss AW. Risks of fine needle puncture—results of a survey in West Germany (German Society of Ultrasound in Medicine survey) [Article in German]. Ultraschall Med 1988; 9: 121–127

[2] Weiss H, Düntsch U. [Complications of fine needle puncture. DEGUM survey II]. Ultraschall Med 1996; 17: 118–130

[3] Fornari F, Civardi G, Cavanna L et al. The Cooperative Italian Study Group. Complications of ultrasonically guided fine-needle abdominal biopsy. Results of a multicenter Italian study and review of the literature. Scand J Gastroenterol 1989; 24: 949–955

[4] Fornari F, Buscarini L. Ultrasonically-guided fine-needle biopsy of gastrointestinal organs: indications, results and complications. Dig Dis 1992; 10: 121–133

[5] Smith EH. Complications of percutaneous abdominal fine-needle biopsy. Review. Radiology 1991; 178: 253–258

[6] Ohlsson B, Nilsson J, Stenram U, Akerman M, Tranberg KG. Percutaneous fine-needle aspiration cytology in the diagnosis and management of liver tumours. Br J Surg 2002; 89: 757–762

[7] Piccinino F, Sagnelli E, Pasquale G, Giusti G. Complications following percutaneous liver biopsy. A multicentre retrospective study on 68,276 biopsies. J Hepatol 1986; 2: 165–173

[8] Frieser M, Lindner A, Meyer S et al. Spectrum and bleeding complications of sonographically guided interventions of the liver and pancreas [Article in German]. Ultraschall Med 2009; 30: 168–174

[9] Padia SA, Baker ME, Schaeffer CJ et al. Safety and efficacy of sonographic-guided random real-time core needle biopsy of the liver. J Clin Ultrasound 2009; 37: 138–143

[10] Riemann B, Menzel J, Schiemann U, Domschke W, Konturek JW. Ultrasound-guided biopsies of abdominal organs with an automatic biopsy system. A retrospective analysis of the quality of biopsies and of hemorrhagic complications. Scand J Gastroenterol 2000; 35: 102–107

[11] Froehlich F, Lamy O, Fried M, Gonvers JJ. Practice and complications of liver biopsy. Results of a nationwide survey in Switzerland. Dig Dis Sci 1993; 38: 1480–1484

[12] Buscarini L, Fornari F, Bolondi L et al. Ultrasound-guided fine-needle biopsy of focal liver lesions: techniques, diagnostic accuracy and complications. A retrospective study on 2091 biopsies. J Hepatol 1990; 11: 344–348

[13] Liang P, Gao Y, Wang Y, Yu X, Yu D, Dong B. US-guided percutaneous needle biopsy of the spleen using 18-gauge versus 21-gauge needles. J Clin Ultrasound 2007; 35: 477–482

[14] Nolsøe C, Nielsen L, Torp-Pedersen S, Holm HH. Major complications and deaths due to interventional ultrasonography: a review of 8000 cases. J Clin Ultrasound 1990; 18: 179–184

[15] Nyman RS, Cappelen-Smith J, Brismar J, von Sinner W, Kagevi I. Yield and complications in ultrasound-guided biopsy of abdominal lesions. Comparison of fine-needle aspiration biopsy and 1.2-mm needle core biopsy using an automated biopsy gun. Acta Radiol 1995; 36: 485–490

[16] Pagani JJ. Biopsy of focal hepatic lesions. Comparison of 18 and 22 gauge needles. Radiology 1983; 147: 673–675

[17] van der Poorten D, Kwok A, Lam T et al. Twenty-year audit of percutaneous liver biopsy in a major Australian teaching hospital. Intern Med J 2006; 36: 692–699

[18] Swobodnik W, Janowitz P, Kratzer W et al. Comparison of ultrasound-controlled fine needle and coarse needle puncture of defined lesions in the abdomen [Article in German]. Ultraschall Med 1990; 11: 287–289

[19] McGill DB, Rakela J, Zinsmeister AR, Ott BJ. A 21-year experience with major hemorrhage after percutaneous liver biopsy. Gastroenterology 1990; 99: 1396–1400

[20] Giorgio A, Tarantino L, de Stefano G et al. Complications after interventional sonography of focal liver lesions: a 22-year single-center experience. J Ultrasound Med 2003; 22: 193–205

[21] Buscarini de E. Review of interventional ultrasound in the abdomen: safety first. Ultraschall Med 2004; 24: 11–15 (EFSUMB Newsletter)

[22] Chuah SY, Moody GA, Wicks AC, Mayberry JF. A nationwide survey of liver biopsy—is there a need to increase resources, manpower and training? Hepatogastroenterology 1994; 41: 4–8

[23] Hatfield MK, Beres RA, Sane SS, Zaleski GX. Percutaneous imaging-guided solid organ core needle biopsy: coaxial versus noncoaxial method. AJR Am J Roentgenol 2008; 190: 413–417

[24] Chevallier P, Ruitort F, Denys A et al. Influence of operator experience on performance of ultrasound-guided percutaneous liver biopsy. Eur Radiol 2004; 14: 2086–2091

[25] Copel L, Sosna J, Kruskal JB, Kane RA. Ultrasound-guided percutaneous liver biopsy: indications, risks, and technique. Surg Technol Int 2003; 11: 154–160

[26] Eiro M, Katoh T, Watanabe T. Risk factors for bleeding complications in percutaneous renal biopsy. Clin Exp Nephrol 2005; 9: 40–45

[27] Di Stasi M, Lencioni R, Solmi L et al. Ultrasound-guided fine needle biopsy of pancreatic masses: results of a multicenter study. Am J Gastroenterol 1998; 93: 1329–1333

[28] Djavan B, Waldert M, Zlotta A et al. Safety and morbidity of first and repeat transrectal ultrasound guided prostate needle biopsies: results of a prospective European prostate cancer detection study. J Urol 2001; 166: 856–860

[29] Atwell TD, Smith RL, Hesley GK et al. Incidence of bleeding after 15,181 percutaneous biopsies and the role of aspirin. AJR Am J Roentgenol 2010; 194: 784–789

[30] Seeff LB, Everson GT, Morgan TR et al. HALT-C Trial Group. Complication rate of percutaneous liver biopsies among persons with advanced chronic liver disease in the HALT-C trial. Clin Gastroenterol Hepatol 2010; 8: 877–883

[31] Tabatabai S, Sperati CJ, Atta MG et al. Predictors of complication after percutaneous ultrasound-guided kidney biopsy in HIV-infected individuals: possible role of hepatitis C and HIV co-infection. Clin J Am Soc Nephrol 2009; 4: 1766–1773

[32] Terjung B, Lemnitzer I, Dumoulin FL et al. Bleeding complications after percutaneous liver biopsy. An analysis of risk factors. Digestion 2003; 67: 138–145

[33] Myers RP, Fong A, Shaheen AA. Utilization rates, complications and costs of percutaneous liver biopsy: a population-based study including 4275 biopsies. Liver Int 2008; 28: 705–712

[34] West J, Card TR. Reduced mortality rates following elective percutaneous liver biopsies. Gastroenterology 2010; 139: 1230–1237

[35] González-Michaca L, Chew-Wong A, Soltero L, Gamba G, Correa-Rotter R. Percutaneous kidney biopsy, analysis of 26 years: complication rate and risk factors; comment [Article in Spanish]. Rev Invest Clin 2000; 52: 125–131

[36] Ishikawa E, Nomura S, Hamaguchi T et al. Ultrasonography as a predictor of overt bleeding after renal biopsy. Clin Exp Nephrol 2009; 13: 325–331

[37] Islam N, Fulop T, Zsom L et al. Do platelet function analyzer-100 testing results correlate with bleeding events after percutaneous renal biopsy? Clin Nephrol 2010; 73: 229–237

[38] Manno C, Strippoli GF, Arnesano L et al. Predictors of bleeding complications in percutaneous ultrasound-guided renal biopsy. Kidney Int 2004; 66: 1570–1577

[39] Shidham GB, Siddiqi N, Beres JA et al. Clinical risk factors associated with bleeding after native kidney biopsy. Nephrology (Carlton) 2005; 10: 305–310

[40] Whittier WL, Korbet SM. Timing of complications in percutaneous renal biopsy. J Am Soc Nephrol 2004; 15: 142–147

[41] Kaw D, Malhotra D. Platelet dysfunction and end-stage renal disease. Semin Dial 2006; 19: 317–322
[42] Boberg KM, Brosstad F, Egeland T, Egge T, Schrumpf E. Is a prolonged bleeding time associated with an increased risk of hemorrhage after liver biopsy? Thromb Haemost 1999; 81: 378–381
[43] Ho SJ, Gemmell R, Brighton TA. Platelet function testing in uraemic patients. Hematology 2008; 13: 49–58
[44] Lehman CM, Blaylock RC, Alexander DP, Rodgers GM. Discontinuation of the bleeding time test without detectable adverse clinical impact. Clin Chem 2001; 47: 1204–1211
[45] Mattix H, Singh AK. Is the bleeding time predictive of bleeding prior to a percutaneous renal biopsy? Curr Opin Nephrol Hypertens 1999; 8: 715–718
[46] Stiles KP, Hill C, LeBrun CJ, Reinmuth B, Yuan CM, Abbott KC. The impact of bleeding times on major complication rates after percutaneous real-time ultrasound-guided renal biopsies. J Nephrol 2001; 14: 275–279
[47] Whittier WL, Korbet SM. Renal biopsy: update. Curr Opin Nephrol Hypertens 2004; 13: 661–665
[48] Cervini P, Hesley GK, Thompson RL, Sampathkumar P, Knudsen JM. Incidence of infectious complications after an ultrasound-guided intervention. AJR Am J Roentgenol 2010; 195: 846–850
[49] Ghent CN. Percutaneous liver biopsy: reflections and refinements. Can J Gastroenterol 2006; 20: 75–79
[50] Hergesell O, Felten H, Andrassy K, Kühn K, Ritz E. Safety of ultrasound-guided percutaneous renal biopsy-retrospective analysis of 1090 consecutive cases. Nephrol Dial Transplant 1998; 13: 975–977
[51] Raaijmakers R, Kirkels WJ, Roobol MJ, Wildhagen MF, Schrder FH. Complication rates and risk factors of 5802 transrectal ultrasound-guided sextant biopsies of the prostate within a population-based screening program. Urology 2002; 60: 826–830
[52] Shigehara K, Miyagi T, Nakashima T, Shimamura M. Acute bacterial prostatitis after transrectal prostate needle biopsy: clinical analysis. J Infect Chemother 2008; 14: 40–43
[53] Simsir A, Kismali E, Mammadov R, Gunaydin G, Cal C. Is it possible to predict sepsis, the most serious complication in prostate biopsy? Urol Int 2010; 84: 395–399
[54] Lange D, Zappavigna C, Hamidizadeh R, Goldenberg SL, Paterson RF, Chew BH. Bacterial sepsis after prostate biopsy—a new perspective. Urology 2009; 74: 1200–1205
[55] Nam RK, Saskin R, Lee Y et al. Increasing hospital admission rates for urological complications after transrectal ultrasound guided prostate biopsy. J Urol 2010; 183: 963–968
[56] Ayar D, Golla B, Lee JY, Nath H. Needle-track metastasis after transthoracic needle biopsy. J Thorac Imaging 1998; 13: 2–6
[57] Chang S, Kim SH, Lim HK, Lee WJ, Choi D, Lim JH. Needle tract implantation after sonographically guided percutaneous biopsy of hepatocellular carcinoma: evaluation of doubling time, frequency, and features on CT. AJR Am J Roentgenol 2005; 185: 400–405
[58] Kosugi C, Furuse J, Ishii H et al. Needle tract implantation of hepatocellular carcinoma and pancreatic carcinoma after ultrasound-guided percutaneous puncture: clinical and pathologic characteristics and the treatment of needle tract implantation. World J Surg 2004; 28: 29–32
[59] Rodgers MS, Collinson R, Desai S, Stubbs RS, McCall JL. Risk of dissemination with biopsy of colorectal liver metastases. Dis Colon Rectum 2003; 46: 454–458; discussion 458–459
[60] Jones OM, Rees M, John TG, Bygrave S, Plant G. Biopsy of resectable colorectal liver metastases causes tumour dissemination and adversely affects survival after liver resection. Br J Surg 2005; 92: 1165–1168
[61] Stigliano R, Marelli L, Yu D, Davies N, Patch D, Burroughs AK. Seeding following percutaneous diagnostic and therapeutic approaches for hepatocellular carcinoma. What is the risk and the outcome? Seeding risk for percutaneous approach of HCC. Cancer Treat Rev 2007; 33: 437–447
[62] Silva MA, Hegab B, Hyde C, Guo B, Buckels JA, Mirza DF. Needle track seeding following biopsy of liver lesions in the diagnosis of hepatocellular cancer: a systematic review and meta-analysis. Gut 2008; 57: 1592–1596
[63] Yu SC, Lo DY, Ip CB, Liew CT, Leung TW, Lau WY. Does percutaneous liver biopsy of hepatocellular carcinoma cause hematogenous dissemination? An in vivo study with quantitative assay of circulating tumor DNA using methylation-specific real-time polymerase chain reaction. AJR Am J Roentgenol 2004; 183: 383–385
[64] Matsuguma H, Nakahara R, Kondo T, Kamiyama Y, Mori K, Yokoi K. Risk of pleural recurrence after needle biopsy in patients with resected early stage lung cancer. Ann Thorac Surg 2005; 80: 2026–2031
[65] Lee C, Bayman N, Swindell R, Faivre-Finn C. Prophylactic radiotherapy to intervention sites in mesothelioma: a systematic review and survey of UK practice. Lung Cancer 2009; 66: 150–156
[66] Agarwal PP, Seely JM, Matzinger FR et al. Pleural mesothelioma: sensitivity and incidence of needle track seeding after image-guided biopsy versus surgical biopsy. Radiology 2006; 241: 589–594
[67] Liebens F, Carly B, Cusumano P et al. Breast cancer seeding associated with core needle biopsies: a systematic review. Maturitas 2009; 62: 113–123
[68] Pérez-Saborido B, de los Galanes SJ, Menéu-Díaz JC et al. Tumor recurrence after liver transplantation for hepatocellular carcinoma: recurrence pathway and prognostic factors. Transplant Proc 2007; 39: 2304–2307
[69] Saborido BP, Díaz JC, de Los Galanes SJ et al. Does preoperative fine needle aspiration-biopsy produce tumor recurrence in patients following liver transplantation for hepatocellular carcinoma? Transplant Proc 2005; 37: 3874–3877
[70] Young AL, Malik HZ, Abu-Hilal M et al. Large hepatocellular carcinoma: time to stop preoperative biopsy. J Am Coll Surg 2007; 205: 453–462
[71] Chee YL, Crawford JC, Watson HG, Greaves M British Committee for Standards in Haematology. Guidelines on the assessment of bleeding risk prior to surgery or invasive procedures. Br J Haematol 2008; 140: 496–504
[72] Jalal DI, Chonchol M, Targher G. Disorders of hemostasis associated with chronic kidney disease. Semin Thromb Hemost 2010; 36: 34–40
[73] Tripodi A, Primignani M, Mannucci PM. Abnormalities of hemostasis and bleeding in chronic liver disease: the paradigm is challenged. Intern Emerg Med 2010; 5: 7–12
[74] Veitch AM, Baglin TP, Gershlick AH, Harnden SM, Tighe R, Cairns S British Society of Gastroenterology. British Committee for Standards in Haematology. British Cardiovascular Intervention Society. Guidelines for the management of anticoagulant and antiplatelet therapy in patients undergoing endoscopic procedures. Gut 2008; 57: 1322–1329
[75] Zuckerman MJ, Hirota WK, Adler DG et al. Standards of Practice Committee of the American Society for Gastrointestinal Endoscopy. ASGE guideline: the management of low-molecular-weight heparin and nonaspirin antiplatelet agents for endoscopic procedures. Gastrointest Endosc 2005; 61: 189–194
[76] Douketis JD, Berger PB, Dunn AS et al. The perioperative management of antithrombotic therapy: American College of Chest Physicians Evidence-Based Clinical Practice Guidelines (8th Edition). Chest 2008; 133: 299S–339S
[77] Vigué B. Bench-to-bedside review: Optimising emergency reversal of vitamin K antagonists in severe haemorrhage - from theory to practice. Crit Care 2009; 13: 209
[78] Klamroth R, Gottstein S, Essers E, Landgraf H. Bridging with enoxaparin using a half-therapeutic dose regimen: safety and efficacy. Vasa 2010; 39: 243–248
[79] Omran H, Hammerstingl C, Paar WD Bonn Registry of Alternative Anticoagulation to Prevent Vascular Events. Perioperative Bridging with Enoxaparin. Results of the Prospective BRAVE Registry with 779 Patients [Article in German]. Med Klin (Munich) 2007; 102: 809–815
[80] Holland LL, Brooks JP. Toward rational fresh frozen plasma transfusion: the effect of plasma transfusion on coagulation test results. Am J Clin Pathol 2006; 126: 133–139

[81] Stanworth SJ, Hyde CJ, Murphy MF. Evidence for indications of fresh frozen plasma. Transfus Clin Biol 2007; 14: 551–556

[82] Stanworth SJ. The evidence-based use of FFP and cryoprecipitate for abnormalities of coagulation tests and clinical coagulopathy. Hematology (Am Soc Hematol Educ Program) 2007: 179–186

[83] Abdel-Wahab OI, Healy B, Dzik WH. Effect of fresh-frozen plasma transfusion on prothrombin time and bleeding in patients with mild coagulation abnormalities. Transfusion 2006; 46: 1279–1285

[84] Sajjad S, Garcia M, Malik A, George MM, Van Thiel DH. Use of recombinant factor VIIa to correct the coagulation status of individuals with advanced liver disease prior to a percutaneous liver biopsy. Dig Dis Sci 2009; 54: 1115–1119

[85] Ozgönenel B, Rajpurkar M, Lusher JM. How do you treat bleeding disorders with desmopressin? Postgrad Med J 2007; 83: 159–163

[86] Agnelli G, Parise P, Levi M, Cosmi B, Nenci GG. Effects of desmopressin on hemostasis in patients with liver cirrhosis. Haemostasis 1995; 25: 241–247

[87] Franchini M. The use of desmopressin as a hemostatic agent: a concise review. Am J Hematol 2007; 82: 731–735

[88] Watson AJ, Keogh JA. Effect of 1-deamino-8-D-arginine vasopressin on the prolonged bleeding time in chronic renal failure. Nephron 1982; 32: 49–52

[89] Crescenzi G, Landoni G, Biondi-Zoccai G et al. Desmopressin reduces transfusion needs after surgery: a meta-analysis of randomized clinical trials. Anesthesiology 2008; 109: 1063–1076

[90] Uppot RN, Harisinghani MG, Gervais DA. Imaging-guided percutaneous renal biopsy: rationale and approach. AJR Am J Roentgenol 2010; 194: 1443–1449

[91] Shemin D, Elnour M, Amarantes B, Abuelo JG, Chazan JA. Oral estrogens decrease bleeding time and improve clinical bleeding in patients with renal failure. Am J Med 1990; 89: 436–440

[92] Hermans C, Altisent C, Batorova A et al. European Haemophilia Therapy Standardisation Board. Replacement therapy for invasive procedures in patients with haemophilia: literature review, European survey and recommendations. Haemophilia 2009; 15: 639–658

[93] Abraham JB, Gamboa AJ, Finley DS et al. The UCI Seldinger technique for percutaneous renal cryoablation: protecting the tract and achieving hemostasis. J Endourol 2009; 23: 43–49

[94] Choi SH, Lee JM, Lee KH et al. Postbiopsy splenic bleeding in a dog model: comparison of cauterization, embolization, and plugging of the needle tract. AJR Am J Roentgenol 2005; 185: 878–884

[95] Fandrich CA, Davies RP, Hall PM. Small gauge gelfoam plug liver biopsy in high risk patients: safety and diagnostic value. Australas Radiol 1996; 40: 230–234

[96] Kamphuisen PW, Wiersma TG, Mulder CJ, de Vries RA. Plugged-percutaneous liver biopsy in patients with impaired coagulation and ascites. Pathophysiol Haemost Thromb 2002; 32: 190–193

[97] Smith TP, McDermott VG, Ayoub DM, Suhocki PV, Stackhouse DJ. Percutaneous transhepatic liver biopsy with tract embolization. Radiology 1996; 198: 769–774

[98] Azlan CA, Mohd Nasir NF, Saifizul AA, Faizul MS, Ng KH, Abdullah BJ. A low cost solution for post-biopsy complications using available RFA generator and coaxial core biopsy needle. Australas Phys Eng Sci Med 2007; 30: 288–291

[99] Pritchard WF, Wray-Cahen D, Karanian JW, Hilbert S, Wood BJ. Radiofrequency cauterization with biopsy introducer needle. J Vasc Interv Radiol 2004; 15: 183–187

[100] Petsas T, Siamblis D, Giannakenas C et al. Fibrin glue for sealing the needle track in fine-needle percutaneous lung biopsy using a coaxial system: Part II—Clinical study. Cardiovasc Intervent Radiol 1995; 18: 378–382

[101] Petsas T, Vassilakos PJ, Dougenis D et al. Fibrin glue for sealing the needle track after percutaneous lung biopsy: Part I—Experimental study. Cardiovasc Intervent Radiol 1995; 18: 373–377

[102] Morello FA, Wright KC, Lembo TM. New suction guide needle designed to reduce the incidence of biopsy-related pneumothorax: experimental evaluation in canine model. Radiology 2005; 235: 1045–1049

[103] Maturen KE, Nghiem HV, Caoili EM, Higgins EG, Wolf JS, Wood DP. Renal mass core biopsy: accuracy and impact on clinical management. AJR Am J Roentgenol 2007; 188: 563–570

[104] Jaffe TA, Nelson RC, Delong DM, Paulson EK. Practice patterns in percutaneous image-guided intraabdominal abscess drainage: survey of academic and private practice centers. Radiology 2004; 233: 750–756

[105] Nolsøe CP, Lorentzen T, Skjoldbye BO, Bachmann Nielsen M. The basics of interventional ultrasound [Article in English, German]. Ultraschall Med 2007; 28: 248–263; quiz 264, 267

[106] Winter TC, Lee FT, Hinshaw JL. Ultrasound-guided biopsies in the abdomen and pelvis. Ultrasound Q 2008; 24: 45–68

[107] Puig J, Darnell A, Bermúdez P et al. Transrectal ultrasound-guided prostate biopsy: is antibiotic prophylaxis necessary? Eur Radiol 2006; 16: 939–943

[108] El-Hakim A, Moussa S. CUA guidelines on prostate biopsy methodology. Can Urol Assoc J 2010; 4: 89–94

[109] Aron M, Rajeev TP, Gupta NP. Antibiotic prophylaxis for transrectal needle biopsy of the prostate: a randomized controlled study. BJU Int 2000; 85: 682–685

[110] Briffaux R, Coloby P, Bruyere F et al. One preoperative dose randomized against 3-day antibiotic prophylaxis for transrectal ultrasonography-guided prostate biopsy. BJU Int 2009; 103: 1069–1073; discussion 1073

[111] Cam K, Kayikci A, Akman Y, Erol A. Prospective assessment of the efficacy of single dose versus traditional 3-day antimicrobial prophylaxis in 12-core transrectal prostate biopsy. Int J Urol 2008; 15: 997–1001

[112] Jeon SS, Woo SH, Hyun JH, Choi HY, Chai SE. Bisacodyl rectal preparation can decrease infectious complications of transrectal ultrasound-guided prostate biopsy. Urology 2003; 62: 461–466

[113] Akay AF, Akay H, Aflay U, Sahin H, Bircan K. Prevention of pain and infective complications after transrectal prostate biopsy: a prospective study. Int Urol Nephrol 2006; 38: 45–48

[114] Kanjanawongdeengam P, Viseshsindh W, Santanirand P, Prathombutr P, Nilkulwattana S. Reduction in bacteremia rates after rectum sterilization before transrectal, ultrasound-guided prostate biopsy: a randomized controlled trial. J Med Assoc Thai 2009; 92: 1621–1626

[115] Park DS, Oh JJ, Lee JH, Jang WK, Hong YK, Hong SK. Simple use of the suppository type povidone-iodine can prevent infectious complications in transrectal ultrasound-guided prostate biopsy. Adv Urol 2009: 750598

[116] Maya ID, Maddela P, Barker J, Allon M. Percutaneous renal biopsy: comparison of blind and real-time ultrasound-guided technique. Semin Dial 2007; 20: 355–358

[117] Al Knawy B, Shiffman M. Percutaneous liver biopsy in clinical practice. Liver Int 2007; 27: 1166–1173

[118] Ahmad M, Riley TR. Can one predict when ultrasound will be useful with percutaneous liver biopsy? Am J Gastroenterol 2001; 96: 547–549

[119] Riley TR. How often does ultrasound marking change the liver biopsy site? Am J Gastroenterol 1999; 94: 3320–3322

[120] Jenssen C, Dietrich CF. Endoscopic ultrasound-guided fine-needle aspiration biopsy and trucut biopsy in gastroenterology - An overview. Best Pract Res Clin Gastroenterol 2009; 23: 743–759

[121] Abbott KC, Musio FM, Chung EM, Lomis NN, Lane JD, Yuan CM. Transjugular renal biopsy in high-risk patients: an American case series. BMC Nephrol 2002; 3: 5

[122] Cluzel P, Martinez F, Bellin MF et al. Transjugular versus percutaneous renal biopsy for the diagnosis of parenchymal disease: comparison of sampling effectiveness and complications. Radiology 2000; 215: 689–693

[123] Shin JL, Teitel J, Swain MG et al. Virology and Immunology Committee of the Association of Hemophilia Clinic Directors of Canada. A Canadian multicenter retrospective study evaluating transjugular liver biopsy in patients with congenital bleeding disorders and hepatitis C: is it safe and useful? Am J Hematol 2005; 78: 85–93

[124] Smith TP, Presson TL, Heneghan MA, Ryan JM. Transjugular biopsy of the liver in pediatric and adult patients using an 18-gauge automated

core biopsy needle: a retrospective review of 410 consecutive procedures. AJR Am J Roentgenol 2003; 180: 167–172

[125] Cresswell AB, Welsh FK, Rees M. A diagnostic paradigm for resectable liver lesions: to biopsy or not to biopsy? HPB (Oxford) 2009; 11: 533–540

[126] Lencioni R, Caramella D, Bartolozzi C. Percutaneous biopsy of liver tumors with color Doppler US guidance. Abdom Imaging 1995; 20: 206–208

[127] Tobin MV, Gilmore IT. Plugged liver biopsy in patients with impaired coagulation. Dig Dis Sci 1989; 34: 13–15

[128] Zins M, Vilgrain V, Gayno S et al. US-guided percutaneous liver biopsy with plugging of the needle track: a prospective study in 72 high-risk patients. Radiology 1992; 184: 841–843

[129] Tung GA, Cronan JJ. Percutaneous needle biopsy of hepatic cavernous hemangioma. J Clin Gastroenterol 1993; 16: 117–122

[130] Nakaizumi A, Iishi H, Yamamoto R et al. Diagnosis of hepatic cavernous hemangioma by fine needle aspiration biopsy under ultrasonic guidance. Gastrointest Radiol 1990; 15: 39–42

[131] Cavanna L, Lazzaro A, Vallisa D, Civardi G, Artioli F. Role of image-guided fine-needle aspiration biopsy in the management of patients with splenic metastasis. World J Surg Oncol 2007; 5: 13

[132] Civardi G, Vallisa D, Bertè R et al. Ultrasound-guided fine needle biopsy of the spleen: high clinical efficacy and low risk in a multicenter Italian study. Am J Hematol 2001; 67: 93–99

[133] Gómez-Rubio M, López-Cano A, Rendón P et al. Safety and diagnostic accuracy of percutaneous ultrasound-guided biopsy of the spleen: a multicenter study. J Clin Ultrasound 2009; 37: 445–450

[134] Kang M, Kalra N, Gulati M, Lal A, Kochhar R, Rajwanshi A. Image guided percutaneous splenic interventions. Eur J Radiol 2007; 64: 140–146

[135] Lucey BC, Boland GW, Maher MM, Hahn PF, Gervais DA, Mueller PR. Percutaneous nonvascular splenic intervention: a 10-year review. AJR Am J Roentgenol 2002; 179: 1591–1596

[136] Tam A, Krishnamurthy S, Pillsbury EP et al. Percutaneous image-guided splenic biopsy in the oncology patient: an audit of 156 consecutive cases. J Vasc Interv Radiol 2008; 19: 80–87

[137] Carson BW, Brown JA, Cooperberg PL. Ultrasonographically guided percutaneous biopsy of gastric, small bowel, and colonic abnormalities: efficacy and safety. J Ultrasound Med 1998; 17: 739–742

[138] Gottlieb RH, Tan R, Widjaja J, Fultz PJ, Robinette WB, Rubens DJ. Extravisceral masses in the peritoneal cavity: sonographically guided biopsies in 52 patients. AJR Am J Roentgenol 1998; 171: 697–701

[139] Heriot AG, Kumar D, Thomas V, Young M, Pilcher J, Joseph AE. Ultrasonographically-guided fine-needle aspiration cytology in the diagnosis of colonic lesions. Br J Surg 1998; 85: 1713–1715

[140] Ledermann HP, Binkert C, Fröhlich E, Börner N, Zollikofer C, Stuckmann G. Diagnosis of symptomatic intestinal metastases using transabdominal sonography and sonographically guided puncture. AJR Am J Roentgenol 2001; 176: 155–158

[141] Marco-Doménech SF, Gil-Sánchez S, Fernández-García P et al. Sonographically guided percutaneous biopsy of gastrointestinal tract lesions. AJR Am J Roentgenol 2001; 176: 147–151

[142] Tombesi P, Postorivo S, Catellani M, Tassinari D, Abbasciano V, Sartori S. Percutaneous ultrasonography-guided core needle biopsy of gastrointestinal lesions: what's its actual role in clinical practice? A retrospective study for safety and effectiveness. Ultraschall Med 2011; 32 (Suppl 1): S62–S67

[143] Tudor GR, Rodgers PM, West KP. Bowel lesions: percutaneous US-guided 18-gauge needle biopsy—preliminary experience. Radiology 1999; 212: 594–597

[144] Farmer KD, Harries SR, Fox BM, Maskell GF, Farrow R. Core biopsy of the bowel wall: efficacy and safety in the clinical setting. AJR Am J Roentgenol 2000; 175: 1627–1630

[145] Ho LM, Thomas J, Fine SA, Paulson EK. Usefulness of sonographic guidance during percutaneous biopsy of mesenteric masses. AJR Am J Roentgenol 2003; 180: 1563–1566

[146] O'Connell MJ, Paulson EK, Jaffe TA, Ho LM. Percutaneous biopsy of periarterial soft tissue cuffs in the diagnosis of pancreatic carcinoma. Abdom Imaging 2004; 29: 115–119

[147] Souza FF, Mortelé KJ, Cibas ES, Erturk SM, Silverman SG. Predictive value of percutaneous imaging-guided biopsy of peritoneal and omental masses: results in 111 patients. AJR Am J Roentgenol 2009; 192: 131–136

[148] Kim KW, Kim MJ, Kim HC et al. Value of "patent track" sign on Doppler sonography after percutaneous liver biopsy in detection of post-biopsy bleeding: a prospective study in 352 patients. AJR Am J Roentgenol 2007; 189: 109–116

[149] Waldo B, Korbet SM, Freimanis MG, Lewis EJ. The value of post-biopsy ultrasound in predicting complications after percutaneous renal biopsy of native kidneys. Nephrol Dial Transplant 2009; 24: 2433–2439

[150] Catalano O, Cusati B, Nunziata A, Siani A. Active abdominal bleeding: contrast-enhanced sonography. Abdom Imaging 2006; 31: 9–16

[151] Ignee A, Baum U, Schuessler G, Dietrich CF. Contrast-enhanced ultrasound-guided percutaneous cholangiography and cholangiodrainage (CEUS-PTCD). Endoscopy 2009; 41: 725–726

[152] Marwah DS, Korbet SM. Timing of complications in percutaneous renal biopsy: what is the optimal period of observation? Am J Kidney Dis 1996; 28: 47–52

[153] Eng M, Vaughan TE, Woo D, Buell JF. Treatment of an extracapsular post-renal biopsy pseudoaneurysm with ultrasound-guided thrombin injection. J Clin Ultrasound 2010; 38: 215–217

[154] Tang Y, Qian NS, Luo W et al. Percutaneous injection of hemostatic agents for active liver hemorrhage. Hepatobiliary Pancreat Dis Int 2010; 9: 402–408

[155] Dewitt J, McGreevy K, Cummings O et al. Initial experience with EUS-guided Tru-cut biopsy of benign liver disease. Gastrointest Endosc 2009; 69: 535–542

[156] Gleeson FC, Clayton AC, Zhang L et al. Adequacy of endoscopic ultrasound core needle biopsy specimen of nonmalignant hepatic parenchymal disease. Clin Gastroenterol Hepatol 2008; 6: 1437–1440

[157] Hollerbach S, Willert J, Topalidis T, Reiser M, Schmiegel W. Endoscopic ultrasound-guided fine-needle aspiration biopsy of liver lesions: histological and cytological assessment. Endoscopy 2003; 35: 743–749

[158] Singh P, Mukhopadhyay P, Bhatt B et al. Endoscopic ultrasound versus CT scan for detection of the metastases to the liver: results of a prospective comparative study. J Clin Gastroenterol 2009; 43: 367–373

[159] Preda A, Van Dijk LC, Van Oostaijen JA, Pattynama PM. Complication rate and diagnostic yield of 515 consecutive ultrasound-guided biopsies of renal allografts and native kidneys using a 14-gauge Biopty gun. Eur Radiol 2003; 13: 527–530

[160] Lefaucheur C, Nochy D, Bariety J. Renal biopsy: procedures, contraindications, complications [Article in French]. Nephrol Ther 2009; 5: 331–339

[161] Remzi M, Marberger M. Renal tumor biopsies for evaluation of small renal tumors: why, in whom, and how? Eur Urol 2009; 55: 359–367

[162] Volpe A, Kachura JR, Geddie WR et al. Techniques, safety and accuracy of sampling of renal tumors by fine needle aspiration and core biopsy. J Urol 2007; 178: 379–386

[163] Walker PD. The renal biopsy. Arch Pathol Lab Med 2009; 133: 181–188

[164] DeWitt J, Gress FG, Levy MJ et al. EUS-guided FNA aspiration of kidney masses: a multicenter U.S. experience. Gastrointest Endosc 2009; 70: 573–578

[165] Zamboni GA, D'Onofrio M, Idili A et al. Ultrasound-guided percutaneous fine-needle aspiration of 545 focal pancreatic lesions. AJR Am J Roentgenol 2009; 193: 1691–1695

[166] Eloubeidi MA, Tamhane A, Varadarajulu S, Wilcox CM. Frequency of major complications after EUS-guided FNA of solid pancreatic masses: a prospective evaluation. Gastrointest Endosc 2006; 63: 622–629

[167] Görg C, Schwerk WB, Bittinger A, Euer B, Görg K. Sonographically guided fine-needle puncture of adrenal tumors [Article in German]. Dtsch Med Wochenschr 1992; 117: 448–454

[168] Kocijancic K, Kocijancic I, Guna F. Role of sonographically guided fine-needle aspiration biopsy of adrenal masses in patients with lung cancer. J Clin Ultrasound 2004; 32: 12–16

[169] Lumachi F, Polistina F, Favia G, D'Amico DF. Extraadrenal and multiple pheochromocytomas. Are there really any differences in pathophysiology and outcome? J Exp Clin Cancer Res 1998; 17: 303–305
[170] Mody MK, Kazerooni EA, Korobkin M. Percutaneous CT-guided biopsy of adrenal masses: immediate and delayed complications. J Comput Assist Tomogr 1995; 19: 434–439
[171] Paulsen SD, Nghiem HV, Korobkin M, Caoili EM, Higgins EJ. Changing role of imaging-guided percutaneous biopsy of adrenal masses: evaluation of 50 adrenal biopsies. AJR Am J Roentgenol 2004; 182: 1033–1037
[172] Welch TJ, Sheedy PF, Stephens DH, Johnson CM, Swensen SJ. Percutaneous adrenal biopsy: review of a 10-year experience. Radiology 1994; 193: 341–344
[173] Quayle FJ, Spitler JA, Pierce RA, Lairmore TC, Moley JF, Brunt LM. Needle biopsy of incidentally discovered adrenal masses is rarely informative and potentially hazardous. Surgery 2007; 142: 497–502; discussion 502–504
[174] Vanderveen KA, Thompson SM, Callstrom MR et al. Biopsy of pheochromocytomas and paragangliomas: potential for disaster. Surgery 2009; 146: 1158–1166
[175] Haseganu LE, Diehl DL. Left adrenal gland hemorrhage as a complication of EUS-FNA. Gastrointest Endosc 2009; 69: e51–e52
[176] Jenssen C, Dietrich CF. Ultrasound and endoscopic ultrasound of the adrenal glands [Article in German]. Ultraschall Med 2010; 31: 228–247, quiz 248–250
[177] Tombesi P, Nielsen I, Tassinari D, Trevisani L, Abbasciano V, Sartori S. Transthoracic ultrasonography-guided core needle biopsy of pleural-based lung lesions: prospective randomized comparison between a Tru-cut-type needle and a modified Menghini-type needle. Ultraschall Med 2009; 30: 390–395
[178] Screaton NJ, Flower CD. Percutaneous needle biopsy of the pleura. Radiol Clin North Am 2000; 38: 293–301
[179] Middleton WD, Teefey SA, Dahiya N. Ultrasound-guided chest biopsies. Ultrasound Q 2006; 22: 241–252
[180] Mathis G, Gehmacher O. Ultrasound-guided diagnostic and therapeutic interventions in peripheral pulmonary masses. Wien Klin Wochenschr 1999; 111: 230–235
[181] Shaham D. Semi-invasive and invasive procedures for the diagnosis and staging of lung cancer. I. Percutaneous transthoracic needle biopsy. Radiol Clin North Am 2000; 38: 525–534
[182] Wang KX, Ben QW, Jin ZD et al. Assessment of morbidity and mortality associated with EUS-guided FNA: a systematic review. Gastrointest Endosc 2011; 73: 283–290
[183] Jenssen C, Alvarez-Sánchez MV, Napoléon B, Faiss S. Diagnostic endoscopic ultrasonography: assessment of safety and prevention of complications. World J Gastroenterol 2012; 18: 4659–4676
[184] Thomas T, Kaye PV, Ragunath K, Aithal G. Efficacy, safety, and predictive factors for a positive yield of EUS-guided Trucut biopsy: a large tertiary referral center experience. Am J Gastroenterol 2009; 104: 584–591
[185] Varela-Lema L, Fernández-Villar A, Ruano-Ravina A. Effectiveness and safety of endobronchial ultrasound-transbronchial needle aspiration: a systematic review. Eur Respir J 2009; 33: 1156–1164
[186] Dietrich CF, Hocke M, Jenssen C. Interventional endosonography [Article in German]. Ultraschall Med 2011; 32: 8–22, quiz 23–25
[187] Kim SJ, Kim SI, Ahn HS, Choi JB, Kim YS, Kim SJ. Risk factors for acute prostatitis after transrectal biopsy of the prostate. Korean J Urol 2010; 51: 426–430
[188] Thomas J, Turner SR, Nelson RC, Paulson EK. Postprocedure sepsis in imaging-guided percutaneous hepatic abscess drainage: how often does it occur? AJR Am J Roentgenol 2006; 186: 1419–1422
[189] Laganà D, Carrafiello G, Mangini M et al. Image-guided percutaneous treatment of abdominal-pelvic abscesses: a 5-year experience. Radiol Med (Torino) 2008; 113: 999–1007
[190] Giorgio A, de Stefano G, Di Sarno A, Liorre G, Ferraioli G. Percutaneous needle aspiration of multiple pyogenic abscesses of the liver: 13-year single-center experience. AJR Am J Roentgenol 2006; 187: 1585–1590
[191] Schwerk WB, Görg C, Görg K, Richter G, Beckh K. Percutaneous drainage of liver and splenic abscess [Article in German]. Z Gastroenterol 1991; 29: 146–152
[192] Tazawa J, Sakai Y, Maekawa S et al. Solitary and multiple pyogenic liver abscesses: characteristics of the patients and efficacy of percutaneous drainage. Am J Gastroenterol 1997; 92: 271–274
[193] Lambiase RE, Deyoe L, Cronan JJ, Dorfman GS. Percutaneous drainage of 335 consecutive abscesses: results of primary drainage with 1-year follow-up. Radiology 1992; 184: 167–179
[194] Jansen M, Truong S, Riesener KP, Sparenberg P, Schumpelick V. Results of sonographically guided percutaneous catheter drainage of intra-abdominal abscesses in surgery [Article in German]. Chirurg 1999; 70: 1168–1171
[195] Tan YM, Chung AY, Chow PK et al. An appraisal of surgical and percutaneous drainage for pyogenic liver abscesses larger than 5 cm. Ann Surg 2005; 241: 485–490
[196] vanSonnenberg E, Ferrucci JT, Mueller PR, Wittenberg J, Simeone JF. Percutaneous drainage of abscesses and fluid collections: technique, results, and applications. Radiology 1982; 142: 1–10
[197] Laméris JS, Hesselink EJ, Van Leeuwen PA, Nijs HG, Meerwaldt JH, Terpstra OT. Ultrasound-guided percutaneous transhepatic cholangiography and drainage in patients with hilar cholangiocarcinoma. Semin Liver Dis 1990; 10: 121–125
[198] Lorenz JM, Funaki B, Leef JA, Rosenblum JD, Van Ha T. Percutaneous transhepatic cholangiography and biliary drainage in pediatric liver transplant patients. AJR Am J Roentgenol 2001; 176: 761–765
[199] Winbladh A, Gullstrand P, Svanvik J, Sandström P. Systematic review of cholecystostomy as a treatment option in acute cholecystitis. HPB (Oxford) 2009; 11: 183–193
[200] Bouza C, López-Cuadrado T, Alcázar R, Saz-Parkinson Z, Amate JM. Meta-analysis of percutaneous radiofrequency ablation versus ethanol injection in hepatocellular carcinoma. BMC Gastroenterol 2009; 9: 31
[201] Livraghi T, Solbiati L, Meloni MF, Gazelle GS, Halpern EF, Goldberg SN. Treatment of focal liver tumors with percutaneous radio-frequency ablation: complications encountered in a multicenter study. Radiology 2003; 226: 441–451
[202] Uppot RN, Silverman SG, Zagoria RJ, Tuncali K, Childs DD, Gervais DA. Imaging-guided percutaneous ablation of renal cell carcinoma: a primer of how we do it. AJR Am J Roentgenol 2009; 192: 1558–1570
[203] Giorgio A, Di Sarno A, de Stefano G et al. Sonography and clinical outcome of viable hydatid liver cysts treated with double percutaneous aspiration and ethanol injection as first-line therapy: efficacy and long-term follow-up. AJR Am J Roentgenol 2009; 193: W186–92
[204] Huo TI, Huang YH, Huang HC et al. Fever and infectious complications after percutaneous acetic acid injection therapy for hepatocellular carcinoma: incidence and risk factor analysis. J Clin Gastroenterol 2006; 40: 639–642
[205] Chen TM, Huang PT, Lin LF, Tung JN. Major complications of ultrasound-guided percutaneous radiofrequency ablations for liver malignancies: single center experience. J Gastroenterol Hepatol 2008; 23: e445–e450
[206] Liang P, Wang Y, Yu X, Dong B. Malignant liver tumors: treatment with percutaneous microwave ablation—complications among cohort of 1136 patients. Radiology 2009; 251: 933–940
[207] Edoute Y, Tibon-Fisher O, Ben Haim S, Malberger E. Ultrasonically guided fine-needle aspiration of liver lesions. Am J Gastroenterol 1992; 87: 1138–1141
[208] Huang GT, Sheu JC, Yang PM, Lee HS, Wang TH, Chen DS. Ultrasound-guided cutting biopsy for the diagnosis of hepatocellular carcinoma—a study based on 420 patients. J Hepatol 1996; 25: 334–338
[209] Shannon BA, Cohen RJ, de Bruto H, Davies RJ. The value of preoperative needle core biopsy for diagnosing benign lesions among small, incidentally detected renal masses. J Urol 2008; 180: 1257–1261; discussion 1261

10 Assistance in Ultrasound Interventions

U. Gottschalk, C. F. Dietrich

10.1 Basic Principles

Ultrasound machines have a long service life. Especially in the outpatient sector, where cost-containment issues may prohibit the acquisition of a new unit, service times of 10 years are not uncommon.

The maintenance of ultrasound machines should include regular cleaning of the air filters. The lighting conditions in the procedure room are a trade-off situation for assisting personnel. On the one hand, positioning the patient requires enough light to avoid damage to surrounding equipment (ultrasound machine, IV pole) and provide a clear view of the patient (drainage tubes, wounds, monitor cables, etc.). On the other hand, the procedure itself requires a darkened room with indirect lighting and spot illumination of the control panel (▶ Fig. 10.1, ▶ Fig. 10.2). Because it takes the eyes up to 2 minutes to adjust to the darkness, bright light should be avoided when one patient leaves the suite and another enters.

The most delicate component of the ultrasound system is the probe (transducer). When not held in the hand of an operator or assistant, the probe should be stowed in the probe holder on the ultrasound machine. A probe should not be left on the patient, bed, or stretcher where it may become damaged. The freeze button should always be pressed before the probe is cleaned. Special cleaning sprays are available that are active against bacteria, fungi, and lipophilic viruses and contain no formaldehyde or phenols (see below).

Ultrasound procedures are classified into several types:

- Diagnostic ultrasound
- Diagnostic interventions
- Therapeutic interventions
- Endosonography

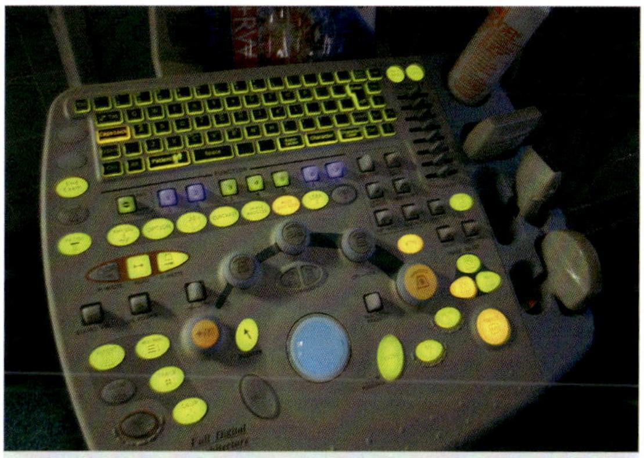

Fig. 10.1 The control panel of a modern ultrasound machine. (The machine should be thoroughly cleaned daily while switched off.)

10.2 Duties of Assisting Personnel

Assisting personnel should prepare the procedure room and the patient, and assist in the administration of local anesthesia, the carrying out of the procedure, provision of postprocedure care, and the early detection of possible complications. The care and maintenance of the ultrasound machine should be regulated within the department and should follow the checklist supplied by manufacturers. An external check of the machine, cables, and probes should be performed daily, however. Ultrasound probes may undergo a three-step treatment process, depending on their intended use.

▶ **Cleaning the probe.** The probe is unplugged from the machine and immersed in water or an enzymatic cleaning solution, always adhering to manufacturer's instructions. The probe is then cleaned mechanically with a

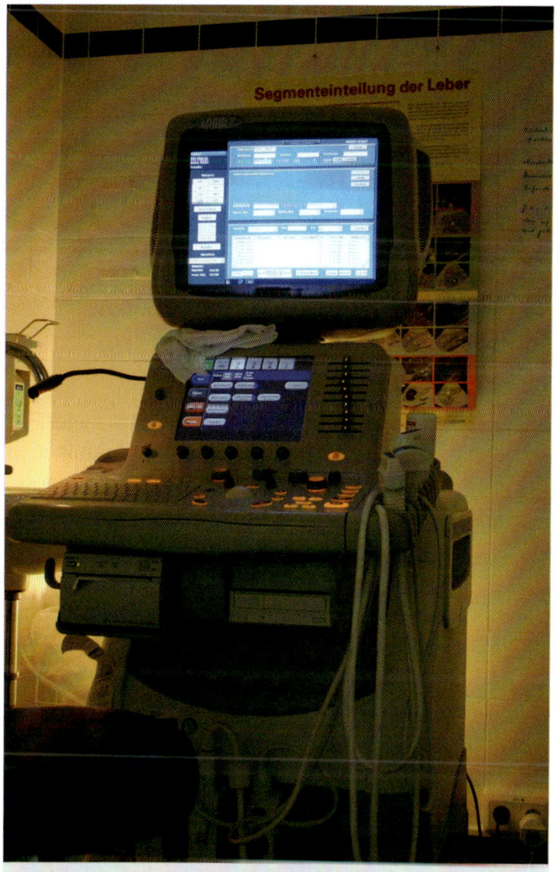

Fig. 10.2 Indirect lighting in an ultrasound examination room.

sponge or cloth, rinsed with water, and dried with a soft cloth.

▸ **Disinfecting the probe.** In this process the probe is either cleaned with a disinfectant wipe or immersed in disinfectant solution prepared according to manufacturer's instructions, then rinsed with sterile water and dried.

▸ **Sterilizing the probe.** The probe is packaged in a suitable pouch. Next, most types of probe undergo ethylene oxide gas sterilization, which is done for 3 hours at a maximum temperature of 55°C and maximum pressure of 8–200 kPa. Once again, manufacturer's instructions should always be followed.

It has become standard practice in many departments to have assisting personnel place peripheral intravenous lines. In difficult situations, venous cannulation can even be performed under ultrasound guidance.[1] European and U.S. rules differ on this matter and can be reviewed on the websites of the European Society of Gastroenterology and Endoscopy Nurses and Associates (www.ESGENA.org) and of the American Society for Gastrointestinal Endoscopy (www.ASGE.org). On the other hand, there is a core set of physician responsibilities that cannot be delegated to nonphysicians because of their technical difficulty, procedural risk, or potential for an unpredictable reaction. But as cost pressures in the health care industry continue to rise in the coming years, it is likely that policies and procedures will be revised[2] and there will be a greater delegation of patient care responsibilities to assisting personnel.

10.3 Diagnostic Ultrasound

The probe used in diagnostic ultrasound is a "noncritical" medical object that comes into contact only with intact skin. The duties of assisting personnel before the actual examination include greeting the patient, checking paperwork, and preparing the examination couch. No assistance is needed during the ultrasound examination, freeing the assisting staff for other duties.[3]

The delegation of limited diagnostic examinations, as in "focused assessment with sonography for trauma" (FAST), has yielded very encouraging results.[4] The overall accuracy of nurse-performed FAST for the detection of free fluid was 95%, with a sensitivity of 84.4% and a specificity of 98.4%. Current developments can be followed by visiting the websites of the Society of Diagnostic Medical Sonography (SDMS, www.sdms.org) and the American Registry of Diagnostic Medical Sonographers (ARDMS, www.ardms.org).

Tele-ultrasound is based on the use of portal ultrasound scanners in emergency settings (Mobile Hospital Emergency Medical System, MHEMS).[5] It is difficult at present to judge the future role of this technology.

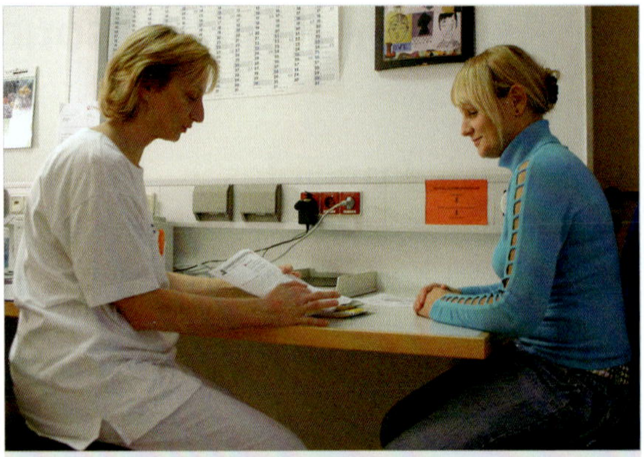

Fig. 10.3 Informed consent is obtained the day before the procedure in a calm, relaxed atmosphere.

10.4 Diagnostic Interventions

Biopsy results will have profound implications for most patients. A patient with a suspected tumor is naturally anxious while awaiting both the biopsy procedure and its results. It is essential, therefore, to establish an atmosphere of trust. An informed patient will be better able to cooperate during the procedure, making it less likely that problems or complications will arise (▸ Fig. 10.3).

A percutaneous biopsy involves contact with blood, and the targeted site is not always sterile, which poses an infection risk for the patient and staff. Biopsy instruments are classified as "critical," meaning that they may come into contact with blood or internal tissues (see Chapter 8). This has led to an increasing use of disposable materials, which are now available in a price range that is competitive with the costs of cleaning, packaging, and sterilization.

If shaving is necessary, it should be done shortly before the procedure. The puncture site should be marked with a water-resistant felt-tip pen so that it will be clearly visible after skin preparation.

The basic materials necessary for a needle biopsy include the following:

- Sterile disposable gown for the operator
- Sterile gloves, swab dish, swabs, gauze pads
- Sterile slit drape for placing over the skin site
- Local anesthetic (syringe and needle)
- Waterproof underpad
- Biopsy needle, plus aspiration syringe if needed
- Histology vessel with formalin or glass microscope slides
- Dressing material

Given the high rates of glove defects that are found after surgical and interventional procedures, doctors and assisting staff should always clean their hands with a hygienic handwash or handrub after the procedure.[6] Conversation during the procedure should be kept to an

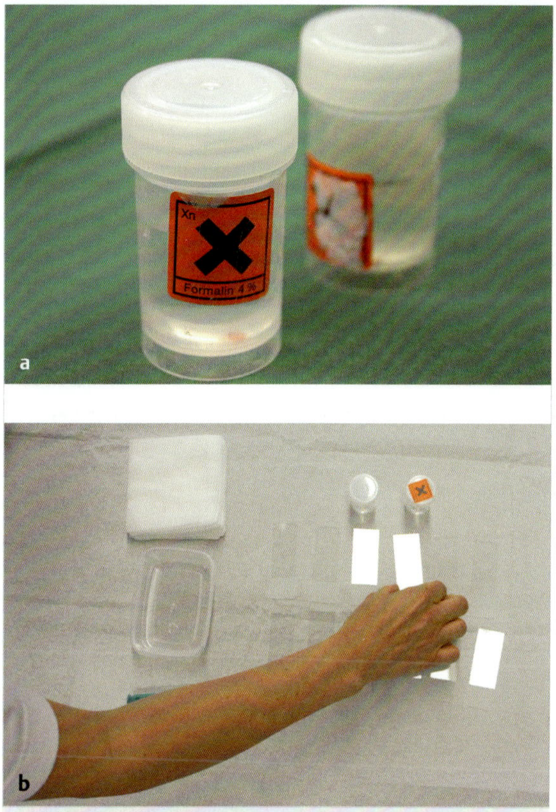

Fig. 10.4 Accessories.
a Containers for histology.
b Glass slides for cytology.

absolute minimum due to the risk of contaminating the sterile field with streptococci.[7]

Care is taken to use sterile swabs and pads. Thin hypodermic needles and 5- or 10-mL syringes are provided for local anesthetic injection. Material for cytology and/or histology is collected, depending on the target site and type of needle used. The following accessories are required (▶ Fig. 10.4):

- **Histology:** formalin container for histology (4% aqueous neutral-buffered solution, possibly 70–96% ethanol). Exposure to light in an unbuffered formalin solution may generate formic acid causing a fall in pH, and this can adversely affect the tissue sample.
- **Cytology:** glass slides for cytology (a dozen or more).

The tray setup should include at least one sterile drape, sterile swabs or gauze pads, a sterile forceps, a container for the prep solution, and a temporary specimen container (▶ Fig. 10.5).

10.5 Therapeutic Interventions

Assisting staff's duties include passing the injectable agent to the operator and observing the patient for

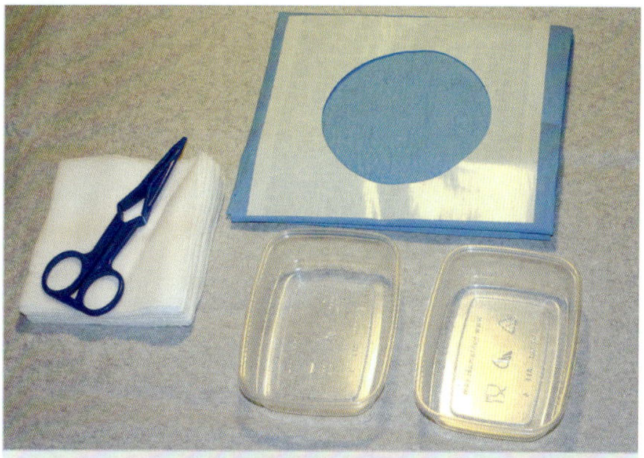

Fig. 10.5 Basic tray setup without local anesthesia or biopsy needle.

unexpected side effects, which should be reported immediately to the physician. A patient care record should be kept for all therapeutic interventions.

10.6 Sedation

The desire of patients for painless procedures has increased in recent years.[8] Occasionally, therefore, it is necessary to sedate the patient during the procedure. Current European S3 guidelines[6,9,10] now allow physicians to delegate patient sedation to assisting personnel (NAPS: nurse-administered propofol sedation). As in trauma ultrasound, this approach has yielded positive results internationally[11] (see Chapter 11). European policies and practices follow the guidelines of the European Society of Gastrointestinal Endoscopy (ESGE), the European Society of Gastroenterology and Endoscopy Nurses and Associates (ESGENA), and the European Society of Anesthesiology (ESA). Administration of oxygen during sedation is strongly advised and should be started before sedation is administered (▶ Fig. 10.6). Dentures are removed and placed in a container labeled with the patient's name (▶ Fig. 10.7). They should never be wrapped in facial tissue, as this often results in lost dentures.

Intravenous sedation is used almost exclusively and requires safe and adequate venous access. The placement of a small-gauge catheter is acceptable only in cases where standard venous access is extremely difficult as a result of chemotherapy or drug abuse (▶ Fig. 10.8).

10.7 Drain Placement

If a large amount of fluid is drawn into the syringe after the placement of a drain, it should not be expelled into a kidney basin. It is better for hygienic reasons to use a collection bag with a three-way stopcock. The tray setup will depend on whether the drain is placed using the direct trocar technique or Seldinger technique (▶ Fig. 10.9). It is helpful to use syringes that lock the plunger in a suction

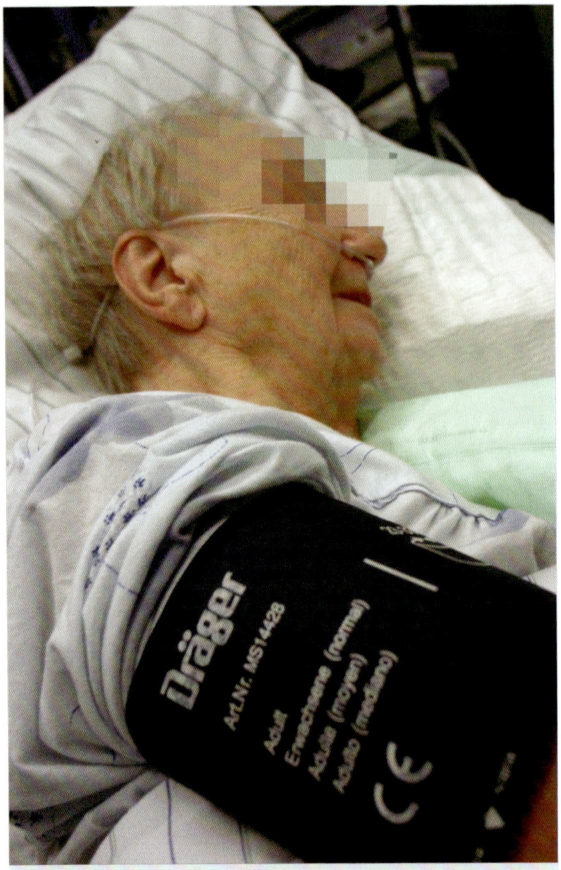

Fig. 10.6 Before the patient is sedated, a blood pressure cuff is placed and supplemental oxygen is delivered by nasal cannula.

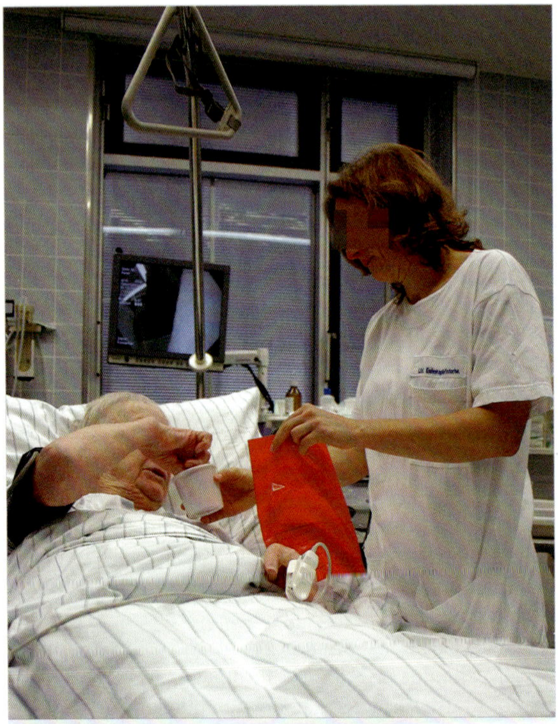

Fig. 10.7 Dentures are placed in a labeled container for safekeeping.

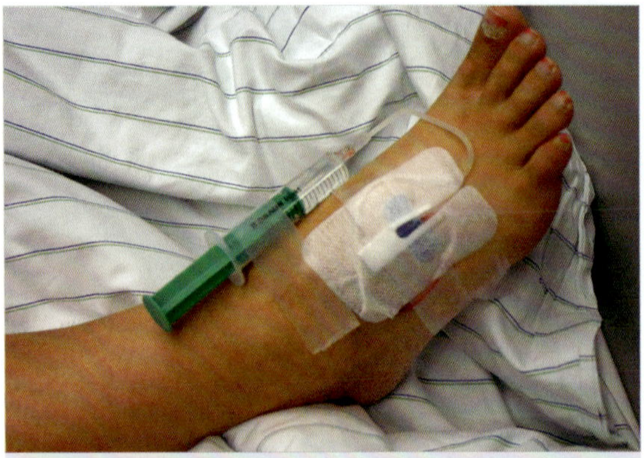

Fig. 10.8 Difficult intravenous access in the upper extremity (as in this drug abuser) may require access at an alternative site.

position to prevent "wiggling" of the puncture needle (► Fig. 10.10).

The outcome of the procedure depends critically upon drain care and maintenance. Drains are not always sutured to the skin or secured with a retention plate. For this reason, the doctor or nurse should personally check the dressing and drain function on the following morning at the latest, and flush the drain with physiologic saline solution if necessary to maintain patency.

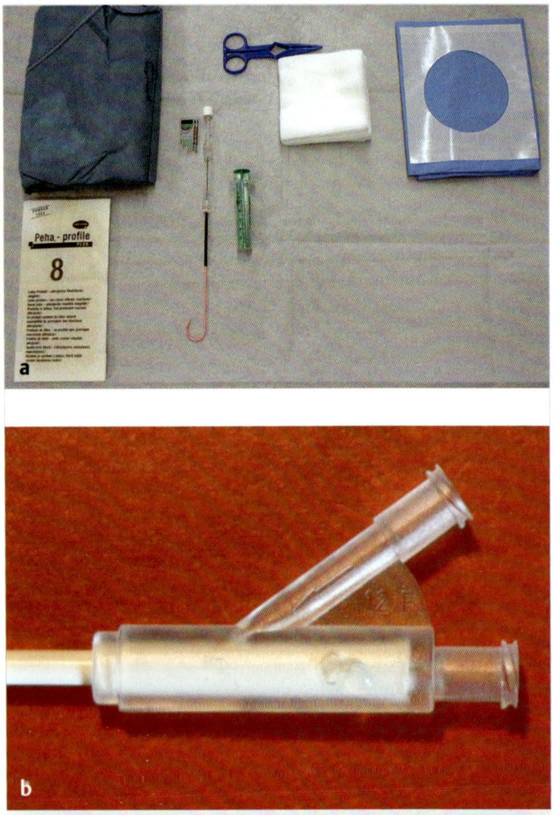

Fig. 10.9 Tray setup with a pigtail drain ready for direct insertion.
a Single-lumen drain.
b Double-lumen drain.

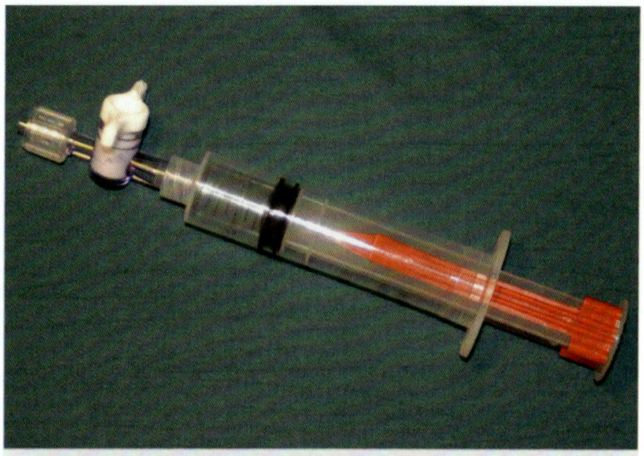

Fig. 10.10 Vacuum syringe.

10.8 Endosonography

As with extracorporeal ultrasound, endosonographic procedures may be purely diagnostic or therapeutic. Each type is an invasive procedure that should be performed by a physician. One assistant is responsible for intravenous sedation and another for passing the endoscope and necessary accessories. Because the cleaning and sterilization of endoscopes, with their numerous channels, is a complex process, we refer the reader to the literature on this subject. Rigid endosonographic probes of the type used in rectal and vaginal examinations are often covered with a sterile, disposable sheath. Probe covers have an average perforation rate of 1 to 9%, however, and so the probes still require disinfection. The use of condoms to reduce costs cannot be recommended.[12] In very complex procedures such as the transgastric drainage of pseudocysts, high-frequency electrocautery is occasionally used as an adjunct. This requires the placement of a neutral electrode (▸ Fig. 10.11).

One difficulty in endosonography is that the endoscopic procedure is done with sedation in a well-darkened room. As a result, instrument passing and patient

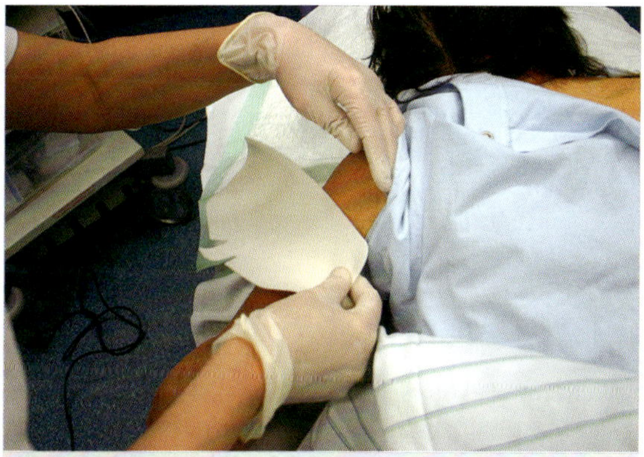

Fig. 10.11 Neutral electrode for the use of high-frequency current.

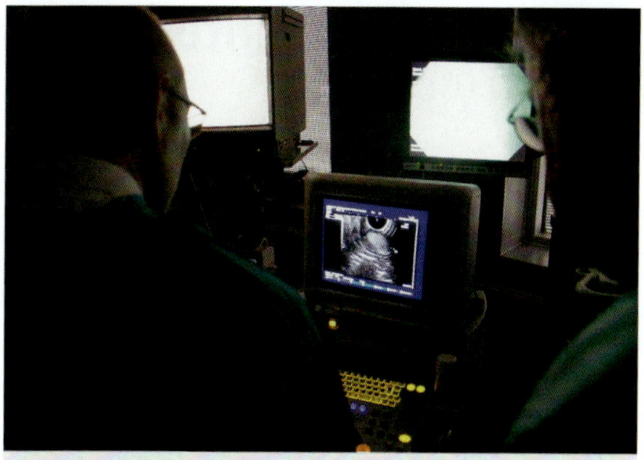

Fig. 10.12 Lighting conditions during endosonography.

observation may prove challenging for assisting personnel (▸ Fig. 10.12).

References

[1] Walker E. Piloting a nurse-led ultrasound cannulation scheme. Br J Nurs 2009; 18-858-859

[2] Nürnberg D, Jung A, Schmieder C, Schmidt M, Holle A. What's the price of routine sonography—results of an analysis of costs and processes in a district hospital [Article in German]. Ultraschall Med 2008; 29: 405–417

[3] Gilman G, Nelson JM, Murphy AT, Kidd GM, Stussy VL, Klarich KW. The role of the nurse in clinical echocardiography. J Am Soc Echocardiogr 2005; 18: 773–777

[4] Bowra J, Forrest-Horder S, Caldwell E, Cox M, D'Amours SK. Validation of nurse-performed FAST ultrasound. Injury 2010; 41: 484–487

[5] Su MJ, Ma HM, Ko CI et al. Application of tele-ultrasound in emergency medical services. Telemed J E Health 2008; 14: 816–824

[6] Riphaus A, Wehrmann T, Weber B et al. Sektion Enoskopie im Auftrag der Deutschen Gesellschaft für Verdauungs- und Stoffwechselerkrankungen e.V. (DGVS). Bundesverband Niedergelassener Gastroenterologen Deuschlands e. V. (Bng). Chirurgische Arbeitsgemeinschaft für Endoskopie und Sonographie der Deutschen Gesellschaft für Allgemein- und Viszeralchirurgie (DGAV). Deutsche Morbus Crohn/Colitis ulcerosa Vereinigung e. V. (DCCV). Deutsche Gesellschaft für Endoskopie-Assistenzpersonal (DEGEA). Deutsche Gesellschaft für Anästhesie und Intensivmedizin (DGAI). Gesellschaft für Recht und Politik im Gesundheitswesen (GPRG). S3-guidelines—sedation in gastrointestinal endoscopy [Article in Danish]. Z Gastroenterol 2008; 46: 1298–1330

[7] Schabrun S, Chipchase L, Rickard H. Are therapeutic ultrasound units a potential vector for nosocomial infection? Physiother Res Int 2006; 11: 61–71

[8] Rex DK, Overley CA, Walker J. Registered nurse-administered propofol sedation for upper endoscopy and colonoscopy: Why? When? How? Rev Gastroenterol Disord 2003; 3: 70–80

[9] Beilenhoff U, Engelke M, Kern-Waechter E et al. Endosk Heute 2009; 22: 237–239

[10] Verschuur EMI, Kuipers EJ, Siersema PD. Nurses working in GI and endoscopic practice: a review. Gastrointest Endosc 2007; 65: 469–479

[11] Vilmann P, Hornslet P, Simmons H, Hammering A, Clementsen P. Propofol sedation administered by nurses for endoscopic procedures [Article in Danish]. Ugeskr Laeger 2009; 171: 1840–1843

[12] Chalouhi GE, Salomon LJ, Marelle P, Bernard JP, Ville Y. Hygiene in endovaginal gynecologic and obstetrical ultrasound in 2008 [Article in French]. J Gynecol Obstet Biol Reprod (Paris) 2009; 38: 43–50

11 Sedation in Interventions

U. Gottschalk, C. F. Dietrich

11.1 Introduction

Almost all percutaneous interventional procedures can be performed under local anesthesia. Sedation may occasionally be indicated for reasons relating to the procedure itself or to the patient.

Endosonography is almost always performed under deep sedation, because it is an endoscopic procedure that requires very steady examination conditions so that small structures can be accurately assessed. In addition, endosonographic procedures may take up to 20 minutes and would be difficult for most patients to tolerate. Although sedation can be administered by the oral, subcutaneous, intramuscular, or intravenous routes in principle, intravenous sedation is the only reasonable option for interventional procedures due to its good short-term controllability.

Sedation in sonographic practice is based on the S3 guideline on sedation for gastrointestinal endoscopy published in 2008.[1] According to this guideline, sedation should always be preceded by a clinical evaluation in which any cardiovascular or respiratory problems are assessed according to ASA (American Society of Anesthesiologists) criteria[2] (▶ Table 11.1). Patients in ASA class III or higher have a markedly increased risk potential for sedation and interventions. The S3 guideline notes that the presence of an anesthesiologist may be desirable for the sedation of patients with a high risk profile. The ASA classification of patients should include a detailed history with questions relating to:

Table 11.1 ASA physical status classification system (classes I–V)

Class	Description
I: Healthy patient	No preexisting diseases
II: Mild systemic disease	Examples: mild asthma, well-controlled seizure disorder, anemia, well-controlled diabetes mellitus, moderate arterial hypertension, obesity
III: Severe systemic disease	Examples: moderately severe to severe asthma, poorly controlled seizure disorder, pneumonia, poorly controlled diabetes mellitus, prior myocardial infarction, pulmonary tuberculosis
IV: Very severe, life-threatening, incapacitating systemic disease	Examples: severe bronchopulmonary dysplasia, sepsis, advanced stage of respiratory, heart, liver or kidney failure, recent myocardial infarction, shock
V: Moribund patient	Death expected within 24 hours

- Diseases of the cardiovascular and respiratory system, stridor, snoring, sleep apnea syndrome
- Prior complications involving the use of sedatives or analgesics, regional and general anesthesia
- Drug allergies, current medications and possible drug interactions
- Time and composition of the most recent meal
- Alcohol, tobacco, and drug use

The history is followed by a physical examination that includes vital signs and auscultation of the heart and lungs.

This practice is analogous to existing guidelines[3–5] and should always be followed. Protective intubation is very rarely necessary during a sonographic procedure.

Sedation, like the procedure itself, requires informed consent. The patient's right of self-determination calls for a timely declaration of consent in which the patient can freely make a decision without time pressure.[6] Informed consent is based on a personal, confidential interview that takes place in a calm atmosphere without distractions or disturbances (see Chapter 3).

11.2 Medications

The agents most often used for procedural sedation are midazolam and propofol. Pethidine and ketanest are less commonly used.[7] With the availability of drug information, it is often asked whether certain types of medications may be administered by nonanesthesiologists. The answer depends in part on personal qualifications such as experience in intensive care medicine, emergency training, or regular service in an ambulance or emergency response vehicle. Thus, nonanesthesiologists may be qualified to work with these agents. The advantages of midazolam are that it induces anterograde amnesia and has an antidote (flumazenil), but it also has a longer duration of action that requires a longer observation period after the procedure.[8–10] Midazolam-induced respiratory depression is reversed approximately 120 seconds after the intravenous administration of flumazenil.[11] Propofol has excellent controllability but does not have an antidote.

11.3 Personnel Requirements

Ideally, intravenous sedation is administered by a specialist in anesthesiology, but this is rarely possible in practice due to staff limitations and cost constraints. Even a physician experienced in critical care medicine is not always available.[1] Studies on nurse-administered propofol sedation (NAPS), although dealing with endoscopic procedures,[12–16] have provided an important basis for expanding the role of assisting personnel. Although many studies were published after the introduction of propofol, the basic principles of sedation guidelines still apply to other agents such as midazolam.[17,18] If a benzodiazepine (midazolam) or pethidine is used for procedural sedation, usually only one intravenous injection is necessary due to the longer duration of action. This calls for qualified, experienced assisting personnel. If a second physician is available who can administer the sedation, that physician will bear the responsibility. In the case of nurse-administered propofol sedation, the examining physician bears the final responsibility.[1]

Ultimately, the involvement of assisting personnel depends on a personal assessment by the responsible physician. There are no legal provisions that cover this issue. Health care professionals involved in sedation, monitoring, and follow-up should participate periodically in structured continuing-education curricula. It should be added that while nurses monitor patients as part of their normal duties, nurses who assume physician activities do so on a voluntary basis, and they are free to refuse those activities without legal ramifications.

11.4 Monitoring Requirements

Because the examining physician is usually unable to give adequate attention to the patient's vital functions during the procedure, one person specially trained and qualified in patient monitoring must be present who can perform this task. Appropriate monitoring devices should be used during sedation, and oxygen saturation should be monitored continuously by pulse oximetry. Propofol sedation may cause significant hypotension and requires that regular blood pressure readings be taken during the procedure. A patient care record that documents the most important parameters should be kept both for legal reasons and for good practice. ECG monitoring is necessary only in certain situations, such as patients with preexisting heart disease. Patient monitoring in endosonography may be particularly difficult because of the darkened room and thus requires specially trained personnel.

11.5 Postprocedure Care

Postinterventional monitoring is necessary to check for potential adverse effects of sedation and to avoid patient injury. The duration of the postinterventional observation period depends on the expected risk.[4,19] Patients may be released from observation when their vital signs are stable and they are fully oriented. This should be a physician-made decision. The following minimal criteria should be met before a patient is discharged home[1,13]:

- The patient is able to walk unaided (if this was possible before the procedure).
- There is little or no pain.
- Oral fluid intake is accomplished without difficulty.
- The patient experiences little or no nausea.
- Adequate follow-up care is available at home.
- If necessary, the physician may remind the patient of typical signs of complications and provide an emergency phone number.
- Patient is accompanied at discharge.

11.6 Complications

The main complication is oxygen desaturation in the blood. Every care team member should be proficient in measures such as increasing the oxygen delivery (*caution* in COPD patients), performing an Esmarch maneuver, and placing a Guedel or Wendel tube. If these measures are insufficient to correct oxygen desaturation, manually assisted ventilation of the patient is indicated. Mask ventilation should be tried first, followed if necessary by intubation. Thus, skills and equipment for intubation and bag ventilation should be available in the examination suite whenever agents such as propofol are used.

11.7 Summary

In summary, it may be said that interventional ultrasound procedures usually take between 5 and 10 minutes, so there is rarely a need for continuous sedation or its delegation to nonphysicians. Although rarely practicable, the presence of a second physician experienced in sedation would be the most favorable scenario. Because procedural sedation is so rarely needed, it is a situation that can usually be planned for. The ESGE (European Society of Gastrointestinal Endoscopy), the ESGENA (European Society of Gastroenterology and Endoscopy Nurses and Associates), and the ESA (European Society of Anesthesiology) published joint recommendations in 2010[20] that can provide excellent guidelines for sedation in interventional ultrasound.

References

[1] Riphaus A, Wehrmann T, Weber B et alSektion Endoskopie im Auftrag der Deutschen Gesellschaft für Verdauungs- und Stoffwechselerkrankungen e.V. (DGVS). Bundesverband Niedergelassener Gastroenterologen Deutschlands e.V. (Bng). Chirurgische Arbeitsgemeinschaft für Endoskopie und Sonographie der Deutschen Gesellschaft für Allgemein- und Viszeralchirurgie (DGAV). Deutsche Morbus Crohn/Colitis ulcerosa Vereinigung e.V. (DCCV). Deutsche Gesellschaft für Endoskopie-Assistenzpersonal (DEGEA). Deutsche Gesellschaft für Anästhesie und Intensivmedizin (DGAI). Gesellschaft für Recht und Politik im Gesundheitswesen (GPRG). S3-guidelines—sedation in gastrointestinal endoscopy [Article in German]. Z Gastroenterol 2008; 46: 1298–1330

[2] Cohen LB, Delegge MH, Aisenberg J et al. AGA Institute. AGA Institute review of endoscopic sedation. Gastroenterology 2007; 133: 675–701

[3] Dripps RD, Lamont A, Eckenhoff JE. The role of anesthesia in surgical mortality. JAMA 1961; 178: 261–266

[4] Faigel DO, Baron TH, Goldstein JL et al. Standards Practice Committee, American Society for Gastrointestinal Endoscopy. Guidelines for the use of deep sedation and anesthesia for GI endoscopy. Gastrointest Endosc 2002; 56: 613–617

[5] Society of Gastroenterology Nurses and Associates. SGNA position statement. Statement on the use of sedation and analgesia in the gastrointestinal endoscopy setting. Gastroenterol Nurs 2004; 27: 142–144

[6] Hochberger J, Maiss J, Hahn EG. The use of simulators for training in GI endoscopy. Endoscopy 2002; 34: 727–729

[7] Riphaus A, Rabofski M, Wehrmann T. Endoscopic sedation and monitoring practice in Germany: results from the first nationwide survey. Z Gastroenterol 2010; 48: 392–397

[8] Kankaria A, Lewis JH, Ginsberg G et al. Flumazenil reversal of psychomotor impairment due to midazolam or diazepam for conscious sedation for upper endoscopy. Gastrointest Endosc 1996; 44: 416–421

[9] Mora CT, Torjman M, White PF. Sedative and ventilatory effects of midazolam infusion: effect of flumazenil reversal. Can J Anaesth 1995; 42: 677–684

[10] Saletin M, Malchow H, Mühlhofer H, Fischer M, Pilot J, Rohde H. A randomised controlled trial to evaluate the effects of flumazenil after midazolam premedication in outpatients undergoing colonoscopy. Endoscopy 1991; 23: 331–333

[11] Carter AS, Bell GD, Coady T, Lee J, Morden A. Speed of reversal of midazolam-induced respiratory depression by flumazenil—a study in patients undergoing upper G.I. endoscopy. Acta Anaesthesiol Scand Suppl 1990; 92: 59–64; discussion 78

[12] Rex DK, Overley CA, Walker J. Registered nurse-administered propofol sedation for upper endoscopy and colonoscopy: Why? When? How? Rev Gastroenterol Disord 2003; 3: 70–80

[13] Riphaus A, Rabofski M, Wehrmann T. Endoscopic sedation and monitoring practice in Germany: results from the first nationwide survey. Z Gastroenterol 2010; 48: 392–397

[14] Schilling D, Rosenbaum A, Schweizer S, Richter H, Rumstadt B. Sedation with propofol for interventional endoscopy by trained nurses in high-risk octogenarians: a prospective, randomized, controlled study. Endoscopy 2009; 41: 295–298

[15] Sieg A. Propofol sedation in outpatient colonoscopy by trained practice nurses supervised by the gastroenterologist: a prospective evaluation of over 3000 cases. Z Gastroenterol 2007; 45: 697–701

[16] Vilmann P, Hornslet P, Simmons H, Hammering A, Clementsen P. [Propofol sedation administered by nurses for endoscopic procedures]. Ugeskr Laeger 2009; 171: 1840–1843

[17] Sipe BW, Rex DK, Latinovich D et al. Propofol versus midazolam/meperidine for outpatient colonoscopy: administration by nurses supervised by endoscopists. Gastrointest Endosc 2002; 55: 815–825

[18] Ulmer BJ, Hansen JJ, Overley CA et al. Propofol versus midazolam/fentanyl for outpatient colonoscopy: administration by nurses supervised by endoscopists. Clin Gastroenterol Hepatol 2003; 1: 425–432

[19] Waring JP, Baron TH, Hirota WK et al. American Society for Gastrointestinal Endoscopy, Standards of Practice Committee. Guidelines for conscious sedation and monitoring during gastrointestinal endoscopy. Gastrointest Endosc 2003; 58: 317–322

[20] Dumonceau JM, Riphaus A, Aparicio JR et al. NAAP Task Force Members. European Society of Gastrointestinal Endoscopy, European Society of Gastroenterology and Endoscopy Nurses and Associates, and the European Society of Anaesthesiology Guideline: Non-anesthesiologist administration of propofol for GI endoscopy. Endoscopy 2010; 42: 960–974

Specific Ultrasound-Guided Procedures:

Abdomen ... 119

Thorax ... 259

Urogenital System ... 273

Other Organ Systems ... 287

Other Applications of Interventional Ultrasound ... 353

Abdomen

12 Indications for Diagnostic Interventions in the Abdomen and Thorax (Liver, Pancreas, Spleen, Kidneys, Lung, Other Sites) . . . 120

13 Diagnostic and Therapeutic Paracentesis of Free Abdominal Fluid . . . 128

14 Fine Needle Aspiration Biopsy and Core Needle Biopsy . . . 138

15 Abscess Drainage . . . 144

16 Percutaneous Sclerotherapy of Cysts . . . 163

17 Interventional Treatment of Echinococcosis . . . 168

18 Local Ablative Procedures; Percutaneous Ethanol and Acetic Acid Injection . . . 179

19 Local Ablative Procedures for Liver Tumors, Radiofrequency Ablation . . . 185

20 Percutaneous Transhepatic Cholangiodrainage . . . 198

21 Percutaneous Gastrostomy . . . 215

22 Interventional Endosonography . . . 224

23 Special Issues Regarding Interventions in the Spleen . . . 254

12 Indications for Diagnostic Interventions in the Abdomen and Thorax (Liver, Pancreas, Spleen, Kidneys, Lung, Other Sites)

H. Kinkel, D. Nuernberg

Focal lesions in abdominal organs are a common finding in routine ultrasound examinations. An ultrasound-guided percutaneous aspiration or biopsy is a simple and safe procedure that allows an experienced operator to obtain material for histologic or cytologic analysis with little risk of complications.[1,2] Besides distinguishing between benign and malignant lesions,[3] this procedure can provide material for immunohistochemical testing that can further differentiate the lesion and direct further management.

12.1 Liver

12.1.1 Diffuse Liver Diseases

In parenchymal diseases of the liver, a histologic examination is crucial for initial evaluation and follow-up (▶ Table 12.1). Neither imaging studies nor serologic tests can accurately quantify disease activity or the fibrotic and cirrhotic changes that will determine the further clinical course. For its simplicity, we prefer the Menghini needle for ultrasound-guided liver biopsies (Hepafix Luer lock, 18 gauge/1.2 mm, needle length 88 mm, 45° bevel; Braun) (see Chapters 2 and 14).

Acute viral hepatitis is usually diagnosed by serologic testing (anti-HAV IgM, anti-HEV IgM; HBsAg, if positive anti-HBc IgM and HBV DNA; anti-HCV, if positive HCV RNA; anti-HDV IgM in acute hepatitis B; EBV IgM in patients with corresponding symptoms; CMV Ab and CMV DNA in immunosuppressed patients). Biopsy confirmation is necessary only if there is another presumed cause of liver damage besides acute viral hepatitis (e.g., a known history of chronic hepatitis with suspected superinfection, known alcohol abuse, autoimmune hepatitis). If the disease takes a fulminating course with impending liver failure, a prompt needle biopsy can be an important prognostic study—for if the rare necrotizing form is identified, liver transplantation will be the only remaining therapeutic option. In patients who show progressive jaundice, a rapid fall in transaminases, hepatic encephalopathy, and

Table 12.1 Indications for core needle biopsy in parenchymal liver diseases

Disease	Abbreviation	Indication for core histology
Acute viral hepatitis	AVH	Fulminating clinical course with impending liver failure
Chronic viral hepatitis	CVH	Grading before treatment and during further course
Autoimmune hepatitis	AIH	For confirmation and follow-up
Primary biliary cirrhosis	PBC	For staging and determining activity
Primary sclerosing cholangitis	PSC	Only in exceptional cases, as in overlap syndrome
Caroli syndrome		Assessment of fibrosis and before liver transplantation
Vanishing bile duct syndrome	VBDS	Essential for confirming diagnosis
Venoocclusive disease	VOD	To confirm diagnosis
Budd–Chiari syndrome	BCS	Biopsy generally is not indicated
Nonalcoholic steatohepatitis	NASH	May be done to confirm diagnosis
Alcoholic steatohepatitis	ASH	For grading of fibrosis and cirrhosis (in selected cases), with coexisting diseases, in preparation for liver transplantation
Hemochromatosis, porphyria, alpha$_1$-antitrypsin deficiency		For grading of fibrosis and cirrhosis
Glycogen storage disease		Biopsy with glycogen analysis, in vitro enzyme assay if needed
Wilson disease		For copper determination in doubtful cases
Drug-induced injury		Biopsy is essential to establish diagnosis
Osteomyelofibrosis	OMF	Detection of extramedullary hematopoiesis

deteriorating clinical status, percutaneous biopsy is contraindicated in cases with coagulation system collapse (Quick value < 50% and platelet count < 50 × 10^9/L) due to the excessive bleeding risk[4] (see Chapters 4 and 9). For the histologic evaluation of necrosis, transjugular liver biopsy is a safer alternative as it substantially reduces the risk of significant bleeding.

Specific diseases that can be investigated by ultrasound-guided biopsy are reviewed in the paragraphs below. Relevant diagnostic tests are shown in parentheses.

Hemochromatosis can be diagnosed serologically (ferritin, transferrin saturation, *HFE* gene mutation chromosome 6—C282Y, H63D, and S65C). The low genetic penetrance requires a liver biopsy if it is suspected that an additional agent is responsible for the liver damage (e.g., nonalcoholic steatohepatitis, NASH). The suspicion of severe fibrosis or cirrhosis should also be investigated by biopsy. This also applies to hepatic porphyria (total porphryins in the urine and stool during an acute attack) and alpha$_1$-antitrypsin deficiency (serum electrophoresis, phenotyping if required). With Wilson disease (ceruloplasmin; may test urinary copper at baseline and with D-penicillamine administration), the diagnosis should be confirmed histologically if tests are inconclusive (▸ Table 12.1). Urinary copper excretion < 100 µg/24 h confirms a positive treatment response. Later in the course of the disease, it may be necessary to perform a repeat liver biopsy to assess the degree of cirrhosis, especially as a prelude to liver transplantation. The glycogen storage diseases require biopsy with a glycogen analysis and, if necessary, an in vitro enzyme activity assay.

Primary biliary cirrhosis (PBC) is diagnosed serologically (anti-mitochondrial antibodies [AMAs]). Histologic evaluation of the activity and stage of the disease has additional prognostic significance (e.g., expand pharmacologic therapy, prepare for liver transplantation) and fully justifies liver biopsy.[5] Autoimmune hepatitis should be consistently investigated by liver biopsy before treatment is initiated and later to evaluate the course. Histologic evaluation is also recommended before treatment is concluded.[6]

While Doppler ultrasound can demonstrate occlusion of the large hepatic veins in Budd–Chiari syndrome, the diagnosis of venoocclusive disease relies entirely on histologic findings.

In chronic hepatitis C and B, the histologic grading of viral hepatitis (e.g., using the Desmet–Scheuer score[7]) provides an additional decision-making criterion for treatment planning, since higher grades of fibrosis would predict a poorer response to interferon therapy. Moreover, evaluation by an experienced pathologist will disclose aspects that may be important in the clinical management of the patient (e.g., changes due to coexisting NASH indicating a need for weight reduction).[8]

In patients with nonalcoholic steatohepatitis (NASH), we routinely perform percutaneous liver biopsy as an aid to differential diagnosis and staging (▸ Table 12.1). Alcohol-induced hepatitis is usually diagnosed from the patient's history and does not consistently require biopsy. If inflammatory hepatitis due to a different cause is suspected (e.g., hepatic involvement by sarcoidosis), liver biopsy may be helpful in exceptional cases—especially if the findings of the presumed disease are inconclusive.

12.1.2 Focal Liver Lesions

Focal liver lesions are a frequent indication for biopsy, due in part to the possibility of metastatic lesions from various tumors. On the other hand, the overall percentage of cases selected for biopsy has fallen by an estimated 5 to 10% due to the high diagnostic accuracy of contrast-enhanced ultrasonography.[9]

Benign Lesions

Hemangioma and focal nodular hyperplasia (FNH) are the most common benign liver lesions and occur predominantly in female patients.[10] Imaging evaluation is adequate in most cases, making it unnecessary to proceed with biopsy (*caution:* FNH is difficult to distinguish from fibrolamellar liver cancer). Liver biopsy is indicated only in patients who have a history of malignancy and equivocal imaging findings. This also applies to the much rarer entity of hepatic adenoma. Larger adenomas should be resected due to the high incidence of rupture (up to 30%).[11] The need for preoperative biopsy should be assessed in consultation with the surgeon.

Malignant Lesions

Metastases

The fine needle aspiration cytology of metastatic lesions in known cancer patients is often sufficient to confirm a malignant histology. But if a primary tumor is not known or the tumor is assumed to have originated in the liver, core needle biopsy may be necessary to establish the tumor histology.

On the initial discovery of liver metastases in the absence of a known primary (CUP syndrome), needle biopsy can provide essential information and should therefore be done liberally and without delay (▸ Fig. 12.1). Immunohistologic staining of the specimen is a very rewarding test.

Primary Liver Tumors

The ultrasound visualization of cholangiocellular carcinoma (CCC) is difficult and often requires the use of sonographic contrast agents. Cytologic-histologic confirmation can be obtained during ERCP (endoscopic retrograde cholangiopancreatography) in tumors that have invaded the biliary tract. Percutaneous biopsy of CCC can also be

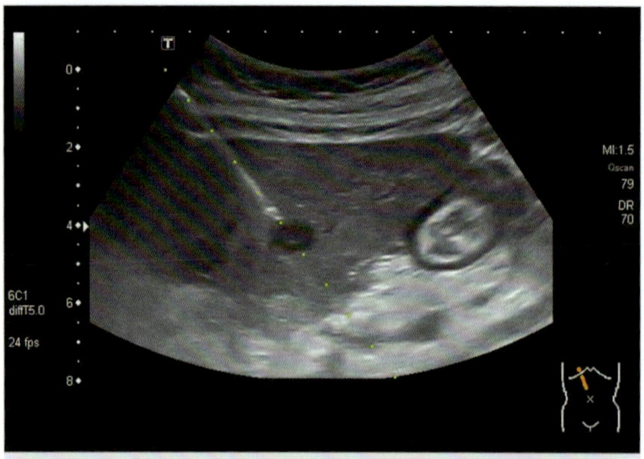

Fig. 12.1 Biopsy of a hepatic metastasis from breast cancer. Metachromatic metastasis. The patient also had a history of renal cell carcinoma.

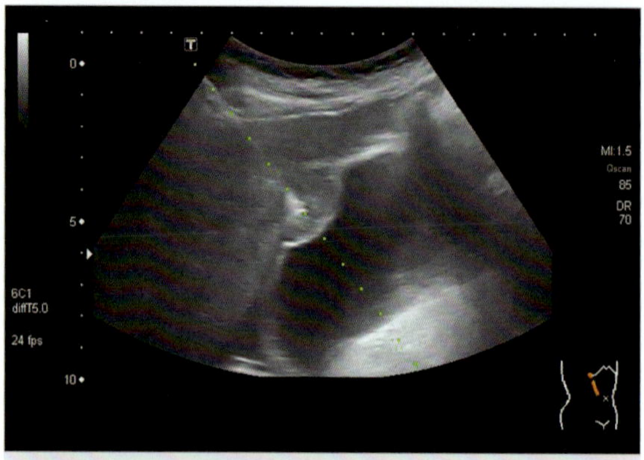

Fig. 12.2 Biopsy of a hepatocellular carcinoma. AFP (alpha-fetoprotein) 73 kU/L, HCC in chronic hepatitis C bordering directly on the gallbladder = liquid structure.

done in a palliative setting,[12,13] in which case we usually perform a fine needle aspiration biopsy.

The cirrhotic liver is an unusual site for metastatic lesions but is a relatively common site for hepatocellular carcinoma (HCC). The friable structure of cirrhotic liver tissue makes it more difficult to retrieve a good-quality tissue core, but it is important for the pathologist to receive an intact core due to the inherent difficulty of distinguishing among regenerative nodules, dysplastic nodules, and well-differentiated hepatocellular carcinoma[11] (▶ Fig. 12.2, ▶ Fig. 12.3).

With contrast-enhanced ultrasound (CEUS), the enhancement kinetics of the contrast agent provide clearer delineation of focal lesions in the cirrhotic liver. If a potentially resectable HCC is suspected, we do not perform a liver biopsy, especially in patients with positive alpha-fetoprotein (AFP).[14,15] If the only treatment options are ablative procedures (see Chapters 18 and 19) or chemotherapy, we biopsy the tumor before treatment. The risks of biopsy in patients with ascites and impaired coagulation are discussed in Chapter 9.

The guidance of liver biopsy by CEUS, with its better delineation of poorly perfused necrotic areas within a focal lesion, results in a better histologic specimen and a more accurate evaluation. For the same reason, it is usually best to target a peripheral site in the lesion for biopsy and avoid highly vascularized areas in larger lesions. This can be facilitated by CEUS.

Liquid Lesions

Liver cysts and biliomas should be biopsied if secondary infection is suspected. Parasitic cysts should be biopsied only in rare cases with equivocal serology. Liver

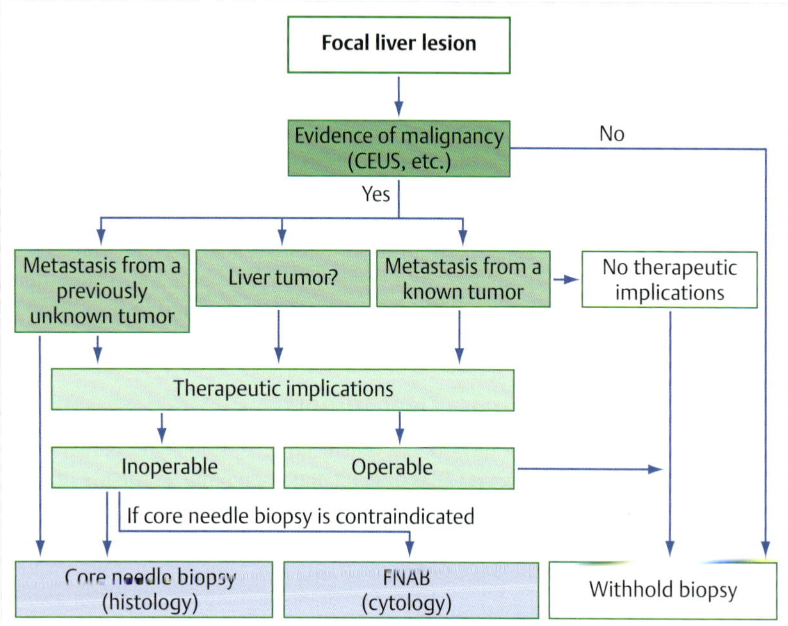

Fig. 12.3 Indications for the benign/malignant differentiation of a focal liver lesion by needle biopsy.

abscesses, which are more common in immunosuppressed patients, should also be biopsied before definitive treatment to obtain material for bacteriologic testing. Fine needle aspiration biopsy is also satisfactory in these cases. Diagnosis and treatment should be performed in one sitting whenever possible. If logistical changes are necessary, such as additional radiologic localization, the examinations should at least be scheduled close together (Chapters 16 and 17).

12.2 Pancreas

Abdominal ultrasound imaging of the pancreas is not always easy, even for experienced operators, due to the retroperitoneal location of the organ posterior to the stomach and bowel. Endosonography (endoscopic ultrasound) can provide excellent visualization of the pancreas, and pancreatic biopsy is increasingly becoming the domain of endosonographic guidance, while the percutaneous technique is rarely practiced today[16,17] (Chapter 22). This applies to pancreatic carcinoma as well as neuroendocrine tumors and gastrointestinal stromal tumors (GIST) in this region. In palliative settings, the tumor should be confirmed prior to chemotherapy (▶ Fig. 12.4, ▶ Fig. 12.5) (Chapter 33). The percutaneous route is still available as an alternative.[18] A potentially operable pancreatic carcinoma is not a primary indication for biopsy. Pancreatic metastasis is a somewhat rare entity that, when suspected (e.g., in patients with a history of RCC), justifies primary investigation by percutaneous biopsy.

In principle, a cystic pancreatic lesion is also an indication for sonographically or endosonographically guided biopsy (▶ Fig. 12.6) (Chapter 22). Pseudocysts, which generally can be positively identified as such based on the history and clinical presentation, should be aspirated with a thin needle under sonographic or endosonographic guidance for recovery of organisms if an infection or abscess is suspected.[19,20]

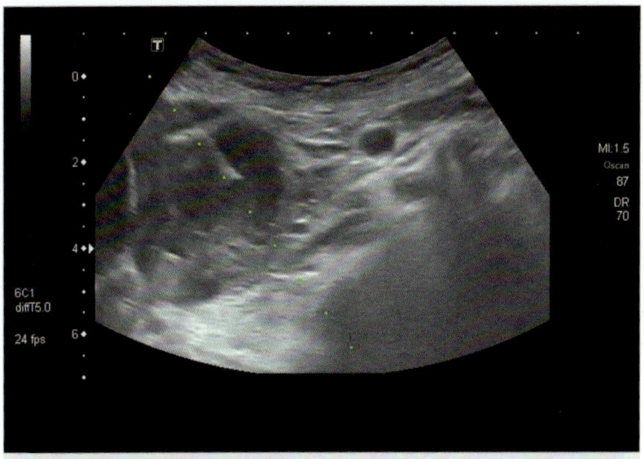

Fig. 12.4 Biopsy of an inoperable pancreatic cancer before palliative chemotherapy.

Discrimination between cystic pancreatic lesions and tumors is difficult to accomplish with ultrasound, just as it is with other imaging procedures (▶ Table 12.2). Endosonographic fine needle aspiration biopsy is helpful in these cases only if the result is positive. If a tumor is suspected in a patient with a history of chronic pancreatitis, surgical treatment is recommended even when not preceded by needle biopsy.[18]

A biopsy needle should not be introduced through the colon or gallbladder. It is safe to pass a needle through the stomach or small intestine. Again, it is occasionally helpful to perform the biopsy under CEUS guidance (see above).

12.3 Spleen

If ultrasound guided spleen biopsy is indicated for the investigation of focal lesions or splenic infiltration by a

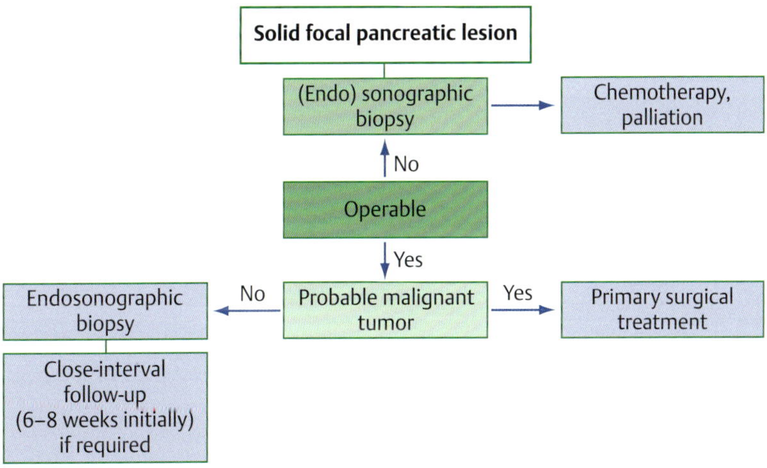

Fig. 12.5 Flowchart for the biopsy of solid pancreatic lesions.

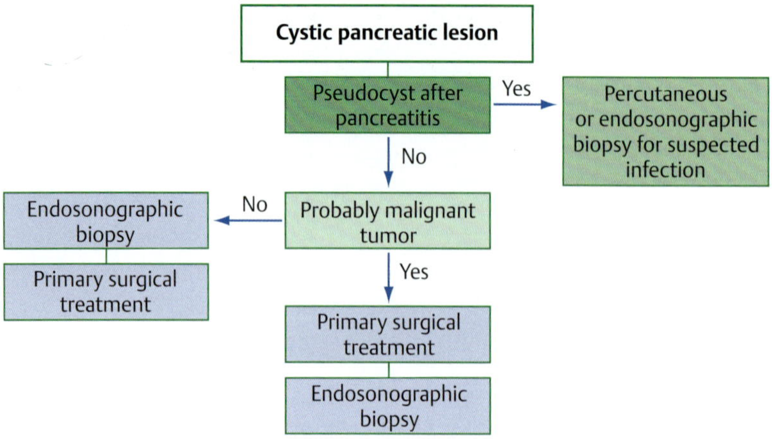

Fig. 12.6 Flowchart for the biopsy of cystic pancreatic lesions.

Table 12.2 Parameters for the diagnosis of cystic pancreatic lesions

Lesion	Cytology	Bacteriology	Lipase	CEA[a]	CA15-3	CA72-4
Pseudocyst	Benign	+	↑↑	→	→	→
Serous cystadenoma	Benign	–	↑	→	→	→
Mucinous cystadenoma	Benign	–	↓	↑	↑	↑
Cystadenocarcinoma	Malignant	–	↓	↑↑	↑↑	↑↑

[a] CEA, carcinoembryonic antigen.

hematologic disease,[21] it should be done strictly with a fine needle to reduce the risk of hemorrhage (Chapter 23).

12.4 Kidneys

Ultrasound-guided biopsy is the procedure of choice for the investigation of parenchymal renal diseases (Chapter 25) and focal renal lesions, although preoperative tumor biopsy is rarely necessary due to the current availability of minimally invasive, organ-conserving surgical techniques.[22–24] Cystic lesions of the kidney can be clearly differentiated with CEUS and then selectively biopsied if required[25,26] (▶ Fig. 12.7). Local ablative therapy, which is increasingly considered as an alternative in geriatric and palliative patients and others, should always be preceded by biopsy to confirm malignancy (Chapter 26).

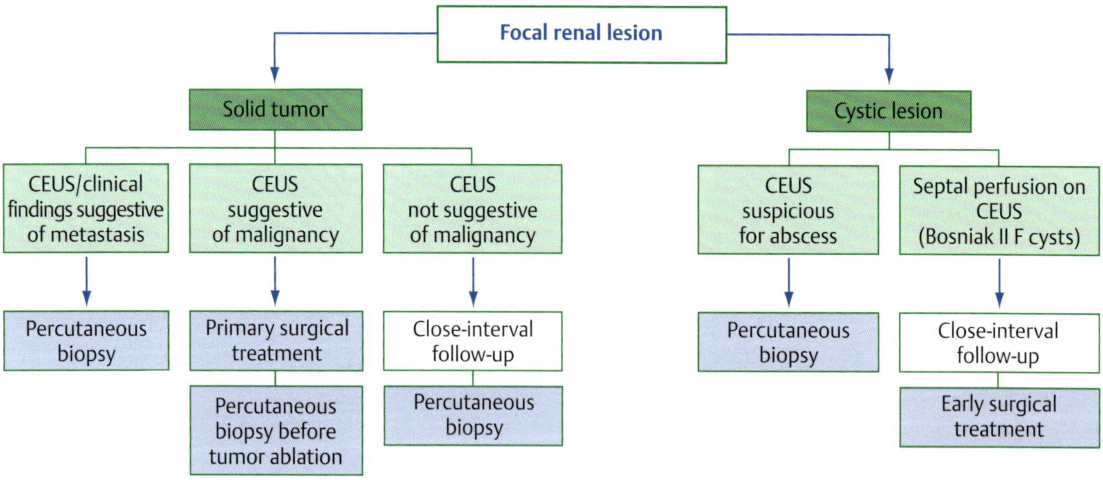

Fig. 12.7 Flowchart for the biopsy of focal renal lesions.

12.5 Lung

Pulmonary lesions can be biopsied with guidance by percutaneous ultrasound, EUS (endoscopic ultrasound) via the transesophageal route, or EBUS (endobronchial ultrasound) via the transbronchial route. CT-guided biopsy as well as mediastinoscopy and thoracoscopy, which are particularly favored by surgeons, should be strictly second-line alternatives.[27–29] Details are described in Chapters 22 and 25.

12.6 Adrenal Gland

The adrenal gland can be consistently defined by percutaneous ultrasound, although endosonography is better for imaging the left adrenal gland. An adrenal mass fortuitously detected by ultrasound in a patient with no tumor history (incidentaloma) is usually benign, adenoma being much more common (up to 80%) than pheochromocytoma. True incidentalomas (no tumor history or hypertension) should be followed with ultrasound and should be biopsied only if they grow larger than 3 to 5 cm. Pheochromocytoma is a relative contraindication to needle biopsy because of the risk of inducing hormone secretion and hypertensive crisis.

The adrenal gland is the fourth most common site of metastatic disease. The tumors that most often metastasize to the adrenal gland are melanoma, lung cancer, breast cancer, stomach cancer, and renal carcinoma. Adrenal metastasis should be excluded in all patients with an underlying malignant disease, and an adrenal mass in a patient with a cancer history should always be investigated by fine needle aspiration biopsy.[30]

Adrenal biopsy should always be preceded by a hormonal evaluation (serum potassium, free catecholamines in 24-hour urine, dexamethasone suppression test, blood pressure monitoring, and serum aldosterone and plasma renin activity in hypertensive patients with a low potassium level).

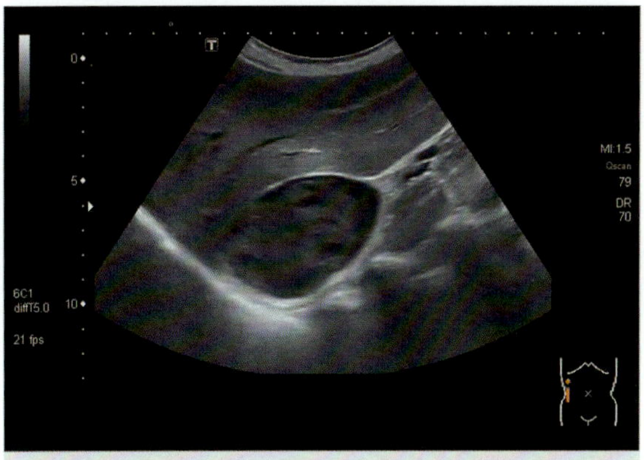

Fig. 12.8 Adrenal metastasis from bronchial carcinoma.

Adrenal biopsy is indicated in patients with adrenal metastases (if it will have therapeutic implications, ▶ Fig. 12.8), an enlarging indeterminate mass (incidentaloma, ▶ Fig. 12.9), suspected lymphomatous infiltration, or in patients who refuse surgery.

12.7 Lymph Nodes

While benign diseases are a relatively frequent cause of enlarged lymph nodes in the adolescent age group and do not require investigation by biopsy, the most common cause of lymph node enlargement in older patients is malignancy. If a malignant lymphoma is suspected, the International Lymphoma Study Group strongly recommends open lymphadenectomy. The German Society of

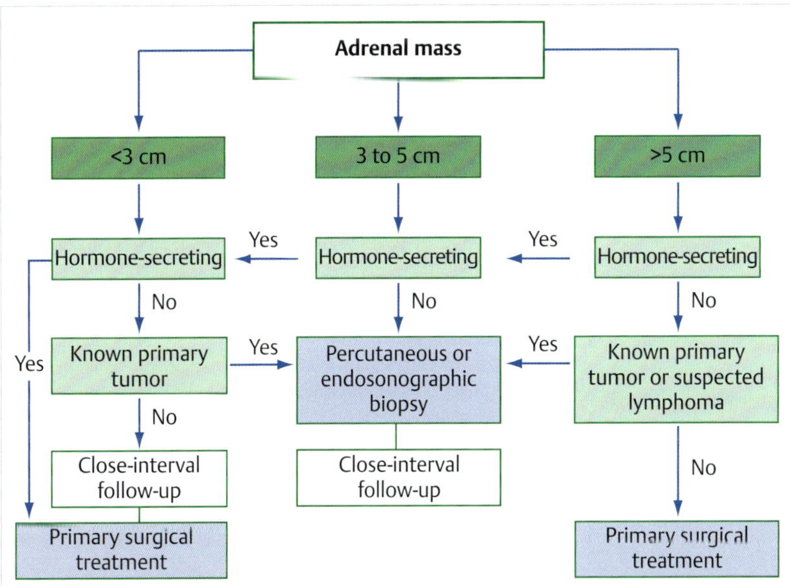

Fig. 12.9 Flowchart for the biopsy of adrenal enlargement. (Source: Nürnberg 2005.[31])

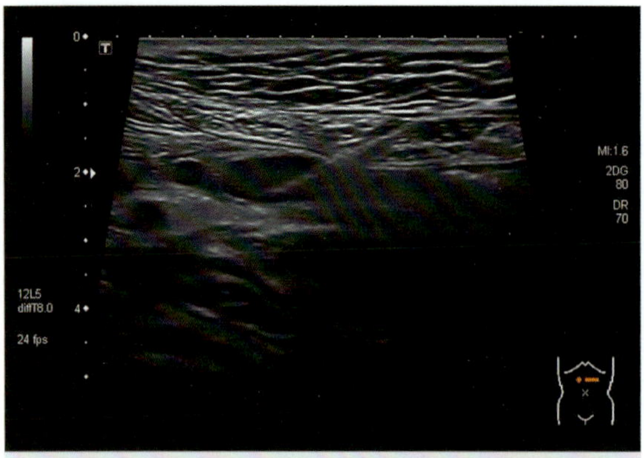

Fig. 12.10 Metachronous lymph node metastases following surgical treatment of gastric carcinoma.

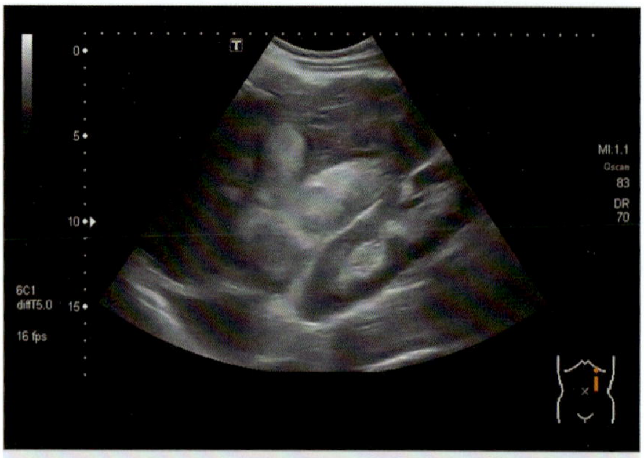

Fig. 12.11 Sarcoma in the area of the left adrenal gland.

Hematology and Oncology favors lymphadenectomy but also allows for percutaneous core needle biopsy. Study protocols for lymphomas also prescribe open lymphadenectomy (lymph node architecture can only be evaluated histologically). Similarly, if Hodgkin disease is suspected, fine needle aspiration is generally considered to provide an inadequate cellular specimen.

Lymph node metastases from solid tumors can be consistently differentiated by fine needle aspiration biopsy (FNAB), and this technique is preferred in patients with a corresponding history (▶ Fig. 12.10). FNAB is usually adequate in patients with metachronous metastases as well.

The percutaneous biopsy of enlarged lymph nodes is generally a safe and uncomplicated procedure.[2,32] Transcolic punctures should be avoided (see Chapter 9).

Practice

If the history and clinical findings suggest a malignant disease, we also favor lymphadenectomy if the lymph node is located at a superficial or favorable site (cervical, axillary, inguinal).

With difficult surgical access (abdominal, retroperitoneal, mediastinal), sonographic or endosonographic biopsy is the preferred initial step.

12.8 Other Lesions

Mesenteric, peritoneal, and subcutaneous masses are another indication for ultrasound-guided biopsy apart from the organ lesions cited above. This particularly applies to patients who would not be good candidates for invasive surgical diagnosis (e.g., geriatric and palliative patients). FNAB has a wide range of indications in these cases, provided it will have therapeutic implications (Chapter 33).

Percutaneous biopsy is appropriate for all gastrointestinal tumors for which endoscopic biopsy is not an option or has been unproductive. On the other hand, preoperative biopsy should be used very sparingly on lesions that are resectable for cure.

If possible, needle biopsy should be avoided if imaging findings are suggestive of a sarcoma[33] (▶ Fig. 12.11).

References

[1] Frieser M, Lindner A, Meyer S et al. Spectrum and bleeding complications of sonographically guided interventions of the liver and pancreas [Article in German]. Ultraschall Med. 2009; 30: 168–174

[2] Weiss H, Düntsch U. Complications of fine needle puncture. DEGUM survey II [Article in German]. Ultraschall Med 1996; 17: 118–130

[3] Seitz K, Stuböck J, Littmann M, Schnitzler S, Seitz G. Histologically proven results of sonographical and computed tomographic tumor diagnosis. Eur J Ultrasound 1996; 4: 43–43

[4] Rifai K, Bahr MJ. Acute liver failure [Article in German]. Internist (Berl) 2003; 44: 58: 5–59–0, 592–598

[5] Lindor KD, Gershwin ME, Poupon R, Kaplan M, Bergasa NV, Heathcote EJ American Association for Study of Liver Diseases. Primary biliary cirrhosis. Hepatology 2009; 50: 291–308

[6] Beuers U, Wiedmann KH, Kleber G, Fleig WE. Therapy of autoimmune hepatitis, primary biliary cirrhosis and primary sclerosing cholangitis. Consensus of the German Society of Digestive System and Metabolic Diseases [Article in German]. Z Gastroenterol 1997; 35: 1041–1049

[7] Desmet VJ, Gerber M, Hoofnagle JH, Manns M, Scheuer PJ. Classification of chronic hepatitis: diagnosis, grading and staging. Hepatology 1994; 19: 1513–1520

[8] Schirmacher P, Fleig WE, Dienes HP Deutsche Gesellschaft fur Pathologie (DGP), Deutsche Gesellschaft fur Verdauungs- und Stoffwechselkrankheiten (DGVS), Kompetenznetz Hepatitis (HepNet). Biopsy diagnosis of chronic hepatitis [Article in German]. Z Gastroenterol 2004; 42: 175–185

[9] Strobel D, Seitz K, Blank W et al. Contrast-enhanced ultrasound for the characterization of focal liver lesions—diagnostic accuracy in clinical practice (DEGUM multicenter trial). Ultraschall Med 2008; 29: 499–505

[10] Nufer M, Stuckmann G, Decurtins M. Benign liver tumors: diagnosis and therapy—a review [Article in German]. Schweiz Med Wochenschr 1999; 129: 1257–1264

[11] Schirmacher P, Longerich T. Highly differentiated liver tumors: recent developments and their diagnostic application [Article in German]. Pathologe 2009; 30 (Suppl 2): 200–206

[12] Khan SA, Davidson BR, Goldin R et al. Guidelines for the diagnosis and treatment of cholangiocarcinoma: consensus document. Gut 2002; 51 (Suppl 6): VI1–9

[13] Anderson CD, Pinson CW, Berlin J, Chari RS. Diagnosis and treatment of cholangiocarcinoma. Oncologist 2004; 9: 43–57

[14] Caselmann WH, Blum HE, Fleig WE et al. Guidelines of the German Society of Digestive and Metabolic Diseases for diagnosis and therapy of hepatocellular carcinoma. German Society of Digestive and Metabolic Diseases [Article in German]. Z Gastroenterol 1999; 37: 353–365

[15] Bruix J, Sherman M Practice Guidelines Committee, American Association for the Study of Liver Diseases. Management of hepatocellular carcinoma. Hepatology 2005; 42: 1208–1236

[16] Boujaoude J. Role of endoscopic ultrasound in diagnosis and therapy of pancreatic adenocarcinoma. World J Gastroenterol 2007; 13: 3662–3666

[17] Gress F, Gottlieb K, Sherman S, Lehman G. Endoscopic ultrasonography-guided fine-needle aspiration biopsy of suspected pancreatic cancer. Ann Intern Med 2001; 134: 459–464

[18] Adler G, Seufferlein T, Bischoff SC et al. S3-Guidelines "Exocrine pancreatic cancer" 2007 [Article in German]. Z Gastroenterol 2007; 45: 487–523

[19] Lerch MM, Stier A, Wahnschaffe U, Mayerle J. Pancreatic pseudocysts: observation, endoscopic drainage, or resection? Dtsch Arztebl Int 2009; 106: 614–621

[20] Huber W, Schmid RM. Acute pancreatitis: evidence based diagnosis and treatment. Dtsch Arztebl Int 2007; 104: A1832–1842

[21] Nuernberg D, Ignee A, Dietrich CF. Ultrasound in gastroenterology—liver and spleen [Article in German]. Z Gastroenterol 2006; 44: 991–1000

[22] Schneider R, Lopau K. What is your diagnosis? Transcutaneous renal biopsy [Article in German]. Dtsch Med Wochenschr 2010; 135: 1247–1249

[23] Ljungberg B, et al. Guidelines on Renal Cell Carcinoma. Arnheim, The Netherlands: European Association of Urology; 2010

[24] Remzi M, Klingler H-Ch, Marberger M. Warum ist eine präoperative bioptische Abklärung einer soliden Nierenraumforderung sinnvoll? J Urogynäkol 2006: 18–19

[25] Warren KS, McFarlane J. The Bosniak classification of renal cystic masses. BJU Int 2005; 95: 939–942

[26] Ignee A, Straub B, Schuessler G, Dietrich CF. Contrast enhanced ultrasound of renal masses. World J Radiol 2010; 2: 15–31

[27] Jenssen C. Diagnostische Endosonographie—state of the art 2009. Endo heute 2009; 22: 89–104

[28] Mathis G, Bitschnau R, Gehmacher O, Dirschmid K. Ultrasound-guided transthoracic puncture [Article in German]. Eur J Ultrasound 1999; 20: 226–235

[29] Schanz S, Kruis W. Endoscopic ultrasound-guided fine-needle aspiration [Article in German]. Dtsch Med Wochenschr 2005; 130: 1957–1961

[30] Allolio B, Fassnacht M, Arlt W. Malignant tumors of the adrenal cortex [Article in German]. Internist (Berl) 2002; 43: 186–195

[31] Nürnberg D. Ultrasound of adrenal gland tumours and indications for fine needle biopsy (uFNB) [Article in German]. Ultraschall Med 2005; 26: 458–469

[32] Urich K. Ultraschallgesteuerte Stanzbiopsien peripherer und abdomineller Lymphknoten. Inaugural-Dissertation Universität Marburg 2008. Available from: http://archiv.ub.uni-marburg.de/diss/z2008/0484/.../dku.pdf

[33] Casali PG, Blay JY ESMO/CONTICANET/EUROBONET Consensus Panel of experts. Soft tissue sarcomas: ESMO Clinical Practice Guidelines for diagnosis, treatment and follow-up. Ann Oncol 2010; 21 (Suppl 5): v198–v203

13 Diagnostic and Therapeutic Paracentesis of Free Abdominal Fluid

D. Nuernberg

Free intra-abdominal fluid collections are generally abnormal and require investigation. Peritoneal fluid collections (ascites) are easy to detect with ultrasound. The fluid appears echo-free, may contain internal echoes, and collects at typical sites between the abdominal organs in the peritoneal cavity.

13.1 Peritoneal Cavity

The peritoneum is the thin serous membrane that covers the abdominal organs (visceral peritoneum) and also lines the abdominal wall (parietal peritoneum). The space between the visceral and parietal peritoneum is the peritoneal cavity. Normally it is only a potential space that is not visible sonographically, but it may become visible under abnormal conditions. An actual space develops only when fluid or some other substance (tumor, gas) occupies the peritoneal cavity, forming an intraperitoneal mass or collection.

13.2 Sites of Predilection for Intra-abdominal Fluid

Fluid tends to gravitate toward dependent sites, i.e., posterior sites in the supine position and lower abdominal sites in an upright position. An awareness of these sites of predilection aids in the identification of fluids and the compartments they occupy (▶ Fig. 13.1). Fluid moves when a patient is repositioned, gravitating toward the lowest level.[1]

Sites of predilection for intra-abdominal fluid collections are:

- Right perihepatic space
- Left perihepatic space
- Right subhepatic space (between the right lobe of the liver and the right kidney = Morison pouch)
- Subphrenic space
- Perisplenic space
- Omental bursa

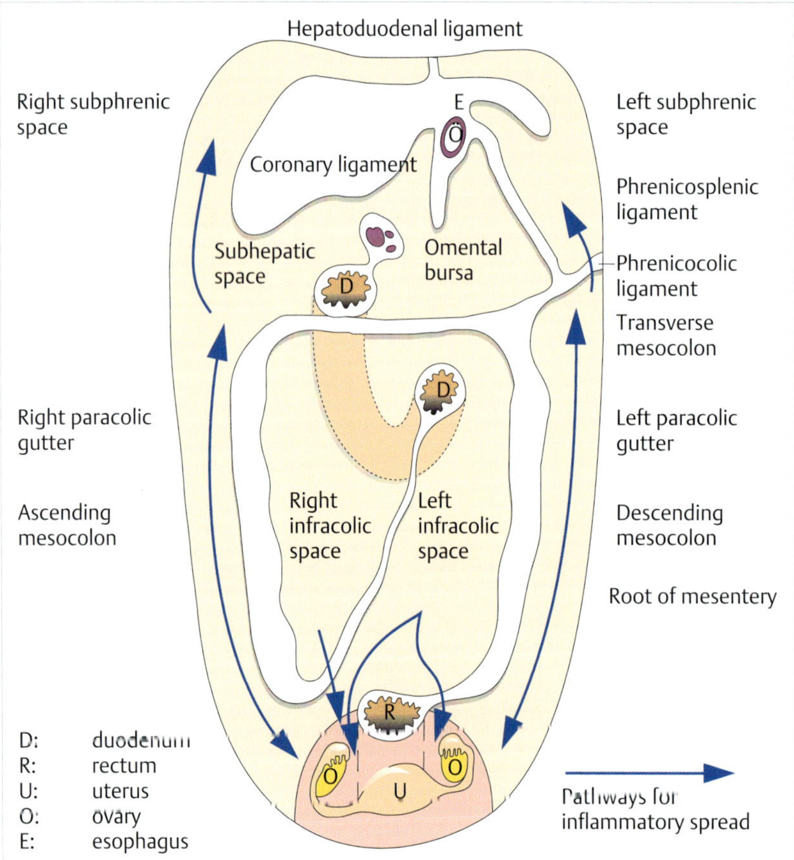

Fig. 13.1 Compartments in the peritoneal cavity. (Source: reference[1].)

Table 13.1 Ultrasound morphology of fluid collections

Echogenicity	Contents	Ultrasound visualization
Echo-free	Transudate	Clear visualization with good evaluation of surroundings
	Exudate	
	Blood (early phase)	
Hypoechoic	Exudate	Clear visualization with moderately good evaluation of surroundings
	Blood (late phase)	
	Bile	
	Pus	
	Chyle	

Source: based on reference[1].

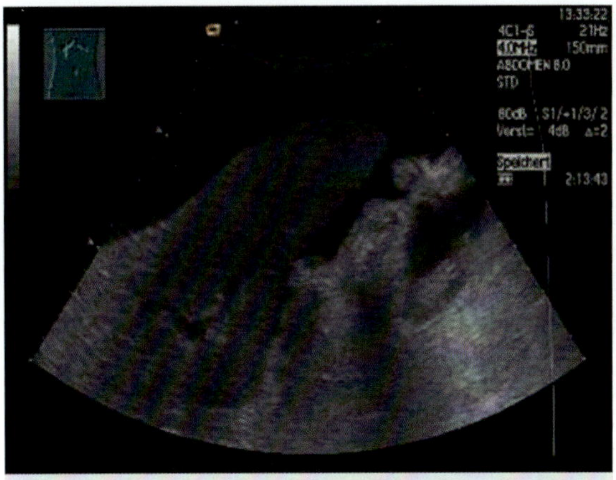

Fig. 13.2 Echo-free ascites: transudate due to decompensated hepatic cirrhosis.

- Cul-de-sac, perivesical space
- Between loops of intestine (separation of bowel loops)

13.3 Pathogenesis and Differential Diagnosis of Ascites

There are various mechanisms of fluid collection within the peritoneal cavity. They include the hypersecretion of serous fluid by the peritoneum and impaired fluid absorption, which may occur in peritonitis, for example. Fluid may also enter the peritoneal cavity as a result of injury to fluid-containing structures. This would include bleeding into the peritoneal cavity (hemoperitoneum), biliary perforation (intraperitoneal bile leak), and gastrointestinal perforation. Intraperitoneal fluid collections may also result from pressure alterations in the venous system (right heart failure, portal hypertension).[2]

Ascites formation has a diverse pathogenesis. Differential diagnosis relies mainly on the history, the clinical presentation, the fluid distribution by ultrasound imaging, ultrasound morphology (▶ Table 13.1), and ultimately on ultrasound-guided fine-needle aspiration biopsy (US-FNAB).

The differential diagnosis of intraperitoneal fluid collections is in ▶ Table 13.2.

13.4 Specific Indications

13.4.1 Transudate

If the intra-abdominal fluid collection is completely echo-free, contains no floating particles or fibrin strands, and shows no wall irregularities, it is most likely a transudate (▶ Fig. 13.2). This means that laboratory testing of the fluid will show a protein content < 30 g/L. Typical examples are found in hepatic cirrhosis and heart failure.

13.4.2 Exudate

If the fluid collection in the abdominal cavity is permeated by fine internal echoes or contains septations, it is most likely an exudate. It is also common for ultrasound to show filamentous structures adherent to the lateral abdominal wall or visceral peritoneum. These fibrin strands often show a classic swaying or undulating motion when the patient is repositioned. Examples of exudative ascites are pancreatogenic ascites and purulent peritonitis. Echogenic ascites is also found in peritoneal carcinomatosis and spontaneous bacterial peritonitis (SBP) in patients with hepatic cirrhosis (▶ Fig. 13.3).

Table 13.2 Differential diagnosis of intraperitoneal fluid

Transudate	Exudate	Blood	Postoperative, traumatic
Hepatic cirrhosis	Peritoneal carcinomatosis	Trauma	Hematoma
Budd–Chiari syndrome	Peritonitis	Iatrogenic	Seroma
Right heart failure	Pancreatitis	Ectopic pregnancy	Bilioma
Inferior vena cava obstruction	Tuberculosis	Coagulopathy	Urinoma
Nephrotic syndrome	Peritoneal dialysis	Ruptured aortic aneurysm	Bowel contents
Mesenteric vein thrombosis	Mesothelioma		Cyst contents
Hypoalbuminemia			Lymphocele (chyloperitoneum)

Source: reference[29].

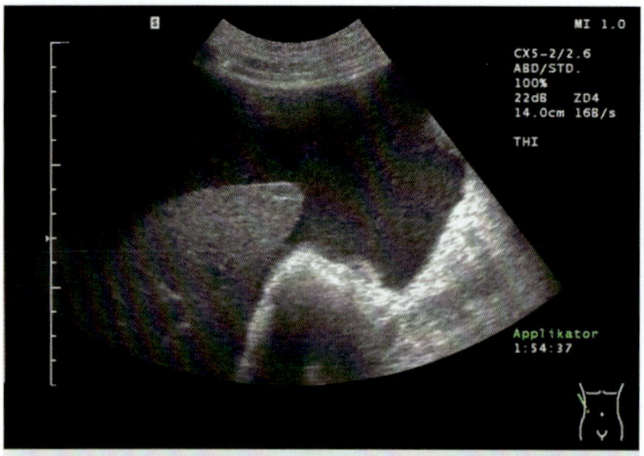

Fig. 13.3 Echogenic ascites in spontaneous bacterial peritonitis.

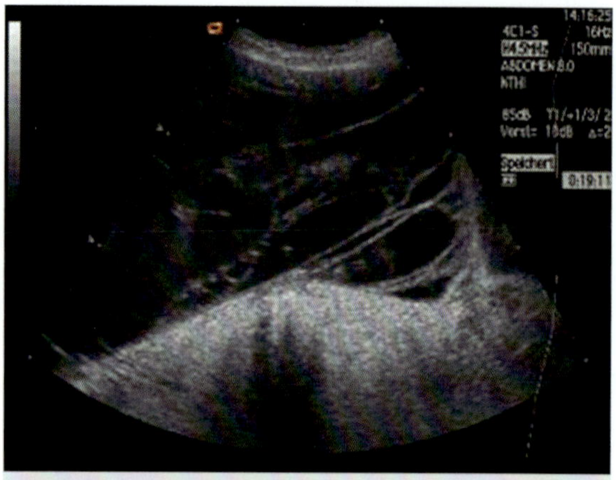

Fig. 13.4 Purulent peritonitis in a patient who had undergone a previous pancreatectomy for chronic pancreatitis.

13.4.3 Cirrhosis

Ascites in portal decompensated hepatic cirrhosis is usually echo-free. The underlying disease is easily diagnosed from the hepatic changes. Irregular liver contours and splenomegaly are the most immediate and reliable signs.

On the other hand, the ascites is found to contain fine, floating internal echoes in up to 20% of cases. Associated findings in pronounced cases may include septa, mural fibrin strands, and partially loculated ascites. Clinically, the ascites is refractory to treatment. These are signs of SBP, one of the most frequent complications of cirrhosis. The diagnosis relies on needle aspiration and fluid analysis (determination of granulocyte count or organism identification). Ascites should be investigated by percutaneous aspiration, at least initially and also later in the course if the ascites is refractory to medical treatment.

13.4.4 Heart Failure

Transudate in decompensated right heart failure is usually a late sign and is observed after or coexisting with pleural effusion (right > left). Besides general clinical manifestations, typical signs at ultrasound are a markedly dilated and stiff inferior vena cava and enlarged hepatic veins (prominent hepatic venous confluence).

13.4.5 Hypoalbuminemia

A protein deficiency (due to varying causes) with a very low plasma albumin level may lead to transudation. This is associated with a detectable thickening of the gallbladder wall (> 3 mm). No changes are observed in the hepatic parenchyma or liver vessels. Laboratory tests further advance the diagnosis.

13.4.6 Peritonitis

Inflammation and infection of the peritoneum may also incite the formation of ascites. Usually this fluid is echogenic and contains fibrin strands and septa (exudate). In cases with moderate hypersecretion due to a viral infection with polyserositis, for example, the ascites may also be echo-free. Severe purulent peritonitis is characterized by echogenic contents and adhesions, matted loops of small bowel, and the frequent presence of gas inclusions (▶ Fig. 13.4).

13.4.7 Peritoneal Carcinomatosis

The malignant ascites that develops in peritoneal carcinomatosis may be echogenic to echo-free. The sonographic criteria for differentiating between benign and malignant ascites are described in ▶ Table 13.3. Notably, no signs of hepatic cirrhosis or portal hypertension are observed, and the detection of a possible primary tumor or metastases may point to the malignant cause.

Echogenic ascites with fine internal echoes, wall irregularities, septa, mesenteric retraction, and solid structures on the peritoneum characterize peritoneal carcinomatosis. Differentiation between benign and malignant ascites is a typical "building block" diagnosis. A single fine-needle aspiration (FNA) provides poor sensitivity (50–60%) in the diagnosis of malignant ascites.[1,3–5] Thus if a tumor is suspected, the cytologic examination should be done more than once (at least three times) or a larger initial fluid volume should be centrifuged for analysis.

13.4.8 Hemoperitoneum

Fresh bleeding into the peritoneal cavity after blunt abdominal trauma, ectopic pregnancy, iatrogenic (interventional) injury, or medication (e.g., anticoagulants) is often echo-free in its initial state. As the hours pass, echogenic internal structures appear in the form of fibrin strands due to initial clotting (▶ Fig. 13.5). The history, clinical presentation, and changing ultrasound findings are diagnostic of intraperitoneal bleeding in 95 to 98% of

Table 13.3 Sonographic differential diagnosis of benign and malignant ascites

Sonographic features	Benign	Malignant
Echogenicity of ascites:		
• Echo-free	++	+
• Internal echoes (echogenic)	+	++
• Septations	+	++
Mobility	Free	Limited
Loculation	Clear	Loculated, encapsulated
Peritoneal borders	Smooth	Irregular, possible mass
Greater omentum	Thin	Thick, rigid
Mesentery	Free	Retracted
Small bowel loops	"Sea anemone" or "climbing vine" pattern	Matted
Bowel wall	Thin, mobile	Thickened, rigid
Bowel–abdominal wall	Free	Adherent
Other signs	Hepatic cirrhosis, pancreatitis, right heart failure	Metastases, tumor mass on bowel, pancreas, uterus, ovaries
Lymph-node and hepatic metastases	None	++

Source: Meckler U. Ultraschall des Abdomens, 3rd ed. Köln: Deutscher Ärzteverlag; 1992:117, with kind permission of Deutscher Ärzteverlag.[27]

cases. In the absence of a volume increase (arrested hemorrhage), ultrasound is suitable for follow-up. Over time the clotted blood becomes more organized and initial reabsorption occurs. Portions of the hematoma may reliquefy in some cases.

13.4.9 Pancreatitis

Exudation into the free abdominal cavity is often observed in the setting of acute or acute recurring pancreatitis. This is more pronounced in necrotizing pancreatitis than in an edematous form. In severe cases all compartments are involved, leading to the complete picture of a pancreatogenic abscess. The abscess may be echo-free, but it is more common to find internal echoes and septa. Fibrin strands are a conspicuous finding on ultrasound (▶ Fig. 13.6). Inflammatory changes in the pancreas itself also contribute to the diagnosis (necrotic changes and other signs of pancreatitis along with typical vascular changes). If the clinical presentation and ultrasound findings in the pancreas are not definitive, FNA will reveal high amylase and lipase levels in the ascites that confirm the pancreatogenic cause.

13.4.10 Other Rare Abdominal Fluid Collections

Tuberculosis

Tuberculous ascites is very rare in Western countries. Its sonographic features resemble those of necrotizing pancreatitis and are characterized by internal echoes, septa, and wall irregularities (▶ Fig. 13.7). A hemorrhagic aspirate is also a suggestive sign.

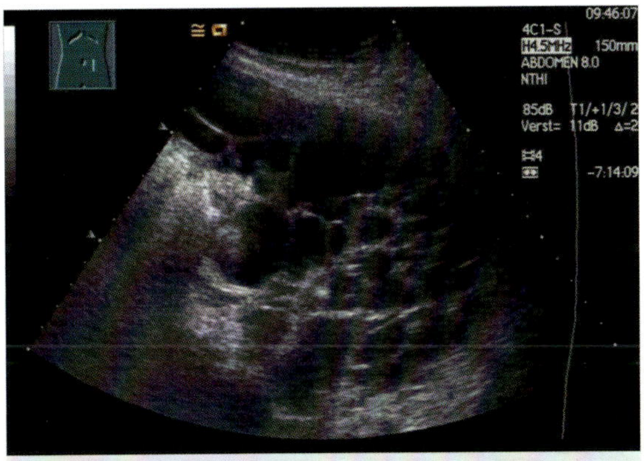

Fig. 13.5 Ascites with internal echoes (fibrin strands and streaks) in the lower abdomen caused by an organizing hemoperitoneum.

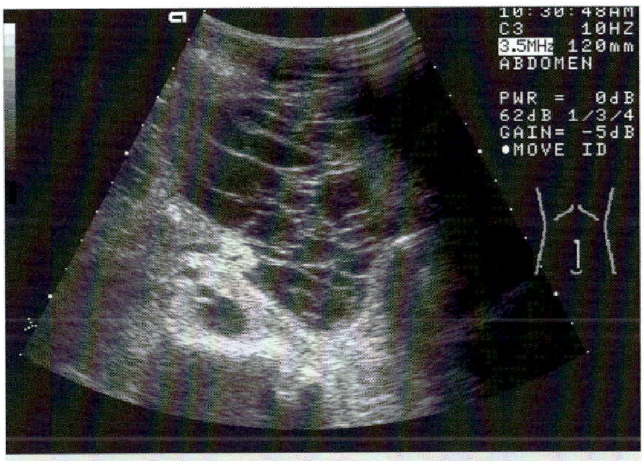

Fig. 13.6 Ascites with internal echoes (fibrin strands and streaks) in the lower abdomen due to necrotizing pancreatitis.

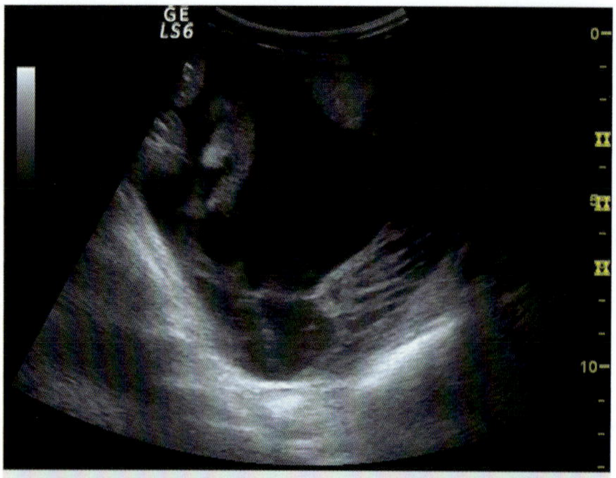

Fig. 13.7 Abdominal tuberculosis in a young woman from Cairo.

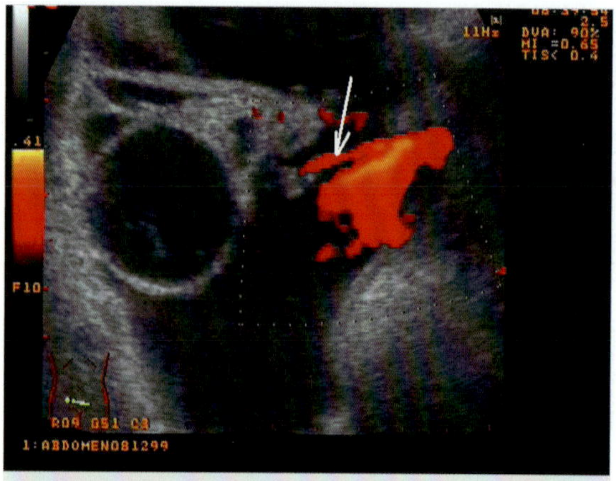

Fig. 13.8 Intraperitoneal urine leak appears as slightly echogenic ascites following a ureteral injury. (Source: reference[26].)

Urinoma, Intraperitoneal Urine Leak

A free intra-abdominal collection of extravasated urine most commonly has an iatrogenic, traumatic, or neoplastic cause. The intra-abdominal fluid usually appears echo-free or slightly echogenic (▶ Fig. 13.8). An acute urine leak is often painful, while a chronic leak is well tolerated for some time.

Intraperitoneal Bile Leak

Gallbladder hydrops or gallbladder empyema may rupture as a rare complication of cholecystolithiasis, causing leakage of bile. A confined perforation is more common than the free leakage of extravasated bile into the abdominal cavity. Other causes may include intraoperative bile duct lesions or intra-abdominal endoscopic injuries. A relatively frequent complication of external PTCD (percutaneous transhepatic cholangiodrainage) for the palliative treatment of a stenosing tumor is bile leakage following the dislodgment of a drain (Chapters 9, 20, 33).

Freshly extravasated bile is initially echo-free. But typical streaks and septations appear within hours, creating the regular stratified pattern that is pathognomonic for a bile leak.[6] Occasional doubtful cases can be resolved by percutaneous aspiration (macroscopic evaluation and bilirubin assay).

Ruptured Cyst

Liver cysts, renal cysts, and pancreatic (pseudo)cysts may rupture into the peritoneal cavity, causing indeterminate ascites. Clinical manifestations may be absent or mild, or the patient may present with significant abdominal pain. A cyst that was missed in previous studies can be detected easily with ultrasound. A ruptured pancreatic pseudocyst in particular may present clinically as an acute abdomen (see Chapters 12 and 22 for the interventional drainage of pancreatic pseudocysts).

Gastrointestinal Perforation

The main imaging feature of a gastrointestinal perforation is the presence of free air in the peritoneal cavity. There may also be evidence of fluid leakage from the perforated stomach or bowel. This fluid is permeated by echoes and shows gas inclusions. It is rarely possible to demonstrate the exact site from which visible gas and fluid have escaped. The fluid collection associated with an upper gastrointestinal perforation is most commonly located around the stomach, in the duodenal region, or around both lobes of the liver. Distal bowel perforations are more often characterized by free gas and air in the lower abdomen (e.g., in diverticulitis).

> **Note**
>
> The combined presence of free gas and free fluid is strongly suggestive of a gastrointestinal perforation.

Chyloperitoneum

Leakage of lymphatic fluid into the peritoneal cavity is a rare event. Possible causes include traumatic and postoperative injuries. Chyloperitoneum is occasionally found in association with malignant lymphoma. Ultrasound in these cases shows a homogeneous ascites that is permeated by fine internal echoes and has a "milky" appearance on needle aspiration. Color Doppler demonstrates color flow during motion. The turbid, yellowish-white lymphatic fluid sampled by fine-needle aspiration permits a spot diagnosis of chyloperitoneum.

Pseudomyxoma peritonei

Pseudomyxoma peritonei is defined as a rare, diffuse, usually low-grade cancer of the peritoneal cavity that presents intraoperatively as large masses of gelatinous

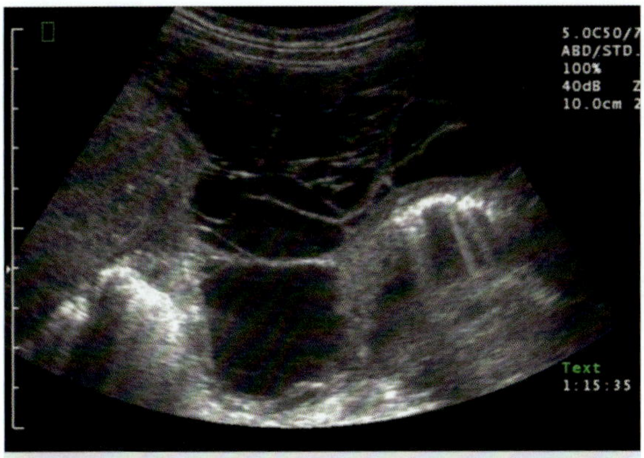

Fig. 13.9 "Ascites" with internal echoes and loculations in the lower abdomen in a patients with pseudomyxoma peritonei (DPAM).

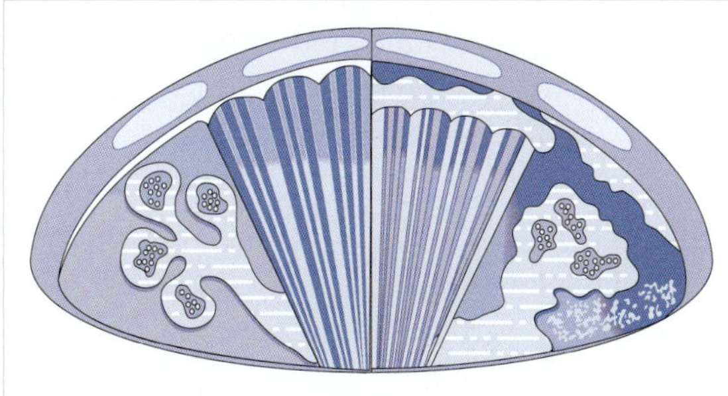

Fig. 13.10 Diagram comparing the ultrasound features of benign and malignant ascites.[27,28] (Source: Meckler U. Ultraschall des Abdomens, 3rd ed. Cologne: Deutscher Ärzteverlag; 1992, with kind permission of Deutscher Ärtzeverlag.)

material on the peritoneum and in the peritoneal cavity ("jelly belly"). Histology can distinguish the prognostically favorable diffuse peritoneal adenomucinosis (DPAM) from aggressive peritoneal mucinous carcinomatosis (PMCA). Ultrasound shows ascites with internal echoes or septations, generally representative of DPAM. Needle aspiration yields a gelatinous material[7] (▶ Fig. 13.9).

The Challenge of Peritoneal Carcinomatosis

With peritoneal carcinomatosis, the peritoneum may be thickened and show irregular borders. Contour irregularities or even tumor masses on the peritoneum are among the signs of advanced peritoneal carcinomatosis. The more pronounced the ascites, the more clearly these irregularities can be seen. Changes on the parietal peritoneum are usually visualized better than changes on the visceral peritoneum.

The peritoneum is a common site for metastatic spread. Eighty percent of all malignant tumors may involve the peritoneum. The most frequent sources are gastrointestinal and gynecologic malignancies. The sonographic diagnosis of peritoneal carcinomatosis is challenging, however. The sensitivity of ultrasound is only 50 to 60%,[3–5] due largely to the fact that peritoneal carcinomatosis is associated with ascites formation in only 50% of cases. The most accurate diagnostic procedure is laparoscopy. Nevertheless, there are several morphologic criteria that are helpful in the sonographic differentiation of malignant and benign ascites (▶ Table 13.3, ▶ Fig. 13.10). Immunocytology offers new capabilities and significantly better results, providing sensitivity rates as high as 92%.[3–6,8–10]

13.5 Differentiating a Localized Fluid Collection from Ascites

Free intra-abdominal fluid requires differentiation from fluid collections that do not communicate with the peritoneal cavity. In the past, these collections were referred to as "pseudoascites." This term is unfortunate in that it refers to structures that are outside the peritoneal cavity and have no access to it. These structures include a large number of liquid masses, some of which are discussed in Chapters 15, 16, and 17). The principal types are as follows:

- Abscess
- Hematoma
- Cysts (liver, kidney, pancreas including pseudocysts, ovary)
- Cystic tumors (e.g., ovarian cystoma and others such as cystadenoma and cystadenocarcinoma)
- Mesothelioma, lymphohemangioma
- Preexisting fluid-filled cavities (urinary bladder, gallbladder including hydrops)
- Aortic aneurysm
- Hydronephrosis
- Bowel obstruction and pyloric stenosis
- Liquid abdominal wall processes

13.6 Practical Issues: How and Where to Aspirate?

The history and clinical information, supplemented by ultrasound findings and distribution pattern, are insufficient in many cases for the accurate classification of ascites. Ultrasound-guided paracentesis is a safe and effective procedure for making a definitive assessment.

Ultrasound guidance avoids injury to vessels that run along the inner abdominal wall (e.g., distended paraumbilical veins) and avoids unproductive aspirations due to malposition of the needle tip. It adds more options to the traditional puncture site in the lower left quadrant of the abdomen (reverse McBurney point). The needle may be inserted anywhere; the operator should choose the shortest possible route that avoids obstacles such as blood vessels, omentum, and bowel.

Generally there is no need for sedation. The procedure may be guided by initial ultrasound imaging without

Table 13.4 Laboratory findings that are helpful in differential diagnosis[11,30–32]

Parameter	Test result	Interpretation
Protein	>30 g/L (3 g/dL)	Exudate
Protein	<30 g/L (3 g/dL)	Transudate
Lipase (amylase)	>>in the serum	Pancreatogenic ascites
Hemoglobin	>>in the serum	Prior hemorrhage
Leukocytes (neutrophils)	>0.50 × 10^9/L (250 µL)	Peritonitis
Tumor cells	+	Malignant ascites
Cholesterol (total)	>1.17 mmol/L (45 mg/dL)	Malignant ascites
LDH	>>in the serum	Malignant ascites
Bacteria	+	Peritonitis, SBP
Tumor markers	>>(in the serum)	Controversial!
Fibronectin	>75 g/L (7.5 mg/dL)	Malignant ascites
Lactate	>4.5 mmol/L	Peritonitis (infectious)

using a transducer during needle insertion, or it may be directed by continuous ultrasound guidance (see Chapter 14). A biopsy transducer is necessary only when targeting a very small fluid collection (a few milliliters). Generous local infiltration with lidocaine solution (2%) is essential. If a drain is to be placed, a more generous amount of local anesthetic should be administered since a stab incision will have to be made. The needle for local anesthesia should be advanced down to the peritoneum while continuously injecting the solution. At the end of the procedure, a trial aspiration should be made with the same syringe to secure the approach, not to collect a sample for laboratory analysis.

Sterile draping is necessary only if a drainage catheter is to be placed. Otherwise it is sufficient to perform an antiseptic skin prep and disinfect the ultrasound probe (see Chapter 8). When dealing with a small fluid collection, the patient should be placed in lateral decubitus or with the upper body elevated to aid the aspiration.

13.7 Diagnostic Paracentesis: Laboratory Tests

When fluid is aspirated, confirming the ultrasound impression of "free fluid," first the specimen is examined grossly to distinguish among transudate/exudate, blood, bile, pus, urine, or chyle. The specimen is then subjected to further cytologic, bacteriologic, and chemical testing.[11]

While one examination is sufficient for performing a chemical analysis, multiple percutaneous aspirations and examinations are often necessary for the cytologic diagnosis of peritoneal carcinomatosis, for example. The sensitivity increases with the number of aspirations. Thus, paracentesis should definitely be repeated in patients with clinical suspicion of a malignant effusion but negative cytology.

Gross examination of the specimen may reveal any of the following:

- Hemorrhagic ascites: pancreatitis, malignant ascites, tuberculosis
- Turbid ascites: infectious peritonitis, spontaneous bacterial peritonitis (SBP), malignant ascites, pancreatitis
- Cloudy, milky ascites: chyloperitoneum
- Yellowish, viscous ascites: intraperitoneal bile leak

The aspirate from malignant ascites consists of exudate, often with a high cholesterol content (▶ Table 13.4). Tumor cells are detected in 50 to 70% of cases. Multiple aspirations and immunocytologic testing can increase the sensitivity of diagnostic paracentesis to 70 to 80%.[3–6,8,9]

Caution

One aspiration is inadequate. Abdominal fluid should be sampled and tested at least two or three times, or a greater initial fluid volume should be collected for centrifugation and analysis.

13.8 Indications for Therapeutic Paracentesis

Therapeutic aspiration and drainage is indicated in the following situations:

- Treatment of ascites in hepatic cirrhosis
- Decompression in hepatic cirrhosis (or pancreatitis)
- Decompression in peritoneal carcinomatosis
- Cytostatic therapy in peritoneal carcinomatosis
- Irrigation and drainage of a bile leak (in a palliative setting)

13.8.1 Treatment of Ascites in Hepatic Cirrhosis: Paracentesis for Symptom Relief in Hepatic Cirrhosis (and Pancreatitis)

Diuretic therapy is at the forefront of treatment recommendations for decompensated hepatic cirrhosis (ascites). A condition in which diuretic therapy is unsuccessful or the ascites is diuretic-resistant (reduced sodium excretion) may be defined as "refractory ascites" (International Ascites Club, 1966) and treated by paracentesis. Other therapeutic options are the insertion of a transjugular intrahepatic portosystemic shunt (TIPS) or surgical shunt procedures. Paracentesis may remove all the ascitic fluid in one tap, or smaller volumes may be drained in multiple sittings, with or without albumin replacement. In total paracentesis, several liters of fluid are drained in one sitting while plasma expanders are simultaneously infused to maintain hemodynamic stability. Small-volume paracentesis may follow various protocols, such as draining 2 liters of fluid every 2 days. An "activation" of fluid mobilization with lasting benefit is observed in approximately 50% of cases.[12]

Moreover, one or two paracentesis sessions are often needed for initial decompression in a patient with dyspnea (due to elevation of the diaphragm) and a feeling of extreme abdominal tension. Paracentesis (usually one session) may also be indicated to relieve the pain and dyspnea associated with a pancreatogenic abscess.

13.8.2 Palliative Paracentesis for Peritoneal Carcinomatosis

Pain, dyspnea, anorexia, malaise, and general debilitation are indications for the palliative decompression of malignant ascites. The goal is the relief of symptoms. The rate of fluid reaccumulation should be noted; continuous drainage is rarely necessary. Palliative paracentesis has several disadvantages, however. It often provides only short-term relief and must be repeated every 6 to 10 days on average. It may also lead to bowel injury, bleeding, peritonitis, or fistula formation. Moreover, repeated taps may cause significant protein depletion (see Hypoalbuminemia above) leading to metabolic disorders and eventual cachexia. Intravenous fluid (e.g., plasma expanders) should be infused during the sessions to avoid hypovolemia as large fluid volumes are removed. The palliative drainage of ascites can be conducted as a bedside procedure in the home (Chapter 33).[13,14]

13.8.3 Cytostatic Therapy of Peritoneal Carcinomatosis (Intraperitoneal Chemotherapy)

Local therapy to reduce secretions is often recommended in palliative settings. In the past, however, this did not become a standard therapy as it was known to induce adhesions that could restrict needle access for further drainage and could itself cause abdominal pain. Intraperitoneal (IP) therapy has repeatedly undergone a renaissance, most recently for metastatic ovarian cancer, which is the most common peritoneal tumor. The German Arbeitsgemeinschaft Gynäkologische Onkologie (AGO) issued the following statement, however, in their guideline of 2009[15]: "While positive data have been published on IP chemotherapy, so far no regimen has been devised that is suitable for routine clinical use, and further studies are needed before IP chemotherapy may be recommended as a standard therapy."

The goal of IP chemotherapy is to deliver high concentrations of cytotoxic agents to the peritoneum. Remission rates of 33 to 85% have been reported. The choice of agents for IP chemotherapy should be based on a slow uptake into the circulation and the ability to elicit a response on IV administration while also inducing tissue fibrosis resulting in a significantly decreased inflow of plasma from tumor and peritoneal vessels. In comparative studies of women with ovarian cancer, IP chemotherapy proved superior to systemic chemotherapy alone in terms of progression-free survival and median overall survival. The combination of systemic and IP chemotherapy was also found to be more effective than intravenous therapy alone.[16–22]

Cytostatic agents used in the treatment of malignant ascites are cisplatin, oxaliplatin, paclitaxel, mitoxantrone, mitomycin, and 5-fluorouracil (5-FU).[23]

Hyperthermic intraperitoneal chemotherapy (HIPEC) is a procedure that was introduced for ovarian cancer treatment. The initially positive results have not been widely confirmed, with the result that this relatively complex therapy has not been incorporated into standard treatment recommendations or routine clinical use.[24]

In summary, the treatment of malignant ascites is characterized by a number of different palliative options, most of which have shown inadequate effectiveness. Moreover, none of these therapeutic approaches has demonstrated efficacy in evidence-based studies, and so there are still no established therapeutic guidelines. Thus, improvements in the treatment of malignant ascites will require new, more powerful studies on the known treatment options in addition to more advanced, validated therapies.[25]

13.8.4 Drainage (with Irrigation) for Bile Leakage (For Example in a Palliative Setting)

Bile leakage into the abdominal cavity may occur in palliative settings as a complication of percutaneous transhepatic cholangiodrainage (PTCD, Chapter 20) due to drain displacement, for example. Paracentesis may be a helpful option in these cases to prevent biliary peritonitis and control pain while avoiding the need for laparotomy. The bile may be removed with a single drain or an inflow–outflow drainage system (▶ Fig. 13.11). A confined gallbladder perforation in palliative or geriatric patients would also be an indication for biliary drainage. The peritoneal cavity can also be irrigated with physiologic saline

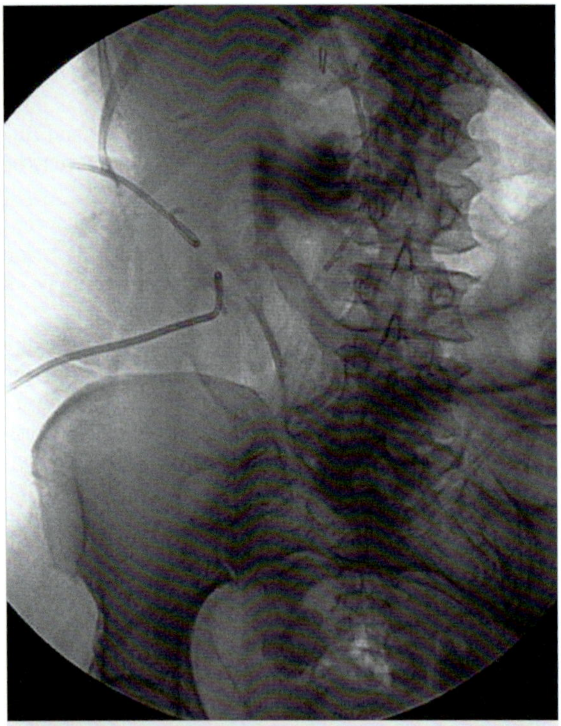

Fig. 13.11 A radiograph showing subhepatic inflow and outflow drains placed for treatment of bile leakage from a common duct injury during endoscopic retrograde cholangiopancreatography (ERCP).

solution when combined with simultaneous antibiotic coverage. This technique uses one drain for inflow and a second drain for outflow, with an irrigation volume of 4 to 6 liters per day.

13.9 Materials

Needles up to 1 mm in diameter are used for diagnostic paracentesis, while larger calibers are used for therapeutic paracentesis. The needle length depends on the abdominal wall thickness; lengths of 6 to 8 cm are usually sufficient. Further details can be found in Chapter 2 (Interventional Materials and Equipment).

Larger-caliber catheter-clad needles like those produced by OptiMed are recommended for therapeutic paracentesis. We use 1.0- to 1.6-mm needles or large, flexible IV catheters (14–18 gauge), and we occasionally use thoracentesis kits from Braun Medical (Pleurofix). In this case as in others, the drain is introduced through a stab incision made after generous local anesthesia (▶ Fig. 13.12). Temporary catheter placement is recommended for larger drainage and aspiration volumes because it is less traumatizing (e.g., pigtail or straight catheter from OptiMed or Pflugbeil). This also simplifies patient care, which may be given continuously or intermittently by assisting personnel.

In selected cases that require repeated punctures at short intervals, it may be necessary to place a drainage catheter for several days. This should be done under antibiotic coverage due to the higher infection rate associated with prolonged catheter placement. The catheter should be secured in place to facilitate ambulation.

The cytostatic agents for IP chemotherapy are always administered through a catheter. To obtain a uniform intraabdominal distribution of the agents, they should be infused with a large fluid volume of physiologic saline solution (1 to 2 L) and left within the abdomen for 1 to 4 hours (some authors state 12 to 24 hours). Mitoxantrone, for example, is administered at a dosage of 1 mg/kg body BW.

13.10 Contraindications, Complications, and Postprocedure Care

Particular care should be taken to avoid the following:

- Excessive protein loss
- Excessive fluid loss (replacement, blood pressure monitoring)

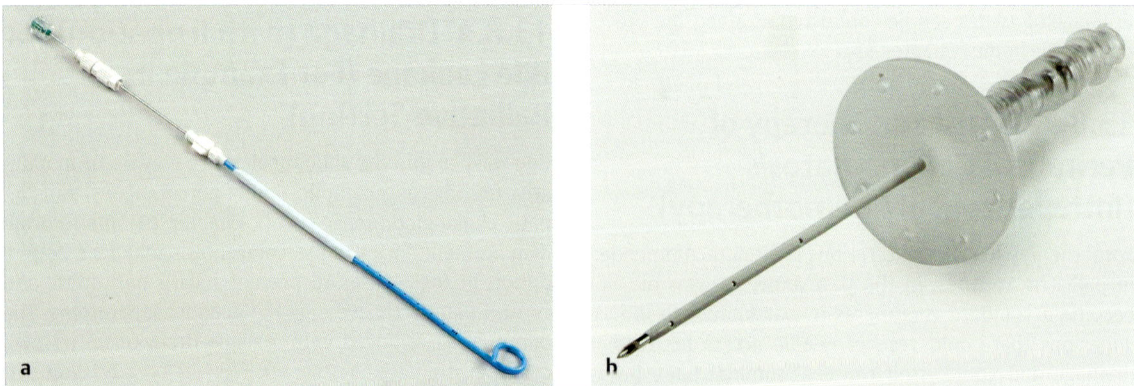

Fig. 13.12 Use of drainage catheters (trocar, 8F to 12F) for the drainage of ascites (Pflugbeil) (a). The Schlottmann paracentesis needle with skin plate is excellent for ascites drainage (Pflugbeil) (b).

- An excessive bleeding risk (particularly note coagulation in cirrhosis and avoid vessels with the needle!)
- Infection (if necessary, give antibiotic prophylaxis for long indwelling times)

References

[1] Nuernberg D. Peritonealraum. In: Schmidt G, Greiner L, Nuernberg D, eds. Sonografische Differenzialdiagnose. Stuttgart: Thieme; 2010

[2] Kremer H, Dobrinski W. Sonographische Diagnostik. Munich: Urban & Schwarzenberg; 1994

[3] Böcking A, Motherby H, Pomjanski N. Treffsicherheit der Ergusszytologie samt adjuvanten Untersuchungsmethoden. Dtsch Arztebl 2000; 97: A-2626/B-2254/C-2096

[4] Metzgeroth G, Kuhn C, Schultheis B, Hehlmann R, Hastka J. Diagnostic accuracy of cytology and immunocytology in carcinomatous effusions. Cytopathology 2008; 19: 205–211

[5] Wiest R, Schölmerich J. Diagnostik und Therapie des Aszites. Dtsch Arztebl 2006; 103(28-29): A-1972/B-1693/C-1637

[6] Lin O. Challenges in the interpretation of peritoneal cytologic specimens. Arch Pathol Lab Med 2009; 133: 739–742

[7] Totkas S, Schneider U, Schlag PM. Surgical and multimodal therapy of pseudomyxoma peritonei [Article in German]. Chirurg 2000; 71: 869–876

[8] Spriggs AI, Boddington MM. Atlas of Serous Fluid Cytopathology. A Guide to the Cells of Pleural, Pericardial, Peritoneal and Hydrocele Fluids. Dordrecht: Kluwer Academic; 1989

[9] Schubert J, Vieth M. Zytologische Befundsicherung durch immunologische Zelldifferenzierung im peritonealen Ergussmaterial. Verdauungskrankheiten 2010; 28: 94–99

[10] Rioux M, Michaud C. Sonographic detection of peritoneal carcinomatosis: a prospective study of 37 cases. Abdom Imaging 1995; 20: 47–51; discussion 56–57

[11] Schölmerich J. Diagnosis and therapy of ascites [Article in German]. Internist (Berl) 1987; 28: 448–458

[12] Gentilini P, Vizzutti F, Gentilini A, Zipoli M, Foschi M, Romanelli RG. Update on ascites and hepatorenal syndrome. Dig Liver Dis 2002; 34: 592–605

[13] Abenhardt W, et al. Manual: Supportive Maßsnahmen und symptomorientierte Therapie. Munich: Tumorzentrum München; 2001

[14] Ross GJ, Kessler HB, Clair MR, Gatenby RA, Hartz WH, Ross LV. Sonographically guided paracentesis for palliation of symptomatic malignant ascites. AJR Am J Roentgenol 1989; 153: 1309–1311

[15] Arbeitsgemeinschaft Gynäkologische Onkologie (AGO). http://www.ago-online.de: Munich: AGO; 2009. Ref type: data file

[16] Alberts DS, Liu PY, Hannigan EV et al. Intraperitoneal cisplatin plus intravenous cyclophosphamide versus intravenous cisplatin plus intravenous cyclophosphamide for stage III ovarian cancer. N Engl J Med 1996; 335: 1950–1955

[17] Armstrong DK, Bundy B, Wenzel L et al. Gynecologic Oncology Group. Intraperitoneal cisplatin and paclitaxel in ovarian cancer. N Engl J Med 2006; 354: 34–43

[18] du Bois A, Lück HJ, Meier W et al. Arbeitsgemeinschaft Gynäkologische Onkologie Ovarian Cancer Study Group. A randomized clinical trial of cisplatin/paclitaxel versus carboplatin/paclitaxel as first-line treatment of ovarian cancer. J Natl Cancer Inst 2003; 95: 1320–1329

[19] Markman M. Intraperitoneal chemotherapy in the management of malignant disease. Expert Rev Anticancer Ther 2001; 1: 142–148

[20] Markman M. Intraperitoneal chemotherapy is appropriate first line therapy for patients with optimally debulked ovarian cancer. Crit Rev Oncol Hematol 2001; 38: 171–175

[21] Markman M. Is there a role for intraperitoneal chemotherapy in the management of ovarian cancer? Oncology (Williston Park) 2001; 15: 93–98; discussion 103–105

[22] Markman M, Liu PY, Wilczynski S et al. Southwest Oncology Group. Gynecologic Oncology Group. Phase III randomized trial of 12 versus 3 months of maintenance paclitaxel in patients with advanced ovarian cancer after complete response to platinum and paclitaxel-based chemotherapy: a Southwest Oncology Group and Gynecologic Oncology Group trial. J Clin Oncol 2003; 21: 2460–2465

[23] Arnold D, Schmoll HJ. Aszites und intraperitoneale Chemotherapie. In: Schmoll HJ, Höffken K, Possinger K, eds. Kompendium Internistische Onkologie. Standards in Diagnostik und Therapie. Berlin: Springer; 2006:1061–1068

[24] Glockzin G, Ghali N, Lang SA, Agha A, Schlitt HJ, Piso P. Peritoneal carcinomatosis. Surgical treatment, including hyperthermal intraperitoneal chemotherapy [Article in German]. Chirurg 2007; 78: 1100, 1102–1106, 1108–1110

[25] Jähne J, Piso P. Peritonectomy and intraperitoneal chemotherapy—new methods in multi-modality therapy of peritoneal carcinosis [Article in German]. Langenbecks Arch Chir Suppl Kongressbd 1998; 115: 1435–1437

[26] Nürnberg D. Competent sonography brings a diagnostic odyssey to an end—a case of seldom genesis of ascites. Ultraschall Med 2008; 29: 461–464

[27] Meckler U. Ultraschall des Abdomens, 3rd ed. Cologne: Deutscher Ärzteverlag; 1992:117

[28] Nuernberg D Peritonealraum. In: Schmidt G, ed. Sonografische Differentialdiagnose. Stuttgart: Thieme; 2002

[29] Rettenmaier G, Seitz KH. Sonographische Differenzialdiagnose. Stuttgart: Thieme; 2000

[30] Thomas L. Diagnostik des Aszites. In: Labor und Diagnose. Frankfurt, M: TH-Books Verlagsgesellschaft; 1998

[31] Runyon BA. Elevated ascitic fluid fibronectin concentration. A nonspecific finding. J Hepatol 1986; 3: 219–222

[32] Gerbes AL, Jüngst D, Xie YN, Permanetter W, Paumgartner G. Ascitic fluid analysis for the differentiation of malignancy-related and nonmalignant ascites. Proposal of a diagnostic sequence. Cancer 1991; 68: 1808–1814

14 Fine Needle Aspiration Biopsy and Core Needle Biopsy

J.-C. Kaemmer, D. Nuernberg

14.1 Historical Background

The first percutaneous needle biopsy with localization by palpation and inspection was documented in 1856 by Albrecht Theodor Middeldorpf (1824–1868) in his "Overview of *Akidopeirastik*, a New Diagnostic Method Using Sharp Pointed Tools."[1] The advent of ultrasonography more than a century later made the diagnostic puncture of small intra-abdominal masses possible. In 1969, Kratochwill performed one of the first ultrasound-guided amniocentesis procedures using a Kretz biopsy transducer and localization by A-mode ultrasound.[2]

Holm and Rasmussen[3] were among the first authors to describe percutaneous biopsies guided by dynamic B-mode ultrasound in the early 1970s. This technique became a safe and established method of tissue sampling for the diagnosis of masses that could be visualized by ultrasonography.

14.2 Description of Biopsy Techniques

14.2.1 What Type of Needle Should Be Used?

Before performing an aspiration or core biopsy, the operator must decide what type of needle to use. Several questions should be answered in making this decision.

Does the Investigation Require a Fine Needle or Core Needle?

A fine needle, defined as a needle less than 1 mm in diameter, is sufficient to sample material for cytologic analysis. A fine needle may also be able to harvest small tissue aggregates when inserted with a slight twisting motion, depending on the consistency of the target site. These tissue aggregates, like blood clots, should be immersed in formalin for histologic processing. This "mini-histology" can result in a more accurate diagnosis[4] (Chapters 5 and 6).

In many cases a cytologic analysis is inadequate, especially in well-differentiated tumors, and a larger specimen is needed for histologic evaluation.[5] Several studies have documented the superiority of a combined histologic-cytologic analysis (fine needle aspiration plus core needle biopsy) over histology and cytology alone (▶ Table 14.1, ▶ Table 14.2). Löschner showed in his study that a combination of fine needle and core needle biopsy increased diagnostic sensitivity, but that the gain depended on the organ biopsied.[6]

How Long is the Needle Path?

We use Chiba needles (0.7-mm), among others, to reach targets located farther from the skin, and we use a 21-gauge needle (green) or 22-gauge needle (black) for more superficial targets (e.g., inguinal lymph nodes).

Even in the case of a palpable superficial mass, the lesion and its surroundings should be evaluated with ultrasound before the biopsy is performed. Time and again, we encounter difficult surroundings that are made clearer by ultrasound, enabling us to sample the lesion with precision. The needle may be inserted after first imaging the lesion with ultrasound and marking the skin, or a short needle may be introduced freehand under continuous ultrasound guidance as in the fine needle aspiration of cervical lymph nodes (▶ Fig. 14.1).

Needle calibers of 21 gauge (green) or 22 gauge (black) are used to harvest cells for cytology, and various types of core needle (≥ 1 mm in diameter) are used for histology (Chapter 2, Interventional Materials and Equipment). Due to the risk of injury to vulnerable structures behind the targeted lesion, we prefer needles that are advanced manually and apply suction at the lesion surface (e.g., Biomol [Enzo], Pflugbeil). The size of the mass is a critical factor in deciding whether to use an automated biopsy device (Section 14.3).

Lesions located deep in the body, such as retroperitoneal lymphomas, require the use of longer biopsy needles, usually in the range of 16 to 22 cm. The insertion

Table 14.1 Prospective sensitivity of combined histologic-cytologic analysis

Organ	Sensitivity (%)		
	CNB	FNA	CNB + FNA
Liver	89.5	81.6	97.4
Kidney	75	83.3	91.7
Pancreas	60	80	90
Lymph nodes	100	90	100

Abbreviations: CNB: core needle biopsy; FNA: fine needle aspiration.
Source: Löschner C. Retrospektive Analyse der ultraschallgestützten diagnostischen Feinnadelpunktion im onkologischen Patientengut eines Versorgungskrankenhauses und prospektive Bewertung der Doppelpunktion. Inauguraldissertation zur Erlangung des akademischen Grades Doktor der Medizin. Rostock; 2008: table 38, p.44, with kind permission of C. Löschner.

Table 14.2 Advantages of combined histologic-cytologic analysis

Author	*n*	Sensitivity (%)		
		FNA	CNB	FNA + CNB
Swobodnik 1990[a]	1213	83	72	Not stated
Buscarini 1990[b]	2091	91	93.5	97.4
Wernecke 1991[c]	180	87	86	94
Tikkakoski 1993[d]	155	86	86	97
Borzio 1994[e]	100	78	81	96
Nürnberg 1997[f]	101	84.5	84.5	95.8

Abbreviations: CNB, core needle biopsy; FNA, fine needle aspiration.

Source: Löschner C. Retrospektive Analyse der ultraschallgestützten diagnostischen Feinnadelpunktion im onkologischen Patientengut eines Versorgungskrankenhauses und prospektive Bewertung der Doppelpunktion. Inauguraldissertation zur Erlangung des akademischen Grades Doktor der Medizin. Rostock; 2008: table 39, p.44, with kind permission of C. Löschner.

[a] Swobodnik W, Janowitz P, Kratzer W, Wechsler JG. Vergleich ultraschallgezielter Fei- und Grobnadelpunktionen bei umschriebenen Läsionen im Abdomen. Ultraschall Med 1990; 11: 287–289.

[b] Buscarini L, Fornari F, Bolondi L et al. Ultrasound guided fine needle biopsy of focal liver leasions: techniques, diagnostic accuray and complications. A retrospectiv study on 2091 biopsies. J Hepatol 1990; 11: 344–348.

[c] Wernecke K, Mertens G, von Bassewitz DB, Peters PE. Möglichkeiten und Grenzen der perkutanen Nadelbiopsie in der histologischen Klassifikation von malignen Tumoren. RoFo 1991; 155: 538–544.

[d] Tikkakoski T, Paivansalo M, Siniluoto T et al. Percutaneous ultrasound-guided biopsy. Fine needle biopsy, cutting needle biopsy, or both? Acta Radiol 1993; 34: 30–34.

[e] Borzio M, Borzio F, Macchi R et al. The evaluation of fine-needle procedures for the diagnosis of focal liver lesions in cirrhosis. J Hepatol 1994; 20(1): 117–121.

[f] Löschner Ch, Nürnberg D, Jung A. Stellenwert und Ergiebigkeit der ultraschall-gezielten Fein- und Grobnadelpunktion in der onkologischen Diagnostik – Vorteil der "Doppelpunktion". Endoskopie heute 1997; 10: 84.

is aided by using a biopsy transducer or a needle guide mounted on the transducer. In this case a guide line is superimposed on the ultrasound image to show the proposed route and depth of needle insertion (▶ Fig. 14.2, ▶ Fig. 14.3). In most cases the progress of the advancing needle can be directly visualized. The more closely the direction of needle insertion approaches the ultrasound beam axis, the less clearly is the needle visualized. If the needle is advanced directly along the beam axis, generally only the needle tip can be seen, appearing as a small, high-amplitude echo produced by an air bubble at the tip. Special bevels have been claimed to improve needle

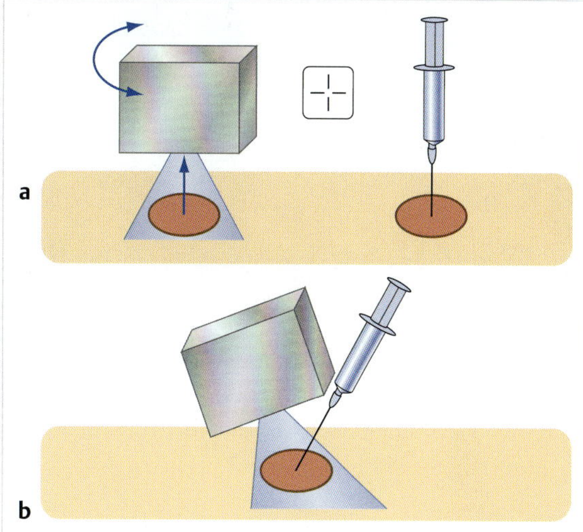

Fig. 14.1
a Principle of the freehand technique. The superficial mass is visualized with ultrasound, and the puncture site is marked on the skin. The needle is inserted without direct ultrasound guidance (e.g., for the aspiration of pleural effusion or ascites).
b Ultrasound-guided technique. The needle is introduced alongside the transducer and is angled slightly for better visualization (see Chapter 27, Interventional Thyroid Ultrasound).

visualization, but in our experience they are rarely effective and need not be purchased.

The guide line in the ultrasound image can be recalibrated on some scanner models, and this should be done periodically. Calibration is aided by comparing the actual needle path in a water bath with the line on the monitor.

If the needle is poorly visualized, a precision biopsy can still be performed based on the path defined by the needle guide and the distance to the lesion measured before the biopsy. It is important to allow for the distance added by the external needle guide.

How Large is the Mass?

Smaller masses located outside of parenchymal organs, such as lymph nodes, should be biopsied with a fine needle or with a full-core needle that is not fired by an automated mechanism (e.g., Biomol [Enzo], Pflugbeil) to avoid injury to structures deep to the targeted lesion.

Any type of needle can be used on smaller lesions located within parenchymal organs (e.g., suspected hepatic metastasis) and on larger masses. The needle selection in these cases will depend largely on the experience of the operator and the desired specimen. (Semi) Automated half-core systems (Trucut needles) are most commonly used in these cases (Chapter 2).

Are There Vessels in the Needle Path?

Before inserting the needle into a mass, the operator should have a clear picture of the blood supply to the

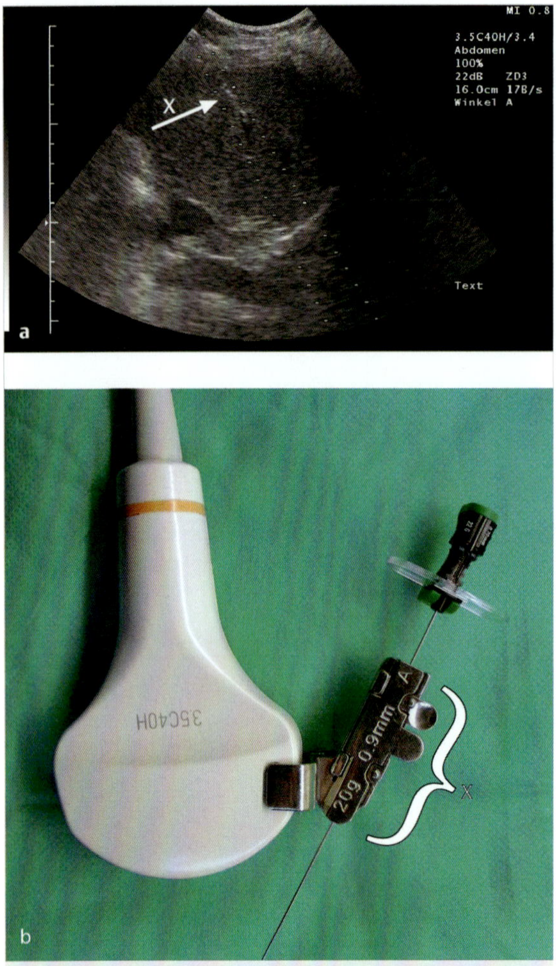

Fig. 14.2
a Transducer with an external needle guide. The target is placed between the guide lines superimposed on the ultrasound image. x = needle echo.
b Transducer (Siemens) with needle guide. x = distance added by the length of the needle guide is taken into account when choosing the needle length.

mass and the location of blood vessels in its immediate vicinity. The puncture of blood vessels should be avoided; bleeding from straight veins may be prolonged and profuse due to the thin vessel wall! Especially with a high-risk biopsy route, the needle caliber should be within the fine needle range.

Is There Bowel in the Needle Path?

In principle, a transgastric or transenteric biopsy route can be used without increasing the complication rate. If the biopsy of a mass through bowel cannot be avoided, only a fine needle (< 1 mm) with a stylet should be used.

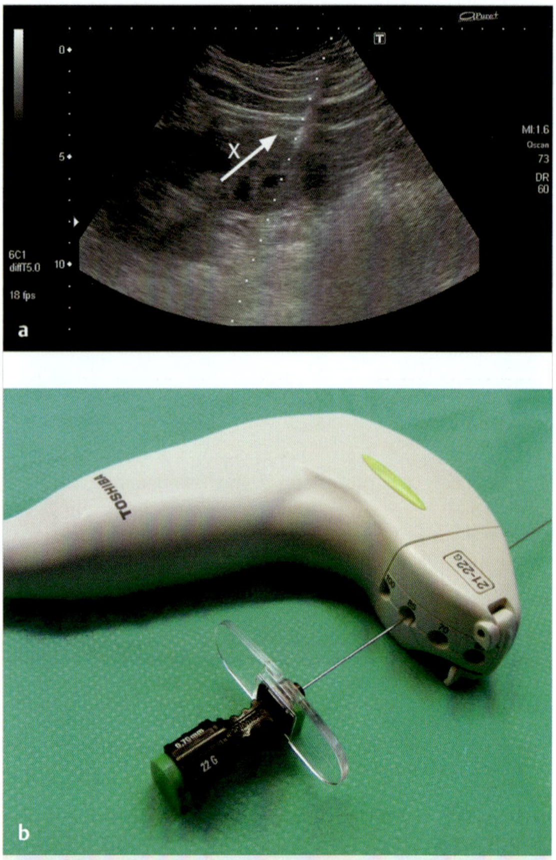

Fig. 14.3 Biopsy transducer.
a Guide lines are superimposed on the B-mode image (here using a 70° needle guide). x = biopsy needle.
b Biopsy transducer (Toshiba) with a choice of four angles for needle insertion.

Blood Vessel or Vulnerable Structure Just Behind a Small Mass?

A (semi)automated biopsy device with an adjustable stroke length up to 4 cm is useful in cases where posterior structures are a concern. With a Trucut needle, the distance from the needle tip to the specimen notch adds 5 to 7 mm to the necessary insertion depth. In some cases a Trucut system can be safely used by altering the angle of needle insertion (▶ Fig. 14.4).

When a biopsy is performed with a fine needle, a full-core needle, or a semiautomated system in which the needle is not fired automatically, the needle is introduced to the surface of the mass and can be manually advanced into the mass, depending on the size of the lesion (▶ Fig. 14.5).

Vascular puncture should be avoided not only due to possible complications but also because blood may be aspirated, rendering the harvested material unsuitable for analysis.

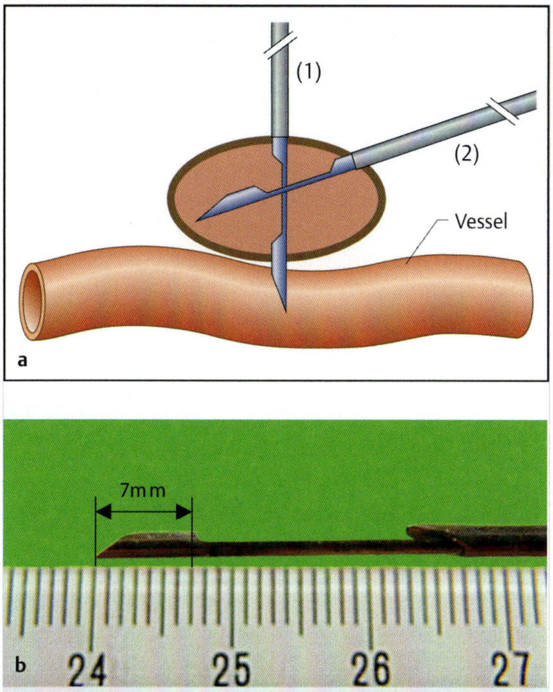

Fig. 14.4
a Trucut needle biopsy of a small mass located just anterior to a large vessel (1). The vessel is spared by altering the biopsy angle (2).
b Material enters the specimen notch 7 mm behind the needle tip.

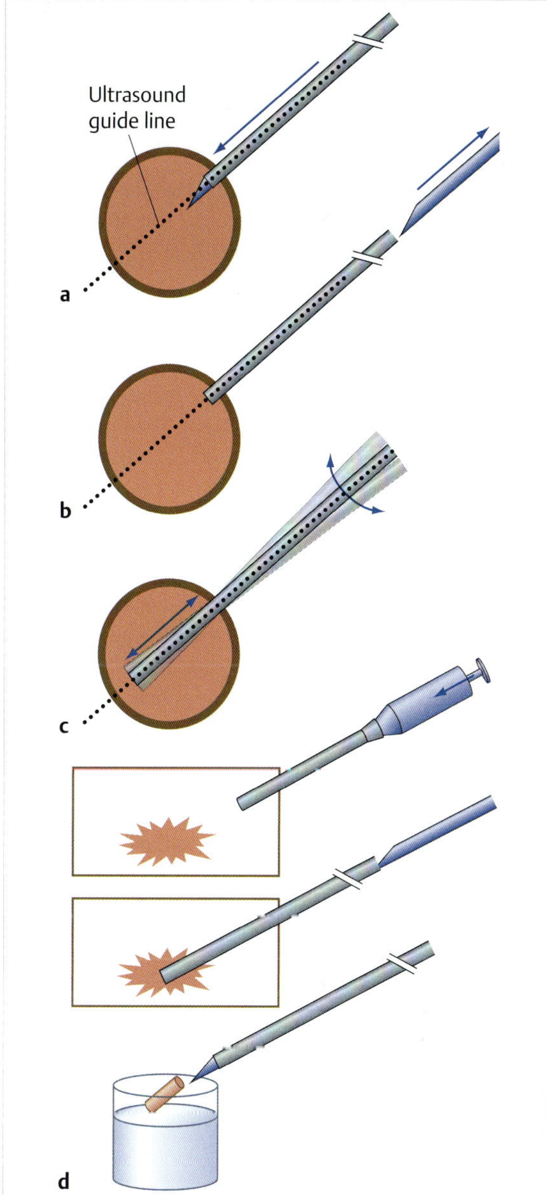

Fig. 14.5 Biopsy technique with a Chiba needle.
a The Chiba needle is advanced to the lesion surface or a few millimeters into the lesion.
b The stylet is removed, leaving the needle in the lesion.
c While suction is applied (with a 5-mL syringe), the needle is repeated moved back and forth ("needling") while slightly changing its direction and also rotating it slightly.
d The needle is withdrawn and connected to an air-filled syringe, and material is expelled onto a glass slide by advancing the plunger and/or reinserting the stylet to clear all aspirate from the needle. Larger fragments and clots are placed in formalin for histologic processing. Material is smeared onto the glass slide and may be air-dried or fixed immediately after smearing, depending on the preference of the cytologist.

14.3 Biopsy Technique for Specific Needle Types

The steps in the procedure are again explained to the patient in a reassuring manner and the patient is comfortably positioned. This is followed by aseptic preparation and sterile draping of the puncture site (Chapters 3, 4, and 8).

Local anesthesia (1% lidocaine) is routinely administered for a core needle biopsy, making sure to infiltrate not just the superficial tissues but also down to the organ capsule. For a fine needle aspiration, local anesthesia would mean one additional stick with a needle of equal caliber and would also obscure the ultrasound image. Local anesthesia may certainly be withheld in selected patients undergoing a fine needle aspiration biopsy. Local anesthesia should be used if multiple needle passes are planned (for a combined histologic-cytologic analysis) or if the patient desires it (Chapter 4).

If the patient desires general sedation, we use midazolam or propofol and basically follow the S3 guidelines for sedation in endoscopy[9] (Chapters 4 and 11).

We sometimes use a Toshiba biopsy transducer, which offers several different guide angles (▶ Fig. 14.3). When an automated system is used, a second examiner would be necessary only for sedation.

The technique for the aspiration and biopsy of superficial lesions is fully described in the chapter on ultrasonography of the thyroid gland (Chapter 27).

14.3.1 Biopsy with the Chiba Needle

Chiba needles are offered by various suppliers (Pflugbeil, Bard, OptiMed, etc.; see Chapter 2). The special bevel designed to improve needle visualization in the ultrasound image does not offer significant advantages in practice.

To prevent cell sampling along the needle tract, the Chiba needle is advanced up to or into the mass with the inner stylet in place. The stylet should be manually stabilized during insertion to keep it from slipping out of the needle. Some firms offer a special lock for this purpose. A holder can also be mounted on the needle to facilitate handling and insertion (▶ Fig. 14.5, ▶ Fig. 14.6).

After the stylet is withdrawn, a 5- to 10-mL syringe is connected to the hub and suction is applied. The needle is moved repeatedly back and forth within the mass while aspiration is maintained. The needle angle may be changed slightly during this "needling" process if desired. Finally the plunger of the syringe is slowly advanced to discontinue the suction. If the suction were released abruptly, the needle could plunge forward or material might be ejected from the needle into the patient's body. On the other hand, suction should not be continued while the needle is being withdrawn from the body, as this could aspirate material into the syringe, where it could be destroyed or become inaccessible for smear preparation.

The harvested material is ejected from the needle with an air-filled syringe onto one or more glass slides and smeared for cytologic analysis. Alternatively, the stylet may be used to expel the aspirate from the needle onto a glass slide. If tissue aggregates or clots are found, they are transferred into a small tube with 4% formalin for histologic processing (microhistology). A lancet is useful for picking up clots and tissue fragments.

14.3.2 Cutting Biopsy with an Otto or Franseen Needle

The biopsy technique is analogous to that with a Chiba needle. These end-cutting biopsy systems[10] are currently available in the fine needle range of 22 gauge (0.7 mm) and smaller. After the stylet is withdrawn, the needle is rotated while aspiration is applied to cut a tissue core from the targeted site. The stylet is then used to expel the tissue core from the needle into formalin solution. Since biopsies with both needles are technically demanding and often result in an inadequate specimen, the Otto and Franseen needles are rarely used today. But an operator who has mastered the technique will be able to obtain good results.

14.3.3 Autovac and BioPince Biopsy Systems

Both of these systems are advanced to the mass under ultrasound guidance. The needle is fired and propelled forward while the stylet stays in place, creating a slight negative pressure inside the cannula The rapid firing action cuts a cylindrical tissue core that is detached with a twisting motion while the suction retains it within the needle. In the BioPince system, the tissue core is secured in the needle by suction and also by a small metal clip. (Make sure the safety button is released from the SAFE to the FIRE position before the firing trigger is pressed.)

The needle stroke length is adjustable: 23 or 40 mm on the Autovac, and 13, 23, or 33 mm on the BioPince. There should be no vulnerable structures within the preset range, as no further corrections can be made once the instrument is fired. The Autovac needle can be reused multiple times. With the BioPince, the metal retaining clip should be closely inspected since multiple uses may cause it to bend and pose a hazard to the patient. Single-use devices are therefore preferred.

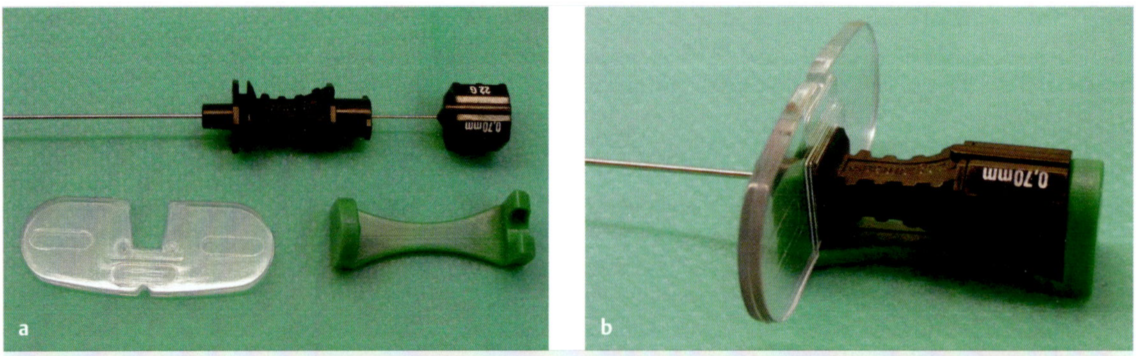

Fig. 14.6 Chiba needle (Pflugbeil).
a Chiba needle with holder and a stopper on the inner stylet (separate parts).
b The parts assembled.

14.3.4 Biomol Biopsy System

The Biomol is similar to the Autovac system, but a major difference is that the stylet of the Biomol needle is withdrawn while the outer cannula stays in place; hence there is no rapid forward propulsion of the needle within the patient's body. After the instrument has been fired, the needle is rotated to excise a cylindrical tissue core. When the instrument is re-cocked after needle removal, the stylet expels the specimen into a formalin container.

14.3.5 Trucut Needles

Trucut needles are available as manual devices, but the semiautomated systems are most widely used. Single-use and reusable models are available (see Chapter 2). The disadvantage of the Trucut needle is the side-notch technique, which does not utilize the full cross-section of the needle. The Vitesse needle (OptiMed) has a narrower bridge at the base of the specimen notch (larger notch circumference) that provides a somewhat greater tissue yield. However, the Vitesse biopsy gun has insufficient power to penetrate all masses—presumably due to the risk of bending or breaking the delicate bridge at the base of the notch—and we have noted a disproportionately high incidence of malfunctions with this device.

Biopsy guns from other manufacturers provide greater power and good cutting properties when used with a standard Trucut needle.

The Trucut needle is loaded into the gun, and the system is closed and cocked (twice) to engage the safety. We can choose between two stroke lengths. The needle is advanced to the mass under ultrasound guidance, the safety is released, and the device is fired, driving the inner stylet into the mass by the preset stroke length. A moment later the outer cannula slides forward, slicing off and capturing tissue that has settled into the specimen notch. It is almost impossible to lose a specimen that has been harvested with a Trucut needle. Cocking the gun again exposes the specimen chamber, allowing us to remove the tissue with a needle or lancet and transfer it to a formalin tube.

14.4 Summary

Almost all structures visible with ultrasound can be sampled with a fine needle at very low risk. When necessary, modern systems can even provide a histologic sample in the fine needle size range. Automated biopsy devices can provide a fast, smooth cut and a better yield with minimal trauma and very little patient discomfort.

References

[1] Middeldorpf A. Ueberblick über die Akidopeirastik, eine neue Untersuchungsmethode mit Hülfe spitziger Werkzeuge. Z Klin Med 1856; 7: 321–330

[2] Kratochwil A. Methods of placenta localization [Article in German]. Wien Klin Wochenschr 1969; 81: 290–293

[3] Holm HH, Kristensen JK, Rasmussen SN, Northeved A, Barlebo H. Ultrasound as a guide in percutaneous puncture technique. Ultrasonics 1972; 10: 83–86

[4] Wildberger JE, Biesterfeld S, Adam GB, Hülsmeier L, Schmitz-Rode T, Günther RW. Refinement of cytopathology of CT-guided fine needle aspiration biopsies with additional histologic examination of formalin-fixed blood-clots [Article in German]. Rofo 2003; 175: 1532–1538

[5] Jain D. Diagnosis of hepatocellular carcinoma: fine needle aspiration cytology or needle core biopsy. J Clin Gastroenterol 2002; 35: S101–S108

[6] Löschner C. Retrospektive Analyse der ultraschallgestützten diagnostischen Feinnadelpunktion im onkologischen Patientengut eines Versorgungskrankenhauses und prospektive Bewertung der Doppelpunktion. Inauguraldissertation zur Erlangung des akademischen Grades Doktor der Medizin. Rostock; 2008:44

[7] Möller K, Papanikolaou IS, Toermer T et al. EUS-guided FNA of solid pancreatic masses: high yield of 2 passes with combined histologic-cytologic analysis. Gastrointest Endosc 2009; 70: 60–69

[8] Welker L, Galle J, Vollmer E. Bronchological bioptic diagnosis of lung cancer—cytology and/or histology? [Article in German]. Pneumologie 2004; 58: 718–723

[9] Riphaus A, Wehrmann T, Weber B et alSektion Enoskopie im Auftrag der Deutschen Gesellschaft für Verdauungs- und Stoffwechselerkrankungen e.V. (DGVS). Bundesverband Niedergelassener Gastroenterologen Deuschlands e. V. (Bng). Chirurgische Arbeitsgemeinschaft für Endoskopie und Sonographie der Deutschen Gesellschaft für Allgemein- und Viszeralchirurgie (DGAV). Deutsche Morbus Crohn/Colitis ulcerosa Vereinigung e. V. (DCCV). Deutsche Gesellschaft für Endoskopie-Assistenzpersonal (DEGEA). Deutsche Gesellschaft für Anästhesie und Intensivmedizin (DGAI). Gesellschaft für Recht und Politik im Gesundheitswesen (GPRG). S3-guidelines—sedation in gastrointestinal endoscopy [Article in German]. Z Gastroenterol 2008; 46: 1298–1330

[10] Otto RC. Indications for ultrasound-guided fine needle puncture under permanent view. 1. Diagnostic puncture [Article in German]. Ultraschall Med 1983; 4: 72–76

15 Abscess Drainage

C. F. Dietrich, A. Ignee, U. Gottschalk

It is important to consider clinical status in ultrasound-guided therapeutic procedures for abscess drainage, and it is equally important to follow a standardized technique. The success rates published for ultrasound-guided abscess drainage vary widely, but a realistic range is 70 to 95%, depending on the patient groups treated.[1–4] Published complication rates also vary widely,[5–16] with a realistic range from < 3 to 15%. A similar range is reported for mortality rates.

A complicated multilocular abscess with difficult drainage access should be managed by a combination of medical and surgical treatment. These severe cases have lower success rates and higher mortality.[17,18]

15.1 Historical Considerations

The drainage of body fluids has been practiced since antiquity. Available materials were quite limited, however. Drainage tubes were often fabricated from lead, which was easy to bend to the desired shape. The development of modern materials was necessary for the creation of effective drainage systems that could remain indwelling for some time. Polyethylene, for example, was discovered by the chemist Hans von Pechmann in 1898 and was first produced industrially by Reginald Gibson and Eric Fawcett in England in 1933. Other historical issues are reviewed in Chapter 2 (Interventional Materials and Equipment).[19,20]

15.2 Preliminary Remarks, Etiology

It is important to identify underlying factors that have major prognostic significance such as underlying malignant diseases, immune defects, diabetes mellitus, or chronic inflammatory bowel diseases treated with immunosuppressant agents. Advanced age is a negative prognostic factor but does not alter the approach to management.

Percutaneous drainage has become the standard treatment for abdominal and pelvic abscesses. Its success rate is high, but there is still a recurrence rate of 5 to 10%. One retrospective analysis found that surgery was avoided in 56% of pelvic abscesses treated by percutaneous drainage. The mean time to recurrence was 51 days (2 to 365 days), and postoperative abscesses were more likely to require further surgery.[3] In another study, experienced interventionalists had a 100% success rate for entering the abscess cavity and a 98% success rate for establishing catheter drainage. Again, however, not all abscesses could be successfully treated by percutaneous drainage alone; surgery was avoided in 88% of the cases.[21]

The differential diagnosis of infectious tropical diseases relies on a combination of serology, detection of eosinophilia, and analysis of IgE levels. The history should include information on possible trips to tropical or subtropical latitudes or endemic regions. Supplemental information should include possible underlying immunosuppression due to HIV infection, for example, or other sexually transmitted diseases.

The following factors and mechanisms may be important in the etiology and pathogenesis of abscess formation:

- Primary versus secondary abscess formation
- Contiguous spread
- Sepsis
- Postoperative or postinterventional abscess formation (after local ablative procedures, embolization, etc.)
- Underlying hepatobiliary disease (mainly involving the liver)
- Underlying acute or chronic inflammatory bowel disease (in which case drainage alone is less likely to be successful)
- Previous trauma
- Predisposition due to weakened host defenses (immunosuppression, HIV infection, diabetes mellitus, advanced age)
- Idiopathic factors

15.3 Selection of Imaging Modality

Ultrasound, conventional radiographic techniques, CT, and MRI are all used as guidance modalities in the interventional treatment of abscesses. Regardless of the modality used, imaging should be contrast-enhanced and should include the whole abdomen because appendicitis with complications, peridiverticulitis, and acute or chronic inflammatory bowel disease are sometimes diagnosed in patients with indeterminate liver lesions.

15.3.1 Ultrasound

Careful attention should be given to the access route in the planning of ultrasound-guided abscess drainage. Adequate guidance requires visualization of the entire route.[22] Drainage should not be done through two body cavities, and liver abscesses should never be drained through the pleural cavity. Other advantages of ultrasound guidance are the real-time display and high resolution. A potential disadvantage is the confined field of view, which limits visualization of the access route.

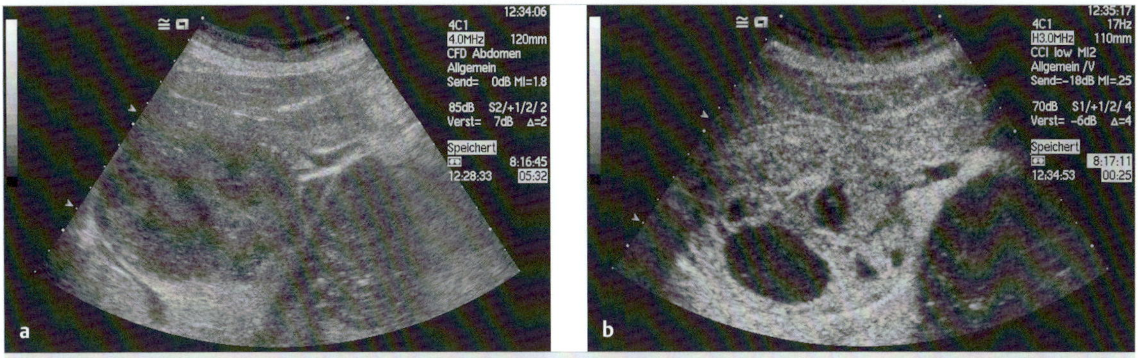

Fig. 15.1 a, b Phlegmonous inflammation with initial liquefaction (liver abscess). The inflammatory process should still be treated medically at this stage because it consists almost entirely of perfused tissue areas and dilated bile ducts (due to biliary disease). The treatment of choice in this case was endoscopic retrograde cholangiography (ERC), sphincterotomy, and stone extraction.

The underlying process giving rise to an abscess is a phlegmonous inflammation. A perifocal reaction is often observed in immunoreactive patients, especially after the administration of a contrast agent (this applies to contrast-enhanced ultrasound as well as contrast-enhanced radiographic methods). Contrast-enhanced ultrasound is the modality of choice for positively distinguishing a phlegmonous inflammation (▶ Fig. 15.1) from an abscess (▶ Fig. 15.2). This is due mainly to the high spatial resolution of ultrasound and the fact that the contrast agent (e.g., SonoVue) remains strictly within the intravascular compartment. The description of the abscess should include the assessment of criteria such as "internal echoes" (vascularization, perfusion) and "loculation."

The detection of intralesional air echoes is helpful in making a diagnosis. Approximately two-thirds of liver abscesses are solitary, depending on the underlying disease, and have an average size of approximately 7 cm when first manifested and diagnosed.[15,26,27]

It should be noted that amoebic abscesses may be isoechoic to surrounding liver and may be identifiable as liquid masses only after contrast administration.

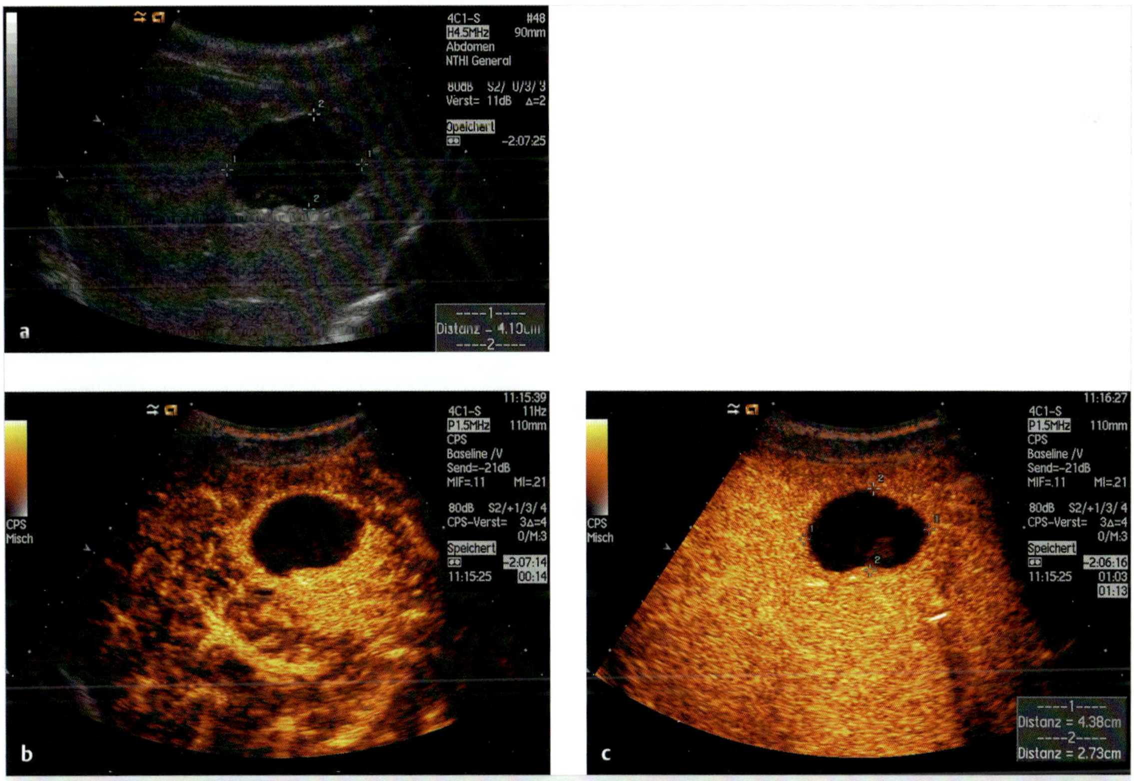

Fig. 15.2 Typical sonographic appearance of an abscess (**a**), which required (single) percutaneous drainage and irrigation (primary drainage). Note the ring pattern of enhancement, which is typical of an abscess (**b, c**).[23–25]

15.3.2 Conventional Radiographic Drainage

Conventional radiography is rarely used today for the guidance of percutaneous abscess drainage, but it may still be helpful as an adjunct to sonographic guidance.

15.3.3 Computed Tomography

Unlike ultrasound contrast agents, the contrast media administered for CT and MRI also diffuse into the interstitium. Because of this, CT and MRI cannot distinguish between perfused and nonperfused areas with the same precision as contrast-enhanced ultrasound.

15.3.4 Magnetic Resonance Imaging

MRI is rarely used as a primary study for abscess diagnosis. Abscesses generally have low signal intensity on T1-weighted images and high signal intensity on T2-weighted images due to their fluid content. Images after IV contrast administration (e.g., gadolinium-DTPA) show peripheral rim enhancement.

15.4 Devices

15.4.1 Drainage Catheters

Which Catheter?

A variety of drainage catheters are available on the market (see Chapter 2) (▶ Fig. 15.3, ▶ Fig. 15.4).

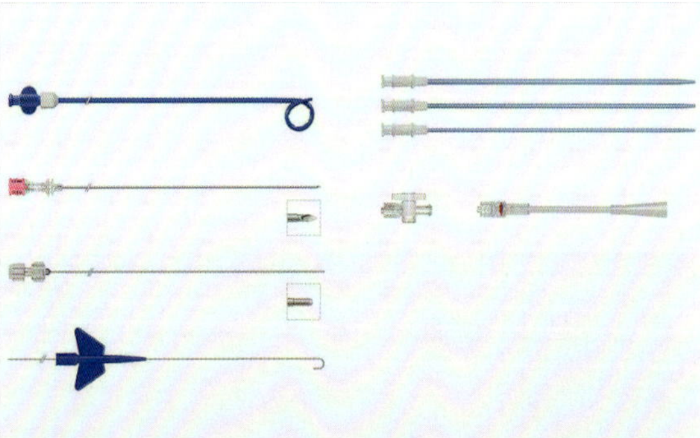

Fig. 15.3 Instrument set for the external drainage of viscous fluids by the Seldinger technique (OptiMed). Materials: OD (soft polyurethane). Components of the set: abscess drainage catheters (diameters 8–16F, lengths 30 and 40 cm). Two-part puncture needle with echogenic tip (diameter 1.3 mm, 17.5 gauge, length 20 cm). Two-part obturator (diameters 1.3–1.8 mm, lengths 33 and 43 cm). Schüller-type catheter exchange wire (diameter 0.035 inch, length 100 cm, 10-cm flexible tip, 3-mm J curve, 40-cm rigid shaft, flexible end). Dilators (diameters 6–18F, length 20 cm). Three-way stopcock. Rotating adapter, male Luer lock.

Trocar or Seldinger Technique

Most drains today are mounted on a blunt trocar when supplied. They consist (from outside to inside) of the catheter itself, made of flexible material, a trocar (a blunt steel cannula), and a sharp puncture needle. The trocar technique is ideal for short access routes that are perpendicular to the skin surface. Catheters in the size range of 10F to14F are recommended in severely ill patients and patients with extensive abscess formation. While the Seldinger technique was once preferred for larger abscesses, it is less commonly used today. The Seldinger technique is preferred in the following situations: difficult access routes, insertions tangential to the skin surface, and large-bore catheters (> 14F). In muscular patients, moreover, it is often difficult to penetrate the anterior abdominal wall with a trocar.

Practice

The trocar technique (8–10F) has proven excellent for the drainage of uncomplicated abscesses in everyday practice.

Considerations on Catheter Size

Drainage catheters are supplied in standard outer diameters ranging from 6F to 16F (see Chapter 2). The choice will depend on the expected consistency of the abscess contents. Catheter diameters smaller than 8F are generally too small to provide adequate drainage and irrigation.

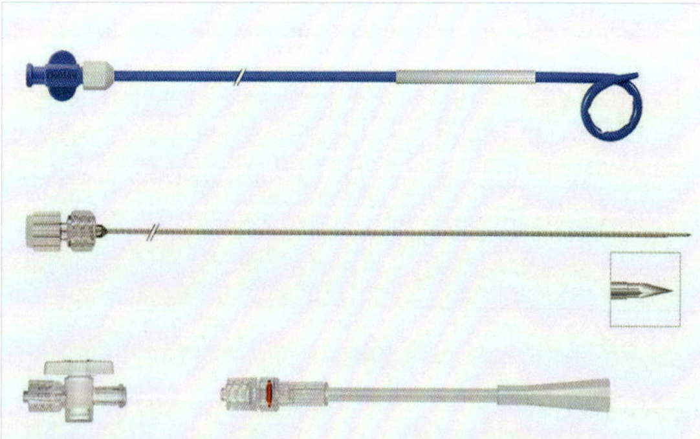

Fig. 15.4 Universal instrument set for the percutaneous drainage of viscous fluids by the trocar technique (OptiMed). Materials: OD (soft polyurethane). Components of the set: abscess drainage catheters (diameters 8–14F, lengths 30 cm). Two-part puncture needle with trocar point. Three-way stopcock. Rotating adapter, male Luer lock.

> **Practice**
>
> The typical size of an abscess drain is 10F. The exact size will depend on the etiology of the abscess, its (potentially difficult) location, viscosity, possible loculation, and the proportion of solid contents.

While small-bore catheters are usually easy to place by direct insertion, larger drains require a bolder approach. If the drain cannot be introduced easily, the tract should be dilated in small increments. This has proven helpful for catheter sizes > 10F. Generally it is sufficient to dilate the tract 2F less than the catheter size. Any slight bleeding that occurs when the dilator is withdrawn should be adequately controlled by pressure from the snug-fitting drainage catheter.

Catheter Properties

Most drainage catheters have a pigtail loop at the distal end and are straightened for insertion. This means that the catheter material must have good "shape memory," and almost all modern materials possess this property. Some manufacturers provide a locking drawstring to stabilize the distal loop.

Other crucial material properties are kink resistance and low surface friction. Because a thin wall is best for optimizing the relationship between outer diameter and inner lumen, special wall structures have been designed. An example is the Navarre universal catheter with its spiral laminated wall construction, which is resistant to kinking and compression despite the thin wall. For deeper insertions, it may be necessary to check the drain placement radiographically, so the catheter must be visible on radiographs. This may be achieved, for example, by adding barium sulfate to the catheter material. Other options are embedding a radiopaque thread in the drain wall or placing a metal ring at the distal end. In most cases, however, drain position will be checked during subsequent special studies in which contrast medium will be used; so isolated visualization of the catheter is not a crucial step. The arrangement of the drainage holes (usually 5 in number) is important in catheter selection. For abscess drainage, all the holes should be in the area of the catheter tip or pigtail. Hydrophilic catheter coatings are helpful in that they facilitate catheter advancement through the tissue. Most catheters have a conical tip with a short or long taper. This feature may adequately dilate the drainage tract, eliminating the need for separate dilators.

The pigtail drain is advanced over the cannula for direct insertion, or it may be slid onto a metal introducer for placement by the Seldinger technique so that the catheter will not distort the guidewire as it tends to reassume its coiled shape. When the catheter is slid onto the introducer, a straightening sleeve (already on the catheter shaft in most cases) is advanced to help prevent damage to the inner wall of the drainage catheter (this is described more fully in Chapter 2). Soft plastic stylets can also be used to straighten the pigtail for insertion.

15.5 Indications

Typical indications for abscess drainage are as follows:

- Hematogenous abscesses in parenchymal organs
- Abscesses secondary to outflow obstruction (e.g., biliary liver abscess)
- Septic embolism (e.g., splenic abscess in endocarditis)
- Complications of Crohn disease[28–30]
- Circumscribed abscess due to anastomotic leakage
- Confined perforation (e.g., in diverticulitis)
- Posttraumatic changes

15.6 Contraindications

Percutaneous abscess drainage may be done as either an elective or an emergency procedure. While an elective drainage procedure should follow the guidelines stated above, there are life-threatening situations in which an increased peri-interventional risk must be accepted. An example would be severe sepsis with multiorgan failure.

Generally valid contraindications to percutaneous abscess drainage include the following:

- Uncooperative patient
- Lack of informed consent
- Quick value (thromboplastin time) < 50%
- Platelet count < 50×10^9/L
- Partial thromboplastin time > 50 seconds
- Inability to visualize the precise abscess location
- Uncertain access route along vulnerable structures

Additional limitations should be noted in cases where pharmacologic obliteration is proposed (e.g., PAIR: puncture–aspiration–injection of alcohol–reaspiration):

- Cyst communicating with the biliary tract
- Cysts in the central nervous system, lung, or urogenital tract
- Calcified cyst (= not an indication)

15.7 Patient Preparation

Because percutaneous abscess drainage is an invasive procedure, the physician should provide the patient with a detailed explanation that includes benefits and possible complications, and informed written consent should be obtained before the procedure (Chapter 3). The patient should be informed of possible surgical alternatives, if they are available. It may be necessary to waive the informed consent requirement in emergency situations (e.g., for septic patients).

15.8 Treatment Options

15.8.1 General

Before a presumed abscess is drained, it is necessary to exclude a possible malignant condition associated with necrotic metastases (for example, larger metastases from neuroendocrine tumors may contain necrotic areas that mimic the ultrasound appearance of an abscess).[31] An echinococcal etiology should also be excluded because of its different therapeutic implications. Ultrasound can reliably diagnose most echinococcal cysts but is not always adequate, and serologic testing may be required (Chapter 17).[32] Tuberculosis of the liver is feared in large portions of Asia and Africa.[33] The treatment of amebic abscesses is usually pharmacologic (see below).

15.8.2 Medical Treatment Options

Pharmacologic treatment strategies may vary, depending on the underlying cause, and are described under specific disease headings.

15.8.3 Surgical Treatment Options

Surgical treatments include open catheter drainage, open surgical drainage, and partial hepatectomy. Surgical treatment has proven effective for large and complex abscesses that are not accessible by other means, multilocular abscesses, and in cases with failed percutaneous treatment.[34]

15.9 Technique of Percutaneous Abscess Drainage

15.9.1 Preparation

Assistants

Assistants prepare for the procedure by laying out the sterile instruments and selecting the necessary drain in consultation with the physician. A highly systematic routine should be followed during the procedure itself, as it involves the drainage of infectious material that may be hazardous to both the patient and staff (▶ Fig. 15.5) (Chapter 10).

A nonsterile assistant should be present for passing any necessary additional materials and monitoring the patient.

Accurate Abscess Localization

Percutaneous abscess drainage always starts with accurate imaging localization of the intended target. If the abscess can be clearly visualized, the drainage route is determined, which also defines the location of the puncture site in the skin. That site is marked with a water-soluble marker.

Skin Preparation

The skin site is aseptically prepared by wiping and spraying, then covered widely with a fenestrated drape.

Sedation

Patient sedation (e.g., with midazolam) is not an absolute requirement but may be helpful in some situations (Chapter 11).

Local Anesthesia

Local anesthesia is usually performed with a 1% local anesthetic solution. The most commonly used agent is 1% lidocaine. It is important to aspirate before injecting the solution since intravascular administration could produce a systemic effect. A subcutaneous or intracutaneous wheal is placed to numb the skin. The hypodermic needle may be 22-gauge (black), 23-gauge (blue), or even 26-gauge (brown) in extremely sensitive patients. Deep analgesia can be produced with somewhat longer needles of 21-gauge (green) or 20-gauge (yellow). An alternative in very obese patients is a 20- or 22-gauge Chiba needle

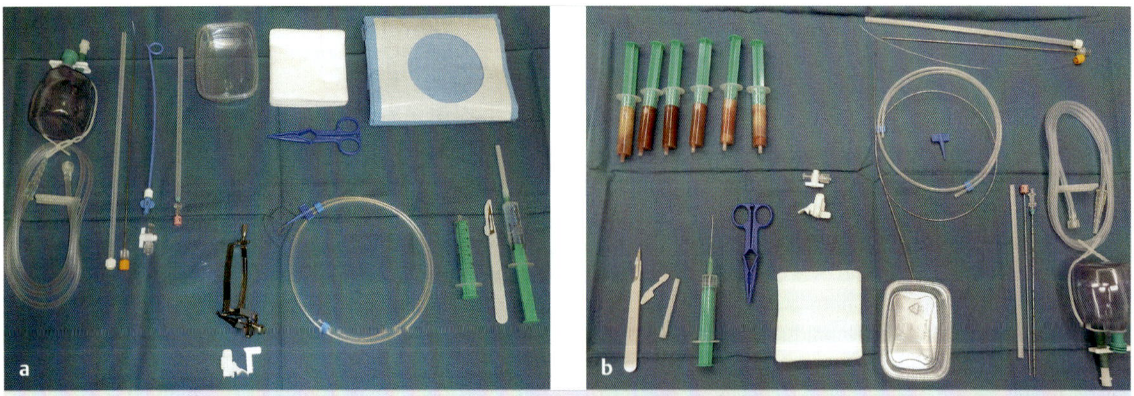

Fig. 15.5 Table setup (a) at the start and (b) at the end of the procedure with the drained abscess contents.

220 mm long, initially using a subcutaneous needle and then changing to a longer needle (green).

15.9.2 Initial Needle Insertion

Because drainage catheters cannot be inserted directly through the skin, an initial stab incision is made with a pointed scalpel. A needle of adequate size is introduced through the incision and advanced into the abscess under ultrasound guidance (▶ Fig. 15.6).

Often the abscess contents are aspirated in an initial step to confirm the diagnosis. This is done with a hollow needle stiffened by a stylet. Regarding needle caliber, 22-gauge needles are generally more difficult to visualize with ultrasound, while 18-gauge needles allow for immediate 0.35-inch wire guidance and can aspirate even viscous abscess contents. A 20-gauge needle (trade-off between the 18- and 22-gauge) is easy to visualize and less traumatizing than an 18-gauge needle but accommodates a smaller wire diameter.

Checking Catheter Placement

Catheter placement can be checked by conventional fluoroscopy. With adequate ultrasound visualization, we also favor sonographic localization aided by the intracavitary instillation of an ultrasound contrast agent (e.g., SonoVue). The direct injection of ultrasound contrast medium through the catheter (diluted at 1–2 drops per 20 mL saline solution) gives excellent visualization of the abscess cavity and the catheter itself, which may be poorly visualized with precontrast ultrasound due to the surface properties of the material. The contrast injection can immediately confirm (▶ Fig. 15.7) or exclude (▶ Fig. 15.8) communication of the abscess cavity with the biliary tract.

It should be noted that both intracavitary and intravenous contrast administration can be combined with real-time ultrasound guidance to confirm complete evacuation of the abscess contents (▶ Fig. 15.9).

As stated earlier, two main techniques are available for catheter insertion. The trocar technique is simpler and less time-consuming, but it involves the primary insertion of a relatively rigid, large-bore instrument, making it difficult to bypass vulnerable structures. The Seldinger technique involves a more subtle initial approach in which a thin needle is passed safely and accurately to the targeted site. After placement of the guidewire, the tract is enlarged with serial dilators.

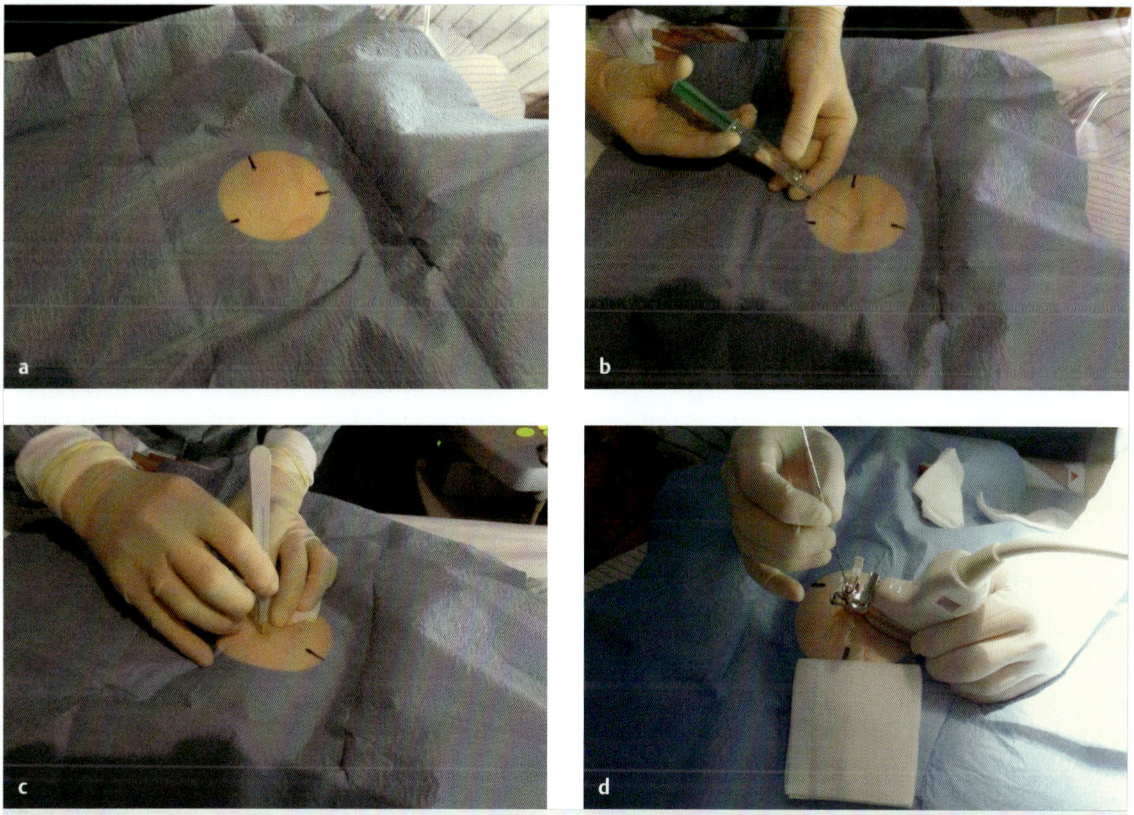

Fig. 15.6 Percutaneous needle insertion.
a Sterile draping of the skin site.
b Local anesthesia.
c Stab incision.
d Ultrasound-guided insertion of the needle into the abscess.

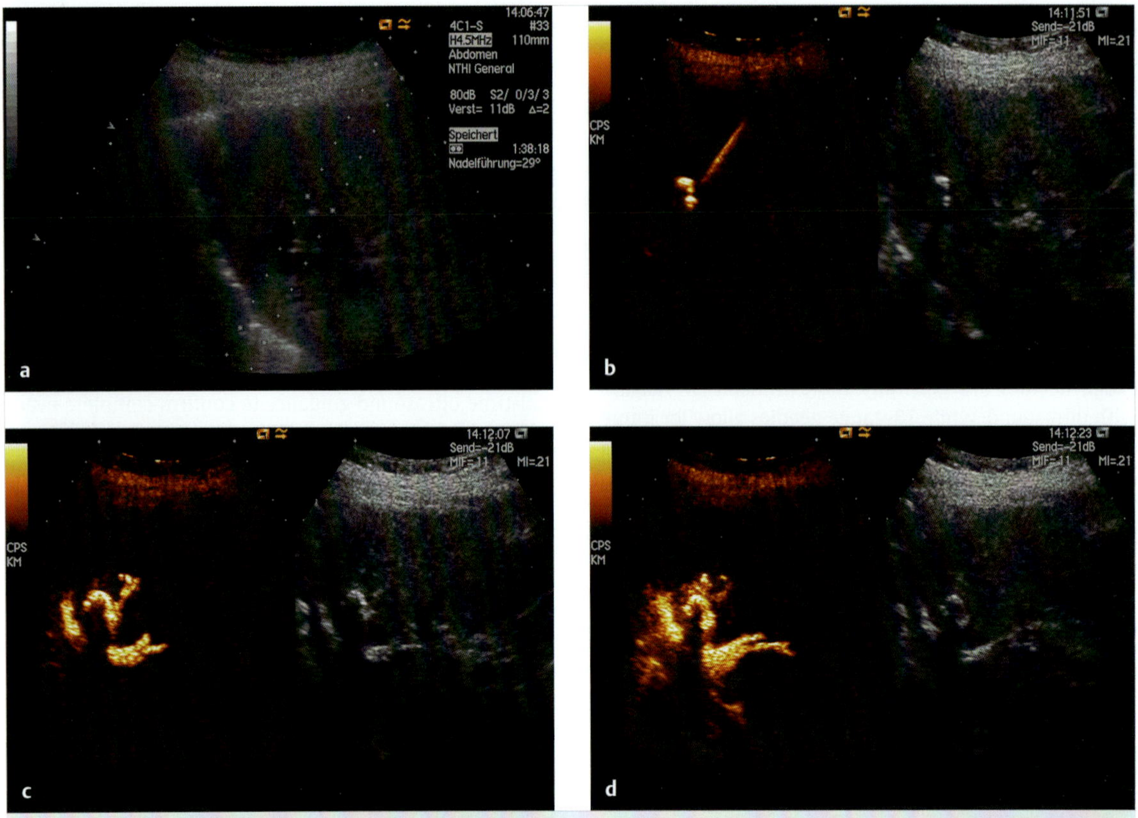

Fig. 15.7 a–d Ultrasound-guided abscess drainage using SonoVue to visualize the abscess cavity. Contrast administration confirms that the abscess communicates with the biliary tract.

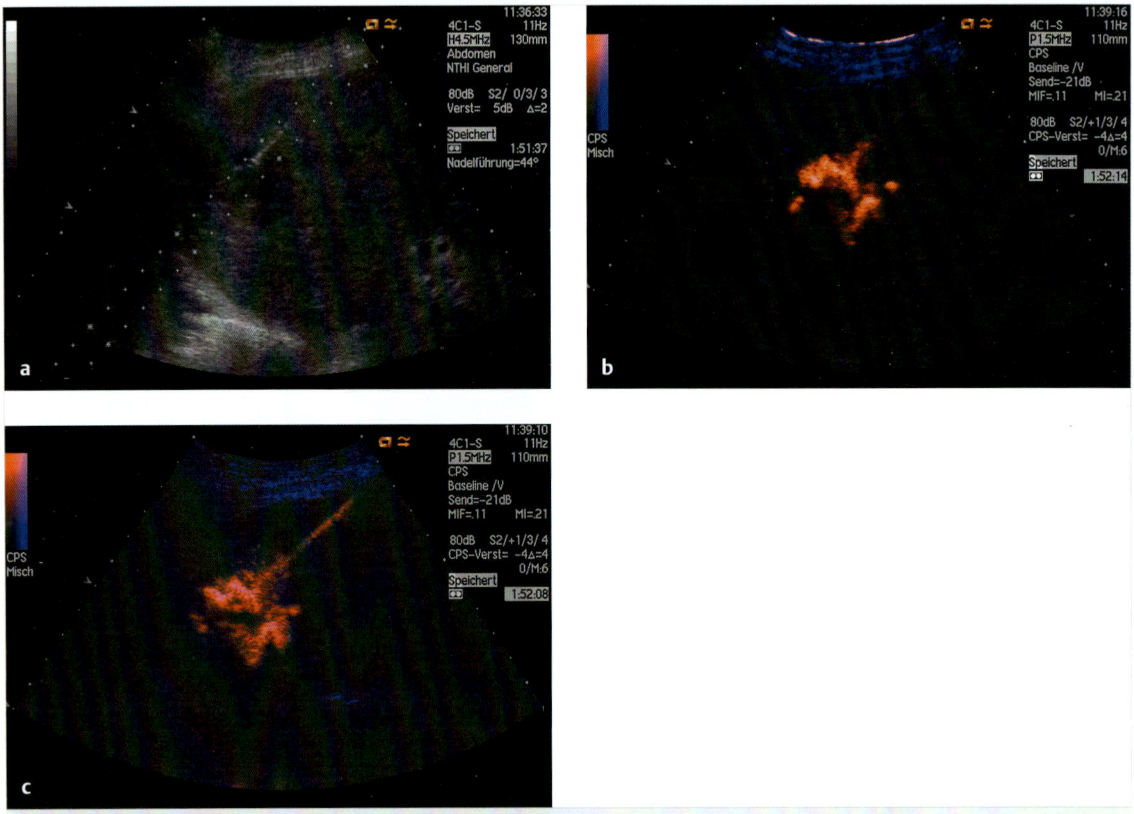

Fig. 15.8 a–c Ultrasound-guided abscess drainage using SonoVue to visualize the abscess cavity. Contrast administration shows that the abscess does not communicate with the biliary tract.

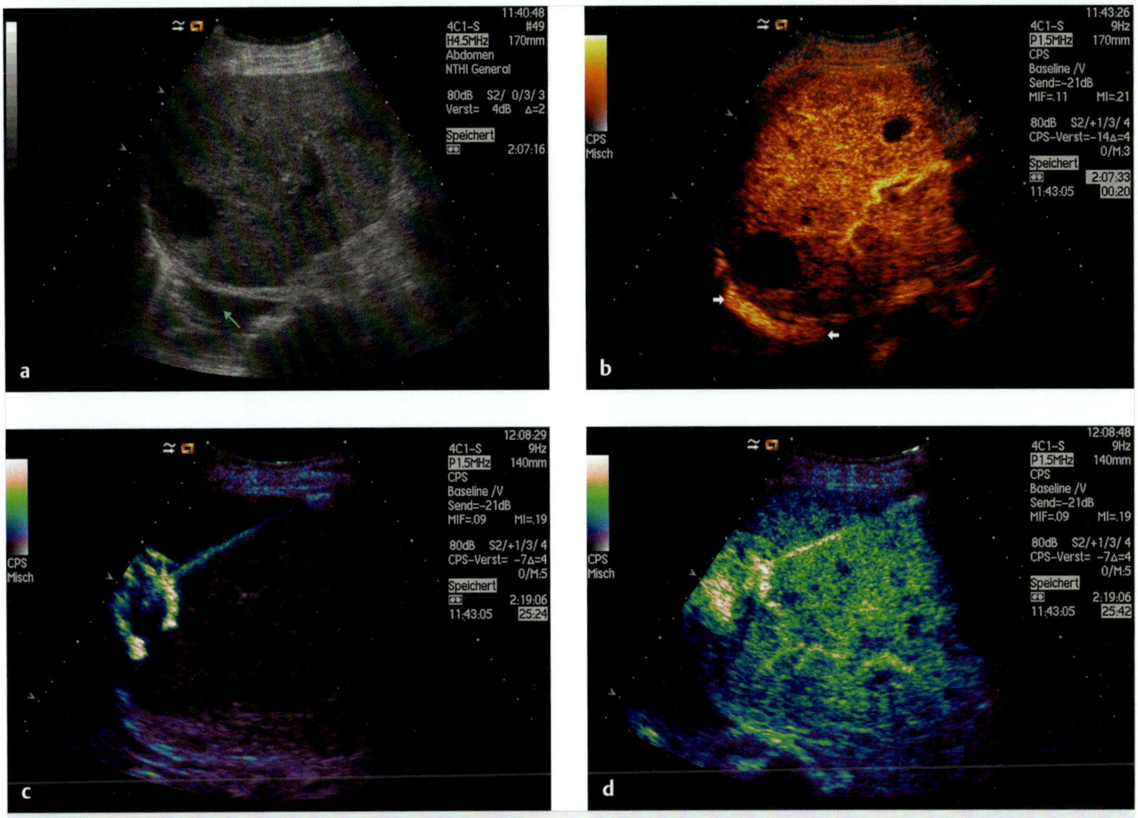

Fig. 15.9 Abscess communicating with the pleural cavity (a, b). Abscess drainage is performed under ultrasound guidance with SonoVue instilled into the abscess cavity (c) and also administered intravenously (d). The latter permits the detection (or exclusion) of any undrained portions of the abscess.

15.9.3 Trocar Technique

Once the operator has decided on the trocar technique, a two- or three-part instrument assembly is inserted directly into the abscess in one step (see Chapter 2). The procedure concludes with removal of the stylet and hollow needle. Contrast medium is then injected to confirm correct catheter placement.

Seldinger Technique

The Seldinger technique begins with the insertion of a fine needle. A 1.1-mm Chiba needle will accommodate a 0.035-inch guidewire. With a thinner needle (e.g., 0.7 mm diameter), a 0.018-inch guidewire is inserted first and the tract is carefully dilated to the size of the larger wire, which is then used for further dilation. These wires are kink-resistant and permit dilation of the needle tract using Seldinger technique. The use of a Lunderquist wire is advantageous in that the highly stable guidewire facilitates passage of the dilator, but the stiffer wire also increases the risk of perforation. Generally, however, there is no need to dilate the tract to 10F, and a drainage catheter with a tapered distal end can be advanced directly over the guidewire and into the abscess. When the guidewire is removed, the catheter reassumes its distal tip shape, which usually consists of a pigtail loop with or without a locking drawstring. Finally the catheter is secured at skin level with a retention plate or sutures (▶ Fig. 15.10).

Needle Aspiration

Quantitative needle aspiration of the abscess contents (with or without irrigation) for decompression purposes is appropriate for abscesses smaller than 5 to 8 cm and is usually worth considering. It can be repeated 1 to 3 days later if necessary. Studies recommend that a drainage catheter should be placed after 2 or 3 needle aspirations if complete evacuation is not achieved. Needle aspiration achieved good results in several studies compared with drain placement for lesions up to 50 mm in size. Arguments made for percutaneous needle aspiration and against catheter drainage are that needle aspiration under ultrasound guidance is technically easier, that the abscess cavity is entered in a very high percentage of cases, and that the great majority of complications are caused by the drainage catheter rather than the initial puncture. (It should be noted that the latter statement is not accepted in general.) Thus, the decision should be made on a case-by-case basis

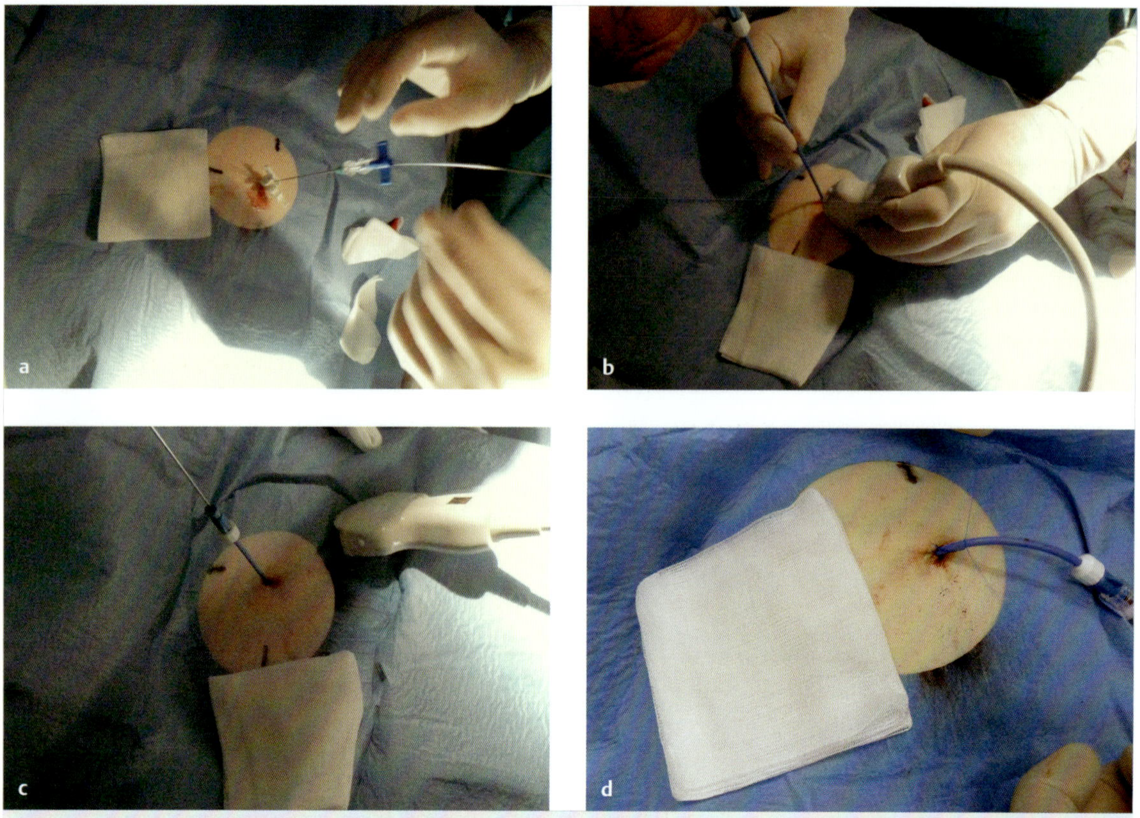

Fig. 15.10 Seldinger technique with a Chiba needle.
a The Chiba needle has been placed, and a guidewire is introduced through the needle.
b The drainage catheter is advanced over the guidewire.
c The guidewire is removed.
d The catheter is secured with sutures.

and depends on factors that include the size, encapsulation, and location of the abscess (e.g., parenchyma abscess, interenteric abscess, retroperitoneal abscess). Some situations, such as multiple liver abscesses, may call for the use of both techniques: catheter drainage and quantitative needle aspiration.

There is a small amount of evidence suggesting that catheter drainage is better for abscesses larger than 50 mm.[35] Other authors report a lower success rate for needle aspirations.[36] One drawback of the published data is that different strategies were employed. The authors who reported an advantage of needle aspiration performed significantly more interventions and used thinner drains (e.g., 8F[6]), while authors who favored catheter drainage abandoned needle aspiration after only two attempts. Interestingly, both procedures required the same length of hospitalization.

Regardless of the drainage procedure used, close-interval imaging follow-up is essential. When a drainage catheter has been placed, success can also be assessed clinically by monitoring the drain output.

Drainage

In contrast to simple needle aspiration, catheters are used for abscess drainage. Once a drain has been placed, it is left indwelling for some time. The drain may irritate neighboring structures and create a portal for ascending infection. Before the needle is inserted, therefore, it is essential to obtain a clear image of the intended target and select the shortest possible drainage route that is still considered safe. The proposed drainage route should avoid intervening blood vessels, and transpleural drainage is a (relative) contraindication. Transsplenic drainage should also be avoided. The drainage of superficial parenchymal abscesses has a higher complication rate. In planning the access route, it is wise to maintain a safety margin of approximately 5 to 10 mm from vessels, bowel, ureters, and nerves.[37] Particular attention should be given to the stage of the abscess (from phlegmonous inflammation to the formation of an abscess membrane).

Combined Procedures, Multiple Abscesses

Given the current interdisciplinary trend, there will be an increasing reliance on combined percutaneous, endoscopic, endosonographic, and laparoscopic approaches in the future. For the present, various endosonographic techniques make it possible to perform ultrasound-guided biopsies transvaginally and through the upper and lower gastrointestinal tract.[38,39] These routes are described in Chapter 22 and are not detailed here. Whenever possible, retroperitoneal lesions should be approached through a posterior route outside the abdominal cavity.

When multiple abscesses have formed in one organ, their communication should be assessed before the procedure. With multiple liver abscesses, for example, it may be necessary to place drains at several sites or use a combination of percutaneous and transpapillary approaches. Moreover, it is important to consider not only the extent of abscess formation but also the sensitivity of the target organ.

Compartment Syndrome

Peritonitis and the less common abdominal compartment syndrome after a spontaneous perforation (or more commonly after endoscopy) may create a life-threatening situation that requires a swift response. Percutaneous drainage can be established at any number of sites in the abdominal cavity, and the route with the lowest risk should be chosen.[40] This decision is aided by preliminary ultrasound to exclude possible collateral vessels in the abdominal wall. The abdominal cavity can be decompressed through an ordinary large-bore IV catheter. When dealing with a superficial abscess (e.g., abdominal wall abscess), ultrasound can direct the placement of soft drainage catheters without tissue injury.[41]

Suture Fixation

Once a catheter has been placed, it can be secured at skin level with a retention plate or suture. We prefer the latter method, in which a U-shaped stitch is passed through the skin approximately 5 to 10 mm from the catheter entry site and the suture material is fixed directly to the skin with three surgical knots. Another knot is tied approximately 10 mm above that point, whereupon the suture is looped around the drainage catheter and tied down, creating a total of three knots (▶ Fig. 15.11).

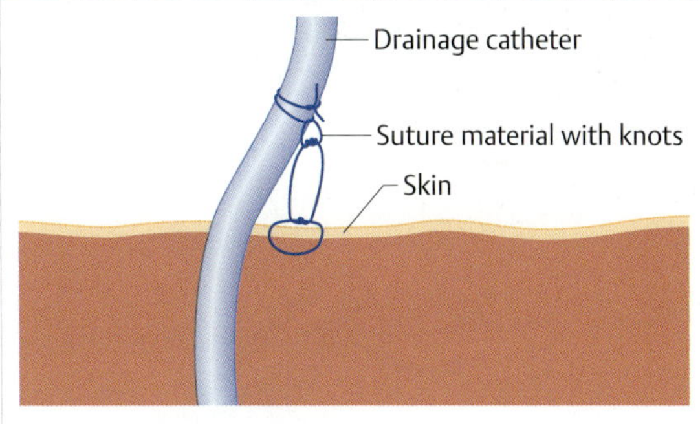

Fig. 15.11 Placement of the suture knots for catheter fixation.

A variety of suture materials may be used. Years ago, sutures and needles were usually supplied separately. Natural silk or catgut (animal intestine) were generally used. Today, modern synthetic materials are used almost exclusively. Suture material was once supplied by the yard in fluid-filled bottles and was cut to the desired size on site, then threaded into a needle. Today the suture material is swaged onto an eyeless needle at the factory to form a unit. Needles are available in various sizes and geometries—straight or curved, round and smooth or triangular with sharp edges, and so on. With "atraumatic" suture material there is no step-off between the needle and suture, and the needle geometry is usually round. Monofilament suture material is used to create a smooth seal at the needle entry site (e.g., for suturing blood vessels). Monofilament sutures are less pliable and more difficult to tie, but their smooth surface is more resistant to bacterial invasion at skin level. Braided (multifilament) suture material is more pliable and easier to tie but has a wicklike surface texture. A trade-off is pseudomonofilament (hybrid) suture material, in which braided suture material is smoothed by a surface coating. Only nonabsorbable suture material should be used for catheter fixation. Two main systems are used for designating suture diameters: the USP system (United States Pharmacopeia) and the metric system (▶ Table 15.1). The nominal suture diameter is always the minimum diameter; the true diameter is usually at the upper end of the millimeter range stated in the table.

Although a needle can be passed through the skin entirely by hand, it is better to use a needle holder when performing the stitch (▶ Fig. 15.12).

Table 15.1 Comparison of suture diameters in the USP system (United States Pharmacopeia) and metric systems

System	Corresponding suture diameters						
USP	7–0	6–0	5–0	4–0	3–0	2–0	1–0
Metric	0.5	0.7	1.0	1.5	2	2.5	3
Millimeter range	0.050 to 0.059	0.070 to 0.079	0.100 to 0.149	0.150 to 0.199	0.200 to 0.249	0.250 to 0.299	0.300 to 0.349

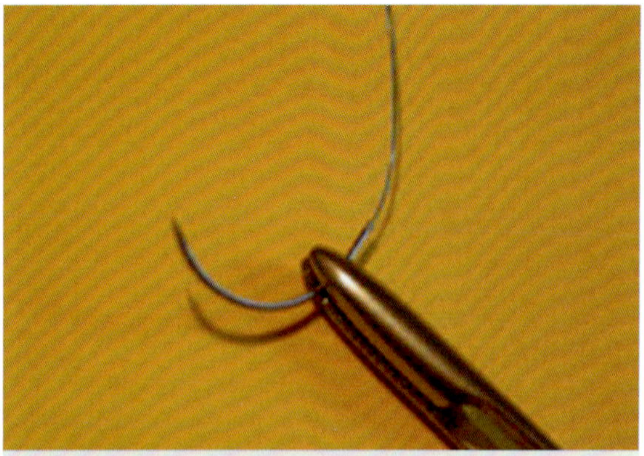

Fig. 15.12 Swaged needle–suture combination gripped in a needle holder.

15.9.4 Irrigation

Initial irrigation is done with sterile saline solution and is continued until clear fluid is returned. Care is taken that the aspirated or drained fluid volume is roughly equal to the volume injected. One possible regimen is to continue irrigating with a volume equal to the size of the abscess cavity, or at least 10 mL of saline solution every 8 or 12 hours.[2] This will also prevent clogging and incrustation of the catheter. Several authors have reported on antibiotic irrigations (gentamycin, tobramycin), and some note the advantages of twice-daily intracavitary infusions of fibrinolytic agents (alteplase), especially in abscesses unsuccessfully drained by initial catheter placement.[42] On the whole, there is no solid evidence to support antibiotic irrigation or fibrinolytic infusion.

15.9.5 Drain Removal

The duration of drainage depends on the number, location, size, and shape of the abscesses. A single needle aspiration and single irrigation have proven satisfactory for abscesses smaller than 8 cm.

The drain may be removed when the patient shows marked improvement in clinical parameters and laboratory values, the catheter output falls to < 10 mL/day, and imaging shows a significant reduction in abscess volume. Drains are usually left in place for 1 to 2 weeks on average, although the exact period will vary from case to case.[43,44] Assessment by B-mode ultrasound is difficult because the collapsed abscess cavity is often isoechoic to surrounding liver tissue. Ultrasound contrast agents are helpful in these cases. Any residual abscess will appear as a contrast void after intravenous contrast administration.

15.9.6 Specimen Processing

Initially, 10 to 20 mL of abscess fluid is collected for bacteriologic and possible cytologic analysis as well as antimicrobial susceptibility testing to allow for specific, systemic antibiotic therapy. The evaluation of pyogenic abscesses does not include serologic tests or tumor factor assays.

15.10 Postprocedure Care

The postprocedure care regimen depends on the specific disease.

15.11 Specific Diseases

15.11.1 Pyogenic Liver Abscess

Epidemiology and Causes

Liver abscesses most commonly develop in a setting of septicemia (e.g. staphylococcal), biliary tract infections (enterobacteria such as *E. coli*, *Klebsiella*, *Bacteriodes* species, and anaerobes), and after invasive procedures. A variety of causative organisms may be involved. Liver abscesses pose a significant threat and still carry a substantial mortality rate of 6 to 14%.[7] Abscesses up to 10 cm in size can be managed relatively easily by percutaneous aspiration and evacuation or catheter drainage. Success rates with these procedures are > 95%.[45] These results may be somewhat better than the 88% success rates reported for the less common splenic abscesses in small groups of patients.[46] The percutaneous treatment of liver abscesses has become a routine procedure in clinical practice and has essentially no procedure-related mortality when adequate drainage is achieved.[47]

Most pyogenic liver abscesses have an ascending biliary cause or result from hematogenous spread via the portal vein and mesenteric veins. Portal venous bacteremia results from inflammatory processes in the region drained by the portal vein, such as diverticulitis, rectal ulcers, pericolic or perianal abscesses, chronic inflammatory bowel diseases, appendicitis, or rare cases of phlegmonous gastritis. The examiner should conduct a specific search for a possible cause. In rare cases, empyemas (e.g., of the gallbladder) or (postoperative) subphrenic abscesses may cause a liver abscess by contiguous spread. An extrahepatic infectious focus is not found in 15 to 60% of patients, however. It must be decided case-by-case whether it is sufficient to aspirate and evacuate an abscess with a large-gauge needle and repeat if necessary, or whether a suction drain should be placed first. Based on available data and our own experience, however, catheter drainage appears to yield a better result and a shorter hospital stay.[36] Available data do not indicate whether very large liver abscesses should be managed by primary surgical treatment, and this is also an individual decision.[48,49] Surgery is definitely the first-line treatment for a ruptured abscess. Today, multilocular abscesses can be treated percutaneously with a success rate of 94%.[50] An important consideration is the degree of multilocularity.

Clinical Features

Cardinal features such as septic fever and abdominal pain and rigidity in the right upper quadrant may be present or may be entirely absent. Jaundice is common in patients with a biliary liver abscess, depending on the underlying cause.

Diagnosis

The diagnosis in typically febrile, septic patients is based on early imaging studies followed by (ultrasound-)guided needle aspiration to obtain material for cultures (pathogen detection, susceptibility testing) and, in selected cases, for cytologic analysis and laboratory tests.

Treatment

Systemic antibiotic therapy is instituted immediately after the abscess is diagnosed and is modified as needed based on antimicrobial susceptibility testing. Local treatment depends on the extent of the pyogenic liver abscess (solitary, multiple) and its size. (Repeated) Ultrasound-guided or CT-guided percutaneous needle aspiration and evacuation of the abscess has proven to be effective. With extensive abscesses, the ultrasound- or CT-guided placement of a (large-bore) drainage catheter may be necessary. Antibiotic therapy alone is generally adequate for the treatment of multiple small abscesses (e.g., approximately 1 cm in size).

Specific Measures

Given the risk of severe septic complications, the abscess should be treated on an inpatient basis in close cooperation with the surgeon. Antibiotic therapy may consist of mezlocillin 4 × 2 g IV or cephalosporins and metronidazole IV (e.g., Ceftriaxon 1 × 2 g/day IV or metronidazole 3 × 0.5 g/day IV) or ciprofloxacin 2 × 0.4 g/day IV. Amoxillin + clavulanic acid (3 × 1.2 g IV) may also be administered in milder cases.

The treatment of pyogenic liver abscesses includes the following steps:

- **Take blood samples before initiating treatment.**
- Intravenous antibiotic therapy (after susceptibility testing): may start mezlocillin at 4 × 2 g/day IV or third-generation cephalosporins and metronidazole IV (e.g., Ceftriaxon 1 × 2 g/day IV or metronidazole 3 × 0.5 g/day IV) or ciprofloxacin 2 × 0.4 g/day IV
- Milder cases may respond to amoxicillin + clavulanic acid 3 × 1/2 g IV
- Ultrasound- or CT-guided needle aspiration and drainage
- With cholangitis due to outflow obstruction: biliary drainage by ERC and transpapillary cholangiodrainage or by percutaneous transhepatic cholangiodrainage (PTCD)
- Nutrition: withhold solid foods during intravenous fluid and electrolyte replacement; introduce light foods as symptoms subside.
- Surgical intervention (if required)

15.11.2 Abscesses in Appendicitis, Peridiverticulitis

While it has not yet been proven that the prophylactic intraoperative placement of a drain in complicated appendicitis will benefit the patient,[51] the percutaneous drainage of abscesses has gained an established role. In the past, these abscesses were considered a definite indication for surgery.[52] Complicated appendicitis is characterized by the presence of a "left-sided abscess," which can be further classified as a high or low left-sided abscess. These lesions require differentiation from a floating (pelvic) abscess and cul-de-sac abscess.[53] It has been shown in children that a single intervention is adequate in over half of cases. Further interventions may be necessary, with an average drain dwell time of 8 days.[12] Meanwhile, the drainage of abscesses after appendicitis has become the most frequent indication for abdominal drainage in pediatric interventional radiology.[54] The goal in many of these interventions should be to avoid repeat laparotomy, and this has been successfully accomplished.[55]

In recent years there have been growing numbers of optimistic reports on endosonographically guided interventions in the treatment of certain abscesses in the upper abdomen, such as omental bursa abscesses.[56] Similar developments are apparent in transvaginal drainage.[57]

In the case of diverticulitis and peridiverticulitis, the goal is to improve the patient to an operable condition. Percutaneous abscess drainage is gaining therapeutic importance in these cases and may even provide definitive treatment in older patients.[11,58,59] Lately it has become clear that percutaneous abscess drainage can reduce the frequency and extent of subsequent surgery and also reduce the need for permanent stomata.[60] Similar trends are noted in inflammatory bowel diseases and especially in Crohn disease.[61]

15.11.3 Liver Abscess in Biliary Disease

A special case is a "sump syndrome" following a side-to-side choledochoduodenostomy or choledochojejunostomy and resulting from an accumulation of bile, plant fibers, or debris in the distal portion of the main bile duct. The dominant features of this condition are right upper quadrant pain, fever, and possible jaundice. It may be complicated by acute cholangitis and/or acute pancreatitis. Ultrasound usually shows a distended extrahepatic bile duct with echogenic contents.[62,63] Surgical intervention should be considered in cases where liver abscesses develop.[64]

The usual initial treatment, however, is percutaneous abscess drainage and biliary tract drainage. Multiple liver abscesses may form as a result of ascending infection. If the abscesses are small, it is reasonable to attempt endoscopic therapy. This is not always sufficient in the long term, however.[65,66] This situation is problematic following hepatocholedochostomy, as there is an approximately 15% incidence of sump syndrome and further surgery should be avoided whenever possible.[67] There have been growing numbers of reports on nonsurgical treatment options for sump syndrome resulting in a reduced need for reoperation.[68] Because most of the patients were elderly and a generally good surgical result in this age group must be weighed against perioperative risks, sonographic endoscopic interventions can provide a definitive treatment option in many cases.[69]

15.11.4 Abscess in Pancreatitis

Abscesses in acute pancreatitis may be localized to the pancreas, may form in extrapancreatic fluid collections, or may occasionally be secondary to biliary tract complications. Specific aspects of the combined percutaneous and endosonographically guided drainage of local abscesses in pancreatitis are described in Chapter 22 owing to their accessibility via the gastrointestinal tract. Although the drainage of pancreatic fluids is associated with a risk of fistula formation, percutaneous drainage still provides an effective treatment in necrotizing pancreatitis. This may require the use of large-bore drains, depending on the consistency of the fluid.[70,71]

Chronic pancreatitis may cause a common duct stricture leading to pyogenic liver abscess.[72]

15.11.5 Liver Abscess in Amebiasis

Epidemiology and Cause

Amebiasis has a worldwide distribution but predominantly affects inhabitants of (or travelers to) the tropics and areas with unsanitary conditions (endemicity of approximately 20 to 30%, transmitted mainly by fecal contamination of water or food). The great majority (> 90%) of infected patients are asymptomatic, and the causative organisms are eliminated. Various species of ameba are known that occur in the human intestine (e.g., *Entamoeba coli*, *Entamoeba polecki*, and *Entamoeba nana*). The only invasive pathogenic species is *Entamoeba histolytica*, which in turn consists of more than 20 subspecies with varying degrees of virulence. Only about half of them can cause liver abscesses.

Clinical Features

Liver abscesses associated with a spiking fever and right upper quadrant pain may develop during or subsequent to amebic colitis (days, weeks, or even years after visiting a tropical area). Some patients may have no intestinal symptoms. These liver abscesses are 7 to 10 times more prevalent in males than females, although intestinal amebiasis affects both sexes equally.

Diagnosis

The diagnosis is confirmed by the detection of magna and minuta forms or cysts in the stool. A single microscopic stool examination has low sensitivity for detecting the parasite, however, and at least three fresh stool samples mixed with saline should be examined to detect the typical motility of vegetative forms. The *stool antigen test* has proved superior to microscopic detection (94% sensitivity and 94% specificity versus 37% and 99%, respectively). Serologic tests of antibody titers (detectable in 92 to 97% of patients after one week) may suggest amebiasis but cannot positively diagnose current disease: up to 25% of the inhabitants in endemic areas are positive for amebic antibodies without having an acute infection. In patients with extraintestinal manifestations such as liver abscess, the parasite can also be identified in histologic sections. Amebas are not detected in abscess contents (aspirated under ultrasound guidance). Trophozoites are microscopically detectable in < 20% of patients when the aspirate includes material from the periphery of the abscess.

Laboratory tests usually show only nonspecific inflammatory markers with elevated ESR, leukocytosis without eosinophilia, anemia, elevated α_1- and α_2-globulins, and hypoalbuminemia. Aminotransferases are elevated in half of patients, alkaline phosphatase in 80%.

General Measures

Good hygienic practices are stressed, with special emphasis on preventing the contamination of food and drinking water by human feces.

Specific Measures

The agent of choice is metronidazole, administered at a dosage of 4 × 500 mg IV or 4 × 400 mg orally (children: 35 –50 mg/kg BW) for 10 days. A luminal agent should also be administered to kill the cysts, such as iodoquinol (diiodohydroxyquinoline) at 3 × 650 mg/day for 20 days, or diloxanide furoate at 3 × 500 mg (pediatric daily dose: 20 mg/kg BW) for 10 days. Patients with a severe intestinal infection may be treated with paromomycin, a poorly absorbed agent that is administered at 25 to 30 mg/kg BW divided into 3 daily doses and taken for one week. Metronidazole may be replaced by tetracycline (4 × 250 mg/day for 10 days) and other more toxic (and therefore less widely used) agents such as dehydroemetine (1.5 mg/kg BW/day [< 90 mg]) or emetine (1 mg/kg BW [< 60 mg] daily) and chloroquine phosphate

(2 × 500 mg/day [= 600 mg base] for the first two days, then 2 × 250 mg/day for 2 weeks).

Unlike pyogenic liver abscesses, amebic abscesses are not drained in most cases and can be successfully managed by medical therapy. Response is monitored clinically and sonographically. Most abscesses are still detectable after the conclusion of medical therapy. This is not a reason to prolong treatment, and any residual findings will generally resolve within a few weeks.

Only large liver abscesses require percutaneous aspiration and drainage ("anchovylike" fluid) to shrink the abscess and promote resolution. Surgical treatment is justified only in rare, exceptional cases.

Thus, the following points should be noted in the treatment of amebic abscesses:

- Emphasize good hygienic practices (e.g., food and drinking water).
- Metronidazole, 4 × 500 mg IV or 3 to 4 × 400 mg orally for 10 days; metronidazole in children: 35 to 50 mg/kg BW Alternative: tinidazole, 2 g daily for 5 days.
- Add a luminal agent such as diloxanide furoate, 3 × 500 mg (pediatric daily dose: 20 mg/kg BW) for 10 days or paromomycin, 25 to 30 mg/kg BW divided into 3 daily doses for 1 week.
- Only large liver abscesses require percutaneous aspiration and drainage.
- Surgical treatment is rarely necessary.

15.11.6 Protozoan Infections with Liver Involvement

A number of protozoans may lead to liver involvement. The treatment options for patients with liver involvement are summarized in ▶ Table 15.2 for various infecting organisms.

15.11.7 Septic (Pyogenic) Abscess with Associated Diseases (Sepsis, Coagulopathies, Ascites)

Systemic infectious complications such as sepsis often lead to significant coagulation disorders. Foremost among them is consumption coagulopathy (disseminated intravascular coagulation), which is associated with a deficiency of antithrombin III. An antithrombin III activity less than 40% signals an increased risk of venous thromboembolism. An increased concentration of prothrombin fragments 1 and 2 is also present. Sepsis may be associated with other organ complications such as acute renal failure and respiratory problems.[73]

The presence of gas in the portal vein is an important warning sign. It is associated with extremely high mortality and is an immediate indication for surgical eradication of the primary focus.[74] But even in other situations, the indication for a surgical or interventional procedure

Table 15.2 Management of protozoan infections with liver involvement

Organism	Diagnosis	Treatment	Remarks
Trematodes	Serology, organ manifestations	Praziquantel is agent of choice	
Schistosomes	Serology, organ manifestations	Praziquantel (e.g., Biltricide), 20 mg/kg BW three times daily for 1 day	Bitter taste, should be swallowed whole without chewing
Clonorchis	Serology	Praziquantel (e.g., Biltricide), 20 mg/kg BW three times daily for 3 days	Bitter taste, should be swallowed whole without chewing
Nematodes	Serology, stool examination, organ manifestations		
Ascaris lumbricoides	Serology, stool examination, organ manifestations	Mebendazole, 100 mg twice daily for 3 days	Alternative is albendazole or pyrantel, single dose of 10 mg/kg BW
Strongyloides stercoralis	Serology, stool examination, organ manifestations	Mebendazole, 200 mg twice daily for 3 days	Alternative is albendazole 400 mg three times daily for 3 days
Cestodes	Serology, organ manifestations		
Echinococcus cysticus	Serology, organ manifestations	Surgery Albendazole, 400 mg twice daily for 4 weeks, then stopped for 2 weeks (total of 3 therapy cycles)	Mebendazole, dose rises in increments to 1.5–3 g/day in three doses, may be continued for years
Echinococcus alveolaris	Serology, organ manifestations		Mebendazole, dose rises in increments to 15–20 mg/kg BW daily, may be continued for years, even for life

Note: Monitor closely for pancytopenia (especially with albendazole).

should always be discussed on an interdisciplinary basis.[70] Fluid collections in the peritoneal cavity may result from a great variety of diseases. The differential diagnosis should include a confined or perforated abscess in the abdominal cavity. Although intraperitoneal tuberculosis is very rare in Western countries, it is also a potential cause. It should be noted that a pulmonary focus is not always present.[75] Ascites per se is a relative contraindication to the drainage of a parenchymal organ.

15.11.8 Infection of Necrotic Tumor Components

When a tumor reaches a certain size, portions of the tumor may undergo spontaneous necrosis. This effect is intensified after radiotherapy, chemotherapy, radiofrequency ablation, or embolization.[76,77] If the necrotic areas become infected, they provide an excellent culture medium with a high risk of colonization by anaerobic organisms. A subphrenic abscess may develop by this mechanism and can be treated by percutaneous aspiration, although primary surgery should be considered for this entity. This decision will be influenced by the general health status of the patient, including quality-of-life issues and life expectancy.[78]

When initial imaging findings are suggestive of a liver abscess or intra-abdominal abscess of unknown cause, it should be considered that the lesion may actually be a degenerating tumor or metastasis and that withholding further diagnostic studies could be disastrous for the patient.[79,80] Because most patients are already immunocompromised as a result of radiation or chemotherapy, the potential need for antibiotic prophylaxis before an interventional procedure should be determined on a case-by-case basis. Patients receiving percutaneous ethanol injection therapy for hepatocellular carcinoma may develop fever in the absence of infection, especially if the tumor is larger than 3 cm. But since many of these patients are immunosuppressed and have advanced hepatic cirrhosis, peri-interventional antibiotics may be utilized on a broad basis.[81] The problem of tumor seeding exists here as in other interventional procedures, but most cases involve an advanced tumor process and an acute situation that warrants immediate action.[82] As in the case of postpancreatic fluid collections, the percutaneous drainage of infected necrosis in pancreatic tumors carries a risk of fistula formation. Transgastric or transduodenal drainage procedures with endosonographic guidance may be an option in these cases.[83] Since many of these patients have already had multiple courses of antibiotic therapy, a serious effort should be made to identify the causative organism based on blood cultures and the analysis of percutaneous aspirate and secretions (including fungal cultures).

If the necrotic cavity is not too large, it may be considered whether spontaneous resolution is likely to occur, or whether obliteration should be attempted by instilling a sclerosing agent or adhesive plug. These treatments carry their own risk of complications.[84]

15.11.9 Liver Abscess after Liver Transplantation

Liver abscess is a rare complication of liver transplantation (▶ Fig. 15.13). It may be causally related to hepatic artery thrombosis, biliary strictures, and diabetes mellitus. Posttransplantation liver abscess is associated with a higher mortality than in patients with healthy livers.[85,86] Because liver transplantation is a major operation that requires intensive care monitoring and immunosuppressant therapy, abscesses tend to be caused by a different spectrum of organisms.[87] Biliary tract reconstruction is a particular risk factor. Anastomotic stenosis leads to cholestasis and secondary cholangitis.[88]

Caution

It is important in these patients to check back with the transplant center, since noninfectious fluid collections rarely require interventional treatment.[89]

15.12 Complications

Pyogenic liver abscess has a significant mortality rate.[2,7,8,50] As in all invasive procedures, abscess drainage may lead to bleeding, perforation, pleural and colon injuries, secondary abscess formation, empyema, and other complications and recurrences.[3] A familiarity with these potential complications and their management is essential. Complications can be subdivided into early and late complications and into direct (intervention-related) and indirect complications (e.g., myocardial infarction).[50]

A prospective study of complications and their management has not yet been published, and a comprehensive assessment cannot be made since most published studies are retrospective. Published data and even prospective (controlled) studies are difficult to compare with one another due to a variety of factors such as age and comorbid conditions (for example, diabetes mellitus, immunosuppression, elderly patients).[6,35,42,81,90–99] One statistical estimate states that a prospective study would require a population of more than 600 and probably more than 1,000 patients with abscesses in order to make a valid analysis.[6]

Bleeding due to vascular injury and hollow viscus injuries with associated air leak can usually be detected (sonographically) during the procedure. A bile leak can be distinguished from brisk bleeding by contrast-enhanced ultrasound. Free air is detected by noting characteristic reverberating echoes between the abdominal wall and

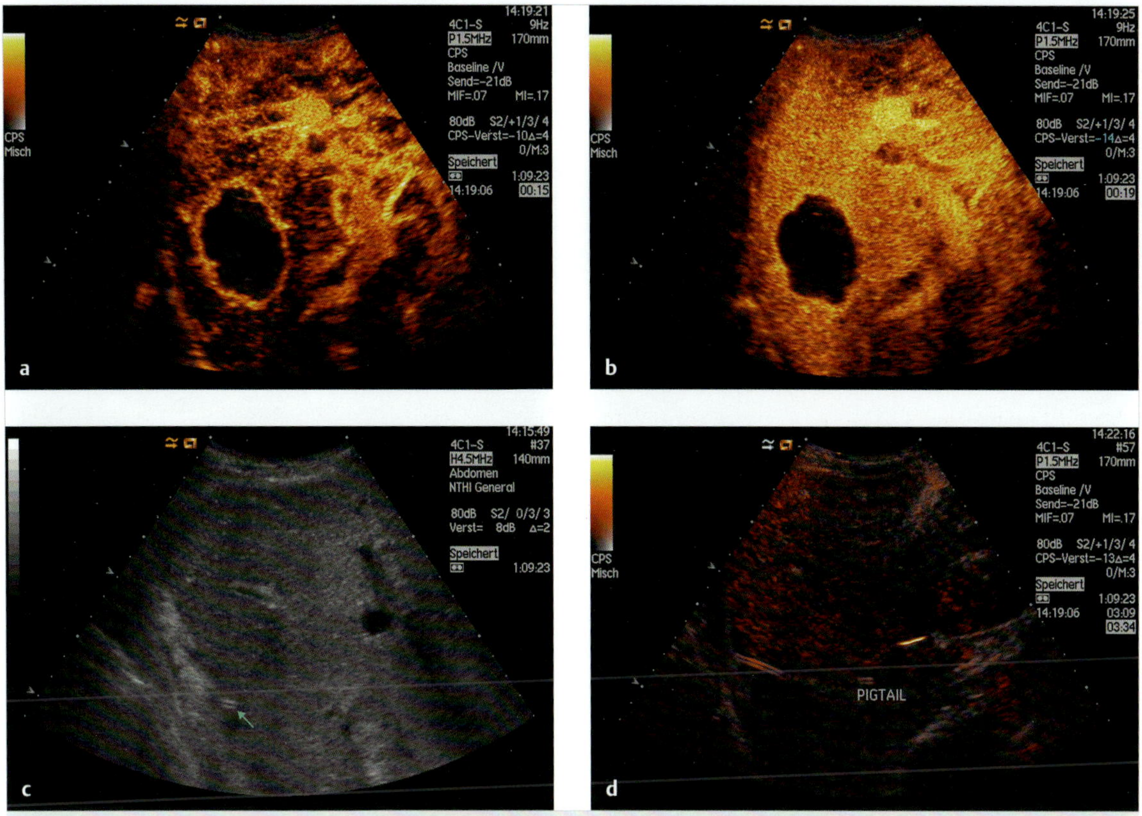

Fig. 15.13 Liver abscess after liver transplantation. Ultrasound demonstrates the abscess in the arterial phase after contrast administration (**a, b**) and assesses drainage (**c, d**), which is most clearly appreciated in the low-MI (mechanical index) mode view (**d**, shown here with a pigtail drain). It should be noted that drainage procedures and especially irrigation should be more intensive in immunosuppressed patients than in immunocompetent patients.

hepatic left lobe in the supine position or along the right side in the left lateral decubitus position. Right shoulder pain is relatively common after liver biopsy; it is a reactive phenomenon cause by nerve irritation and requires only temporary analgesic therapy. The puncture of a pyogenic focus consistently leads to bacteremia. This condition is often manifested by postinterventional chills, and the patient should be informed of this possibility before the procedure. Concomitant antibiotic therapy is required.

15.13 Irrigation

Regular (manual) irrigation of the drains is essential. Flushing with physiologic saline solution should be continued until the return is clear. This may have to be done several times daily and on several consecutive days, depending on the fluid consistency and placement site. Because abscess contents are usually viscous, a continuous irrigation system cannot generate enough flow to mobilize the contents. Double-lumen irrigation catheters should also be avoided because the total luminal area is relatively small. Single-lumen, large-bore drainage catheters are more effective than multilumen drains with a small inner diameter.

The question of possible drain displacement can be resolved by B-mode ultrasound, air insufflation, or post-contrast fluoroscopy. A recent study also described the injection of diluted ultrasound contrast medium (0.2–20 mL saline solution).[100]

15.14 Sequelae

Liver abscesses may resolve without sequelae, but in some cases postresolution images may show confusing parenchymal changes as illustrated in ▶ Fig. 15.14.

15.15 Ultrasound-Guided Gallbladder Drainage and Other Indications

Two indications are important in this context: the litholysis of cholesterol stones, which is rarely practiced any longer owing to the availability of laparoscopic cholecystectomy, and acute interventions for gallbladder

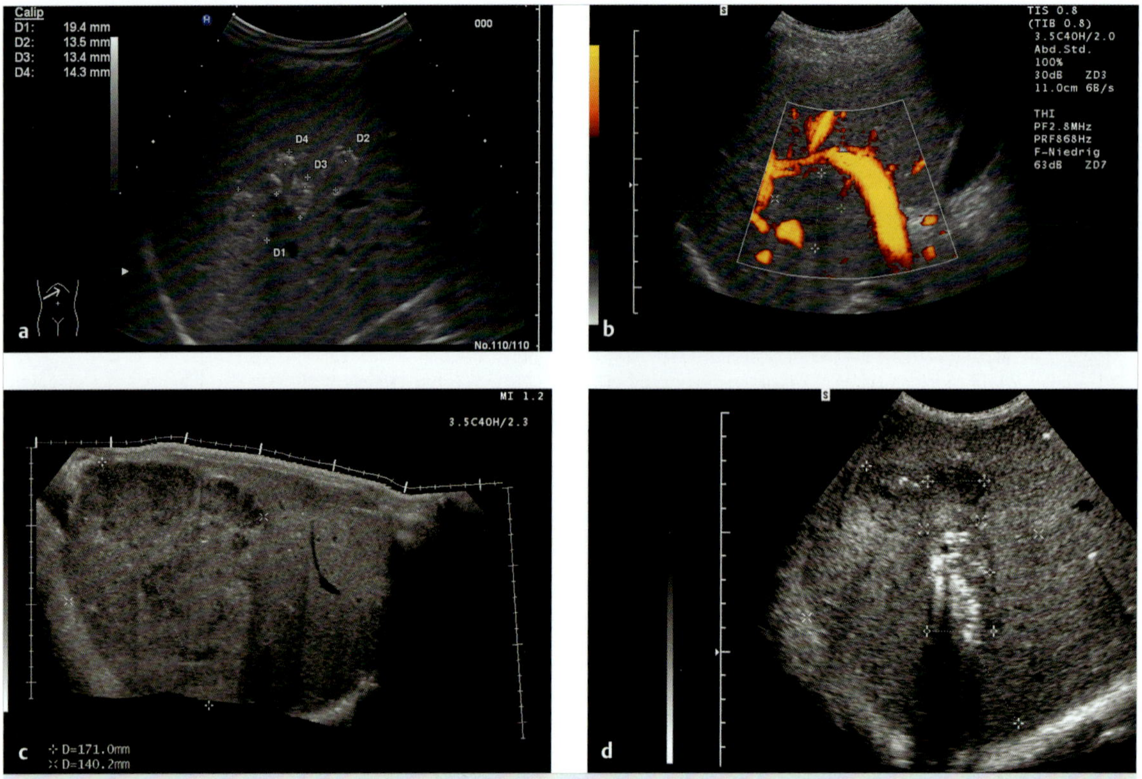

Fig. 15.14 Healed liver abscess after cholangitis (**a**), old amebic abscess (**b**), and large pyogenic liver abscess occupying the entire hepatic right lobe (**c**, panoramic image). An enlarged view after resolution (**d**) shows extensive scarring.

empyema in inoperable patients. The second indication pertains almost exclusively to elderly patients who cannot tolerate surgery or general anesthesia due to multimorbid conditions or have become seriously debilitated by their acute illness. Drainage in these cases may help restore the patients to an operable state and may even provide definitive treatment in some cases. If the only goal is to drain clear bile or introduce irrigating fluid, small-bore catheters of 4–6F are adequate. If pus is present, it may be necessary to use a larger drainage catheter. The gallbladder should not be approached through the free abdominal cavity due to risk of leakage, and the transhepatic approach has become standard. We recommend using the trocar technique since 8 to 9F drains can easily penetrate the inflamed gallbladder wall. This technique also eliminates the risk of a wire penetrating through the gallbladder wall into the abdominal cavity.

References

[1] Gervais DA, Hahn PF, O'Neill MJ, Mueller PR. Percutaneous abscess drainage in Crohn disease: technical success and short- and long-term outcomes during 14 years. Radiology 2002; 222: 645–651

[2] Gee MS, Kim JY, Gervais DA, Hahn PF, Mueller PR. Management of abdominal and pelvic abscesses that persist despite satisfactory percutaneous drainage catheter placement. AJR Am J Roentgenol 2010; 194: 815–820

[3] Gervais DA, Ho CH, O'Neill MJ, Arellano RS, Hahn PF, Mueller PR. Recurrent abdominal and pelvic abscesses: incidence, results of repeated percutaneous drainage, and underlying causes in 956 drainages. AJR Am J Roentgenol 2004; 182: 463–466

[4] vanSonnenberg E, Wittich GR, Goodacre BW, Casola G, D'Agostino HB. Percutaneous abscess drainage: update. World J Surg 2001; 25: 362–369; discussion 370–372

[5] Buckley BT, Goodwin M, Boardman P, Uberoi R. Percutaneous abscess drainage in the UK: A national survey and single centre study. Clin Radiol 2006; 61: 55–64; discussion 53–54

[6] Yu SC, Ho SS, Lau WY et al. Treatment of pyogenic liver abscess: prospective randomized comparison of catheter drainage and needle aspiration. Hepatology 2004; 39: 932–938

[7] Mohsen AH, Green ST, Read RC, McKendrick MW. Liver abscess in adults: ten years experience in a UK centre. QJM 2002; 95: 797–802

[8] Wong WM, Wong BC, Hui CK et al. Pyogenic liver abscess: retrospective analysis of 80 cases over a 10-year period. J Gastroenterol Hepatol 2002; 17: 1001–1007

[9] Massarweh NN, Park JO, Farjah F et al. Trends in the utilization and impact of radiofrequency ablation for hepatocellular carcinoma. J Am Coll Surg 2010; 210: 441–448

[10] Marin D, Ho LM, Barnhart H, Neville AM, White RR, Paulson EK. Percutaneous abscess drainage in patients with perforated acute appendicitis: effectiveness, safety, and prediction of outcome. AJR Am J Roentgenol 2010; 194: 422–429

[11] Whiteoak S, Khan O, Allen SC. Perforated colonic diverticulum in old age: surgical or medical management? Br J Hosp Med (Lond) 2009; 70: 699–703

[12] McCann JW, Maroo S, Wales P et al. Image-guided drainage of multiple intraabdominal abscesses in children with perforated appendicitis: an alternative to laparotomy. Pediatr Radiol 2008; 38: 661–668

[13] Lencioni RA, Allgaier HP, Cioni D et al. Small hepatocellular carcinoma in cirrhosis: randomized comparison of radio-frequency thermal ablation versus percutaneous ethanol injection. Radiology 2003; 228: 235–240

[14] Di Stasi M, Buscarini L, Livraghi T et al. Percutaneous ethanol injection in the treatment of hepatocellular carcinoma. A multicenter survey of evaluation practices and complication rates. Scand J Gastroenterol 1997; 32: 1168–1173

[15] Chou FF, Sheen-Chen SM, Chen YS, Chen MC. Single and multiple pyogenic liver abscesses: clinical course, etiology, and results of treatment. World J Surg 1997; 21: 384–388; discussion 388–389

[16] Schwerk WB. Ultrasonically guided percutaneous puncture and analysis of aspirated material of cystic pancreatic lesions. Digestion 1981; 21: 184–192

[17] Vogl TJ, Estifan F. Pyogenic liver abscess: interventional versus surgical therapy: technique, results and indications [Article in German]. Rofo 2001; 173: 663–667

[18] Olak J, Christou NV, Stein LA, Casola G, Meakins JL. Operative vs percutaneous drainage of intra-abdominal abscesses. Comparison of morbidity and mortality. Arch Surg 1986; 121: 141–146

[19] Gottschalk U, Ignee A, Dietrich CF. Ultrasound guided interventions, part 1, diagnostic procedures [Article in German]. Z Gastroenterol 2009; 47: 682–690

[20] Gottschalk U, Ignee A, Dietrich CF. Ultrasound-guided interventions and description of the equipment [Article in German]. Z Gastroenterol 2010; 48: 1305–1316

[21] Gray R, Leekam R, Mackenzie R, St Louis EL, Grosman H. Percutaneous abscess drainage. Gastrointest Radiol 1985; 10: 79–84

[22] Abdelouafi A, Ousehal A, Ouzidane L, Kadiri R. Ultrasonography in the diagnosis of liver abscesses. Apropos of 32 cases [Article in French]. Ann Radiol (Paris) 1993; 36: 286–292

[23] Claudon M, Cosgrove D, Albrecht T et al. Guidelines and good clinical practice recommendations for contrast enhanced ultrasound (CEUS) —update 2008. Ultraschall Med 2008; 29: 28–44

[24] Dietrich CF. Comments and illustrations regarding the guidelines and good clinical practice recommendations for contrast-enhanced ultrasound (CEUS)—update 2008. Ultraschall Med 2008; 29 (Suppl 4): S188–S202

[25] Dietrich CF, Schreiber-Dietrich D, Schuessler G, Ignee A. Contrast enhanced ultrasound of the liver—state of the art [Article in German]. Dtsch Med Wochenschr 2007; 132: 1225–1231

[26] Carrillo , Nañez L, Cuadra Urteaga JL, Canelo-Aybar C, Pintado , Caballero S, Gil , Fuentes M. Liver abscess: clinical, imaging and management features in a 5 year study in the Arzobispo Loayza National Hospital [Article in Spanish]. Rev Gastroenterol Peru 2010; 30: 46–51

[27] Khan R, Hamid S, Abid S et al. Predictive factors for early aspiration in liver abscess. World J Gastroenterol 2008; 14: 2089–2093

[28] Dietrich CF. Significance of abdominal ultrasound in inflammatory bowel disease. Dig Dis 2009; 27: 482–493

[29] Hirche TO, Russler J, Schröder O et al. The value of routinely performed ultrasonography in patients with Crohn disease. Scand J Gastroenterol 2002; 37: 1178–1183

[30] Veloso FT, Teixeira AA, Saraiva C, Carvalho J, Maia J, Fraga J. Hepatic abscess in Crohn's disease. Hepatogastroenterology 1990; 37: 215–216

[31] Mörk H, Ignee A, Schuessler G, Ott M, Dietrich CF. Analysis of neuroendocrine tumour metastases in the liver using contrast enhanced ultrasonography. Scand J Gastroenterol 2007; 42: 652–662

[32] Dietrich CF, Mueller G, Beyer-Enke S. Cysts in the cyst pattern. Z Gastroenterol 2009; 47: 1203–1207

[33] Barreiros AP, Braden B, Schieferstein-Knauer C, Ignee A, Dietrich CF. Characteristics of intestinal tuberculosis in ultrasonographic techniques. Scand J Gastroenterol 2008; 43: 1224–1231

[34] Hemming A, Davis NL, Robins RE. Surgical versus percutaneous drainage of intra-abdominal abscesses. Am J Surg 1991; 161: 593–595

[35] Zerem E, Hadzic A. Sonographically guided percutaneous catheter drainage versus needle aspiration in the management of pyogenic liver abscess. AJR Am J Roentgenol 2007; 189: W138–42

[36] Rajak CL, Gupta S, Jain S, Chawla Y, Gulati M, Suri S. Percutaneous treatment of liver abscesses: needle aspiration versus catheter drainage. AJR Am J Roentgenol 1998; 170: 1035–1039

[37] Kos S, Jacob L. Perkutane Abszessdrainagen. Radiologe up2date 2008; 8: 107–131

[38] Roy D, Kulkarni A, Kulkarni S, Thakur MH, Maheshwari A, Tongaonkar HB. Transrectal ultrasound-guided biopsy of recurrent cervical carcinoma. Br J Radiol 2008; 81: 902–906

[39] Mathevet P, Dargent D. Role of ultrasound guided puncture in the management of ovarian cysts [Article in French]. J Gynecol Obstet Biol Reprod (Paris) 2001; 30 (Suppl): S53–S58

[40] Vikrama KS, Shyamkumar NK, Vinu M, Joseph P, Vyas F, Venkatramani S. Percutaneous catheter drainage in the treatment of abdominal compartment syndrome. Can J Surg 2009; 52: E19–E20

[41] Sacks BA, Vine HS, Bartek S, Palestrant AM. Postoperative abscess drainage in patients with established sinus tracks or drains. Radiology 1982; 142: 537–538

[42] Cheng D, Nagata KT, Yoon HC. Randomized prospective comparison of alteplase versus saline solution for the percutaneous treatment of loculated abdominopelvic abscesses. J Vasc Interv Radiol 2008; 19: 906–911

[43] Akinci D, Akhan O, Ozmen MN et al. Percutaneous drainage of 300 intraperitoneal abscesses with long-term follow-up. Cardiovasc Intervent Radiol 2005; 28: 744–750

[44] Bergert H, Kersting S, Pyrc J, Saeger HD, Bunk A. Therapeutic options in the treatment of pyogenic liver abscess [Article in German]. Ultraschall Med 2004; 25: 356–362

[45] Schwerk WB, Görg C, Görg K, Richter G, Beckh K. Percutaneous drainage of liver and splenic abscess [Article in German]. Z Gastroenterol 1991; 29: 146–152

[46] Schwerk WB, Görg C, Görg K, Restrepo I. Ultrasound-guided percutaneous drainage of pyogenic splenic abscesses. J Clin Ultrasound 1994; 22: 161–166

[47] Andersson R, Forsberg L, Hederstrom E, Hochbergs P, Bengmark S. Percutaneous management of pyogenic hepatic abscesses. HPB Surg 1990; 2: 185–188

[48] Tan YM, Chung AY, Chow PK et al. An appraisal of surgical and percutaneous drainage for pyogenic liver abscesses larger than 5 cm. Ann Surg 2005; 241: 485–490

[49] Chung YF, Tan YM, Lui HF et al. Management of pyogenic liver abscesses - percutaneous or open drainage? Singapore Med J 2007; 48: 1158–1165, quiz 1165

[50] Liu CH, Gervais DA, Hahn PF, Arellano RS, Uppot RN, Mueller PR. Percutaneous hepatic abscess drainage: do multiple abscesses or multiloculated abscesses preclude drainage or affect outcome? J Vasc Interv Radiol 2009; 20: 1059–1065

[51] Allemann P, Probst H, Demartines N, Schäfer M. Prevention of infectious complications after laparoscopic appendectomy for complicated acute appendicitis—the role of routine abdominal drainage. Langenbecks Arch Surg 2011; 396: 63–68

[52] Dobremez E, Lavrand F, Lefevre Y, Boer M, Bondonny JM, Vergnes P. Treatment of post-appendectomy intra-abdominal deep abscesses. Eur J Pediatr Surg 2003; 13: 393–397

[53] Nather K, Ochsner A. Der linksseitige Abszess bei Appendicitis. Langenbecks Arch Surg 1924; 188: 114–123

[54] Hogan MJ. Appendiceal abscess drainage. Tech Vasc Interv Radiol 2003; 6: 205–214

[55] Shuler FW, Newman CN, Angood PB, Tucker JG, Lucas GW. Nonoperative management for intra-abdominal abscesses. Am Surg 1996; 62: 218–222

[56] Imazu H, Kawahara Y, Koyama S, Tajiri H. Endoscopic ultrasound-guided transgastric drainage for omental bursa abscess complicating appendicitis with diffuse peritonitis. Endoscopy 2008; 40 (Suppl 2): E249

[57] vanSonnenberg E, D'Agostino HB, Casola G, Goodacre BW, Sanchez RB, Taylor B. US-guided transvaginal drainage of pelvic abscesses and fluid collections. Radiology 1991; 181: 53–56

[58] Durmishi Y, Gervaz P, Brandt D et al. Results from percutaneous drainage of Hinchey stage II diverticulitis guided by computed tomography scan. Surg Endosc 2006; 20: 1129–1133
[59] Men S, Akhan O, Köroğlu M. Percutaneous drainage of abdominal abcess. Eur J Radiol 2002; 43: 204–218
[60] Singh B, May K, Coltart I, Moore NR, Cunningham C. The long-term results of percutaneous drainage of diverticular abscess. Ann R Coll Surg Engl 2008; 90: 297–301
[61] Wiesmayr M, Bankier A, Fleischmann D, Karnel F. Percutaneous drainage of intra-abdominal abscesses in Crohn disease [Article in German]. Aktuelle Radiol 1994; 4: 184–187
[62] Hawes DR, Pelsang RE, Janda RC, Lu CC. Imaging of the biliary sump syndrome. AJR Am J Roentgenol 1992; 158: 315–319
[63] Miros M, Kerlin P, Strong R, Hartley L, Dickey D. Post-choledochoenterostomy 'sump syndrome'. Aust N Z J Surg 1990; 60: 109–112
[64] Hiura A, Kim EC, Ikehara T, Matsumura Y, Mishima K, Ishida I. Hepatic abscess as a complication of the sump syndrome. J Hepatobiliary Pancreat Surg 2000; 7: 231–235
[65] Hallstone A, Triadafilopoulos G. "Spontaneous sump syndrome": Successful treatment by duodenoscopic sphincterotomy. Am J Gastroenterol 1990; 85: 1518–1520
[66] Rumans MC, Katon RM, Lowe DK. Hepatic abscesses as a complication of the sump syndrome: combined surgical and endoscopic therapy. Case report and review of the literature. Gastroenterology 1987; 92: 791–795
[67] Demirel BT, Kekilli M, Onal IK et al. ERCP experience in patients with choledochoduodenostomy: diagnostic findings and therapeutic management. Surg Endosc 2011; 25: 1043–1047
[68] Ell C, Boosfeld C, Henrich R, Rabenstein T. Endoscopic treatment of the "sump syndrome" after choledochoduodenostomy: a new technique using an amplatzer septal occluder. Z Gastroenterol 2006; 44: 1231–1235
[69] Marbet UA, Stalder GA, Faust H, Harder F, Gyr K. Endoscopic sphincterotomy and surgical approaches in the treatment of the 'sump syndrome'. Gut 1987; 28: 142–145
[70] Bruennler T, Langgartner J, Lang S et al. Outcome of patients with acute, necrotizing pancreatitis requiring drainage-does drainage size matter? World J Gastroenterol 2008; 14: 725–730
[71] Habscheid W, Burghardt W, Lackner K. Percutaneous drainage of recurrent peripancreatic fluid collections in acute pancreatitis. A case report [Article in German]. Z Gastroenterol 1989; 27: 690–692
[72] Cunningham SC, Napolitano LM. Pyogenic liver abscess complicating biliary stricture due to chronic pancreatitis. Surg Infect (Larchmt) 2004; 5: 188–194
[73] Fukuchi T, Morisawa Y. A case of cat-scratch-induced Pasteurella multocida infection presenting with disseminated intravascular coagulation and acute renal failure [Article in Japanese]. Kansenshogaku Zasshi 2009; 83: 557–560
[74] Yajima Y, Ohhira S, Meguro S, Shibuya D, Miyazaki A, Sakurada H. A case of gas-containing liver abscess complicated with endotoxin shock and DIC [Article in Japanese]. Nippon Shokakibyo Gakkai Zasshi 1993; 90: 1602–1605
[75] Cheung HY, Siu WT, Yau KK, Ku CF, Li MK. Acute abdomen: an unusual case of ruptured tuberculous mesenteric abscess. Surg Infect (Larchmt) 2005; 6: 259–261
[76] Tejirian T, Heaney A, Colquhoun S, Nissen N. Laparoscopic debridement of hepatic necrosis after hepatic artery chemoembolization. JSLS 2007; 11: 493–495
[77] de Baère T, Roche A, Amenabar JM et al. Liver abscess formation after local treatment of liver tumors. Hepatology 1996; 23: 1436–1440
[78] Yokoi Y, Suzuki S, Sakaguchi T et al. Subphrenic abscess formation following superselective transcatheter chemoembolization for hepatocellular carcinoma. Radiat Med 2002; 20: 45–49
[79] Yeh TS, Jan YY, Jeng LB, Chen TC, Hwang TL, Chen MF. Hepatocellular carcinoma presenting as pyogenic liver abscess: characteristics, diagnosis, and management. Clin Infect Dis 1998; 26: 1224–1226
[80] Warshauer DM, Criado E, Woosley JT, Grimmer DL. Infarcted appendiceal carcinoid. CT appearance mimicking appendiceal abscess. Clin Imaging 1991; 15: 182–184
[81] Huo TI, Huang YH, Huang HC et al. Fever and infectious complications after percutaneous acetic acid injection therapy for hepatocellular carcinoma: incidence and risk factor analysis. J Clin Gastroenterol 2006; 40: 639–642
[82] Giorgio A, Tarantino L, de Stefano G et al. Complications after interventional sonography of focal liver lesions: a 22-year single-center experience. J Ultrasound Med 2003; 22: 193–205
[83] Kolvenbach H, Hirner A. Infected pancreatic necrosis possibly due to combined percutaneous aspiration, cystogastric pseudocyst drainage and injection of a sclerosant. Endoscopy 1991; 23: 102–105
[84] Görich J, Brensing KA, Kunze V et al. Percutaneous drainage of refractory necrotizing tumors: experience in 9 patients [Article in German]. Rofo 1995; 163: 527–531
[85] Nikeghbalian S, Salahi R, Salahi H et al. Hepatic abscesses after liver transplant: 1997–2008. Exp Clin Transplant 2009; 7: 256–260
[86] Tachopoulou OA, Vogt DP, Henderson JM, Baker M, Keys TF. Hepatic abscess after liver transplantation: 1990–2000. Transplantation 2003; 75: 79–83
[87] Chen H, Zhang Y, Chen YG, Yu YS, Zheng SS, Li LJ. Sepsis resulting from Enterobacter aerogenes resistant to carbapenems after liver transplantation. Hepatobiliary Pancreat Dis Int 2009; 8: 320–322
[88] Alsharabi A, Zieniewicz K, Michałowicz B et al. Biliary complications in relation to the technique of biliary reconstruction in adult liver transplant recipients. Transplant Proc 2007; 39: 2785–2787
[89] Akin K, Ozturk A, Guvenc Z, Isiklar I, Haberal M. Localized fluid collections after liver transplantation. Transplant Proc 2006; 38: 627–630
[90] Tani M, Kawai M, Hirono S et al. A prospective randomized controlled trial of internal versus external drainage with pancreaticojejunostomy for pancreaticoduodenectomy. Am J Surg 2010; 199: 759–764
[91] Spradlin NM, Wise PE, Herline AJ, Muldoon RL, Rosen M, Schwartz DA. A randomized prospective trial of endoscopic ultrasound to guide combination medical and surgical treatment for Crohn's perianal fistulas. Am J Gastroenterol 2008; 103: 2527–2535
[92] Zerem E, Salkic N, Imamovic G, Terzić I. Comparison of therapeutic effectiveness of percutaneous drainage with antibiotics versus antibiotics alone in the treatment of periappendiceal abscess: is appendectomy always necessary after perforation of appendix? Surg Endosc 2007; 21: 461–466
[93] Oliver I, Lacueva FJ, Pérez Vicente F et al. Randomized clinical trial comparing simple drainage of anorectal abscess with and without fistula track treatment. Int J Colorectal Dis 2003; 18: 107–110
[94] Abraham N, Doudle M, Carson P. Open versus closed surgical treatment of abscesses: a controlled clinical trial. Aust N Z J Surg 1997; 67: 173–176
[95] Tang CL, Chew SP, Seow-Choen F. Prospective randomized trial of drainage alone vs. drainage and fistulotomy for acute perianal abscesses with proven internal opening. Dis Colon Rectum 1996; 39: 1415–1417
[96] Widjaya P, Bilić A, Babić Z, Ljubicić N, Bakula B, Pilas V. Amoebic liver abscess: ultrasonographic characteristics and results of different therapeutic approaches. Acta Med Iugosl 1991; 45: 15–21
[97] Schouten WR, van Vroonhoven TJ. Treatment of anorectal abscess with or without primary fistulectomy. Results of a prospective randomized trial. Dis Colon Rectum 1991; 34: 60–63
[98] Lang EK, Paolini RM, Pottmeyer A. The efficacy of palliative and definitive percutaneous versus surgical drainage of pancreatic abscesses and pseudocysts: a prospective study of 85 patients. South Med J 1991; 84: 55–64
[99] Singh JP, Kashyap A. A comparative evaluation of percutaneous catheter drainage for resistant amebic liver abscesses. Am J Surg 1989; 158: 58–62
[100] Ignee A, Baum U, Schuessler G, Dietrich CF. Contrast-enhanced ultrasound-guided percutaneous cholangiography and cholangiodrainage (CEUS-PTCD). Endoscopy 2009; 41: 725–726

16 Percutaneous Sclerotherapy of Cysts

C. F. Dietrich, B. Braden

16.1 Percutaneous Sclerotherapy of Liver Cysts

16.1.1 Epidemiology and Etiology

The incidence of liver cysts is age-dependent and was up to 5% in our study of 20,000 consecutive patients. Other authors have reported similar values of 1 to 3%.[1,2]

Liver cysts with a multifactorial cause may consist of cystic dilatations of intralobular bile ducts, which are more common in females (von Meyenburg anomalies), or may be an expression of congenital changes. A polycystic liver has a high association with renal cysts (75%, again depending on age). Associations with cysts in other organs are much less common. A small percentage of patients have coexisting anomalies (e.g., spina bifida).

Symptoms are rare and usually do not appear until the fourth or fifth decade of life. However, palpable organ enlargement may create a pressure sensation; compression of the gastrointestinal tract, veins (peripheral edema), and portal venous vessels (signs of portal hypertension); and other problems that may require treatment. Spontaneous or trauma-induced rupture (or intracystic hemorrhage) may be a source of unexplained pain.

16.1.2 Symptoms

Liver cysts are asymptomatic in most patients. The most common symptom is pain, which may be accompanied by abdominal distention after meals. Other symptoms are dyspepsia and weight loss. Small meals can help to prevent undesired excessive gastric filling. Cyst infection and intracystic hemorrhage occasionally occur. Biliary tract obstruction has been observed in isolated cases.

16.1.3 Indications

The need for treatment depends on the symptoms, the size of the cyst (> 50–100 mm), and the risk of rupture (large superficial cysts). Asymptomatic cysts generally are not treated. Exceptions are small subcapsular cysts located at sites exposed to mechanical stresses (beneath the ribs or sternum), which may occasionally cause complaints. Other causes of pain should be excluded (gastritis, ulcer disease, cholelithiasis, pancreatitis, vertebragenic pain, etc.). It is important to recognize an atypical gallbladder location, segmental biliary tract dilatation, or portal vein thrombosis prior to interventional treatment, especially in patients with a polycystic liver. The diagnosis and treatment of cystic pancreatic lesions are described in Chapter 22.[3]

16.1.4 Contraindications

Interventional treatment is contraindicated in patients with positive echinococcal serology, who would require PAIR (puncture–aspiration–injection of alcohol–reaspiration, see Chapter 17) or some other preliminary treatment.[4] Planned liver transplantation is another relative contraindication.

16.1.5 Interventional Materials and Equipment

Necessary materials and equipment are described in Chapters 2 and 15 and in the text.[5] The following are required:

- Local anesthesia (standard technique)
- Various drainage sets are available such as a nephrostomy set (OptiMed), 6.6F (2.2 mm) with a metal wire and dilator
- Sclerosing agent of choice: 1% polidocanol (Aethoxysklerol, Kreussler Pharma), Reg. No. A 1122–2
- Adhesive tape for catheter fixation
- Suture material (generally unnecessary): Ethicon Mersilene green, FSL 30 mm 3/8c (Johnson & Johnson)

16.1.6 Sclerosing Agents

As described for other interventions, cysts can be sclerosed with 96% alcohol,[6] 1% polidocanol (preferred for its local anesthetic properties, less painful than alcohol), or 10% (to 30%) NaCl solution. Tetracycline, doxycycline, and minocycline are common pleurodesis agents that may also be considered[7,8]; 50% acetic acid has been used for renal cysts.[9]

16.1.7 Treatment Options

Surgical interventions are available for the symptomatic reduction of liver cyst size (by cyst fenestration or resection), although there is a potential for significant postoperative complications.[10] Another treatment option is ultrasound-guided percutaneous cyst aspiration followed by the instillation of a sclerosing agent.

16.1.8 Technique for Percutaneous Sclerotherapy of a Liver Cyst

Skin Preparation and Local Anesthesia

Skin preparation and local anesthesia follow standard protocols described elsewhere in this book (e.g., Chapter 15).

Cyst Aspiration and Drain Insertion

A Chiba needle (20 gauge, 220 mm) is introduced into the cyst under ultrasound guidance and advanced into the distal third of the cyst, stopping short of the far wall.[11] The trocar is removed to permit a diagnostic aspiration. When an adequate sample has been collected, a 0.018-inch metal guidewire with a soft tip is inserted into the cyst and coiled 1 to 3 times to secure its placement. The needle is removed, leaving the wire inside the cyst, and the tract is dilated over the wire (using the dilator contained in the set) to accommodate a 6F (or 5F) catheter, which is passed deep into the cyst with a slight twisting motion. When it has been confirmed that the catheter is inside the cyst with its tip on the far wall, the wire is removed. The catheter may now be fixed to the skin with adhesive tape (or sutures), depending on further intended measures.

Generally the cyst contents will drain spontaneously through the 6F catheter, which is left indwelling for several hours or overnight. Alternatively, the cyst contents may be completely evacuated with syringes and the aspirated volume measured. If the fluid is clear or amber-colored, it is highly unlikely that the cyst communicates with the biliary tract. One aliquot should be routinely collected for cytologic analysis (blood count [cell count], microbiology, and biluribin level are optional). A yellowish or dark-greenish tint suggests a biliary communication and cause; these cysts should be aspirated and drained and the bilirubin level determined. The optional instillation of radiopaque contrast medium (or SonoVue [Bracco][12]) may be done to exclude a connection with the biliary tree. Contrast medium should not enter the bile ducts; if it does, sclerotherapy is contraindicated. A feared complication is sclerosing cholangitis, which has been observed following the intracystic injection of scolicidal solution.[13] Biliary tract communication will cause cysts to refill within a remarkably short time, often in a matter of hours or days.

Brown or reddish-brown cyst contents suggest an (old) intracystic hemorrhage. Other types of discoloration will additionally require bacteriologic testing if a prior infection is suspected. Complicated cysts should be copiously irrigated with sterile 0.9% NaCl before they are sclerosed with 1% polidocanol, which reportedly has slight bactericidal activity.

16.2 Sclerotherapy Technique

Before sclerotherapy, correct drain placement is confirmed by administering 10 to 20 mL of 0.9% NaCl and reaspirating under ultrasound guidance (▶ Fig. 16.1). Next the sclerosing agent is administered. In the case of polidocanol, for example, the solution is instilled over 15 to 60 minutes followed by reaspiration. If reaspiration is unsuccessful, it can be facilitated by respiratory maneuvers, coughing, position changes, repositioning (retraction or rotation) of the drain, or the immediate infusion of 0.9% NaCl into the cyst to dilute its contents. The drain is removed following complete evacuation (or after about 2 hours).

The most commonly used sclerosing agent is ethanol (96%), with 1% polidocanol available as an alternative. The amount of sclerosing agent should be approximately one-third of the estimated cyst volume. The agent is retained in the cyst for 30 to 120 minutes. The longer the sclerosing time (retention time, reinjections), the lower the recurrence rate but the higher the complication rate in this inherently benign disease. The recurrence rate is 10 to 30% based on data in the literature, but the true rate is probably higher. Sclerotherapy may be repeated within a few days (at least 2–3 days later) with a somewhat higher associated risk. Fever, tachycardia, and other autonomic and cardiovascular symptoms are observed in rare cases.

16.2.1 Follow-up Care

No general rules have been established. In patients free of complaints, we schedule an initial sonographic follow-up at 3 to 6 months. Besides size and consistency, ultrasound signs of successful sclerotherapy include the presence of threadlike internal echoes and peripheral regressive scarring with accentuated wall echoes.

Acute or delayed complaints should be promptly evaluated to exclude complications (hemorrhage, infection, pleural effusion). Active bleeding can be controlled by the (repeat) injection of 1% polidocanol.

16.2.2 Prognosis

The long-term results of sclerotherapy depend on the original indication, comorbid conditions, and other evaluated criteria (pain, cyst size). A few reports have been published on the prognosis of cyst sclerotherapy. Imaging shows an absence of cyst recurrence in 50 to 75% of cases (71% in one multicenter observational study). A similar percentage of cases show a significant, 50% reduction in cyst diameter (29% in one multicenter observational study).[6]

16.3 Percutaneous Sclerotherapy of Renal Cysts

16.3.1 Summary of the Literature

A total of 118 patients with 132 cysts were followed for a mean period of 25.8 months. No evidence of a residual cyst was found in 56% of the cysts treated by percutaneous sclerotherapy. In 30% of cases the cyst had a residual volume of < 10%. After sclerotherapy, only 4

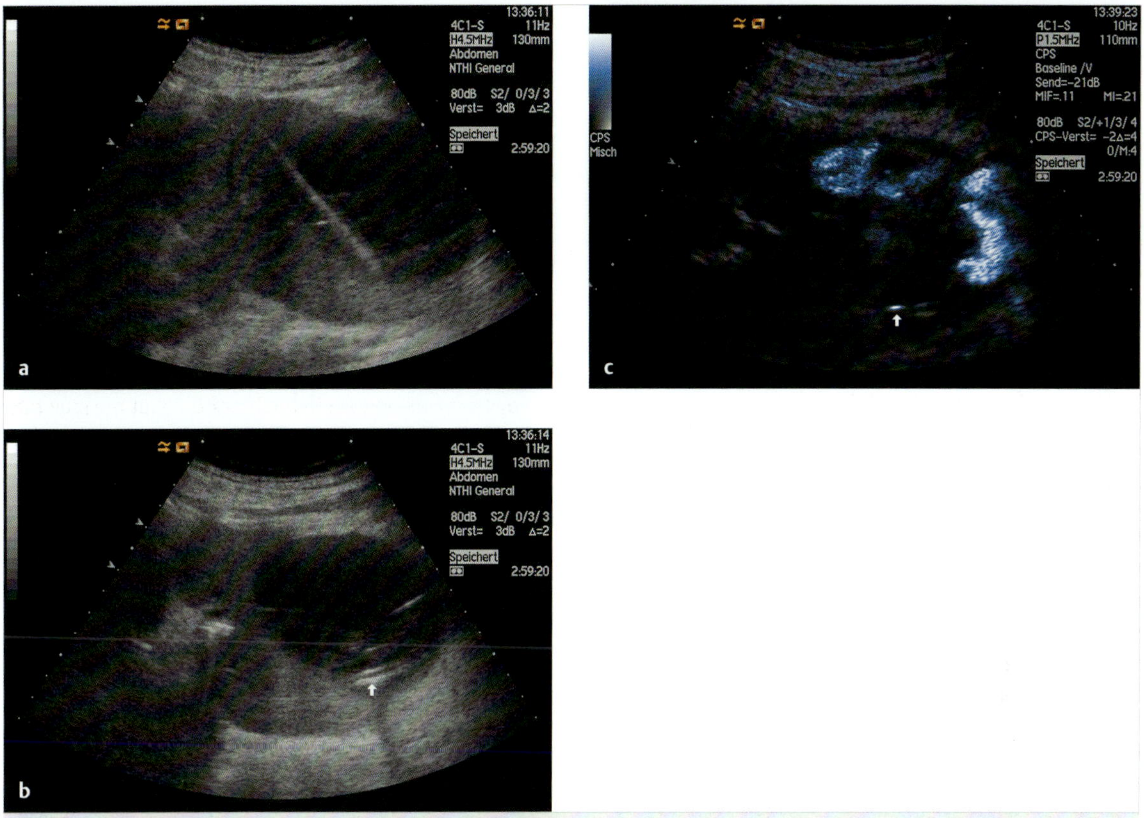

Fig. 16.1 The technique for inserting a needle into a cyst is basically the same as in abscess drainage, except that a catheter of smaller caliber (5F or 6F) is used.
a The needle is passed into the cyst through adjacent liver tissue.
b A 6F drain is placed.
c Contrast medium is instilled to check catheter position (arrow).

patients (3.4%) had no change in the severity of their pretreatment symptoms. The morbidity of the procedure was 9%. None of the patients required surgical reintervention, and the average hospitalization time was 1.06 days. The percutaneous sclerotherapy of uncomplicated renal cysts with polidocanol has a high success rate.[14]

16.3.2 Epidemiology, Differential Diagnosis, and Classification

Renal cysts are found in up to 50% of autopsies and are detectable with a similar frequency at ultrasound. A simple (typical) cyst is easily recognized by its sonographic features: round and echo-free with thin walls, smooth margins, edge shadows, and distal acoustic enhancement. Generally this finding has no further diagnostic or therapeutic implications. With atypical cysts that do not display all of the above criteria for renal cysts, it is necessary to exclude pyelocalyceal dilatation and cystic renal tumors.

Cystic renal masses include simple cysts (▶ Table 16.1), localized cystic diseases such as tubular retention cysts in inflammatory pyelonephritic or vascular renal diseases, segmental cystic dysplasia, benign cystic nephroma ([papillary] cystadenoma), polycystic kidney disease, nephronophthisis, cysts in the setting of tuberous sclerosis and von Hippel–Lindau syndrome, and acquired renal cysts in dialysis patients. There are renal carcinomas and pediatric Wilms tumors that may have cystic components. These lesions require differentiation from benign cystic nephroma, which may grow very large, and from

Table 16.1 Modified Bosniak classification of cystic renal lesions

Category	Features
I: Simple (typical) cyst	Thin wall, no septa, no calcifications, no solid components, no enhancement
II: Minimally complex cyst	Thin wall, thin-walled septa (< 1 mm), fine wall calcifications, no solid components at ultrasound (CT: 50–90 HU possible), no enhancement
III: Indeterminate cystic mass	Thick, irregular cyst walls or septa with enhancement, variable calcification
IV: Cystic renal cell carcinoma	Thick, irregular cyst walls or septa with enhancement, variable calcification, perifocal enhancement

segmental dysplasia, a partial renal developmental anomaly with cystic features.

The following findings make it necessary to exclude other masses, especially neoplasms:

- Thick or irregular septa
- Course wall irregularities
- Absence of secondary cyst criteria (acoustic enhancement, edge shadows)
- High or mixed echogenicity of the cyst contents

The simple renal cysts described above may change their echogenicity as a result of secondary intracystic bleeding or ascending infection.

Minimally complex cysts are also mostly benign, although they may harbor a cystic tumor. Based on experience to date, contrast-enhanced ultrasound is better than CT for identifying a minimally complex cyst[15,16] (▶ Table 16.1).

A Bosniak type III indeterminate cystic mass requires definitive investigation because enhancement suggests a neoplasm and a malignant tumor is diagnosed in approximately 50% of cases. The only exception to this rule is a nonenhancing cyst with smooth margins, coarse calcifications, and no internal septa. A wait-and-see approach is acceptable for that type of cyst.

In polycystic kidney disease, both kidneys show cystic enlargement and may extend from the diaphragm into the lesser pelvis. Pronounced cysts that are confined to one kidney in children may indicate multicystic renal dysplasia. In the follow-up of polycystic kidney disease, attention should be given to the possible development of secondary malignant changes. Contrast-enhanced techniques have proved very helpful in making this assessment.[15,16]

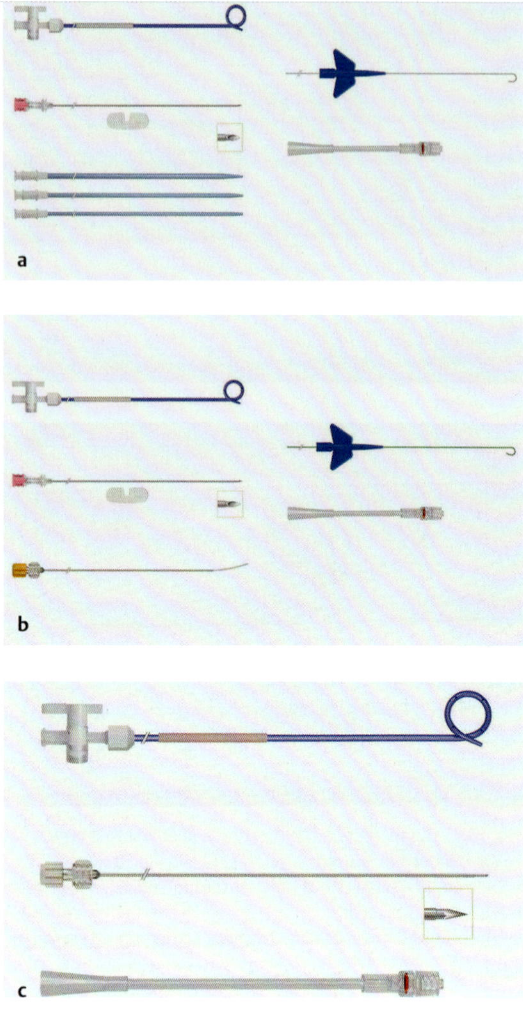

Fig. 16.2 Nephrostomy sets (for external drainage of urine and fluids; available from OptiMed and other suppliers).
a Classic Seldinger technique. Set components: pigtail catheter with attached two-way stopcock (diameters of 7–16F, lengths 30 cm). Two-piece puncture needle with echogenic tip (diameter 1.3 mm, 17.5 gauge, length 20 cm). Schüller-type catheter exchange wire (diameter 0.035 in., length 90 cm, 10-cm flexible tip, 3-mm J curve, 40-cm rigid shaft, flexible end). Dilators (diameters of 6–18F, length 20 cm). Rotating adapter, male Luer lock.
b Special nephrostomy set. Puncture set for drainage catheter placement using Seldinger technique. The obturator allows catheter insertion without perforation. Set components: pigtail catheter with attached two-way stopcock (diameters of 7–9F, lengths 30 cm). Two-piece puncture needle with echogenic tip (diameter 1.3 mm; 17.5 gauge, length 20 cm). Two-part obturator with round blunt plastic introducer (1.2–1.3 mm in diameter). PTFE guidewire, coated (diameter 0.035 in., length 100 cm, flexible tip, 3-mm J curve). Rotating adapter, male Luer lock.
c Set for nephrostomy tube insertion by the trocar technique. Set components: pigtail catheter with attached two-way stopcock (diameters of 7–9F, lengths 30 cm). Two-piece puncture needle with trocar point (1.2–1.4 mm in diameter, 16–17.5 gauge, length 33 cm). Rotating adapter, male Luer lock.

16.3.3 Technique

Following a standard skin prep and local anesthesia, a thin percutaneous nephrostomy tube (5F) is introduced and positioned under ultrasound guidance (▶ Fig. 16.2).

The cyst contents are completely evacuated and the collected volume is measured. Samples are sent for cytologic analysis and creatinine determination. Interpretation: The creatinine concentration in the cyst should not be higher than the patient's serum creatinine level. Radiopaque contrast medium is instilled to exclude communication with the renal pelvis and collecting system: the contrast medium should not opacify the collecting system.

16.3.4 Sclerosing Agents

The most widely used sclerosing agent for renal cysts, as for liver cysts, is 96% ethanol. (Another option is 1% polidocanol, which may be preferable owing to its local anesthetic and bactericidal properties.) The ethanol dosage is approximately one-third the estimated cyst volume (or 20–50% of the cyst volume, based on experience), or approximately 100 mL. Acetic acid has also been used. The agent is retained in the cyst for 30 to 120 min. The longer the sclerosing time, the lower the recurrence rate but the higher the complication risk is also true for renal cysts. A recurrence rate of 10–30% has been reported in studies, but might be higher in practice. Sclerotherapy may be repeated with a somewhat higher associated risk.

16.4 Alternative Procedures

Laparoscopic cyst removal and retroperitoneoscopic renal exposure are second-line options owing to the relative simplicity of the ultrasound-guided technique. The ureter in proximity to the cyst should be identified to minimize the risk of injury. The cyst is unroofed close to the renal parenchyma (much as in other laparoscopic cyst treatments), leaving behind the floor of the cyst.

16.5 Special Issues Relating to Splenic Cysts

It is rare to find simple, epithelialized splenic cysts that require treatment. It is more common to encounter complex splenic cysts whose differential diagnosis will direct treatment planning. Indeterminate solid tumors should be investigated by ultrasound-guided splenic biopsy as described in Chapter 23. Splenectomy is indicated in these cases. The procedure described for the liver may be appropriate in selected cases, although the authors have had no experience with this procedure when applied to the spleen.

16.6 Special Issues Relating to Pancreatic Cysts

The treatment of pancreatic pseudocysts and peripancreatic fluid collections is described in Chapter 22.[3]

References

[1] Schwerk WB, Braun B. Ultrasound in the diagnosis of cystic lesions of the liver (author's transl) [Article in German]. Z Gastroenterol 1978; 16: 24–31

[2] Linhart P, Bönhof JA, Baqué PE, Pering C. Ultrasound in diagnosis of benign and malignant liver tumors [Article in German]. Zentralbl Chir 1998; 123: 119–123

[3] Beyer-Enke SA, Hocke M, Ignee A, Braden B, Dietrich CF. Contrast enhanced transabdominal ultrasound in the characterisation of pancreatic lesions with cystic appearance. JOP 2010; 11: 427–433

[4] Dietrich CF, Mueller G, Beyer-Enke S. Cysts in the cyst pattern. Z Gastroenterol 2009; 47: 1203–1207

[5] Gottschalk U, Ignee A, Dietrich CF. Ultrasound-guided interventions and description of the equipment [Article in German]. Z Gastroenterol 2010; 48: 1305–1316

[6] Montorsi M, Torzilli G, Fumagalli U et al. Percutaneous alcohol sclerotherapy of simple hepatic cysts. Results from a multicentre survey in Italy. HPB Surg 1994; 8: 89–94

[7] vanSonnenberg E, Wroblicka JT, D'Agostino HB et al. Symptomatic hepatic cysts: percutaneous drainage and sclerosis. Radiology 1994; 190: 387–392

[8] Yoshida H, Onda M, Tajiri T et al. Long-term results of multiple minocycline hydrochloride injections for the treatment of symptomatic solitary hepatic cyst. J Gastroenterol Hepatol 2003; 18: 595–598

[9] Seo TS, Oh JH, Yoon Y et al. Acetic acid as a sclerosing agent for renal cysts: comparison with ethanol in follow-up results. Cardiovasc Intervent Radiol 2000; 23: 177–181

[10] Soravia C, Mentha G, Giostra E, Morel P, Rohner A. Surgery for adult polycystic liver disease. Surgery 1995; 117: 272–275

[11] Gottschalk U, Ignee A, Dietrich CF. Ultrasound guided interventions, part 1, diagnostic procedures [Article in German]. Z Gastroenterol 2009; 47: 682–690

[12] Ignee A, Baum U, Schuessler G, Dietrich CF. Contrast-enhanced ultrasound-guided percutaneous cholangiography and cholangiodrainage (CEUS-PTCD). Endoscopy 2009; 41: 725–726

[13] Taranto D, Beneduce F, Vitale LM, Loguercio C, Del Vecchio Blanco C. Chemical sclerosing cholangitis after injection of scolicidal solution. Ital J Gastroenterol 1995; 27: 78–79

[14] Brunken C, Pfeiffer D, Tauber R. Long term outcome after percutaneous sclerotherapy of renal cysts with polidocanol [Article in German]. Urologe A 2002; 41: 263–266

[15] Ignee A, Straub B, Brix D, Schuessler G, Ott M, Dietrich CF. The value of contrast enhanced ultrasound (CEUS) in the characterisation of patients with renal masses. Clin Hemorheol Microcirc 2010; 46: 275–290

[16] Ignee A, Straub B, Schuessler G, Dietrich CF. Contrast enhanced ultrasound of renal masses. World J Radiol 2010; 2: 15–31

17 Interventional Treatment of Echinococcosis

C. F. Dietrich, M. Hocke

Echinococcosis (hydatid disease) is a zoonotic infection caused by flatworms of the class Cestoda. The dog tapeworm (*Echinococcus granulosus* or *cysticus*; cystic echinococcosis) and fox tapeworm (*Echinococcus multilocularis* or *alveolaris*; alveolar echinococcosis) can cause parasitisms in humans. Two other species that are pathogenic to humans (*Echinococcus vogeli* and *Echinococcus oligarthus*) are confined to Central and South America and are very rare. An improved understanding of hydatid disease and advances in imaging technology have revolutionized the diagnosis, treatment, and prognosis of cystic echinococcosis. This does not apply equally to alveolar echinococcosis, which unfortunately continues to be a diagnostic and therapeutic "chameleon."

Cystic echinococcosis—the main topic of this chapter—is generally diagnosed by an imaging study (ultrasound or possibly CT) combined with serologic techniques (ELISA and confirmation tests). A WHO working group has assembled the various classification systems to provide a summary of morphologic findings that are relevant to treatment. The WHO guidelines and recommendations for establishing a uniform approach to the diagnosis and treatment of echinococcosis have been published.[1–3]

17.1 Echinococci: Types and Epidemiology

17.1.1 *Echinococcus granulosus*

Echinococcus granulosus (the dog tapeworm) is the main causative agent of acquired parasitic (cystic) liver disease in Europe. Its prevalence increases markedly from northern to southern latitudes (▶ Fig. 17.1). The incidence of symptomatic cystic echinococcosis varies considerably worldwide and, depending on the region, ranges from < 1 per 100,000 population and year (estimated 0.5/100,000 in Germany) to 198 per 100,000 a percentage range/prevalence in certain regions based on living habits, as in northwest Kenya (Turkana) in Africa.[4–7] Obviously there is a high percentage of unreported, asymptomatic cases in which the parasites produce no clinical manifestations. The cycle of transmission through dogs and sheep explains why endemic cystic echinococcosis is most prevalent in sheep-raising regions: Anatolia (Turkey), Eastern Europe, (southern) Mediterranean countries (North Africa, Asia Minor) and South America. By contrast, cystic echinococcosis is a rare disease in Central and Northern

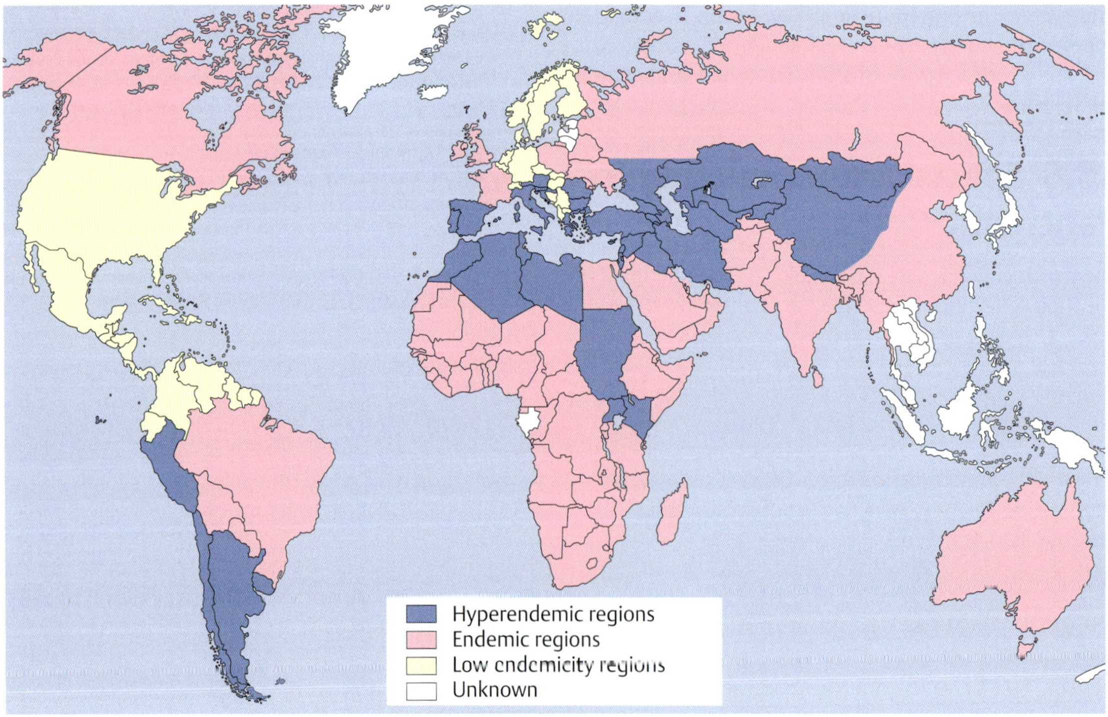

Fig. 17.1 Worldwide distribution of cystic echinococcosis. (Source: reference[42].)

Europe and is diagnosed almost exclusively in guest workers and immigrants (and rarely in travelers).

17.1.2 *Echinococcus multilocularis*

Unlike the dog tapeworm, whose larva grows by expansion, the larva of *Echinococcus multilocularis* (fox tapeworm) grows by infiltrating and destroying surrounding tissues (▶ Fig. 17.2). What may look like a cyst is actually a central necrotic zone within the parasitic tissue. As with the dog tapeworm, infection is acquired by the gastrointestinal route and the larvae are deposited chiefly in the liver. The geographical regions most commonly affected in Central Europe are Baden-Württemberg, Bavaria, Tyrolia, Kärnten, Styria, and Switzerland. The field mouse is a common intermediate host.

The clinical manifestations of alveolar echinococcosis result less from mass effects than from hepatic complications such as cholestasis or chronic cholangitis. Itching, skin rash, and night sweats are typical associated symptoms. Alveolar echinococcosis is most often confused with hepatocellular carcinoma, but forms that mimic hepatic cirrhosis have also been described. Abscess formation is not uncommon, especially after the initiation of treatment. The disease may also present with pyloric stenosis, obstructive jaundice, or portal hypertension.

Because *Echinococcus multilocularis* is not suitable for ultrasound-guided interventional treatment due to its exophytic growth and relatively solid consistency, that entity will not be discussed further in this chapter. The only treatment options are surgical removal or albendazole therapy (▶ Fig. 17.2).

Caution

Echinococcus multilocularis is not suitable for ultrasound-guided percutaneous treatment.

17.2 Clinical Manifestations

Symptoms in echinococcosis depend on the location and size of the cyst (generally must be > 8 cm in the liver, considerably smaller in other organ systems [brain, eye]) and may result from complications. Large cysts may cause compression with an associated feeling of abdominal fullness, epigastric pain, or nausea. Cyst rupture may have a spontaneous, traumatic, or iatrogenic cause (due to puncture or drug-induced involution) and may or may not incite an allergic reaction or occasional anaphylaxis. Other possible complications are fistula formation between hydatid cysts and bile ducts (or bronchi), for example, and symptoms due to secondary obstruction and inflammation (cholangitis, bronchitis). Spontaneous fractures have been reported due to skeletal involvement and erosive hemorrhage due to vascular infiltration. A feared complication is dissemination of the parasite into the abdominal or thoracic cavity from a ruptured cyst. Apparently it is much more common for the cysts to undergo spontaneous involution and transformation to an inactive, calcified state.

Any of the following complications may arise from cystic echinococcosis:

- Cyst rupture (spontaneous, traumatic or iatrogenic), with or without secondary dissemination
- Fistula formation
- Obstruction and inflammation

17.3 Diagnosis

17.3.1 Three Main Diagnostic Criteria

The diagnosis of echinococcosis is based on the history (nationality, exposure risk), imaging findings, and serologic testing.

17.3.2 Laboratory Parameters

Abnormal laboratory parameters reflect organ involvement and its complications and are often unhelpful in making a diagnosis. Liver function and cholestasis indicator enzymes may be abnormal in patients with hepatic involvement. Significant eosinophilia is rarely observed (< 10% of cases) and, in contrast to the diagnosis of helminthiases, is not a helpful finding.

17.3.3 Serologic and Molecular Biologic Tests

ELISA test systems and the indirect hemagglutination antibody test (IHAT) are sensitive screening tests that are usually combined and can confirm a positive Western blot with high specificity.

17.4 Imaging Studies, Staging of Disease

The value of imaging studies depends on the location of the cyst. Ultrasonography is the imaging modality of choice for the diagnosis of abdominal cystic echinococcosis and its follow-up, while CT is indispensable for evaluating the lung and bone. The sonomorphologic staging classification described below can be applied to most organ systems.

17.4.1 Historical Background

Various classification systems have been published.[8–13] In 1981 Gharbi developed a classification of hydatid

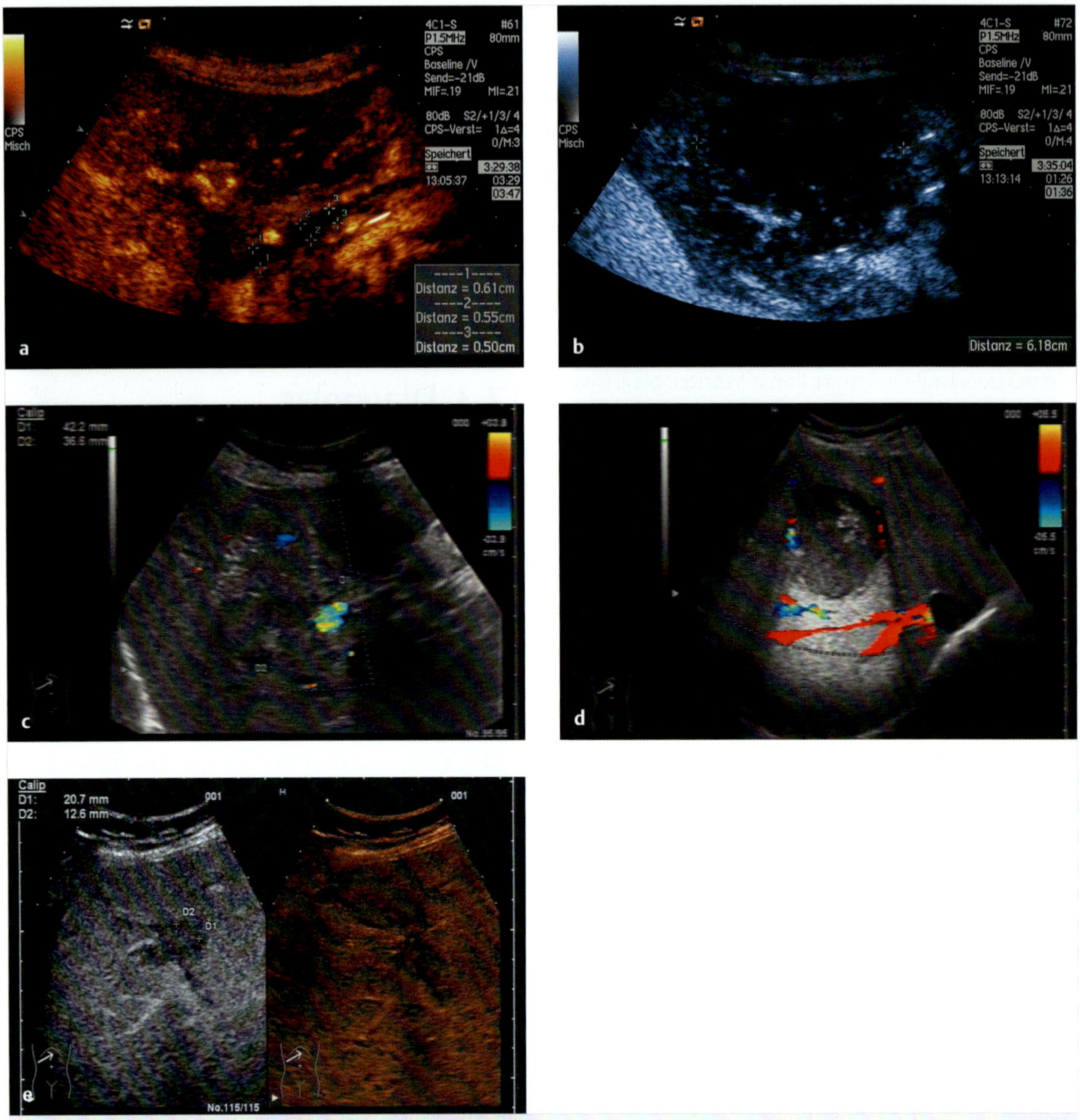

Fig. 17.2 *Echinococcus multilocularis.*
a, b Larva of *Echinococcus multilocularis* (fox tapeworm) infiltrating its surroundings. With contrast-enhanced ultrasound, the left lobe of the liver shows less enhancement while portions of the liver show no vascularity. The left hepatic artery is occluded and is visible between the markers. Similar changes are found in cholangiocellular carcinoma, which may also be associated with liver infarction in some cases.
c–e Later image sequence documents response to pharmacologic therapy.
c Ultrasound scan of the hepatic right lobe shows an echogenic, inhomogeneous mass at the center of the lobe displacing the surrounding vessels, consistent with untreated *Echinococcus multilocularis*. Indistinguishable from a tumor mass by ultrasound.
d Appearance of the same finding after 2 months of albendazole therapy. Note the inflammatory peripheral hypervascularity of the lesion with complete central liquefaction due to dead parasites.
e Same site after 6 months of therapy. Ultrasound shows a significantly smaller mass with a nonenhancing area in the portal venous phase after contrast administration. The lesion is no longer visible in an unenhanced scan.

morphology[10] that has been modified several times over the years.

A *Gharbi type I cyst* is a pure fluid collection that is difficult to distinguish from other types of epithelial liver cyst. It is the most common lesion (50–80%, depending on the study population), and its morphology is that of a "normal" cyst without internal septa or echoes (hydatid sand). The cyst contains fertile protoscolices. The main difficulty lies in distinguishing it from an epithelialized cyst.

The hallmark of *Gharbi type II cyst* morphology is a split wall with separation of the membranes, which may fill the interior of the cyst producing a "water lily sign" on ultrasound. The cyst is fertile and is basically a spot diagnosis on ultrasound images. Ultrasound is definitely superior to other modalities at this stage for depicting the fine details of the cyst wall and contents. The more membranes and hydatid sand there are in the cyst, and the more difficult the scanning conditions or poorer the equipment, the greater the likelihood that this stage will be mistaken for an abscess or neoplasm. The detection of hydatid sand is aided by moving the patient to a lateral decubitus or standing position.

The *Gharbi type III cyst* is characterized by daughter cysts with internal septa and the possible presence of degenerated solid material. The septa eventually produce a honeycomb pattern with undulating membranes. This stage is called the transitional stage because live parasitic tissue undergoes regressive changes that may occur spontaneously or in response to host defenses or drug therapy. Typical features are a "cyst within a cyst" pattern (www.EFSUMB.org[14]), hydatid sand, and stippled contrast enhancement in the surroundings, which becomes more distinct from stage I to stage III.

The *Gharbi type IV cyst* has a very heterogeneous echo pattern with mixed high- and low-amplitude echoes (regressive changes due to scarring). Characteristic ultrasound signs of an inactive lesion include a collapsing, somewhat flattened, elliptical cyst shape (correlating with low intracystic pressure) and detachment of the germinal layer from the cyst wall (water lily sign). Other signs include coarse intracystic echoes and initial calcification of the cyst wall (see type V). It may be difficult in some cases to exclude the complex late stage of an abscess. This stage is much less typical than stages II and III.

A *Gharbi type V cyst* has a calcified wall and contents. This stage reflects mixed expansile changes (perifocal reaction) and regressive scar contraction showing highly variable echogenicity with a calcified wall and internal structures. The calcified rim may create an "eggshell" appearance on CT, which can also be demonstrated sonographically.

Similar morphologic changes may develop in the lung, in bone, and rarely in the brain.

17.4.2 Morphologic and Functional Classification Systems

An improved morphologic and functional classification takes into account not only imaging characteristics but also the biological behavior of the parasites—viable (fertile) protoscolices (Garbhi types I and II) versus inactive, nonviable (infertile) parasitic cysts that have undergone degenerative and regressive changes (Garbhi types IV and V). The transitional stage (Garbhi type III) cannot be uniquely classified in terms of its biological behavior. It is significant that one lesion may show various developmental stages. The evolution of cyst morphology takes 5 to 10 years to reach the regressive, calcified end stage. It has been found, however, that calcifications may also be observed during the initial (viable) stage. It became necessary to unite the different staging classifications into a uniform system.

Vivid descriptions of pathognomonic ultrasound signs have been published in the literature but should be discarded in favor of a precise nomenclature. The double membrane has been described as the "double line sign"; mobile echogenic cyst contents as hydatid sand or a "snowstorm" pattern; separation of the endocyst as the "water lily sign"; and multiple internal septa as a rosette sign or honeycomb pattern.

17.4.3 WHO Classification

The WHO classification published in 2001[1,3] not only describes the stages of cyst evolution but also subdivides echinococcal cysts into three groups to aid in clinical viability assessment and follow-up (▶ Table 17.1). This WHO ultrasound classification of cystic echinococcosis compares the sonomorphologic classifications of Gharbi, Perdomo, and Caremani,[15] correlates them with the WHO stages, and provides a clinical subdivision of echinococcal cysts into three groups—active, involuting, and inactive—that are useful for treatment planning and follow-up (column 5).

As ▶ Table 17.1 indicates, cysts in group 2 are already undergoing involution; it is uncertain whether they are still active and only follow-ups can determine this. Group 3 cysts, on the other hand, are usually inactive because they consist mainly of degenerated forms. The subdivision of cysts into three groups is useful both for planning treatment and evaluating response.

Group 1: Active Cysts

Cyst in the group 1 category (CL and CE 1 stages) are echo-free at ultrasound and often show relative distal acoustic enhancement. They represent viable juvenile echinococcal cysts that have growth potential. The structure is nicely displayed in the macrophotograph (▶ Fig. 17.3).

Table 17.1 WHO classification of cystic echinococcosis

Expanded classifications			WHO stages in the 2001 classification[1,3]	Clinical classification
Gharbi 1981[9]	Perdomo 1988[11]	Caremani 1997[8,14]		
Type I	Type 1 a		CL Univesicular cysts	Group 1 Active group Growing cysts
	Type 1 a, b, c Type 2 a	Type I b Type III a	CE 1 Hydatid sand, double line sign	
Type III	Type 3	Type II a, b	CE 2 Multivesicular cyst, rosette or honeycomb pattern	Group 2 Involutional stage Viable protoscolices likely present
Type II	Type 2 b	Type III b	CE 3 Univesicular cysts with detached endocyst, "water lily" sign from floating membrane	
Type III	Type 4	Type IV	Multivesicular cyst with signs of solid transformation	
Type IV	Type 5 a, b, c	Type V a, b Type VI	CE 4 Heterogeneous echo pattern with solid cyst contents; no evidence of daughter cysts	Group 3 Inactive group Degenerated cyst showing partial or complete calcification; (probably) no viable protoscolices
Type V	Type 6 a, b	Type VII a, b	CE 5 Partial to complete calcification	

Nonspecific "cystic lesions" (CL) are indistinguishable from dysontogenetic cysts by conventional B-mode ultrasound. In our experience, contrast-enhanced ultrasound shows typical perifocal enhancement in the surrounding liver parenchyma, enabling a more confident and specific early diagnosis.[16] Imaging with a high-frequency transducer is helpful for demonstrating initial foci of irregular, circumscribed wall thickening (still without a double membrane), which are interpreted as the precursor stage of a split wall. The conventional view is that a definable double membrane (double line sign) signals progression to a stage CE 1 morphology (▶ Fig. 17.4, ▶ Fig. 17.5).

CE 1 cysts contain a layer of sediment called hydatid sand. This material consists of brood capsules that have detached from the germinal membrane. CE 1 cysts occasionally contain a definable double membrane (double line sign) formed by separation of the endocyst from the pericyst along the laminated membrane.

CE 2 cysts contain multivesicular daughter cysts that occupy all or part of the mother cyst, creating a rosette or honeycomb pattern.

Group 2: Involuting Cysts

Cysts in group 2 are undergoing an involutional process characterized by loss of hypoechoic and echo-free components and a reduction in size (CE 3; ▶ Fig. 17.6). Univesicular cysts with a detached endocyst (water lily sign, sometimes subclassified as WHO stage CE 3a) are distinguished from multivesicular cysts with solid transformation of the cystic contents (rosette or honeycomb pattern, sometimes subclassified as WHO stage CE 3b).

Group 3: Inactive Cysts

Echogenic contents become increasingly dominant in the cyst matrix. Internal canalicular structures are still observed. Daughter cysts are no longer detectable by stage CE 4. Stage CE 5 is marked by complete solid transformation in the form of complete or segmental calcification, although calcifications may be observed at any stage (▶ Fig. 17.7).

Contrast-enhanced Ultrasonography

Contrast-enhanced ultrasound (CEUS) is not yet represented in the WHO classification. In our experience, CEUS is reasonably effective in distinguishing hydatid cysts from neoplasms and dysontogenetic cysts. Additionally, it displays perifocal inflammatory reactions as nodular zones of ring enhancement.[16,17] Published experience with CEUS in the diagnosis of echinococcosis is limited, but to date we have been able to evaluate more than 50 patients. The absence of contrast enhancement excludes a neoplasm.[16]

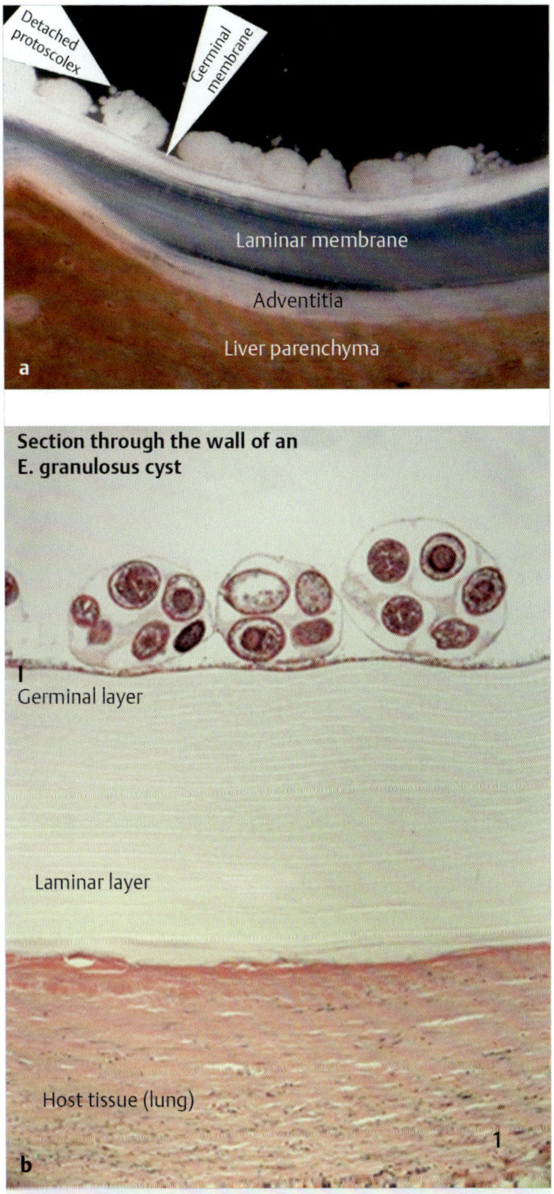

Fig. 17.3 Wall structure of a live echinococcal cyst. Macrophotograph of the wall of an echinococcal cyst in the liver parenchyma (**a**) and histologic section of an echinococcal cyst from the lung (**b**). The germinal layer is topped by brood capsules that contain mature protoscolices (future heads of adult tapeworms). (Source: Reproduced with kind permission of Professor H. M. Seitz, Bonn, Germany.)

Computed Tomography

When imaged by computed tomography (CT), typical cystic echinococcosis displays the size and shape features described for ultrasound in addition to fluid-equivalent (homogeneous) attenuation values. As cysts evolve to older stages, they show an increasingly dense rim while their internal structure and surroundings acquire a more inhomogeneous and tumorlike (hypodense) appearance.

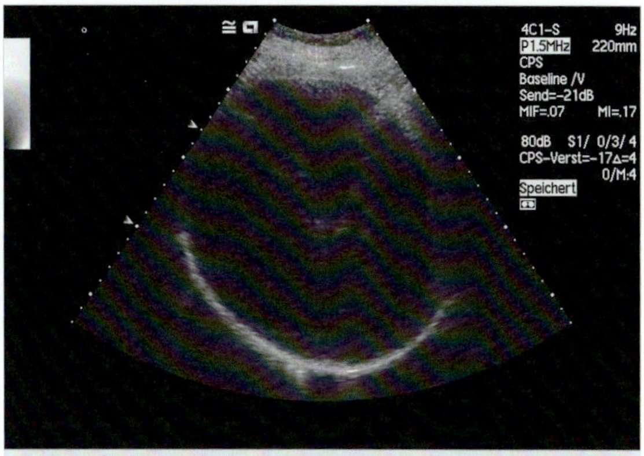

Fig. 17.4 Group 1 echinococcal cyst (CL, cystic lesion). The echinococcal cyst does not have a distinct double membrane.

Ultrasound permits a more accurate assessment of fine details. An important advantage of (unenhanced!) CT is its ability to detect calcifications. Involutional signs and perifocal enhancement are sometimes observed. As in contrast-enhanced ultrasound, CT contrast administration is a crucial aid in the differential diagnosis of focal liver lesions.[16–20] CT can also be used in the PAIR treatment of echinococcal cysts.[15,21]

Magnetic Resonance Imaging

Magnetic resonance imaging (MRI) is better than CT for characterizing the internal structures of echinococcal cysts (except for calcifications).[22,23] The cyst fluid in viable early stages has low signal intensity in T1-weighted sequences and high signal intensity in T2-weighted sequences.[24] Higher T1-weighted signal intensities are also caused by involutional processes but do not have prognostic significance in terms of "complicated cysts." The detection of a hypointense rim is considered characteristic, but there is disagreement as to what it represents. The detaching endocyst is often (but not always!) hypointense in all sequences and is most clearly appreciated in T2-weighted sequences owing to its high contrast with the hydatid fluid.[25]

Pitfalls

Calcifications are by no means pathognomonic for echinococcosis, as they may be found in association with neoplasms and other diseases. Calcifications are not only observed in inactive cyst stages CE 4 and CE 5 but may already be present in cysts of group 1 and group 2.[19]

17.5 Treatment

Procedures used in the treatment of cystic echinococcosis differ as a result of local health care factors and the marked differences in prevalence and clinical experience between developing countries (high prevalence, extensive

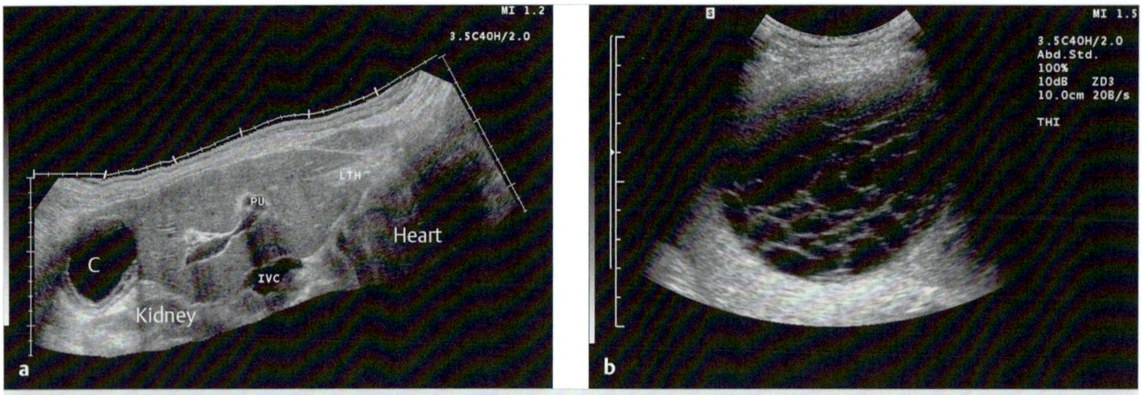

Fig. 17.5 Group 1 echinococcal cysts.
a Panoramic ultrasound scan shows a type CE 1 echinococcal cyst (C) with a definable double membrane.[16] The kidney, heart, inferior vena cava (IVC), umbilical part of the portal vein (PV) and ligamentum teres of the liver (LTH) are also shown.
b Honeycomb pattern in a type CE 2 echinococcal cyst.

experience, scant resources) and industrialized countries (low prevalence, little experience, extensive resources). Ideally, patients should be managed by a highly experienced interdisciplinary team.[26–28]

Four main treatment options are available for cystic echinococcosis: surgery, interventional treatment, drug treatment, and best supportive care. Not all echinococcal cysts require treatment. Fully consolidated and calcified lesions (stage CE 4 and CE 5) should be followed at yearly intervals in a watch-and-wait approach.

Evidence-based criteria for an individualized, stage-specific approach to treatment would be desirable but have not yet been adequately evaluated. Thus, current treatment recommendations for cystic echinococcosis continue to be expert recommendations (level III evidence)[29] and are explained below (▶ Table 17.2).

17.5.1 Surgical Treatment Options

Endocystectomy with aspiration of the cyst contents, unroofing of the cyst, and complete removal of the endocyst lining the pericyst is the most widely practiced surgical treatment. Any remaining viable membrane elements and protoscolices can be destroyed with protoscolicidal solutions (96% alcohol, 20% saline solution). A cystobiliary fistula should be excluded by testing the cyst contents for bilirubin (and if necessary by cystography; see also PAIR below). Other surgical options include pericystectomy (resection of the parasitic cyst with a margin of surrounding liver tissue) and segmental hepatectomy. Perioperative drug treatment (agent of choice: albendazole) is mandatory to prevent spreading of the parasites. A favorable reduction of the "cyst pressure" has also been postulated.

Complicated echinococcal cysts (e.g., cystobiliary fistula, obstructive cholangitis and bacterial infection [with or without abscess formation] in the liver, or cystobronchial fistulas in the lung) are usually treated surgically.[30]

17.5.2 Drug Treatment Options

Benzimidazoles are the agents of choice for echinococcosis and are often combined with a surgical procedure or PAIR. The WHO recommends drug treatment in the following situations:

1. Cases where surgery is contraindicated due to inoperability or comorbidity
2. Presence of multiple cysts in two or more organs
3. Multiple small liver cysts or cysts located at poorly accessible sites
4. Peritoneal echinococcal cysts
5. Previous incomplete surgical intervention or recurrence
6. Prevention of spontaneous rupture or following trauma or cyst aspiration

Medical treatment with albendazole alone (formerly: mebendazole) is successful in 30 to 50% of cases.[1,26,31–34]

Mebendazole was the first effective benzimidazole despite its poor oral availability of < 10%. The recommended dosage is 40 to 50 mg/kg BW per day taken in three separate doses after meals (not to exceed 6 g daily). It was recommended that mebendazole therapy be continued for at least 3 to 6 months.

Albendazole is more effective than mebendazole because it has a more favorable pharmacokinetic profile including active metabolites, resulting in a higher serum level and fluid concentration. Albendazole is taken at a daily dosage of 10 to 15 mg/kg BW in two separate doses (generally 400 mg twice a day) and is continued for 3 to 6 months. Due to its presumed toxicity and safety concerns, albendazole was initially taken intermittently in a cycle of 4 weeks followed by 2 weeks of not taking the drug (obsolete today). More recent experience shows that this intermittent dosing is no longer necessary and that continuous use does not significantly increase the risk of side effects.

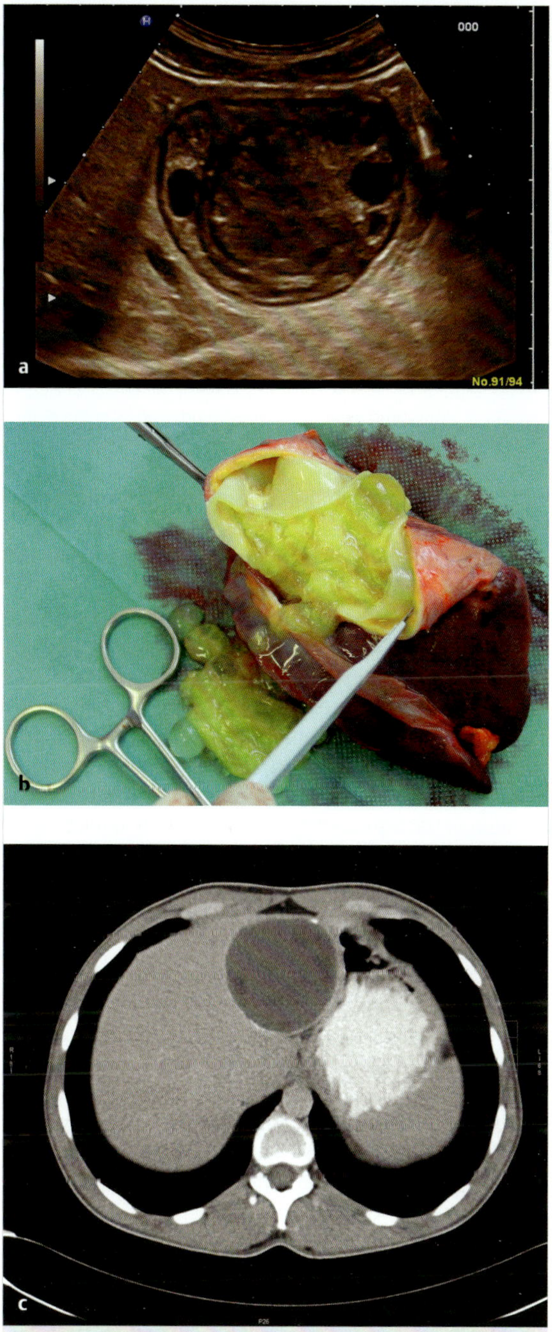

Fig. 17.6 Group 2 echinococcal cysts[7] (www.EFSUMB.org).
a Type CE 3 echinococcal cyst with solid transformation and daughter cysts.
b Surgical specimen.
c Corresponding CT scan. (Source: reprinted from Macpherson CN, Wachira TM, Zeyhle E, Romig T, Macpherson C. Hydatid disease: research and control in Turkana, IV. The pilot control programme. Trans R Soc Trop Med Hyg 1986;80(2):196–200; with permission from Elsevier.)

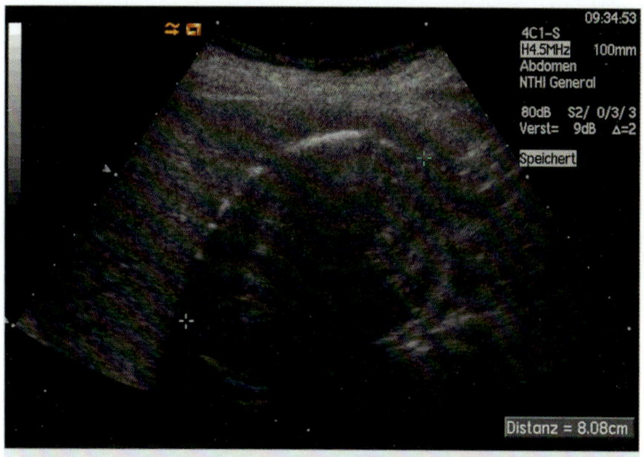

Fig. 17.7 Group 3 echinococcal cyst. Ultrasound shows complete solid transformation of a type CE 5 echinococcal cyst with canalicular inner structures and a calcified cyst wall and matrix.

Table 17.2 Stage-specific treatment recommendations for uncomplicated cystic echinococcosis. The various therapeutic procedures are described in the text

WHO stage	Recommended treatment[a]
CE 1	PAIR and drug therapy with albendazole if the cyst is > 5 cm. Albendazole therapy alone if the cyst is < 5 cm.
CE 2	Surgical treatment. Possible alternative: large-bore catheter intervention with peri-interventional albendazole.
CE 3a	PAIR and drug therapy with albendazole if the cyst is > 5 cm. Albendazole therapy alone if the cyst is < 5 cm.
CE 3b	Surgical treatment. Possible alternative: large-bore catheter intervention with peri-interventional albendazole.
CE 4 or 5	Observation

[a] PAIR, puncture, aspiration, injection, reaspiration.

The WHO originally recommended that the drug level be measured after 2 weeks on albendazole and after 4 weeks on mebendazole and then rechecked every 3 months, both to avoid toxicity and to ensure that drug levels have not fallen too low. The drug level for mebendazole is 250 nmol/L 4 hours after morning dosing, and for albendazole it is 650 to 3000 nmol/L. It has been found, however, that the blood levels do not require monitoring and this is rarely practiced any longer.

17.5.3 Local Ablative Procedures: PAIR

PAIR (puncture, aspiration, injection, reaspiration) involves the percutaneous puncture of echinococcal cysts, aspiration of the cyst contents, the injection of protoscolicidal agents (e.g., 20% saline or 96% alcohol) to destroy the germinal membrane, and reaspiration 15 to 20 minutes later. PAIR

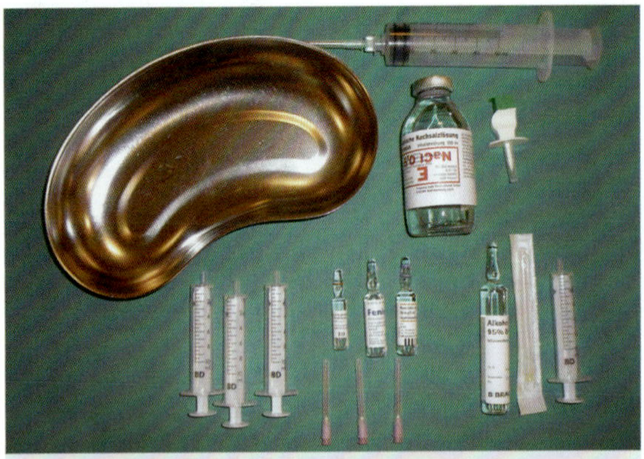

Fig. 17.8 Instrument setup for PAIR permits rapid access to ranitidine, prednisolone, and dimetindene maleate (Fenistil) along with injection syringes and drawing needles. On the right: an ampule with 95% alcohol and a 22-gauge puncture needle. At top: waste receptacle and aspirating syringe with Luer lock connector.

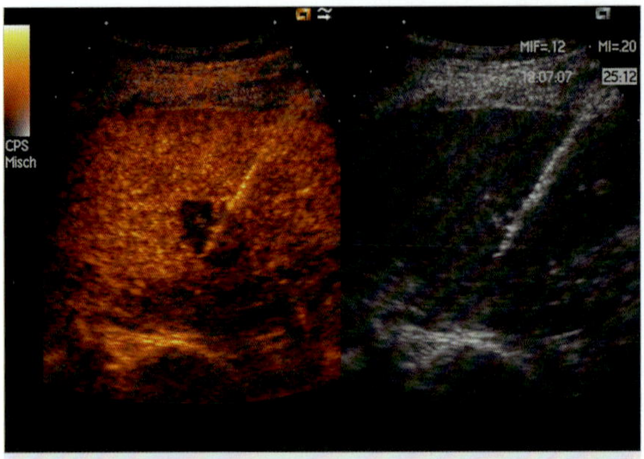

Fig. 17.9 Ultrasound view of the needle positioned in the cyst.

was introduced in the 1980s. Modifications have been described (large-bore catheter intervention).

PAIR is recognized by the WHO as an alternative to surgery and drug treatment. It has a low complication rate in properly selected cases along with low failure and recurrence rates. Two randomized clinical studies on PAIR have been published to date.[35,36] Radiofrequency therapy has not become established for this indication.[37]

PAIR for Echinococcal Liver Cysts

Preparations

General preparations include written informed consent and routine blood work. The following specific measures should be done before the intervention:

- Check the indication and establish the diagnosis by serologic testing.
- Identify the WHO stage based on sonographic criteria. Optional studies: CT, MRI, MRC(P) (magnetic resonance cholangio[pancreato]graphy), ERC(P) (endoscopic retrograde cholangio[pancreato]graphy).
- Check the safety of the percutaneous route and confirm adequate cyst coverage by liver parenchyma.
- Provide albendazole coverage at 400 mg twice a day (10–15 mg/kg BW per day) the day before the procedure, or at least 4 hours before the intervention.

Monitoring During the Intervention

ECG, pulse oximetry (desirable).

Technique

Following local anesthesia, a percutaneous needle is introduced into the cyst (e.g., 22-gauge needle set [Uni-Dwell, Bard, Angiomed]). The needle is used with a Luer lock fitting, syringes, an Erlanger extension, and a three-way stopcock (▶ Fig. 17.8, ▶ Fig. 17.9).

The indication for cyst aspiration and instillation of 95% ethanol is based on the microscopic detection of viable protoscolices and the exclusion of a cystobiliary fistula. For this reason, 10 mL of cystic fluid is aspirated for immediate evaluation (pathognomonic criteria: clear fluid with corpuscular elements [hydatid sand, endocyst membrane parts]). A helpful tool is on-site staining with May–Grünwald-Giemsa stain and microscopic examination for viable/nonviable differentiation. The detection of bilirubin in the aspirated cyst fluid, either visually or with a commercially available reagent strip (e.g., Multistix, Siemens Healthcare Diagnostics), confirms that the cyst communicates with the biliary tree and would contraindicate PAIR.

The cyst fluid is aspirated as completely as possible (▶ Fig. 17.10), followed by the instillation of 95% ethanol (e.g., 95% alcohol concentrate, Braun Melsungen). The three-way stopcock and extension should be removed before the agent is injected, as the concentrated alcohol would attack the plastic material. The agent is left in the cyst for 15 to 20 minutes and then completely reaspirated. The patient is monitored for the next 24 hours.

Follow-Up

Ultrasound follow-ups should be scheduled the day after the procedure (free fluid visible?) and at 4 weeks, 3 months, and every 6 months thereafter. Drug therapy with albendazole should be continued for at least 4 weeks, both to treat the primary lesion and to prevent secondary echinococcosis.

PAIR for Cysts at Other Locations

Studies have been published on the interventional treatment of echinococcal cysts at various sites: liver (54%), peritoneum (39%), kidneys (1%), spleen (1%), lung (0.4%),[37] muscle/soft tissues (0.3%), spinal column (0.2%), and other organs (pancreas, breast, heart,[38] 0.1% each).[28]

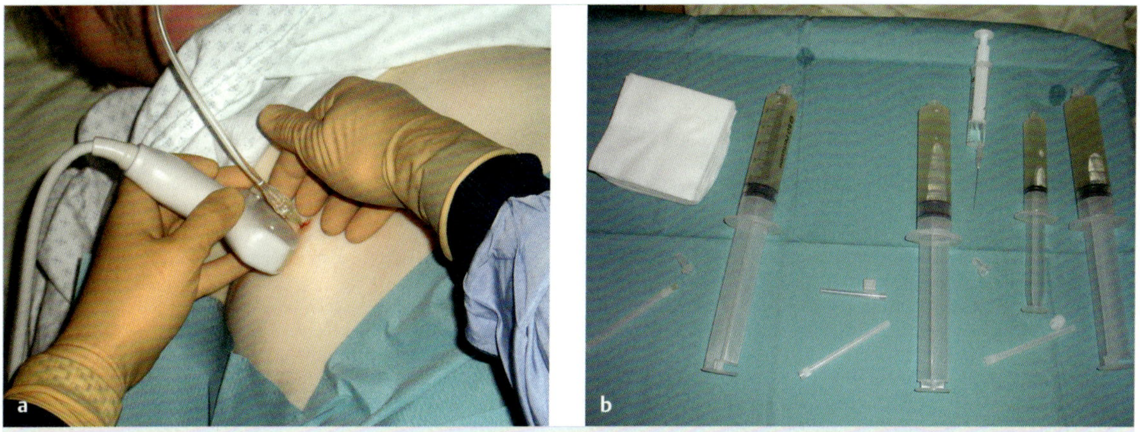

Fig. 17.10 Drainage catheter (a) and syringes with aspirated fluid (b).

Risks and Management of Side Effects

The main risks of percutaneous interventions are anaphylactic shock[39] (→ provide necessary emergency medications [H_1 and H_2 blockers, intravenous corticosteroids]), dissemination (→ confirm > 1 cm coverage by liver parenchyma, preinterventional drug treatment), and sclerosing cholangitis induced by the scolicidal fluid (→ exclude cystobiliary fistula before the intervention).

Anaphylactic Reaction

If an anaphylactic reaction occurs during the procedure, it should be treated with high-dose prednisolone (150 mg IV) and H_1 and H_2 antagonists (e.g., Fenistil [dimetindene maleate], 1 ampule IV, or Ranitic [ranitidine], one 100-mg ampule IV). Concurrent IV fluid administration (isotonic saline, other electrolyte solutions, Ringer lactate) may be necessary. Some cases may require hemodynamic stabilization with catecholamines. The patient should be monitored in the ICU for the next 24 hours.

Febrile Reaction

The febrile reaction that occurs in the days following PAIR is immunologic in nature. Often it is difficult to distinguish clinically from superinfection, so treatment with a broad-spectrum antibiotic is sometimes necessary.

Open Questions

At present there is no standard protocol for using a specific catheter or needle to aspirate the cyst and instill the scolicidal agent. The dosage of the agent is not standardized, nor is the optimum duration of drug therapy before (at least 4 hours before PAIR) and after the procedure (at least 4 weeks).

17.5.4 Endoscopic Retrograde Cholangiography

Endoscopic retrograde cholangiography (ERC) is used in both the diagnosis and treatment of cystobiliary fistulas. It can confirm both the location of the fistula and the cause of biliary obstruction.[40,41] MR cholangiography is less sensitive than ERC and cannot be used for interventional procedures.[23,42]

References

[1] Pawlowski ZS, Eckert J, Vuitton DA et al. WHO/OIE Manual on Echinococcosis in Humans and Animals: a Public Health Problem of Global Concern. In: Eckert J, Gemmell M, Meslin FX, Pawlowski ZS, eds. Paris: Office International des Epizooties (OIE); 2001:20–72

[2] WHO Informal Working Group on Echinococcosis. Guidelines for treatment of cystic and alveolar echinococcosis in humans. Bull World Health Organ 1996; 74: 231–242

[3] WHO Informal Working Group. International classification of ultrasound images in cystic echinococcosis for application in clinical and field epidemiological settings. Acta Trop 2003; 85: 253–261

[4] Njoroge EM, Mbithi PM, Gathuma JM et al. A study of cystic echinococcosis in slaughter animals in three selected areas of northern Turkana, Kenya. Vet Parasitol 2002, 104: 85–91

[5] Njoroge EM, Mbithi PM, Gathuma JM, Wachira TM, Magambo JK, Zeyhle E. Application of ultrasonography in prevalence studies of hydatid cysts in goats in north-western Turkana, Kenya and Toposaland, southern Sudan. Onderstepoort J Vet Res 2000; 67: 251–255

[6] Gathura PB, Kamiya M. Echinococcosis in Kenya: transmission characteristics, incidence and control measures. Jpn J Vet Res 1990; 38: 107–116

[7] Macpherson CN, Wachira TM, Zeyhle E, Romig T, Macpherson C. Hydatid disease: research and control in Turkana, IV. The pilot control programme. Trans R Soc Trop Med Hyg 1986; 80: 196–200

[8] Caremani M, Benci A, Maestrini R, Rossi G, Menchetti D. Abdominal cystic hydatid disease (CHD): classification of sonographic appearance and response to treatment. J Clin Ultrasound 1996; 24: 491–500

[9] Caremani M, Benci A, Maestrini R, Accorsi A, Caremani D, Lapini L. Ultrasound imaging in cystic echinococcosis. Proposal of a new sonographic classification. Acta Trop 1997; 67: 91–105

[10] Gharbi HA, Hassine W, Brauner MW, Dupuch K. Ultrasound examination of the hydatic liver. Radiology 1981; 139: 459–463

[11] Lewall DB, McCorkell SJ. Hepatic echinococcal cysts: sonographic appearance and classification. Radiology 1985; 155: 773–775

[12] Perdomo R, Alvarez C, Geninazzi H et al. Early diagnosis of hydatidosis by ultrasonography. Lancet 1988; 1: 244

[13] Perdomo R, Alvarez C, Monti J et al. Principles of the surgical approach in human liver cystic echinococcosis. Acta Trop 1997; 64: 109–122

[14] Dietrich CF, Mueller G, Beyer-Enke S. Cysts in the cyst pattern. Z Gastroenterol 2009; 47: 1203–1207

[15] Hosch W, Junghanss T, Werner J, Düx M. Imaging methods in the diagnosis and therapy of cystic echinococcosis [Article in German]. Rofo 2004; 176: 679–687

[16] Dietrich CF, Schreiber-Dietrich D, Schuessler G, Ignee A. Contrast enhanced ultrasound of the liver—state of the art [Article in German]. Dtsch Med Wochenschr 2007; 132: 1225–1231

[17] Claudon M, Cosgrove D, Albrecht T et al. Guidelines and good clinical practice recommendations for contrast enhanced ultrasound (CEUS) —update 2008. Ultraschall Med 2008; 29: 28–44

[18] Trojan J, Hammerstingl R, Engels K, Schneider AR, Zeuzem S, Dietrich CF. Contrast-enhanced ultrasound in the diagnosis of malignant mesenchymal liver tumors. J Clin Ultrasound 2010; 38: 227–231

[19] Mörk H, Ignee A, Schuessler G, Ott M, Dietrich CF. Analysis of neuroendocrine tumour metastases in the liver using contrast enhanced ultrasonography. Scand J Gastroenterol 2007; 42: 652–662

[20] Dietrich CF. Comments and illustrations regarding the guidelines and good clinical practice recommendations for contrast-enhanced ultrasound (CEUS)—update 2008. Ultraschall Med 2008; 29 (Suppl 4): S188–S202

[21] Hosch W, Kauffmann GW, Junghanss T. Cystic liver lesions with unspecified upper abdominal pain [Article in German]. Radiologe 2005; 45: 924–928

[22] Hosch W, Junghanss T, Stojkovic M et al. Metabolic viability assessment of cystic echinococcosis using high-field 1 H MRS of cyst contents. NMR Biomed 2008; 21: 734–754

[23] Hosch W, Stojkovic M, Jänisch T et al. MR imaging for diagnosing cysto-biliary fistulas in cystic echinococcosis. Eur J Radiol 2008; 66: 262–267

[24] Ağildere AM, Aytekin C, Coşkun M, Boyvat F, Boyacioğlu S. MRI of hydatid disease of the liver: a variety of sequences. J Comput Assist Tomogr 1998; 22: 718–724

[25] Kalovidouris A, Gouliamos A, Vlachos L et al. MRI of abdominal hydatid disease. Abdom Imaging 1994; 19: 489–494

[26] Stojkovic M, Zwahlen M, Teggi A et al. Treatment response of cystic echinococcosis to benzimidazoles: a systematic review. PLoS Negl Trop Dis 2009; 3: e524

[27] Brunetti E, Junghanss T. Update on cystic hydatid disease. Curr Opin Infect Dis 2009; 22: 497–502

[28] Junghanss T, da Silva AM, Horton J, Chiodini PL, Brunetti E. Clinical management of cystic echinococcosis: state of the art, problems, and perspectives. Am J Trop Med Hyg 2008; 79: 301–311

[29] Kish MA Infectious Diseases Society of America. Guide to development of practice guidelines. Clin Infect Dis 2001; 32: 851–854

[30] Brunetti E, Kern P, Vuitton DA. Writing Panel for the WHO-IWGE. Expert consensus for the diagnosis and treatment of cystic and alveolar echinococcosis in humans. Acta Trop 2010; 114: 1–16

[31] Filice C, Pirola F, Brunetti E, Dughetti S, Strosselli M, Foglieni CS. A new therapeutic approach for hydatid liver cysts. Aspiration and alcohol injection under sonographic guidance. Gastroenterology 1990; 98: 1366–1368

[32] Gargouri M, Ben Amor N, Ben Chehida F et al. Percutaneous treatment of hydatid cysts (*Echinococcus granulosus*). Cardiovasc Intervent Radiol 1990; 13: 169–173

[33] Mueller PR, Dawson SL, Ferrucci JT, Nardi GL. Hepatic echinococcal cyst: successful percutaneous drainage. Radiology 1985; 155: 627–628

[34] Salama H, Farid Abdel-Wahab M, Strickland GT. Diagnosis and treatment of hepatic hydatid cysts with the aid of echo-guided percutaneous cyst puncture. Clin Infect Dis 1995; 21: 1372–1376

[35] Khuroo MS, Wani NA, Javid G et al. Percutaneous drainage compared with surgery for hepatic hydatid cysts. N Engl J Med 1997; 337: 881–887

[36] Khuroo MS, Dar MY, Yattoo GN et al. Percutaneous drainage versus albendazole therapy in hepatic hydatidosis: a prospective, randomized study. Gastroenterology 1993; 104: 1452–1459

[37] Brunetti E, Filice C. Radiofrequency thermal ablation of echinococcal liver cysts. Lancet 2001; 358: 1464

[38] Heye T, Lichtenberg A, Junghanss T, Hosch W. Cardiac manifestation of cystic echinococcosis: comparison of dual-source cardio-computed tomography and cardiac magnetic resonance imaging and their impact on disease management. Am J Trop Med Hyg 2007; 77: 875–877

[39] Köppen S, Wejda B, Dormann A, Seesko H, Huchzermeyer H, Junghanss T. Anaphylactic shock caused by rupture of an echinococcal cyst in a 25-year-old asylum seeker from Georgia [Article in German]. Dtsch Med Wochenschr 2003; 128: 663–666

[40] Magistrelli P, Masetti R, Coppola R et al. Value of ERCP in the diagnosis and management of pre- and postoperative biliary complications in hydatid disease of the liver. Gastrointest Radiol 1989; 14: 315–320

[41] Ozaslan E, Bayraktar Y. Endoscopic therapy in the management of hepatobiliary hydatid disease. J Clin Gastroenterol 2002; 35: 160–174

[42] Ignee A, Baum U, Schuessler G, Dietrich CF. Contrast-enhanced ultrasound-guided percutaneous cholangiography and cholangiodrainage (CEUS-PTCD). Endoscopy 2009; 41: 725–726

18 Local Ablative Procedures; Percutaneous Ethanol and Acetic Acid Injection

C. F. Dietrich, B. Braden, M. Hocke

Local ablative injection therapies (e.g., percutaneous ethanol injection) have become established routine procedures for the treatment of hepatocellular carcinoma. They compete with surgical resection and other local ablative procedures such as radiofrequency ablation (RFA)[1] and laser-induced thermotherapy (LITT), which are discussed separately in Chapter 19.

18.1 Basic Considerations

18.1.1 What Tumors Are Suitable for Local Ablative Procedures?

Percutaneous ethanol injection (PEI) and percutaneous acetic acid injection (PAI) have yielded very favorable results for (primary) hepatocellular carcinoma but not for metastases from other tumors. This is explained by the cirrhotic transformation of the liver resulting in a predominantly arterial blood supply to the cirrhotic tissue and the frequent encapsulation of hepatocellular carcinoma.[2–8] Only a few studies have been published on local ablative injection therapies for metastatic lesions due to the disappointing results.[9–12]

Note

PEI has become an established therapy for hepatocellular carcinoma but not for metastases.

18.1.2 Radiofrequency Ablation or Percutaneous Ethanol Injection?

Studies to date have not shown a definite survival advantage of radiofrequency thermoablation (RFA or RFTA) over PEI,[5] although reports have repeatedly noted a certain trend in that direction. Thus, the local injection of alcohol and other agents should continue to play a key role in the treatment of hepatocellular carcinoma. Remarkably, much more costly local ablative procedures are still being recommended to patients—perhaps uncritically in some cases.

The literature comparing RFA and PEI, and the somewhat contradictory results of published findings, will be explored in more detail in Chapter 19.

18.1.3 Ethanol or Acetic Acid Injection?

Most interventionalists have more experience with ethanol than with acetic acid, with the result that PEI is favored at most centers. The differences between the two therapies appear to be marginal.[13–15] It has been suggested that PAI requires fewer injections and smaller injection volumes than PEI to achieve the same response, but this is no more than a reported trend.[16,17]

18.1.4 Single or Multiple Sessions?

Both PEI and PAI can be administered in a single- or multiple-session regimen.[8,18–20] The advantage of single-session treatment is that in regions and countries with limited health care facilities, definitive treatment can be provided in one visit to the doctor for patients unable to make repeated visits. The advantage of multiple treatment sessions is that they probably yield a better result. It has been found that the injection of large ethanol volumes (100 mL or more) may induce the decompensation of cardiopulmonary diseases such as coronary heart disease or pulmonary hypertension, and therefore these conditions should be excluded before treatment.[21]

18.2 Indications

Local ablative procedures can be used as a bridging strategy in patients on a waiting list for a liver transplant or if liver transplantation is contraindicated due to age, comorbidity, or other documentable causes and the risk of surgical treatment (resection) outweighs the potential survival benefit.[22–24] Local ablative procedures are appropriate for small, solitary tumors. The prognosis of these lesions is excellent with PEI and is comparable to that following tumor resection. But there are other factors that would weaken the indication for local ablative therapy: a number of tumors are multifocal when first diagnosed in unscreened cases, tumors are often associated with local satellite lesions, and invasion of the portal vein and hepatic veins may occur early in the course of the disease —although data suggest that this invasion does not affect survival after PEI.[25]

Solitary, well-circumscribed tumors up to 3 cm in size (n = up to 3) are an established indication for local ablation by PEI and PAI. A solitary lesion up to 50 mm in size is an established indication in patients with Child class A or B hepatic cirrhosis. Child class C patients may also benefit in selected cases, depending on the degree of tumor differentiation.[26] Tumor invasion of the portal vein or its side branches is not a contraindication to local ablative therapy.

18.2.1 Considerations on Hepatocellular Carcinoma

It is important to consider the pathogenesis of a hyperregenerative liver nodule, a dysplastic nodule with a low or high grade of dysplasia, well-differentiated hepatocellular carcinoma, and poorly differentiated forms (G1 to G4) since different nodular lesions have different prognostic implications.

Factors Determining Prognosis

It has been known for some time that the prognosis of hepatocellular carcinoma depends on the size of the tumor at the time of initial diagnosis,[27,28] and this has been confirmed by treatment outcomes in recent large studies.[3–6,29]

Hepatocellular carcinoma in a Child class C cirrhotic liver appears to have less prognostic importance than in a Child–Pugh class A liver. This is because the tumor itself does not greatly affect the inherently poor prognosis of the advanced liver disease.[26] Multifocal hepatocellular carcinomas should be excluded with the highest possible certainty before local ablative therapy.

Histologic Confirmation

We require histologic confirmation of the tumor before proceeding with local ablative treatment. This confirmation is essential for oncologic reasons in most palliative treatment settings. Other, noninvasive diagnostic criteria have been proposed for the prevention of tumor cell seeding, especially before liver transplantation. According to guidelines, a hypervascular tumor > 20 mm is considered to be hepatocellular carcinoma when identified by one contrast-enhanced study (CT, MRI, ultrasound). For tumors 10 to 20 mm in size, two contrast-enhanced studies are required (combined if necessary with elevated AFP levels).[29–31] Tumors smaller than 10 mm can be followed at 3 months.

18.3 Contraindications

Besides general contraindications relating to coagulation status (coagulation disorders and platelet dysfunction) and lack of informed consent, a local ablative procedure may be contraindicated due to comorbidity, poor prognosis, or short life expectancy < 3 months. Bleeding time should be determined if the coagulation status is unclear.

Another contraindication is ascites, because free fluid increases the complication rate and ascites during diuretic therapy is an unfavorable prognostic factor.

Advanced pulmonary hypertension and coronary heart disease are particularly important comorbid conditions, since the injection of large amounts of alcohol may occasionally cause cardiovascular deterioration in these patients.

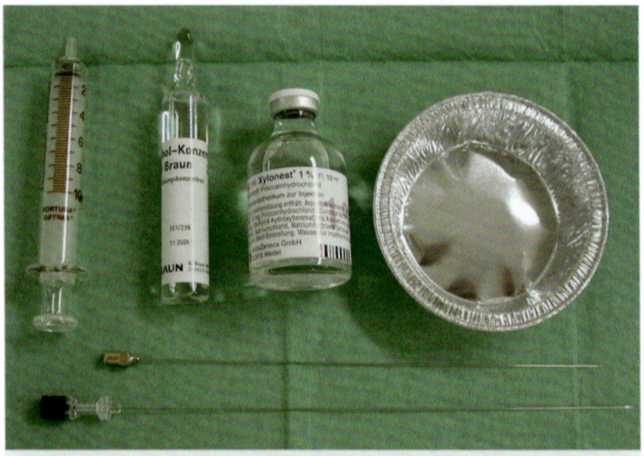

Fig. 18.1 Tray setup includes sterile 0.7-mm injection needles with a long bevel (2 mm), 95% or 96% alcohol, and 10-mL syringes.

18.4 Practical Aspects

18.4.1 Materials and Equipment

► **Basic materials.** Sterile injection needles 0.7 mm in diameter with a long bevel (2 mm), 95% or 96% alcohol, and 10-mL syringes (► Fig. 18.1).

► **Special materials.** 20-gauge special injection needle, length 20 cm (Peter Pflugbeil), 95% ethanol (Braun Melsungen).

► **What type of needle?.** Alcohol-resistant material should be used. Various needle types have been used ranging from a simple yellow No. 1 needle to No. 2 needles and needles with multiple side holes (Otto needle) that can provide better dispersal (20-gauge special injection needle, 20 cm, Peter Pflugbeil). There is no hard evidence for the superiority of specific needle types, however.

18.4.2 Preparations

Standard protocols for skin preparation and local anesthesia for percutaneous procedures should be followed (see Chapter 8). If necessary, local anesthesia may be supplemented by sedation (e.g., with diazepam in patients with liver damage; Chapter 11). Piritramide is widely preferred over pethidine for analgesia, although there are no study data to support this preference.

General anesthesia is most commonly used for single-shot techniques because the larger injected alcohol volume may cause significant (and sometimes uncontrollable) local pain reactions.[18]

18.4.3 Technique

Needle Insertion

Before the needle is introduced, local anatomy is scrutinized with ultrasound and color Doppler is used to exclude blood vessels in the needle path.

Following standard skin prep and local anesthesia, the needle is advanced into the tumor under ultrasound guidance using freehand technique, a biopsy transducer, or a side-mounted needle guide. The needle tip is initially placed against the *far tumor border* and then slowly withdrawn to create a uniform dispersal of the injected agent. This technique also creates shadowing artifacts caused by tiny air bubbles present in the alcohol collection (▶ Fig. 18.2).

Painful alcohol along the liver capsule may be a problem with tumors close to the liver surface. This can be prevented by applying slight suction during needle retraction or, less elegantly, by flushing the needle with isotonic saline solution proximal to the tumor to ensure that alcohol does not come into contact with the liver capsule.

How Much Alcohol is Injected?

The average injected volume varies between 1 and 40 mL depending on the tumor size. When multiple sessions are planned, the treatments can be repeated up to 10 times at intervals of 2 to 3 days (this may be done on an ambulatory basis). With single-shot techniques, a greater alcohol volume is injected into the generally larger tumor, and the treatment may be repeated as needed at intervals

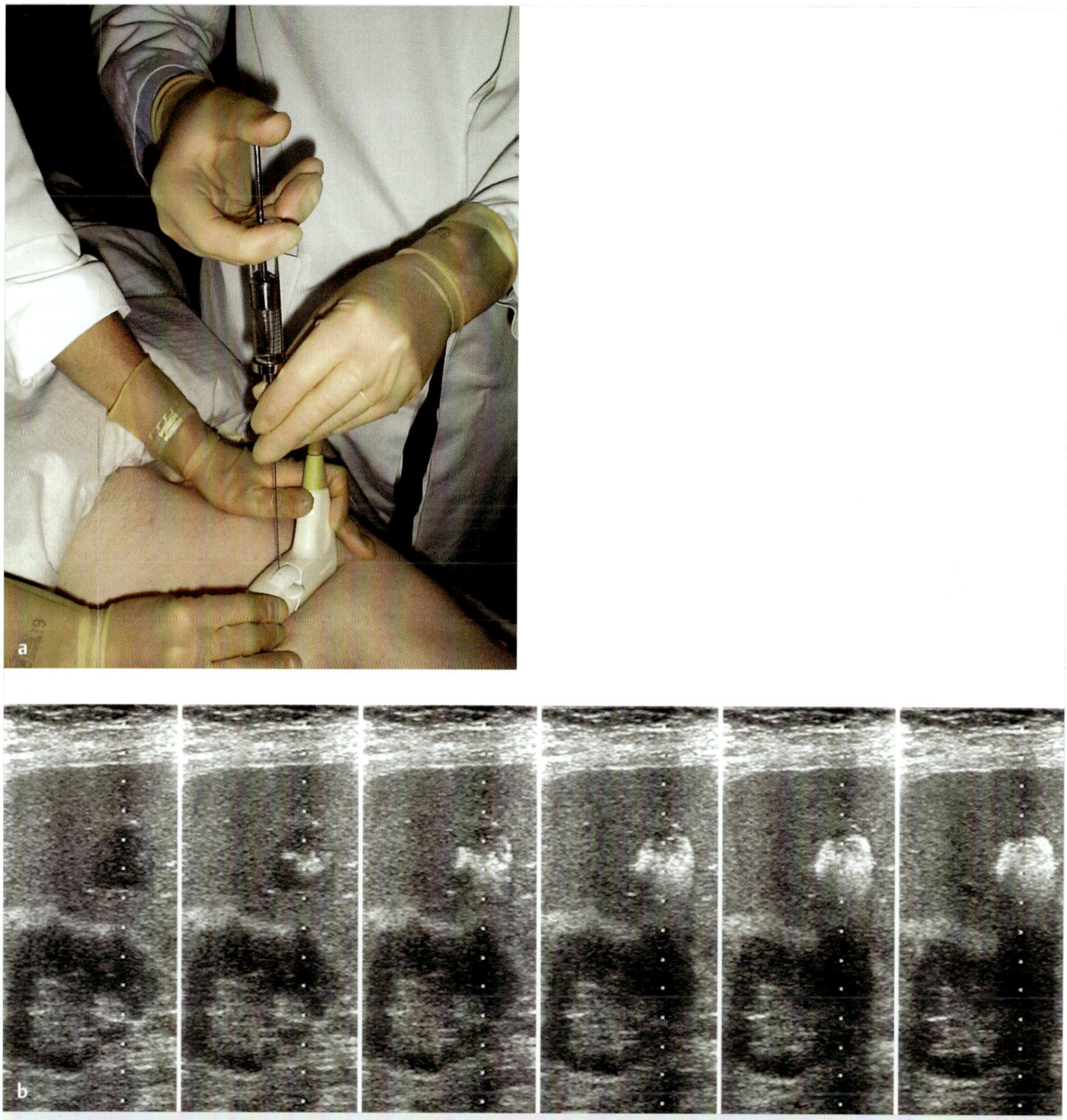

Fig. 18.2 Alcohol is injected into the tumor (**a**). Ultrasound scans document good distribution of the agent (**b**). (Source: Reproduced with kind permission of Professor J. Bleck, Stendal, Germany.)

of 6 to 8 weeks.[18] Inpatient treatment has proven favorable for complication management and adjuvant pain therapy. The administered alcohol volume generally equals the estimated spherical volume of the target tumor and may be up to 100 mL or more.[18,21]

Large alcohol volumes should be administered under sedation or general anesthesia. When general endotracheal anesthesia is used, the respiratory position can be controlled to facilitate optimum needle placement. With a successful high-volume alcohol injection, tiny air bubbles in the solution should obscure the sonographic tumor image for the first 5 to 10 minutes after the procedure. Good tumor visualization shortly after ablation suggests that local ethanol spillage has occurred, resulting in poorer treatment response.

18.5 Follow-up Care, Complications, and Prognosis

18.5.1 Follow-up Care

The aim of follow-up care in the immediate postinterventional period is to exclude bleeding and pleural effusion. Patients treated with alcohol volumes < 10 mL should be monitored for 1 to 3 hours; patients treated with 10 to 100 mL require 24 hours observation. Antibiotic prophylaxis is advisable (e.g., ceftriaxone [Rocephin, Hoffmann-La Roche], 2 g IV), although a benefit has not been documented in studies.

18.5.2 Complications

Severe complications are rare and occur in approximately 1% of patients; comorbidity is a factor.[2,18,21,32,33] A feared complication is bleeding due to the accidental puncture of collateral vessels at the liver capsule or in intraperitoneal septa. Other possible complications are bile leakage and peri- and postinterventional pain from the injected alcohol.

Follow-up examinations should exclude complications such as ascites formation, pleural effusion, portal vein thrombosis, liver infarction, infection, and abscess formation. The synthetic function of the liver may show a transient decline of up to 20% following high-volume ethanol injection. The group of Bleck and Gebel identified stable serum cholinesterase (CHE) after PEI as a prognostic indicator.[18]

When PEI is done palliatively, the seeding of tumor cells along the needle track will not affect prognosis.

High-volume alcohol injections may cause decompensation of pulmonary hypertension, and coronary heart disease may progress to myocardial infarction. High-risk patients with preexisting cardiopulmonary disease should be monitored after single-shot PEI in a protocol that includes repeated pulmonary pressure measurements.

Marked elevation of blood alcohol levels has been observed in isolated cases.

18.5.3 Monitoring of Treatment Response

Ultrasound follow-ups, preferably using sonographic contrast agents, should be scheduled at 3-month intervals to exclude recurrent or metachronous tumor. Immediate postinterventional follow-up by contrast-enhanced ultrasound (or on the day following the intervention) is optional (▶ Fig. 18.3). Its value is disputed due to edema formation.

B-mode ultrasound signs of a positive response are tumor shrinkage, the formation of a sharply demarcated capsule, and calcifications. Contrast-enhanced ultrasound has proven superior to conventional B-mode criteria.[29]

Determination of alpha fetoprotein (AFP) is optional and depends on the baseline value. It may provide a useful follow-up parameter, at least in patients with elevated baseline levels. It should be noted that only about 70% of patients are found to have elevated AFP levels.

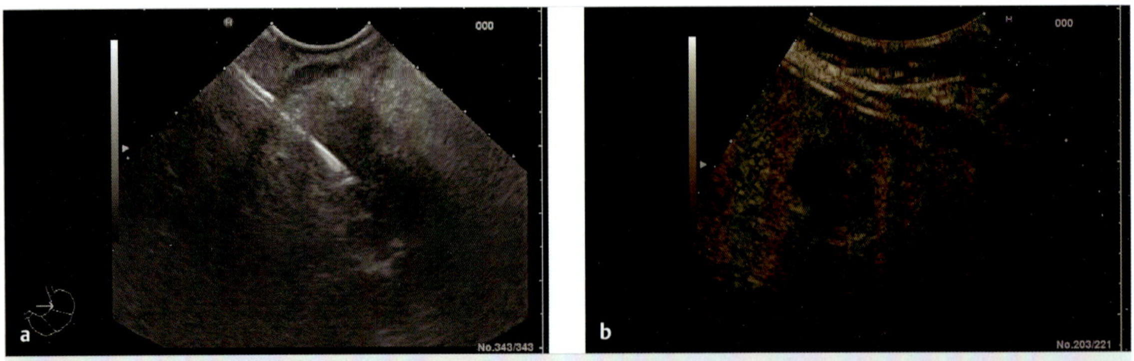

Fig. 18.3 Treatment and postinterventional follow-up.[29,30]
a Procedure.
b Postinterventional follow-up by contrast-enhanced ultrasound (here, on the day following the procedure) documents treatment response by showing central necrosis and peripheral hyperemia.

18.5.4 Factors That Determine Prognosis

In a multivariant regression analysis, the following parameters were associated with a positive effect on long-term survival > 3 years after the initiation of treatment:

- A tumor number of 5 nodules or less ($P = 0.01$, odds ratio 11.1, confidence interval 3.3 to 22.3)
- Tumors up to 50 mm in size ($P = 0.04$, odds ratio 6.1, confidence interval 1.3 to 17.5)
- Absence of ascites before treatment ($P = 0.03$, odds ratio 12.2, confidence interval 4.7 to 30.3)

The AFP level, fever, Child–Pugh class, Okuda stage, detection of portal vein thrombosis, and complications of PEI did not affect long-term survival. Changes in serum cholinesterase after treatment < 1 mU/mL and the treatment modality (combination of TACE [transarterial chemoembolization] and PEI) were marginally significant ($P = 0.05$).[18]

18.6 Summary

Although RFA ablation appears to be superior to PEI in published reports, PEI continues to be the most widely and effectively used locoregional treatment modality throughout the world. Laser-induced treatments and microwave techniques are of minor importance, at least for the present.

References

[1] Hasegawa K, Kokudo N, Makuuchi M et al. Comparison of resection and ablation for hepatocellular carcinoma: a cohort study based on a Japanese nationwide survey. J Hepatol 2013; 58: 724–729

[2] Germani G, Pleguezuelo M, Gurusamy K, Meyer T, Isgrò G, Burroughs AK. Clinical outcomes of radiofrequency ablation, percutaneous alcohol and acetic acid injection for hepatocelullar carcinoma: a meta-analysis. J Hepatol 2010; 52: 380–388

[3] Kuang M, Lu MD, Xie XY et al. Ethanol ablation of hepatocellular carcinoma Up to 5.0 cm by using a multipronged injection needle with high-dose strategy. Radiology 2009; 253: 552–561

[4] Lencioni R. Loco-regional treatment of hepatocellular carcinoma. Hepatology 2010; 52: 762–773

[5] Lencioni RA, Allgaier HP, Cioni D et al. Small hepatocellular carcinoma in cirrhosis: randomized comparison of radio-frequency thermal ablation versus percutaneous ethanol injection. Radiology 2003; 228: 235–240

[6] Livraghi T. Single HCC smaller than 2 cm: surgery or ablation: interventional oncologist's perspective. J Hepatobiliary Pancreat Sci 2010; 17: 425–429

[7] Livraghi T, Meloni F, Di Stasi M et al. Sustained complete response and complications rates after radiofrequency ablation of very early hepatocellular carcinoma in cirrhosis: Is resection still the treatment of choice? Hepatology 2008; 47: 82–89

[8] Meloni F, Lazzaroni S, Livraghi T. Percutaneous ethanol injection: single session treatment. Eur J Ultrasound 2001; 13: 107–115

[9] Giorgio A, Tarantino L, Mariniello N et al. [Ultrasonography-guided percutaneous ethanol injection in large an/or multiple liver metastasis]. Radiol Med (Torino) 1998; 96: 238–242

[10] Stang A, Fischbach R, Teichmann W, Bokemeyer C, Braumann D. A systematic review on the clinical benefit and role of radiofrequency ablation as treatment of colorectal liver metastases. Eur J Cancer 2009; 45: 1748–1756

[11] Chin K, Mangat K. Radiofrequency ablation of colorectal liver metastases in a transplanted liver. Cardiovasc Intervent Radiol 2009; 32: 1114–1116

[12] Becker D, Hänsler JM, Strobel D, Hahn EG. Percutaneous ethanol injection and radio-frequency ablation for the treatment of nonresectable colorectal liver metastases – techniques and results. Langenbecks Arch Surg 1999; 384: 339–343

[13] Huo TI, Huang YH, Wu JC, Lee PC, Chang FY, Lee SD. Comparison of percutaneous acetic acid injection and percutaneous ethanol injection for hepatocellular carcinoma in cirrhotic patients: a prospective study. Scand J Gastroenterol 2003; 38: 770–778

[14] Ohnishi K. Comparison of percutaneous acetic acid injection and percutaneous ethanol injection for small hepatocellular carcinoma. Hepatogastroenterology 1998; 45 (Suppl 3): 1254–1258

[15] Ohnishi K, Yoshioka H, Ito S, Fujiwara K. Prospective randomized controlled trial comparing percutaneous acetic acid injection and percutaneous ethanol injection for small hepatocellular carcinoma. Hepatology 1998; 27: 67–72

[16] Huo TI, Huang YH, Chiang JH et al. Survival impact of delayed treatment in patients with hepatocellular carcinoma undergoing locoregional therapy: is there a lead-time bias? Scand J Gastroenterol 2007; 42: 485–492

[17] Huo TI, Huang YH, Wu JC, Lee PC, Chang FY, Lee SD. Persistent retention of acetic acid is associated with complete tumour necrosis in patients with hepatocellular carcinoma undergoing percutaneous acetic acid injection. Scand J Gastroenterol 2004; 39: 168–173

[18] Dettmer A, Kirchhoff TD, Gebel M et al. Combination of repeated single-session percutaneous ethanol injection and transarterial chemoembolisation compared to repeated single-session percutaneous ethanol injection in patients with non-resectable hepatocellular carcinoma. World J Gastroenterol 2006; 12: 3707–3715

[19] Hori T, Nagata K, Hasuike S et al. Risk factors for the local recurrence of hepatocellular carcinoma after a single session of percutaneous radiofrequency ablation. J Gastroenterol 2003; 38: 977–981

[20] Livraghi T, Benedini V, Lazzaroni S, Meloni F, Torzilli G, Vettori C. Long term results of single session percutaneous ethanol injection in patients with large hepatocellular carcinoma. Cancer 1998; 83: 48–57

[21] Kielstein JT, Hesse G, Bahr MJ et al. Procedure-related pulmonary hypertension in patients with hepatocellular carcinoma undergoing percutaneous ethanol injection—role of ethanol, hemolysis, asymmetric dimethylarginine, and the nitric oxide system. Crit Care Med 2009; 37: 1483–1485

[22] Ruzzenente A, Capra F, Pachera S et al. Is liver resection justified in advanced hepatocellular carcinoma? Results of an observational study in 464 patients. J Gastrointest Surg 2009; 13: 1313–1320

[23] Yao FY, Hirose R, LaBerge JM et al. A prospective study on downstaging of hepatocellular carcinoma prior to liver transplantation. Liver Transpl 2005; 11: 1505–1514

[24] Nanashima A, Tobinaga S, Masuda J et al. Selecting treatment for hepatocellular carcinoma based on the results of hepatic resection and local ablation therapy. J Surg Oncol 2010; 101: 481–485

[25] Dettmer A, Kirchhoff TD, Gebel M et al. Combination of repeated single-session percutaneous ethanol injection and transarterial chemoembolisation compared to repeated single-session percutaneous ethanol injection in patients with non-resectable hepatocellular carcinoma. World J Gastroenterol 2006; 12: 3707–3715

[26] Ueno S, Tanabe G, Nuruki K et al. Prognosis of hepatocellular carcinoma associated with Child class B and C cirrhosis in relation to treatment: a multivariate analysis of 411 patients at a single center. J Hepatobiliary Pancreat Surg 2002; 9: 469–477

[27] Ebara M, Okabe S, Kita K et al. Percutaneous ethanol injection for small hepatocellular carcinoma: therapeutic efficacy based on 20-year observation. J Hepatol 2005; 43: 458–464

[28] Ebara M, Hatano R, Fukuda H, Yoshikawa M, Sugiura N, Saisho H. Natural course of small hepatocellular carcinoma with underlying cirrhosis. A study of 30 patients. Hepatogastroenterology 1998; 45 (Suppl 3): 1214–1220

[29] Claudon M, Cosgrove D, Albrecht T et al. Guidelines and good clinical practice recommendations for contrast enhanced ultrasound (CEUS) - update 2008. Ultraschall Med 2008; 29: 28–44

[30] Dietrich CF. Comments and illustrations regarding the guidelines and good clinical practice recommendations for contrast-enhanced ultrasound (CEUS)—update 2008. Ultraschall Med 2008; 29 (Suppl 4): S188–S202

[31] Leoni S, Piscaglia F, Golfieri R et al. The impact of vascular and nonvascular findings on the noninvasive diagnosis of small hepatocellular carcinoma based on the EASL and AASLD criteria. Am J Gastroenterol 2010; 105: 599–609

[32] Da Ines D, Buc E, Petitcolin V et al. Massive hepatic necrosis with gastric, splenic, and pancreatic infarctions after ethanol ablation for hepatocellular carcinoma. J Vasc Interv Radiol 2010; 21: 1301–1305

[33] Frieser M, Lindner A, Meyer S et al. [Spectrum and bleeding complications of sonographically guided interventions of the liver and pancreas]. Ultraschall Med 2009; 30: 168–174

19 Local Ablative Procedures for Liver Tumors, Radiofrequency Ablation

C. F. Dietrich, T. Albrecht, T. Bernatik, A. Ignee

Local ablative procedures for the treatment of liver tumors are classified as follows:

- Percutaneous injection of ethanol, acetic acid, or other agents
- Heat-based techniques
  - Radiofrequency thermoablation, RFA
  - Microwave ablation
  - Laser-induced thermotherapy (LITT)
- High-intensity focused ultrasound (HIFU)
- Cryoablation (generally done surgically due to the larger diameter of the probes)[1–3]

RFA is the most widely used of the above modalities and will be the focus of this chapter.

RFA can be performed percutaneously under general anesthesia with endotracheal intubation or under local anesthesia plus sedation. The placement of the applicator and the progress of treatment are monitored by ultrasound, CT, or MRI. The choice of imaging modality depends on availability and tumor visibility. RFA can also be performed in the setting of an open or laparoscopic operation under general anesthesia and with intraoperative ultrasound guidance.

19.1 Concepts (Curative, Palliative, Multimodal)

The local ablation of liver tumors is usually done with curative intent. This applies mainly to small hepatocellular carcinomas (HCC) up to 5 cm in size as well as colorectal tumors metastatic to the liver, also up to 5 cm (4 cm) in size (details below). The decision for local ablation over resection should take into account patient age, comorbidity, parenchymal reserve, and the tumor distribution in the liver weighed against the invasiveness of the procedure.

Palliative reduction of tumor mass is done for metastatic neuroendocrine tumors, for example, and is repeatedly tried on other tumor entities such as liver metastases of breast cancer. Thus, multimodal palliative local ablation is routinely employed even in patients with predominant liver metastases.[4–6] On the other hand, the principle of tumor mass reduction has been generally acknowledged and specified in guidelines only for certain tumor entities, e.g., for symptom control in neuroendocrine cancers and for symptom relief (pain and pressure) in carcinoid liver metastases.[7–14]

Local ablative treatments can be effectively combined with other procedures for both curative and palliative intent. The combination of surgical resection and ablative treatment for localized colorectal metastases with an unfavorable bilobular distribution is practiced at many centers with curative intent.

19.1.1 Hepatocellular Carcinoma

The treatment options for hepatocellular carcinoma in a cirrhotic liver are liver transplantation, partial hepatectomy, local ablative therapies, transarterial chemoembolization (TACE), radioembolization (selective internal radiation therapy [SIRT], etc.) and, in advanced stages, chemotherapy with sorafenib (Nexavar, Bayer HealthCare Pharmaceuticals).

The favorable results of percutaneous ethanol injection for HCC are attributable to the hard perifocal reaction (hepatic cirrhosis), encapsulation, and decreased portal venous blood flow causing less washout of the ethanol. However, several recent studies comparing PEI and RFA have shown that RFA yields better long-term results and requires fewer treatment sessions.[15–17] As a result, PEI has been replaced by RFA at most European centers.

The 5-year survival rates following RFA in a selected cohort with small, well-differentiated HCC are as high as 80% in our patients, although the rates in most cases were < 45%.[1,2] Two controlled, randomized studies have shown that the RFA of solitary HCCs up to 5 cm in size, or as many as three HCCs up to 3 cm in size, is comparable to surgical resection in terms of survival rates at 3 and 4 years while having a lower procedure-related mortality.[18,19] Given the significantly lower costs and invasiveness of ablation, it may be considered superior to resection in patients with localized HCC. This is particularly true in patients with preexisting portal hypertension, which is a relative contraindication to surgery. A particular advantage of ablation is that it is a parenchyma-sparing procedure. This is of major benefit in HCC patients, most of whom have a cirrhotic liver.

New multipolar ablative techniques involving the simultaneous use of several ablation probes (see below) can achieve reasonably good tumor control rates of 85% even with large HCCs up to 9 cm in diameter.[20]

Treatment concepts and protocols for hepatocellular carcinoma have been published by numerous authors and summarized, for example, in the stage-oriented treatment recommendations of the Barcelona Clinic Liver Cancer (BCLC) staging system and other systems.[21,22] The literature may be consulted for details on the differences between recommendations.[23–25]

19.1.2 Colorectal Carcinoma

In patients with colorectal metastases confined to the liver, liver resection according to S3 guidelines is indicated as a potentially curative treatment whenever an R0 resection of all metastases is technically feasible.[26,27] The 5-year survival rates after partial hepatectomy range from 25 to 45%. Approximately 70% of patients will develop a recurrence (usually intrahepatic) after the resection.[26]

Local ablative procedures with curative intent have played a growing role in the management of colorectal liver metastases in recent years. RFA may be performed alone or may be combined with resection, depending on the size of the lesions. Several cohort studies in recent years, some involving several hundred patients, have shown that RFA can not only achieve permanent local devitalization of liver metastases but can also provide 5-year survival rates of 24 to 43%.[28–30] These results are comparable to those of partial hepatectomy. This is all the more remarkable when we consider that RFA patients generally have a poorer long-term prognosis, due in part to their higher comorbidity than candidates for resection. On the other hand, the rate of intralesional recurrence, which is approximately 15% even in experienced hands using current aggressive ablative techniques (see below), is higher than the rate of surgical margin recurrence after resection (< 5–10%). But given the fact that approximately 70% of patients will develop new metastases anyway, the higher intralesional recurrence rate may have no more than a minor impact on long-term survival.

On the critical side, it should be noted that no controlled, randomized data are available on the comparison of resection and local ablative procedures. This is also reflected in current guidelines, which unfortunately do not offer any treatment recommendations.[26,27,31,32] At the same time, no controlled, randomized data have yet been published on the resection of liver metastases, which is nevertheless considered the gold standard.

> **Practice**
>
> Ultrasound-guided interventional procedures should be integrated into an overall oncologic concept, and interdisciplinary oncologic consultation is essential.
>
> The combination of minimally invasive interventional procedures with chemotherapeutic treatment strategies should be considered.

19.2 Selection of Imaging Modality (Ultrasound, CT, MRI)

Ultrasonography has established itself as the first-line imaging modality for local ablative procedures on the liver (except for LITT[33] and intraoperative cryoablation). Contrast-enhanced ultrasound is used after the intervention to evaluate response. Prerequisites are that the lesions must be accessible and clearly visible by ultrasound. CT (or MRI) is the preferred imaging modality in all cases where ultrasound guidance is not possible or is subject to significant limitations. Local expertise and personal experience should be considered in determining the modality of choice. In all cases, contrast-enhanced imaging should be used during the intervention to confirm effective treatment.

The advantages of ultrasonography are its real-time capability, making it easier to control than the static modalities of CT and MRI, its high spatial resolution, and its availability. Ultrasound has proven particularly advantageous in the puncture of subdiaphragmatic liver lesions (in which the needle is angled cephalad), as it can safely avoid accidental puncture of the pleura and lung.

19.3 Indications

Ultrasound-guided tissue ablation (e.g., of liver tumors and renal neoplasms) is technically feasible in all cases where ultrasound can define a safe access route to the lesion.

The number of tumors, their locations, and preferably their histology (grade) should be known prior to treatment so that complete tumor ablation can be accomplished in one or more steps.

19.3.1 Number of Tumors

The maximum number of tumors that can reasonably be ablated is not clearly defined but ranges from 3 to 5 at most centers.

19.3.2 Tumor Size

Again, there is no established standard for the maximum tumor size that can be ablated. The maximum size of ablatable tumors is generally in the range of 4 to 5 cm. New techniques such as the simultaneous or consecutive use of multiple ablation probes and stereotactically guided RFA can successfully treat tumors up to 10 cm in diameter.[20,34,35] Because a single ablation needle can produce necrotic zones no larger than about 2 to 3 cm (depending on the application system), multineedle systems have been introduced that can produce zones as large as 7 cm with simultaneous use. Consecutive needle use can produce even larger ablation volumes. Tumors larger than 2 cm require multineedle ablation to destroy the tumor along with a safety margin of at least 5 to 10 mm.[36,37]

19.3.3 Tumor Location

Attention must be given to vulnerable structures that border directly on the tumor or ablation zone. This particularly applies to the small intestine and colon, which are highly thermosensitive. Thermally induced bowel perforation is a feared complication of RFA. The stomach, gallbladder, and diaphragm are less thermosensitive, and tumors in proximity to these structures can generally be ablated without difficulty. The ultrasound-guided intraperitoneal injection of glucose solution to separate hollow organs from the liver surface before ablation is an established method of avoiding thermal injury (saline solution is contraindicated due to its electrical conductivity). The RFA of lesions that border directly on central bile ducts is contraindicated due to the risk of thermal injury.

Close proximity to large hepatic vessels is also problematic because these vessels are efficient heat eliminators, potentially leading to incomplete ablation or local recurrence. This problem can be solved by the concomitant, transient embolization of arterial branches supplying the liver, causing a temporary reduction in blood flow.[38] Nevertheless these procedures lack a stable evidence base.

19.4 Contraindications

The contraindications to local ablation are the same as the general contraindications to interventional procedures based on the risk and benefit for the individual patient, giving particular attention to the age, comorbidity, and desires of the patient. Acetylsalicylic acid use is no more than a relative contraindication. Clopidogrel should be discontinued before the intervention if at all possible.

The use of monopolar systems is contraindicated by cardiac pacemakers and implanted defibrillators, which must be turned off prior to ablation. Bipolar systems are safe to use in patients with active pacemakers.

Status post biliary–enteric anastomosis is a relative contraindication, as this would predispose to abscess formation in the zone of thermal necrosis. If it is decided to proceed with RFA regardless of the anastomosis, antibiotic prophylaxis should be given (see below).

Contraindications relating to tumor location were discussed in the previous section.

19.5 Preparations

19.5.1 Antibiotic Prophylaxis

Antibiotic prophylaxis with a third-generation cephalosporin (e.g., ceftriaxone, 2 g IV) or agents with a comparable spectrum can be given as a (single) bolus 30 to 60 minutes before the intervention. While this has been recommended by some authors, it is not a widely adopted practice. Prophylaxis is mandatory in patients who have had a previous biliary–enteric anastomosis or papillotomy (see above).

19.5.2 Local Anesthesia, Sedation, Sedation/Analgesia, and General Anesthesia

There is no consensus as to whether RFA should be performed under sedation, sedation/analgesia, or general anesthesia with endotracheal intubation. Nevertheless, many centers have come to favor general anesthesia, especially when treating larger tumors with multiple probes and long ablation times, because these interventions are very painful. Advantages of general anesthesia are greater patient comfort and better control of the intervention, including significantly better control of respiration during needle insertions. One disadvantage is the higher logistical cost.

Local anesthesia and sedation/analgesia follow the principles described elsewhere in this book (Chapter 11).

19.5.3 Treatment Planning

Treatment planning takes into account the size (diameter) and location of the tumor (liver segment; adjacent vessels; at-risk structures such as bowel, bile ducts, or heart), the proposed access route, and the target position of the electrodes. Preinterventional CT or MR images are usually available and should be consulted to assist planning. The patient should be placed in an optimum position; left lateral decubitus is often advantageous for lesions in the hepatic right lobe. Key considerations are the number, type, and (recommended) spacing of the electrodes, power settings, and energy levels (taking into account dosimetry tables).

In ultrasound-guided RFA using multiple probes, it should be noted that the placement of the ultrasound transducer for inserting additional probes may be hampered by probes that have already been placed. This should be anticipated at the planning stage and avoided by suitable placement strategies.

The ablation should be planned and carried out to destroy all the tumors and in addition > 5 mm (preferably > 10 mm) of normal liver parenchyma on all sides. This is necessary to avoid high rates of intralesional recurrence.[37] Accurate planning and positioning of the ablation needles is the basis for successful RFA.

19.6 Materials

19.6.1 Standard Materials

The characteristics of standard ablation systems available on the market are listed in ▶ Table 19.1. An RF generator

Table 19.1 Characteristics of ablation systems currently on the market (various combinations are possible)[49,50]

Characteristic	Description
Needle type	Smooth needle Multiple needles in one shaft Retractable multiple-tined needles Retractable coiled electrode
Mode of current application	Monopolar Bipolar (one probe), smooth or retractable Bipolar (between multiple probes)
Cooling	Not cooled Liquid-cooled through two channels Cluster-cooled
Surface	No openings Multiple side holes for fluid outflow
Control	Impedance-controlled Resistance-controlled Temperature-controlled
Current delivery	Continuous Dose alternating Consecutive between the electrodes Simultaneous to the electrodes

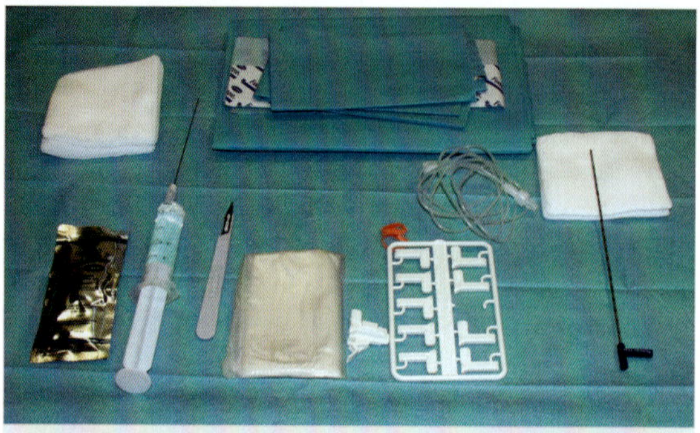

Fig. 19.2 The materials necessary for RFA are laid out on a sterile table (see text for details). The setup includes sterile sponges, draping material, sterile ultrasound gel, a transducer sheath and needle holder, and an RFA needle with irrigation system.

(from Celon/Olympus) is illustrated in ▶ Fig. 19.1. The recommended instrument setup for RFA is shown in ▶ Fig. 19.2.

19.6.2 Basic Principle

The principle of RFA involves mechanisms in which energy at a frequency of, say, 350 kHz and a power of 4 to 40 W (up to 250 W in bipolar and multipolar systems) is converted to heat within the tissue. In this principle, the tissue forms part of a high-frequency, low-resistance electrical circuit that includes a grounding pad applied to the skin (▶ Fig. 19.3).

This mechanism is like that of monopolar electrocoagulation (microarc-free “soft” coagulation), which has been applied surgically for many years. Heating occurs chiefly in the area where high-frequency fields and high-frequency currents are most concentrated. The energy transfer of high-frequency currents diminishes with the square of distance, while the heat generated at the targeted site increases linearly with the application time.

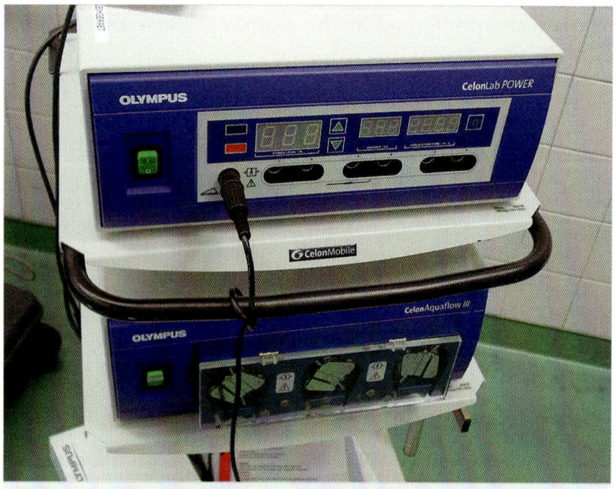

Fig. 19.1 RF generator (Celon/Olympus).

In a favorable case, the high-frequency current produced by the power control unit flows through the pathologic tissue located at the distal end of the applicator, heating the tissue to temperatures up to 100°C. This is sufficient to cause coagulation (denaturing) and necrosis of the affected tissue. The size of the ablated tissue volume depends on the applicators used, the amount of energy applied, and local tissue anatomy. The coagulated necrotic tissue is subsequently broken down and converted to scar tissue by endogenous mechanisms in the body. In this way a tumor can be completely destroyed in properly selected cases.

19.6.3 Monopolar versus Bipolar and Multipolar Systems

Monopolar systems employ a neutral electrode (grounding pad) that is applied to the body surface. The current flows between the ablation probe in the tumor and the

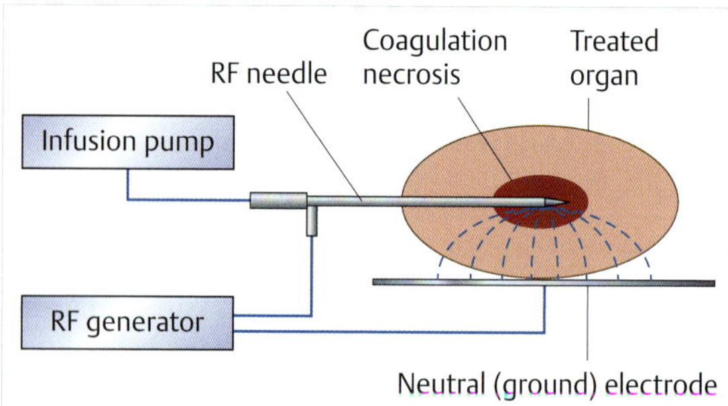

Fig. 19.3 The treated tissue is part of a high-frequency, low-resistance electrical circuit that includes a grounding pad.

neutral electrode, generating heat that is distributed concentrically around the probe.

A newer concept is bipolar RFA. In this system both electrodes are mounted close together on one probe so that all current flow occurs directly between the two probe electrodes; a neutral electrode is not required.[39] This arrangement has a number of advantages, including the fact that ablation can be performed with an active cardiac pacemaker in place, provided the ablation zone is not closely adjacent to the pacemaker. Bipolar systems also eliminate the danger of skin burns from the neutral electrode in monopolar systems. The bipolar system from Celon Medical Instruments permits the simultaneous use of up to six probes. In this system both electrodes on one probe are connected so that the probe acts as a single electrode; the six electrodes are alternately powered by the generator to coagulate all the tissue surrounding the electrodes. This multipolar mode can produce zones of tumor necrosis up to approximately 7 to 8 cm in diameter in one sitting.

A monopolar system is also available in which up to three electrodes can be used at one time in an alternating mode.

19.6.4 Needle Applicators

Needle applicators are 1 to 2 mm in diameter and have an active electrode of variable length (e.g., 20–40 mm) at their distal end (▶ Fig. 19.4) (Chapter 2).

The shaft of the needle applicator is insulated with Teflon or other insulating material. The active electrode contains a tiny cavity system that is perfused by a continuous liquid stream (▶ Fig. 19.5). The continuous perfusion protects the electrodes from overheating (optimum temperature: 80°C) and prevents complete drying or charring of the tissue in contact with the probe. In this way it preserves conductivity at the target site even during prolonged ablation. The needle applicator is connected to a high-frequency generator.

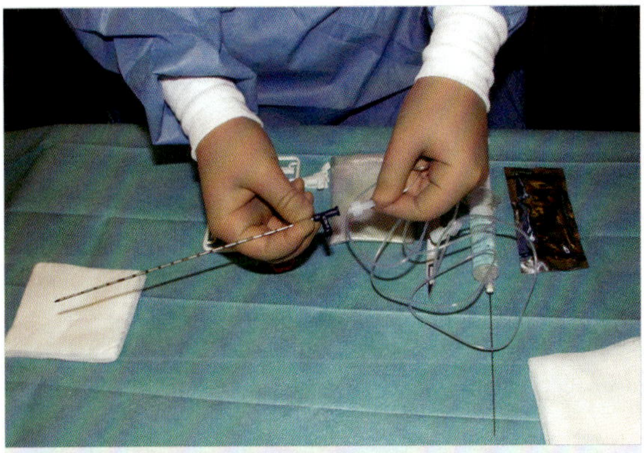

Fig. 19.4 Example of a needle applicator.

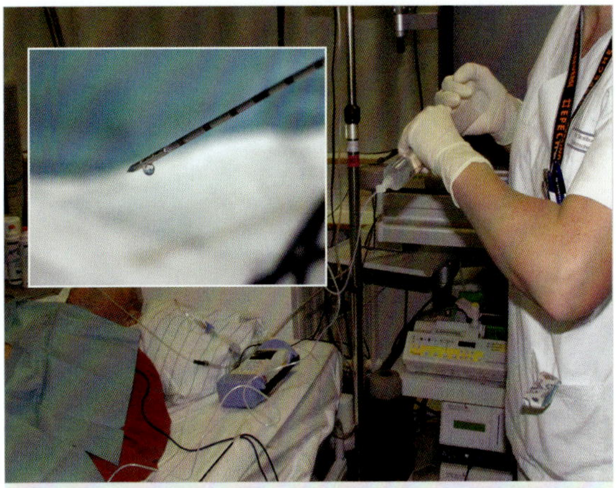

Fig. 19.5 The active electrode contains a tiny cavity system that is perfused by a continuous liquid stream.

19.6.5 Control and Temperature Measurement

Modern systems allow for continuous temperature measurement by an integrated thermal sensor in the needle tip. An autoregulation mechanism adjusts the power output to prevent overheating, evaporation, and charring at the treated site. Other systems are impedance-controlled, meaning that the power output of the generator is regulated by the tissue resistance in order to achieve the highest possible energy transfer while preventing premature drying.

Power is typically applied at approximately 40 W per ablation needle. Higher power settings have not resulted in shorter procedure times or larger ablation volumes. The needle systems are disposable, nonreusable products.

19.6.6 Flow Rate of Needle Perfusion

The flow rate in the ablation needle, at least nominally, is 80 mL/h as recommended by the manufacturer. With modern needle applicators, the flow rate of the perfusor can be adjusted on the basis of impedance changes, resulting in a bolus perfusion range of 80 to 500 mL/h.

19.7 Technique

An intercostal or subcostal approach may be used. Intervening bowel should be excluded. Transpleural puncture should also be avoided, noting that the pleural recess extends approximately 2 cm caudally past the inferior border of the lung.

19.7.1 Patient Positioning

The patient's position should remain unchanged throughout the maneuver. Hence the ultrasound-guided access

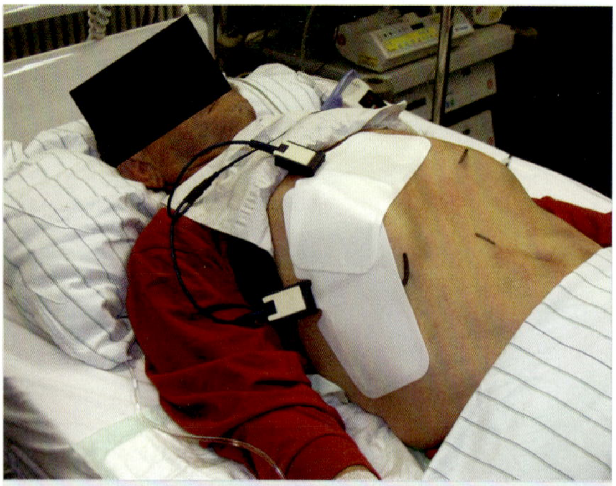

Fig. 19.6 Patient positioning.

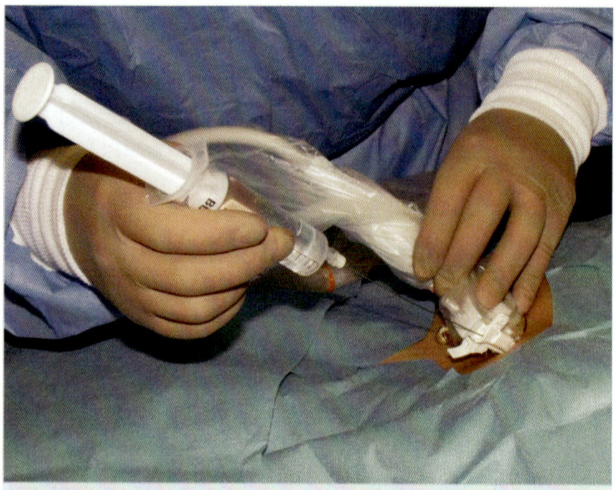

Fig. 19.7 Local anesthesia.

route should be established before the intervention. The procedure may take several hours in some cases, so the patient should be comfortably positioned. Left lateral decubitus may be optimum for sonographic access (see above and ▶ Fig. 19.6).

The needle should be introduced with the lungs at functional residual capacity, and the potential for slight needle deviation during inspiration and expiration should be considered.

19.7.2 (Local) Anesthesia

Local anesthetic should be infiltrated over a large area (if necessary, under ultrasound guidance) after raising an intracutaneous wheal. The subperitoneal tissue and liver capsule should be generously infiltrated to ensure adequate anesthesia of this very painful region (▶ Fig. 19.7).

For relatively large tumors in close proximity to portal vein branches, some operators also infiltrate intrahepatic tissue areas with local anesthetic since the interaction with portal vein branches may cause pain.

The RF needle, which is generally 1 to 2 mm in diameter, can be advanced more easily through a small stab incision, which may be deepened somewhat into connective tissue structures (▶ Fig. 19.8).

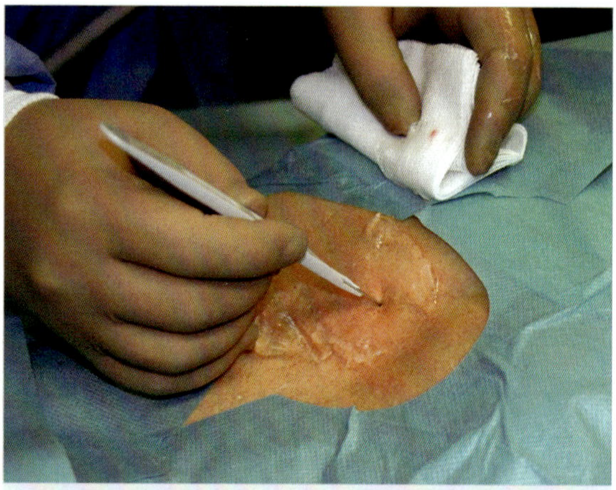

Fig. 19.8 Stab incision.

19.7.3 Probe Insertion

Radiofrequency probes (▶ Fig. 19.9, ▶ Fig. 19.10) that are cooled by continuous irrigation and possess open needle holes should be flushed ("flooded") with isotonic saline solution before insertion to prevent trapped air from obscuring the field of view. Needles in which the fluid leaves after cooling using a separate outflow channel (closed cooling system) do not require that maneuver. In a favorable case, a protective layer of liver tissue (> 10 mm) should be present between the liver surface and tumor, although recent techniques have been developed for ablating lesions that abut the liver surface.

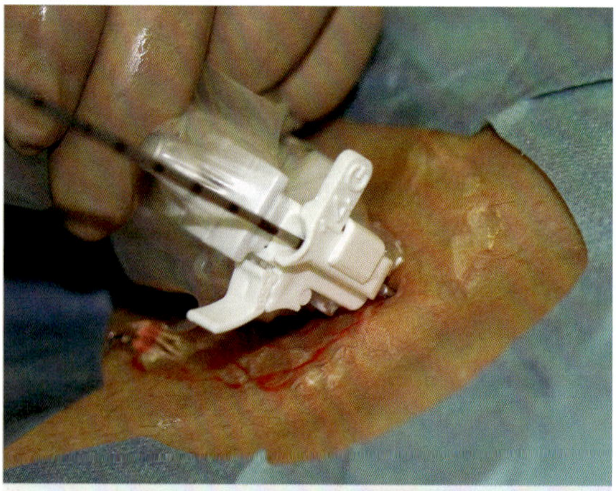

Fig. 19.9 Puncture process with application and advancement of the electrode.

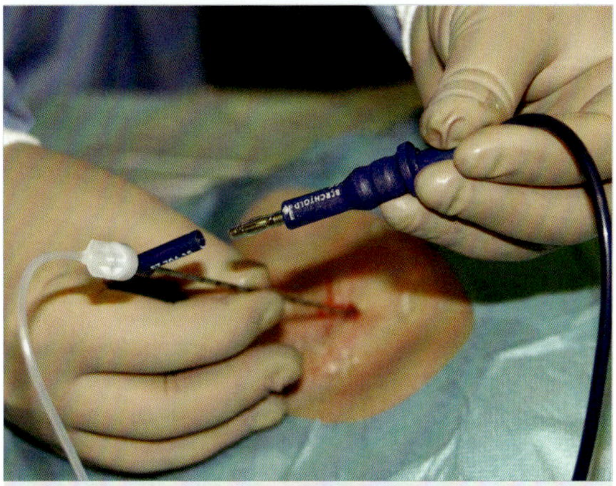

Fig. 19.10 The electrode is connected to the electrical circuit.

In the treatment of (larger) tumors, the ablation process should start at the far side of the tumor rather than its center, because the coagulated area will obscure vision. It has proven helpful to subdivide larger tumors into quadrants or spherical segments. Further treatment proceeds in the distal-to-proximal direction, working toward the transducer. In this process the needle may be progressively withdrawn at short intervals or it may be completely withdrawn into the abdominal wall and redeployed to the desired area. It must be taken into account that a three-dimensional spherical volume is treated, demanding repositioning above and below the initial ablation plane.

19.7.4 Techniques for Specific Systems

Below we describe the technique for an ablation system that we use. Other systems are equally good.

Table 19.2 Shaft and electrode lengths in the Celon system

Shaft lengths	Electrode lengths
100 mm	20/30/40 mm
150 mm	20/30/40 mm
200 mm	20/30/40 mm
250 mm	30/40 mm

CelonPOWER System

The CelonPOWER System (Olympus) was the first bipolar and multipolar ablation system for minimally invasive tumor treatment using radiofrequency-induced thermotherapy (RFITT). The system is equipped with the patented RCAP (resistance-controlled automatic power) automatic power control. By means of microprocessor-controlled evaluation of the time–resistance curve, the RCAP mode determines the maximum power uptake of the tissue, adapted to the momentary treatment status, and automatically adjusts the power control unit.

The regular shaft diameter is 15 gauge (1.8 mm). Thicker diameters are used for intraoperative needles (up to 2.1 mm). Possible shaft and electrode lengths are listed in ▶ Table 19.2

Positioning the Applicators

The percutaneous technique follows the general guidelines for interventional procedures, including draping, that are described in Chapter 10.

The injection of a protective barrier to separate the liver capsule from nearby gastrointestinal organs is necessary to avoid thermal injury to adjacent bowel (▶ Fig. 19.11). The protective medium may consist of dextrose solution (or saline solution for bipolar or multipolar technology). Air is another option, but we do not use it because it creates troublesome ultrasound artifacts.

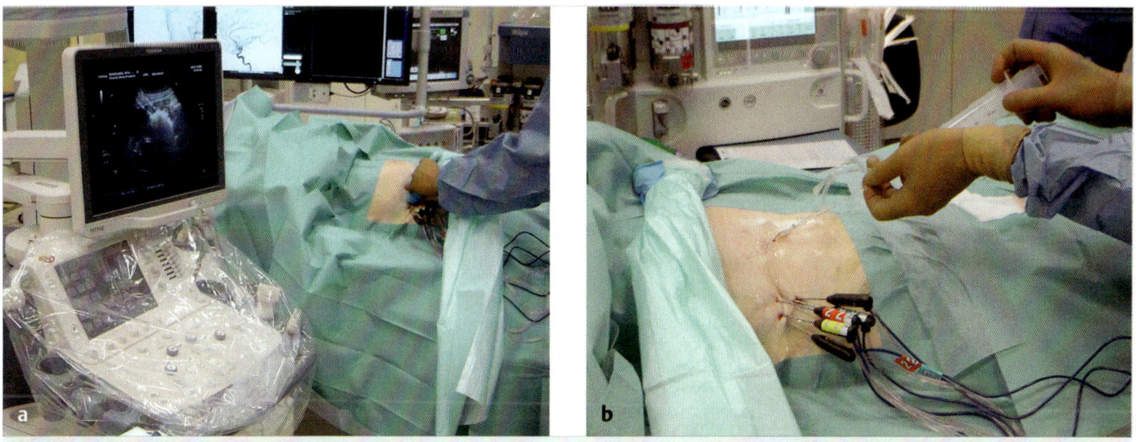

Fig. 19.11
a Typical sterile setup for ultrasound-guided multipolar RFA, in this case using five probes.
b Five percent glucose is injected through a preplaced ultrasound-guided catheter in the peritoneum to separate bowel loops from the subcapsular liver tumor.

The applicators are positioned according to the criteria described above. It may be necessary to reposition the applicator during the procedure. If the applicator tip has already "touched" the tumor, it should be activated as it is withdrawn to prevent intrahepatic seeding of tumor cells. Details on necessary system settings are presented below (Track Ablation).

Cables and hoses are connected according to user instructions. For treatment with multiple applicators, imaging should be used to check the distances between the applicators at the level of the insulators (at the center of the active electrode lengths) and compare the results with the specified treatment plan. The distance between the active electrodes is 10 to 30 mm depending on the desired ablation volumes and applied energy. Greater distances should be avoided as they may prevent confluence of the thermonecrosis zones.

RFA Technique

First the peristaltic pump is activated. The recommended power (in watts) is set in accordance with the Celon dosimetry table. For example, if three T40 electrodes (length 40 mm) are used and the recommended setting is 1 W per millimeter active electrode length, the power should be set to 120 W.

Next the generator is activated by pressing the foot switch. Once the desired energy transfer or coagulation volume has been reached, the process is halted by releasing the foot switch or pressing it again.

It may be necessary to reposition the applicators by slowly withdrawing them by a specified distance in order to achieve complete ablation. (Note: withdraw the applicator by no more than 75% of the electrode length; e.g., 3 cm for a T40 applicator). It may also be necessary to redeploy the applicators in a lateral direction to achieve complete ablation.

Track Ablation (to Avoid Tumor Seeding and Bleeding)

For track ablation a setting without needle cooling is used. Maximum temperature, resulting in carbonization of tissue, occurs causing complete destruction of the tissue close to the tract. The peristaltic pump is switched off, then the reset button is pressed briefly to deactivate the automatic power control mode (RCAP). The recommended power is set in watts in accordance with the Celon dosimetry table. For example, if a T40 electrode is used and the recommended power setting is 1 W per millimeter active electrode length, the power should be set to 40 W when the applicator is withdrawn.

With the applicator in the original position, the power control unit is activated until the rise in impedance (acoustic signal) triggers an automatic stop (pulsed tone), at which point the foot switch is released.

The applicator should be withdrawn to a length that is approximately 75% of the active electrode length (e.g., 3 cm for a T40 applicator), and the generator is restarted with the foot switch until the auto-stop is triggered. The exposure will last only a few seconds, depending on the situation.

This process is repeated until the active electrode is close to the skin surface. (*Caution:* activating the generator while the active electrode is at skin level may burn the skin.)

The track ablation procedure described above is repeated for the withdrawal of all additional applicators.

19.8 Assessing the Efficacy of Treatment

The extent of the necrotic zone cannot be clearly determined during the ablation process but it can be estimated by noting the size of the echogenic tissue zone around the electrode tip (▶ Fig. 19.12).

This provides a very imprecise estimate, however. With larger tumors, the necrotic zones produced in the individual sessions should overlap to a considerable degree, even if this increases the procedure time. In everyday practice, the necrotic zones are consistently found to be smaller than initially estimated. As an example, when a power of 40 W is applied for 15 minutes, the apparent necrotic zone will often measure 2 to 3 cm instead of the desired 3 to 4 cm.

Intraoperative use of the applicators is illustrated in ▶ Fig. 19.13 and ▶ Fig. 19.14.

Assessing the efficacy of treatment during the intervention is crucial for successful RFA. The intervention should not be concluded until the operator can confirm complete destruction of the tumor along with an adequate safety margin of surrounding liver tissue. In the case of ultrasound- or CT-guided RFA, this requires contrast-enhanced imaging confirmation during and immediately after the ablation (▶ Fig. 19.15). Only

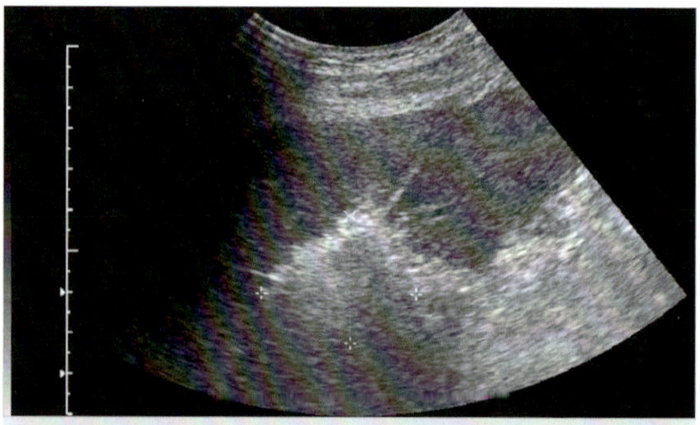

Fig. 19.12 Ultrasonography during the ablation. The necrotic zone is not clearly visualized during the ablation process, but it can be estimated from the echogenic tissue zone that forms around the electrode tip.

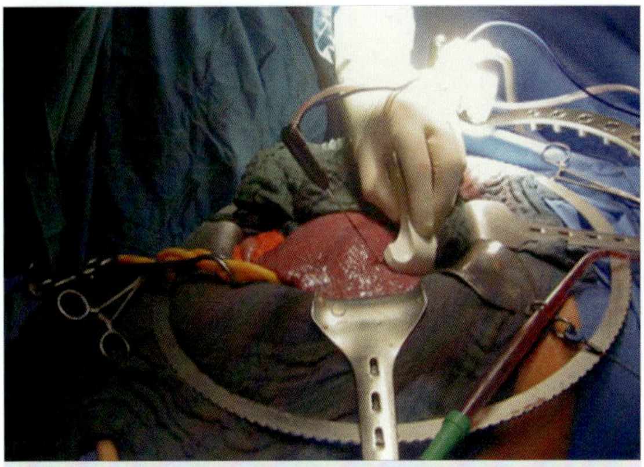

Fig. 19.13 Intraoperative probe application under ultrasound guidance.

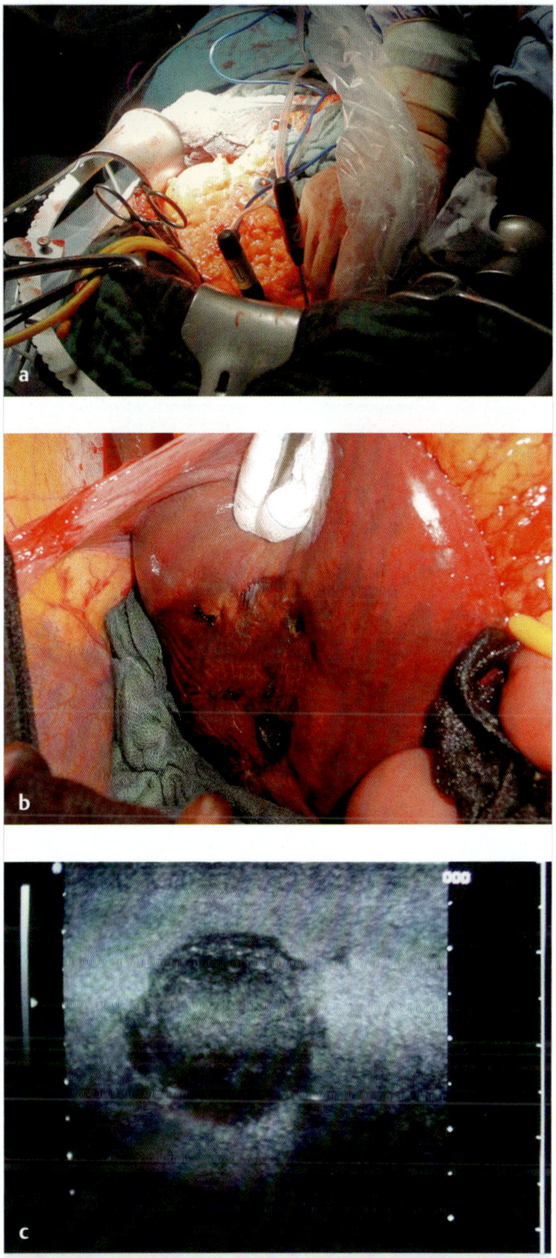

Fig. 19.14
a RF applicator in situ.
b Intraoperative view of the coagulation zones associated with different needle tracks.
c Ultrasound image to evaluate response.
(Source: Image **b** reproduced with kind permission of Professor G. Müller, Bad Mergenheim, Germany.)

contrast-enhanced imaging can define the presence and size of the necrotic zone and evaluate its exact position.

One problem in ultrasound-guided RFA is that significant gas generation occurs, obscuring vision of the ablated area. But most of the gas should be absorbed within 10 to 15 minutes after the generator is switched off, providing a clearer view of the site. While this view is often still limited, it is generally adequate for obtaining a contrast-enhanced image of the ablation zone. This post-treatment view is obtained with the probes still deployed to facilitate any repositioning and reablation that may be needed. This phase of the procedure should be performed with utmost care and precision and should be repeated if necessary until all residual tumor has been destroyed.

▶ Fig. 19.16 illustrates the sequence of a radiofrequency ablation.

19.9 Complications and Aftercare

19.9.1 Complications

Bleeding, infection, fistula formation, and tumor seeding are addressed in a separate chapter (see Chapter 9). Acute bleeding is rarely observed because small vessels are destroyed by coagulation and surrounding vessels are thrombosed. After the intervention, the patient should be positioned with the treated side down to restrict respiratory movements on that side.

Thrombosis of the hepatic veins, which could theoretically lead to pulmonary embolism, is observed very rarely. Infectious complications are also rare but may range from local infections with abscess formation to sepsis.

Tumor seeding of the needle track has been observed mainly in percutaneous ethanol injections.[40–45] On closer analysis of the literature, we note that larger needle diameters are associated with a higher risk of tumor seeding. But track ablation is always performed at the conclusion of RFA, and this significantly reduces the likelihood of tumor seeding. There have been only a few published case reports describing this complication after RFA. More details on the risk of complications can be found in Chapter 9.

It has been postulated that tumor growth may be stimulated by an incomplete ablation that leaves behind gross

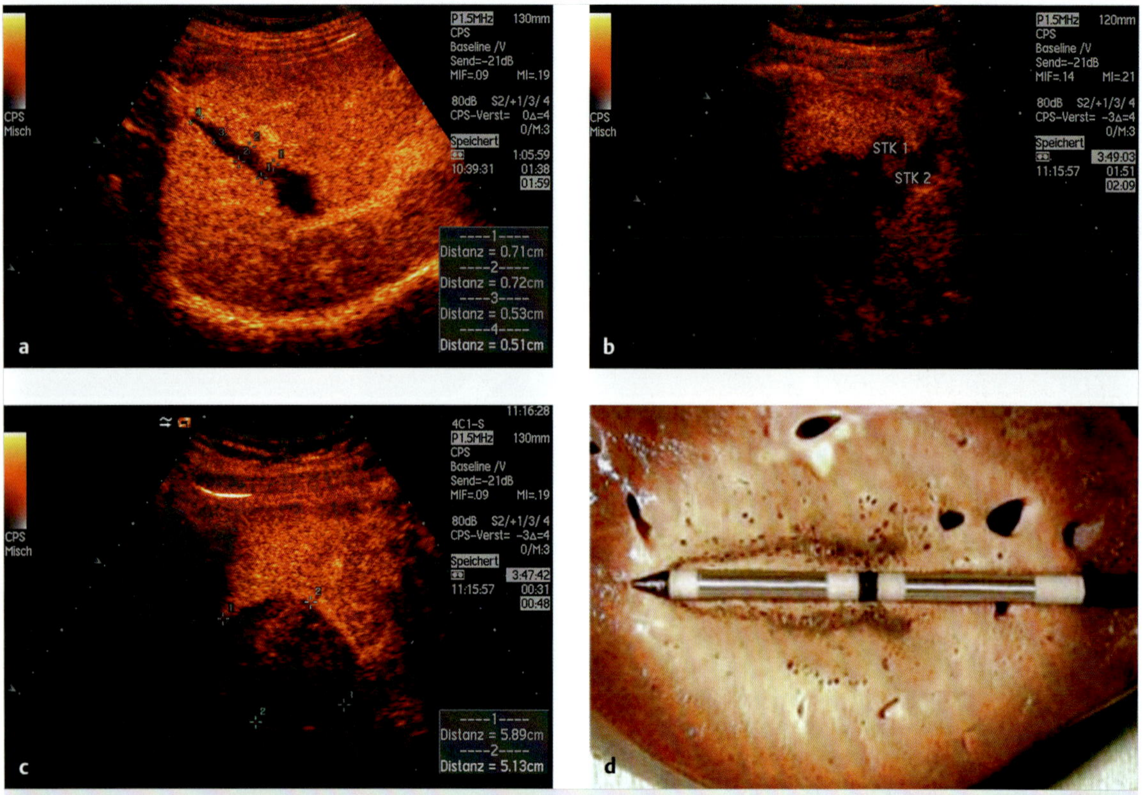

Fig. 19.15 Evaluating tumor response. (**a**, **b**) Contrast-enhanced ultrasound is a useful tool, even intraoperatively, for defining the necrotic zone around the needle, illustrated here for a single-needle system (**a**) and two-needle system (**b**). The operator should be familiar with possible artifacts (**c**). Coagulation necrosis demonstrated in a porcine liver (**d**).

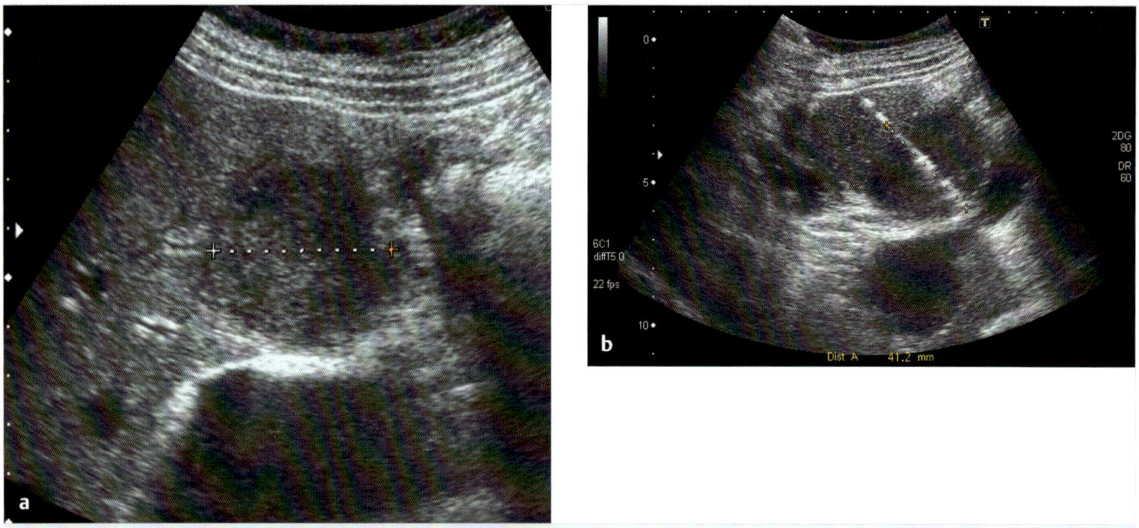

Fig. 19.16 The sequence of steps in radiofrequency ablation. Ultrasound demonstrates a liver metastasis 38 mm in diameter (**a**). Five probes are introduced (**b–f**). With the start of ablation, increasing gas generation occurs at the treatment site (**d**) until the lesion is completely obscured by shadowing (**e**). Approximately 10 minutes after ablation is completed, the gas is partially absorbed and the lesion can again be seen (**f**). The efficacy of the ablation is assessed 15 minutes later by CEUS (SonoVue) with the probes still in place. The necrotic zone measures 47 mm; this confirms complete destruction of the tumor and an adequate surrounding tissue margin. Gas artifacts are still visible in the lesion (**g**). Corresponding external photographic views of the procedure are also shown (**h**, **i**).

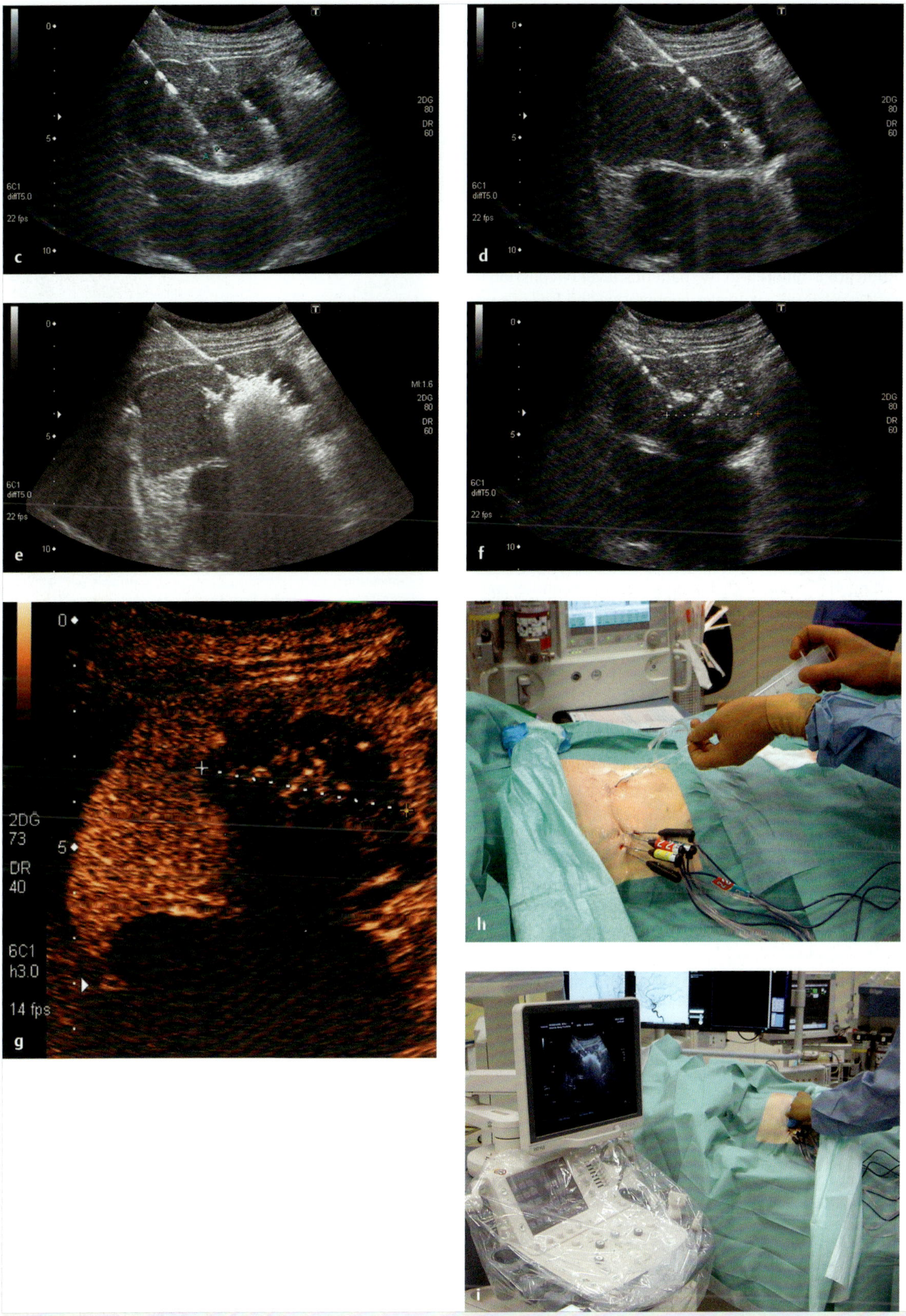

Fig. 19.16 (continued) The sequence of steps in radiofrequency ablation.

residual tumor.[46] There is no definitive answer to this question at present. The therapeutic goal should always be to achieve complete tumor destruction, however, and this is the most effective way of addressing these concerns.

19.9.2 Postinterventional Care

Several minutes after the applicators have been removed, a final ultrasound survey should be performed to exclude hemorrhage. An experienced operator can detect a possible pneumothorax at this time.[47]

Aftercare is tailored to the patient's level of consciousness. A patient who is awake, cooperative and free of pain should be positioned in lateral decubitus with the treated side down and the forearm over the puncture site (as an adjunct or alternative to a sand bag). This position is maintained for 30 minutes to 2 hours. We recommend a shorter period of immobilization that is easily monitored, followed by comfortable positioning in bed (limited bed rest with toilet visits allowed, preferably waiting until 2 to 3 hours after the procedure). A once-common recommendation was to obtain a routine blood count at 4 hours, but this is pointless since active bleeding would not produce any blood count changes by that time. Active bleeding will produce clinical manifestations and is confirmed by ultrasonography (see Management of Complications in Chapter 9).

19.9.3 Clinical Aftercare and Follow-up

Patients require close imaging follow-up after thermoablation and, if necessary, a tumor marker assay. In our follow-up regimen, the patient is reexamined at 24 hours and then every 3 months for the first year, increasing to 6-month intervals thereafter. One goal is the early detection of possible locoregional recurrence; another is the detection or exclusion of new tumors. It is essential that both entities be caught while still treatable. As a rule, very early recurrences can be successfully managed by ablation or resection, so it is essential to use the best modality available. This would be contrast-enhanced MRI or CT, with contrast-enhanced ultrasound as an alternative.[9,48]

References

[1] Kudo M. Radiofrequency ablation for hepatocellular carcinoma: updated review in 2010. Oncology 2010; 78 (Suppl 1): 113–124

[2] Zhou Y, Zhao Y, Li B et al. Meta-analysis of radiofrequency ablation versus hepatic resection for small hepatocellular carcinoma. BMC Gastroenterol 2010; 10: 78

[3] Livraghi T. Single HCC smaller than 2 cm: surgery or ablation: interventional oncologist's perspective. J Hepatobiliary Pancreat Sci 2010; 17: 425–429

[4] Abdalla EK, Vauthey JN. Colorectal metastases: resect or ablate? Ann Surg Oncol 2006; 13: 602–603

[5] Abdalla EK, Vauthey JN, Ellis LM et al. Recurrence and outcomes following hepatic resection, radiofrequency ablation, and combined resection/ablation for colorectal liver metastases. Ann Surg 2004; 239: 818–825; discussion 825–827

[6] Abdalla EK. Commentary: Radiofrequency ablation for colorectal liver metastases: do not blame the biology when it is the technology. Am J Surg 2009; 197: 737–739

[7] Ploeckinger U, Kloeppel G, Wiedenmann B, Lohmann R representatives of 21 German NET Centers. The German NET-registry: an audit on the diagnosis and therapy of neuroendocrine tumors. Neuroendocrinology 2009; 90: 349–363

[8] Auernhammer CJ, Jauch KW, Hoffmann JN. Liver metastases from neuroendocrine tumours of the gastroenteropancreatic system—therapeutic strategies [Article in German]. Zentralbl Chir 2009; 134: 410–417

[9] Dietrich CF. Comments and illustrations regarding the guidelines and good clinical practice recommendations for contrast-enhanced ultrasound (CEUS)—update 2008. Ultraschall Med 2008; 29 (Suppl 4): S188–S202

[10] Madoff DC, Gupta S, Ahrar K, Murthy R, Yao JC. Update on the management of neuroendocrine hepatic metastases. J Vasc Interv Radiol 2006; 17: 1235–1249, quiz 1250

[11] Atwell TD, Charboneau JW, Que FG et al. Treatment of neuroendocrine cancer metastatic to the liver: the role of ablative techniques. Cardiovasc Intervent Radiol 2005; 28: 409–421

[12] Aschoff AJ, Brambs HJ. Local radiofrequency ablation of liver lesions—possibilities and limitations [Article in German]. Z Gastroenterol 2005; 43: 47–56

[13] Plöckinger U, Wiedenmann B. Neuroendocrine tumours of the gastrointestinal tract [Article in German]. Z Gastroenterol 2004; 42: 517–527

[14] Siperstein AE, Berber E. Cryoablation, percutaneous alcohol injection, and radiofrequency ablation for treatment of neuroendocrine liver metastases. World J Surg 2001; 25: 693–696

[15] Lin SM, Lin CJ, Lin CC, Hsu CW, Chen YC. Radiofrequency ablation improves prognosis compared with ethanol injection for hepatocellular carcinoma < or =4 cm. Gastroenterology 2004; 127: 1714–1723

[16] Shiina S, Teratani T, Obi S et al. A randomized controlled trial of radiofrequency ablation with ethanol injection for small hepatocellular carcinoma. Gastroenterology 2005; 129: 122–130

[17] Lencioni RA, Allgaier HP, Cioni D et al. Small hepatocellular carcinoma in cirrhosis: randomized comparison of radio-frequency thermal ablation versus percutaneous ethanol injection. Radiology 2003; 228: 235–240

[18] Lü MD, Kuang M, Liang LJ et al. Surgical resection versus percutaneous thermal ablation for early-stage hepatocellular carcinoma: a randomized clinical trial [Article in Chinese]. Zhonghua Yi Xue Za Zhi 2006; 86: 801–805

[19] Chen MS, Li JQ, Zheng Y et al. A prospective randomized trial comparing percutaneous local ablative therapy and partial hepatectomy for small hepatocellular carcinoma. Ann Surg 2006; 243: 321–328

[20] Seror O, N'Kontchou G, Ibraheem M et al. Large (> or=5.0-cm) HCCs: multipolar RF ablation with three internally cooled bipolar electrodes—initial experience in 26 patients. Radiology 2008; 248: 288–296

[21] Llovet JM, Di Bisceglie AM, Bruix J et al. Panel of Experts in HCC-Design Clinical Trials. Design and endpoints of clinical trials in hepatocellular carcinoma. J Natl Cancer Inst 2008; 100: 698–711

[22] Bruix J, Sherman M. American Association for the Study of Liver Diseases. Management of hepatocellular carcinoma: an update. Hepatology 2011; 53: 1020–1022

[23] Lencioni R, Llovet JM. Modified RECIST (mRECIST) assessment for hepatocellular carcinoma. Semin Liver Dis 2010; 30: 52–60

[24] Korean Liver Cancer Study Group and National Cancer Center, Korea. Practice guidelines for management of hepatocellular carcinoma 2009 [Article in Korean]. Korean J Hepatol 2009; 15: 391–423

[25] Kudo M, Okanoue T. Japan Society of Hepatology. Management of hepatocellular carcinoma in Japan: consensus-based clinical practice

manual proposed by the Japan Society of Hepatology. Oncology 2007; 72 (Suppl 1): 2–15

[26] Schmiegel W, Reinacher-Schick A, Arnold D et al. Update S3-guideline "colorectal cancer" 2008 [Article in German]. Z Gastroenterol 2008; 46: 799–840

[27] Schmiegel W, Pox C, Reinacher-Schick A et al. Federal Committee of Physicians and Health Insurers. S3 guidelines for colorectal carcinoma: results of an evidence-based consensus conference on February 6/7, 2004 and June 8/9, 2007 (for the topics IV, VI and VII). Z Gastroenterol 2010; 48: 65–136

[28] Knudsen AR, Kannerup AS, Mortensen FV, Nielsen DT. Radiofrequency ablation of colorectal liver metastases downstaged by chemotherapy. Acta Radiol 2009; 50: 716–721

[29] Gillams AR, Lees WR. Radio-frequency ablation of colorectal liver metastases in 167 patients. Eur Radiol 2004; 14: 2261–2267

[30] Lee WS, Yun SH, Chun HK et al. Clinical outcomes of hepatic resection and radiofrequency ablation in patients with solitary colorectal liver metastasis. J Clin Gastroenterol 2008; 42: 945–949

[31] Altendorf-Hofmann A, Scheele J. A critical review of the major indicators of prognosis after resection of hepatic metastases from colorectal carcinoma. Surg Oncol Clin N Am 2003; 12: 165–192, xi

[32] Morise Z, Sugioka A, Fujita J et al. Does repeated surgery improve the prognosis of colorectal liver metastases? J Gastrointest Surg 2006; 10: 6–11

[33] Vogl TJ, Naguib NN, Eichler K, Lehnert T, Ackermann H, Mack MG. Volumetric evaluation of liver metastases after thermal ablation: long-term results following MR-guided laser-induced thermotherapy. Radiology 2008; 249: 865–871

[34] Bale R, Widmann G, Haidu M. Stereotactic radiofrequency ablation. Cardiovasc Intervent Radiol 2011; 34: 852–856

[35] Chen MH, Yang W, Yan K et al. Large liver tumors: protocol for radiofrequency ablation and its clinical application in 110 patients—mathematic model, overlapping mode, and electrode placement process. Radiology 2004; 232: 260–271

[36] Burdio F, Mulier S, Navarro A et al. Influence of approach on outcome in radiofrequency ablation of liver tumors. Surg Oncol 2008; 17: 295–299

[37] Mulier S, Ni Y, Jamart J, Ruers T, Marchal G, Michel L. Local recurrence after hepatic radiofrequency coagulation: multivariate meta-analysis and review of contributing factors. Ann Surg 2005; 242: 158–171

[38] Ritz JP, Lehmann K, Isbert C, Roggan A, Germer CT, Buhr HJ. Effectivity of laser-induced thermotherapy: in vivo comparison of arterial microembolization and complete hepatic inflow occlusion. Lasers Surg Med 2005; 36: 238–244

[39] Frericks BB, Ritz JP, Roggan A, Wolf KJ, Albrecht T. Multipolar radiofrequency ablation of hepatic tumors: initial experience. Radiology 2005; 237: 1056–1062

[40] Cedrone A, Rapaccini GL, Pompili M, Grattagliano A, Aliotta A, Trombino C. Neoplastic seeding complicating percutaneous ethanol injection for treatment of hepatocellular carcinoma. Radiology 1992; 183: 787–788

[41] Ozdil B, Akkiz H, Sandikçi M, Keçe C, Coşar A. Giant subcutaneous HCC case occurring after percutaneous ethanol injection. Turk J Gastroenterol 2009; 20: 301–302

[42] Chang S, Kim SH, Lim HK et al. Needle tract implantation after percutaneous interventional procedures in hepatocellular carcinomas: lessons learned from a 10-year experience. Korean J Radiol 2008; 9: 268–274

[43] Livraghi T, Lazzaroni S, Meloni F, Solbiati L. Risk of tumour seeding after percutaneous radiofrequency ablation for hepatocellular carcinoma. Br J Surg 2005; 92: 856–858

[44] Bolondi L, Gaiani S, Celli N, Piscaglia F. Tumor dissemination after radiofrequency ablation of hepatocellular carcinoma. Hepatology 2001; 34: 608–611, author reply 610–611

[45] Di Stasi M, Buscarini L, Livraghi T et al. Percutaneous ethanol injection in the treatment of hepatocellular carcinoma. A multicenter survey of evaluation practices and complication rates. Scand J Gastroenterol 1997; 32: 1168–1173

[46] Ruzzenente A, Manzoni GD, Molfetta M et al. Rapid progression of hepatocellular carcinoma after radiofrequency ablation. World J Gastroenterol 2004; 10: 1137–1140

[47] Dietrich CF, Hirche TO, Schreiber D, Wagner TO. Sonographie von pleura und lunge [Article in German]. Ultraschall Med 2003; 24: 303–311

[48] Claudon M, Cosgrove D, Albrecht T et al. Guidelines and good clinical practice recommendations for contrast enhanced ultrasound (CEUS) - update 2008. Ultraschall Med 2008; 29: 28–44

[49] Gottschalk U, Ignee A, Dietrich CF. Ultrasound guided interventions, part 1, diagnostic procedures [Article in German]. Z Gastroenterol 2009; 47: 682–690

[50] Gottschalk U, Ignee A, Dietrich CF. Ultrasound-guided interventions and description of the equipment [Article in German]. Z Gastroenterol 2010; 48: 1305–1316

20 Percutaneous Transhepatic Cholangiodrainage

C. F. Dietrich, B. Braden, X. W. Cui, A. Ignee

20.1 Basic Principles

Several basic methods are available for accessing the bile ducts through an interventional, nonoperative approach:

- Endoscopic retrograde cholangiography
- Percutaneous transhepatic cholangiography and drainage
- Endosonographically guided cholangiography and drainage (EUS-CD), which is discussed in Chapter 22

Today, diagnostic indications have become less important than therapeutic indications owing to the quality of imaging procedures such as EUS and magnetic resonance cholangiopancreaticography (MRCP). Endoscopic retrograde cholangiography (ERC) has become the procedure of first choice at most centers. Percutaneous transhepatic cholangiography is generally used if ERC fails for some reason or will very likely be unsuccessful. Endosonographically guided cholangiography and drainage (EUS-CD) has not yet become widely established and is practiced at only a few select centers.

Percutaneous transhepatic cholangiography (PTC) and percutaneous transhepatic cholangiodrainage (PTCD) are procedures for visualizing (by contrast injection) and treating (by drainage, dilatation, and other means) the extra- and intrahepatic biliary tree. The combination of endoscopic and percutaneous techniques is called the rendezvous technique. Rapid technical advances and refinements in instrumentation have constantly expanded interventional capabilities. PTC offers particular advantages over endoscopic drainage techniques in the hilar region and in the management of intrahepatic strictures.[1–3]

Surgery is the treatment of choice for biliary tract tumors that are amenable to primary curative treatment.

Treatment in the palliative setting (inoperable patient or high comorbidity) should be symptom-oriented. Biliary obstruction is managed by primary endoscopic treatment or alternative drainage procedures (PTCD, EUS-CD). These procedures require a shorter hospital stay than surgery. Today, even patients with benign biliary tract diseases may consistently be managed nonsurgically as a result of technical advances and growing experience with interventional techniques.

Ultrasound-guided PTC(D), with its capacity for real-time imaging in three dimensions, can provide a higher success rate and a significantly smaller number of failed attempts, especially for beginners.[4–6] It has also been shown that the added use of color Doppler ultrasound can further reduce complication rates.[7] Remarkably, however, ultrasound-guided percutaneous techniques have not become established at all institutions, especially those that continue to rely on radiography. Other arguments in favor of ultrasound guidance are a decrease in fluoroscopy time and less radiation exposure to patients and staff. The accidental puncture, for example, of the gallbladder or other cystic structures will certainly become less frequent, despite the lack of "hard" controlled data to support this claim.

The success of the procedure depends on the individual experience of the operator, the quality of the equipment, and patient-specific factors. A "two-person technique" is helpful during the placement of a drain.

20.2 Indications

In principle, endoscopic retrograde cholangiopancreatography (ERCP) has become the standard procedure and is superior to percutaneous transhepatic cholangiodrainage in its success rates and side effects, especially in nondilated bile ducts. PTC and PTCD are indicated in cases where a simpler and less risky[8,9] endoscopic procedure is not feasible for diagnosis and treatment (e.g., inaccessibility following the creation of a biliary–enteric anastomosis, a Billroth II operation, gastrectomy, hepaticojejunostomy, a Roux-en-Y choledochojejunostomy with a failed afferent limb, duodenal diverticula, etc.), or cases in which endoscopic approaches have failed (e.g., unpassable stenosis). If we include centers with experienced operators and access to specialized equipment (papillotomes and balloon-based forward-viewing enteroscopes), we find that the endoscopic approach is likely to be successful in < 70% of patients who have postsurgical anatomical changes in the gastrointestinal tract.[10] Some centers employ PTC as their primary technique for extensive hilar tumors owing to its higher success rates.

Patient selection criteria are very similar to those for endoscopic procedures (location and extent of the biliary tract obstruction and its drainage):

- Cholangiolithiasis (intra- or extrahepatic)
- Neoplasms
- Congenital anomalies
- Immune-related diseases (e.g., primary sclerosing cholangitis [PSC]) and their sequelae,[11,12] also bacterial (secondary sclerosing) cholangitis

Other indications are postoperative and other posttraumatic changes such as bile leaks and complications after liver transplantation. Biliary tract imaging may also be necessary to detect or exclude a communication in patients requiring abscess drainage or the local ablative treatment of a parasitic disease (e.g., puncture aspiration–injection of alcohol–reaspiration [PAIR], Chapter 17). Today the indication for PTC is almost always therapeutic

—the decompression of an obstructed biliary tract—and drainage procedures are most frequently performed.[13]

20.2.1 Endoscopic Retrograde or Percutaneous Approach

If surgery is not indicated in a patient with malignant obstructive jaundice, it must be decided whether to proceed with the endoscopic retrograde or percutaneous implantation of a drain or stent. Stanley (1986) compared percutaneous and endoscopic techniques alone and combined with surgical intervention and emphasized the lower rate of bleeding complications, higher patient acceptance, and avoidance of an extracorporeal catheter system as the advantages of endoscopic retrograde treatment.[14]

In 1987, Speer recommended endoscopic retrograde stenting via the papilla of Vater as a primary treatment for elderly patients in poor general health. A randomized study comparing endoscopic and percutaneous stent insertion for malignant occlusive jaundice found that the endoscopic retrograde approach was associated with a significantly higher regression of bilirubinemia and a significantly lower 30-day mortality rate.[15]

20.2.2 Rendezvous Technique

Sommer (1987) reported on the combined use of endoscopic and percutaneous approaches in the "rendezvous" technique, also viewing the placement of an internal biliary drain as the treatment of choice for malignant common duct strictures no longer curable by surgery. Here a thin drainage is placed through the liver into the duodenum for the endoscopic access and a guidewire is placed over the papilla and grasped with an endoscopic forceps. Then a prosthesis can be placed over this wire to achieve biliary drainage. In a significant proportion of patients the endoscopic access is possible without transhepatically placed wire shortly after removing the PTC drain since the papilla has been slightly dilated and can be intubated easily. With this technique, a stent can be placed even after Billroth II surgery or with a duodenal diverticulum restricting endoscopic papillary access, and long proximal stenoses can be crossed and stented.[16] In 1985, Shorvon described a successful papillotomy using the rendezvous technique in 10 of 11 cases where endoscopic technique had failed due to large duodenal diverticula or a prior Billroth II gastrectomy.[17] Another advantage of the rendezvous technique, noted by Hauenstein, is the ability to place a large-bore endoprosthetic stent without painful dilatation of the percutaneous transhepatic tract.[18,19] Indications for the percutaneous implantation of biliary drains are listed in ▶ Table 20.1.

20.3 Contraindications

PTCD has the same contraindications as any liver puncture. Lack of informed consent, comorbidity that affects prognosis, coagulation disorders (Quick prothrombin < 50%, PTT > 50 seconds), and thrombopenia ($< 50 \times 10^9$/L) should be corrected prior to the intervention. The presence of ascites (decompensated hepatic cirrhosis with neoplasia) may necessitate preliminary fluid drainage if conservative therapies are unsuccessful

Table 20.1 Indications for the percutaneous implantation of biliary drains

State/Intention	Situation
Preoperative when endoscopic retrograde approach is not possible	• Acute cholangitis with existing or impending sepsis • Precise localization of an obstruction, possibly with histologic confirmation of the tumor and peripheral tumor boundaries (Klatskin tumors) to assess local operability (cholangioscopy) • *Comment:* Posthepatic jaundice with dilated intrahepatic bile ducts and bilirubin levels > 85.52 µmol/L (5 mg/dL) is no longer considered an indication for ERCP/PTCD to improve general patient status prior to surgery[62–66]
Curative	• Stone extraction when endoscopic retrograde approach is not possible: ◦ Dormia basket passed under fluoroscopic guidance or through the working channel of a cholangioscope ◦ Contact lithotripsy with a piezoelectric probe through the working channel of a cholangioscope • Temporary drainage and splinting for iatrogenic bile duct injury or for postoperative or inflammatory stenosis • Afterloading intracavitary radiation treatment of proximal bile duct carcinoma (Klatskin tumor)
Palliative	• Severe pruritus • Cholangitis with existing or impending sepsis • Quality-of-life improvement enabling patients to return home sooner • Improvement of digestion • Confirm a tumor and exclude an inflammatory cause • Exclude the possibility of a curative procedure • Temporary drainage in cases treatable and potentially curable by chemotherapy or radiation (e.g., lymphoma)

(Chapter 13). Ascites is associated with an increased risk of biliary peritonitis and hemorrhage. Contrast allergy is considered a relative contraindication and, if the procedure is definitely required, calls for suitable premedication with corticosteroids and antihistamines (e.g., 150 mg prednisolone, H_1 and H_2 blockers) following adequate informed consent. Contraindications should be viewed as relative in septic patients and when no alternatives are available.

20.4 Materials and Equipment

20.4.1 Description of Materials

The following are required:

- Fluoroscopy unit
- Sterile gloves, gown, and drapes
- Sterile ultrasound probe covers
- Sterile table with sufficient sponges
- Hypodermic needle, 22 gauge, 0.7 mm diameter, length 3 cm (Braun Melsungen)
- Large supply of 5-mL, 10-mL, and 20-mL syringes, assorted syringe volumes for different fluids to avoid confusion: e.g., local anesthetic (5-mL syringes), 0.9% isotonic saline solution (10-mL syringes), and radiographic contrast medium (20-mL syringes)
- Local anesthetic such as 1% prilocaine hydrochloride
- Radiographic contrast medium such as Conray 30 (Mallinckrodt Medical), 50 mL
- Sterile dishes for 0.9% NaCl
- One three-way stopcock
- Saline solution, 50 mL
- Skin prep solution such as octenidene (Octenisept, Schuelke), scalpel (pointed), needle holders, scissors, forceps, dressing and sponge holding forceps
- Hollow needles with stylet (e.g., Chiba needles), 20 gauge and/or 22 gauge
- Wire, 60 to 90 cm, 0.018-inch, soft with very soft tip
- Wire, 90 cm, 0.035-inch, stiff with soft tip
- Insertion catheter, 5F or 6F, straight, mounted on blunt metal cannula
- Dilators, 8F and 10F
- Internal/external drainage catheter; 8F, 10F or 12F, with pigtail and side holes for long-term drainage (e.g., Biliary Plus drain, Peter Pflugbeil)
- Collecting bag
- Suture material, Mersilene 0 MH plus, 36 mm 1/2 c, polyester (Ethicon)
- Dressing material

▸ **Puncture needles.** Suitable types: 22-gauge Chiba needle, diameter 0.7 mm, length 22 mm, disposable (Pajunk); 20-gauge puncture needle (1.1 mm), length 20 cm; 18-gauge puncture needle (1.3 mm), length 20 cm with inserted movable trocar (Pajunk). It should be noted that 20-gauge needles deliver a better steering and ultrasound visibility despite the 22-gauge needle being the standard version. In the standard procedure a blind puncture technique is used, demanding several needle passes. US-PTCD is frequently performed with 1 or 2 needle passes.

▸ **Guidewires.** The classic standard guidewires for PTCD are 0.018-inch, length 60 cm for changing from the puncture needle to the insertion set, and 0.035-inch, length 90 cm. Guidewires longer than 90 cm are more cumbersome to handle (Chapter 22). Other guidewires are available for special applications: straight, 0.018-inch, nitinol, platinum tip, length 120 cm (OptiMed); Terumo guidewire, curved, 0.035-inch, flexible 10-mm tip, length 180 cm (Terumo Europe); stiff guidewire, Bardselect Ultra-Torque GW (Black Wire), 0.035-inch, flexible 8-cm tip, length 145 cm (Bard Angiomed). The usage of uncoated wires in puncture needles is recommended to avoid shearing of the coating.

▸ **Insertion set.** PTC drainage set loop catheter, length 40 cm, 6F (2 mm) or 7F (2.33 mm) (Bard Angiomed); 6F or 20201 051 (7F) bile duct initial puncture set with platinum marker, catheter diameter 6F, catheter length 20 cm, guidewire 0.018-inch, length 80 cm (OptiMed) or Dilplus metal dilator with 5F Teflon catheter, length 27 cm (Peter Pflugbeil).

▸ **Dilators.** 6F to 10F dilators (e.g., Bard Angiomed); Nimura bile duct dilator, 8F to 16F, length 60 cm (Peter Pflugbeil).

▸ **Drainage sets.** 8F to18F with side holes, length 34 cm (distance from skin 7.5 cm) with connecting tube, sealing cap and skin plate (Peter Pflugbeil). Other sets for PTCD are available from various suppliers (Cook Medical, Endoflex, and many others). The sets usually include a puncture needle, two wires, a dilator, and a PTCD catheter (angled ring catheter with a pigtail end and multiple side holes). Generally the catheters are available in sizes from 7F to 10F (or 12F). Some companies also offer introducer drains, usually consisting of a 5F catheter with a straight end that can function as a sheath. We have had good results with the Pflugbeil system, in which the Teflon catheter is mounted on a blunt metal dilator allowing for uncomplicated insertion of the drain. The sheath material also allows it to remain indwelling for some time. When the drains are placed under ultrasound guidance, it is helpful to choose the best introducing cannula for that purpose. A 20-gauge cannula with an echogenic tip is ideal, while a standard 22-gauge cannula is often difficult to image with ultrasound. We prefer to assemble a customized set. Ours consists of a 20F Chiba needle plus a 60-cm-long 0.018-inch guidewire, a 90-cm-long 0.035-inch guidewire, two dilators (8F and 10F, each 20 cm long), a 10F Biliary Plus angled drainage catheter (30 cm,

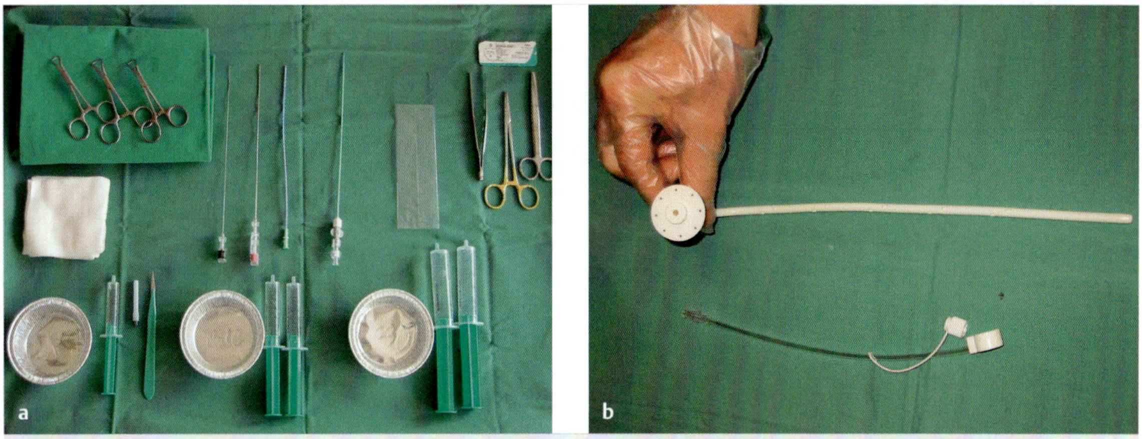

Fig. 20.1
a Materials required for percutaneous transhepatic cholangiography and drainage (PTCD).
b Munich drain (Peter Pflugbeil), size 12F.

24 side holes, pigtail with 9.5-cm perforated distal end), and a Dilplus Teflon catheter (27 cm, 5F) mounted on a metal dilator (Peter Pflugbeil).

Materials necessary for percutaneous transhepatic cholangiography and drainage (PTCD) are illustrated in ▶ Fig. 20.1.

20.5 Technique

Three basic methods of biliary tract drainage are available and can be combined with one another as needed:

- Purely external percutaneous biliary drainage
- Combined internal and external drainage
- Placement of an endoprosthesis or stent without necessity of percutaneous tract for internal drainage of the bile ducts

A combined approach can lengthen survival time by approximately 3 months over external drainage alone, but the real breakthrough came with the introduction of large-bore endoprosthetic stents.[19]

Biliary stenting has the following advantages over external catheter drainage:

- Greater drainage efficiency due to the larger lumen
- No bile loss from the enterohepatic circulation
- Better patient tolerance
- No problems with drain migration or dislodgment
- No need for daily flushing with NaCl
- Less risk of contamination from duodenal juice in the bile ducts, no aspiration of duodenal juice
- Preservation of papillary function, also with respect to the pancreatic duct

PTCD is a percutaneous procedure that includes the following basic steps. A percutaneous needle is introduced into a bile duct and contrast medium is injected. Next a sheath is inserted into the bile duct, with or without additional contrast injection (cholangiography); the papilla is crossed and permanent drainage is established (drain placement).

These steps may be completed in one intervention or in multiple stages. Analogous to surgical treatment, a multistage approach is advisable in critically ill patients. In a septic patient, for example, primary external drainage is done to decompress the bile ducts. Once the patient has improved clinically, internal drainage can be established.

The complete procedure is outlined below:

1. Benefits (target parameters, indications) are weighed against risks (risk factors and contraindications) taking into account possible alternatives (endoscopic treatment, including EUS-CD, and surgery). The steps in the procedure are described and informed consent is obtained.
2. Preinterventional imaging results are reviewed (conventional sonography, ERC attempts, MRCP), and an optimum access route is identified.
3. Coagulation status is assessed (see under Contraindications above); blood typing is optional according to individual patient risk.
4. Preinterventional antibiotic therapy is planned (to select a suitable antibiotic that is excreted in the bile, such as ceftriaxone or ciprofloxacin).
5. Current endocarditis guidelines are reviewed.
6. The patient is adequately fasted before the procedure (generally 6 hours).
7. Instrument and equipment setups are prepared.
8. Standard sedation/analgesia is prepared with propofol (e.g., initial additional bolus of midazolam, 1–2.5 mg IV), fractionated during continuous pulse oximetry, circulatory monitoring, and assessment of consciousness (level of sedation; see Chapters 11 and 22). Analgesic use is optional but is widely practiced (e.g., meperidine hydrochloride [pethidine], 50 mg, or another morphine derivative).

9. The patient is positioned supine on the fluoroscopy table.
10. The puncture site is localized with ultrasound (right intercostal, epigastric).
11. Local anesthesia is administered and the skin incision is made.
12. The needle is introduced under ultrasound guidance.
13. Bile is sampled (optional).
14. Contrast injection and fluoroscopy are carried out and documented.
15. A 0.018-inch guidewire is introduced.
16. A sheath is inserted (e.g., Dilplus, Peter Pflugbeil) to exchange for a 0.035-inch catheter, and access is secured for further manipulations (internalization).
17. The needle tract is dilated with Seldinger technique up to or up to 2F less than the proposed drain size.
18. The percutaneous biliary drain is placed and its placement is documented.
19. The incision is sutured and dressed.
20. The drainage setup is completed.
21. Postinterventional monitoring protocol after sedation/analgesia is implemented.
22. Drain care is recommended (flushed several times daily, at least twice, and output is recorded; in case of internal–external drainage, decision for complete internal drainage or external drainage).
23. Further interventional management is planned including internalization of drainage (or long-term drainage with drain changes at approximate 3-month intervals), metal stent insertion, lithotripsy (may include cholangioscopy), and other procedures such as photodynamic therapy or brachytherapy.

20.5.1 Patient Positioning

The patient position and equipment setup are illustrated in ▶ Fig. 20.2.

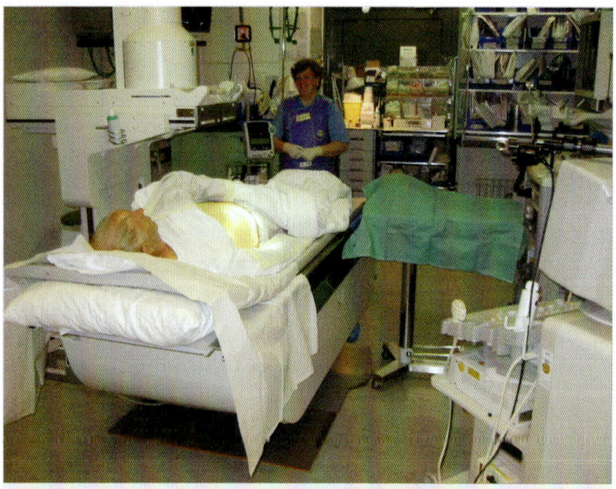

Fig. 20.2 Patient positioning and equipment setup (ultrasound scanner, fluoroscopy unit, monitoring unit, instrumentation). The instrument stand, ultrasound scanner, C-arm fluoroscopy unit, and operator stool are shown.

20.5.2 Needle Insertion and Drainage

Puncture Site and Access Route

The location of the puncture site conforms to drainage requirements (left or right lobe of the liver). The puncture site may be intercostal (10th–11th intercostal space); right anterolateral (just anterior to the midaxillary line, usually caudal to the 10th rib), for drainage of the right hepatic duct and its anterior and posterior side branches; or epigastric (subcostal) for drainage of the left hepatic duct. The angle of needle insertion (horizontal and slightly cephalad) should ensure that the needle tip will enter a peripheral bile duct at an approximately parallel (tangential) angle. Color Doppler imaging is helpful for avoiding the undesired puncture of portal vein branches.

Needle Orientation for Conventional PTCD

For an intercostal approach directed toward the porta hepatis, the needle is oriented roughly horizontal to the radiography table (and perhaps angled slightly cephalad), aiming it toward the contralateral shoulder or the transverse process of the T12 (or L1) vertebral body.[20] With an epigastric approach, the needle is directed toward the porta hepatis while angled approximately 30° to 50° to the table surface.

Local Anesthesia

Local anesthetic is infiltrated down to the liver capsule (22-gauge needle with 10 mL of 1% prilocaine hydrochloride). The needle is introduced along the superior border of the lower rib to avoid injury to intercostal nerves and vessels (▶ Fig. 20.3).

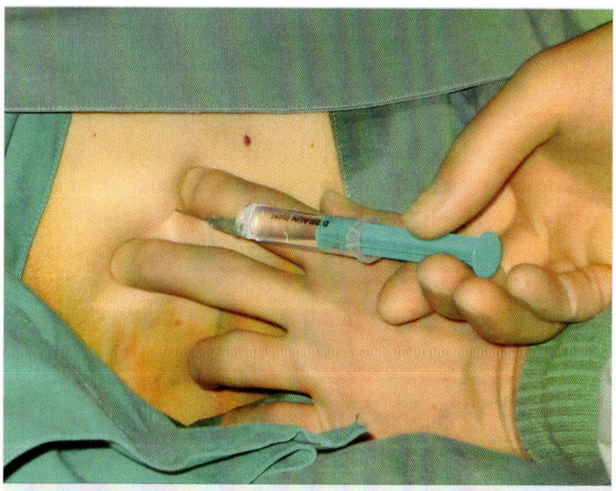

Fig. 20.3 A stab incision is made following local anesthesia.

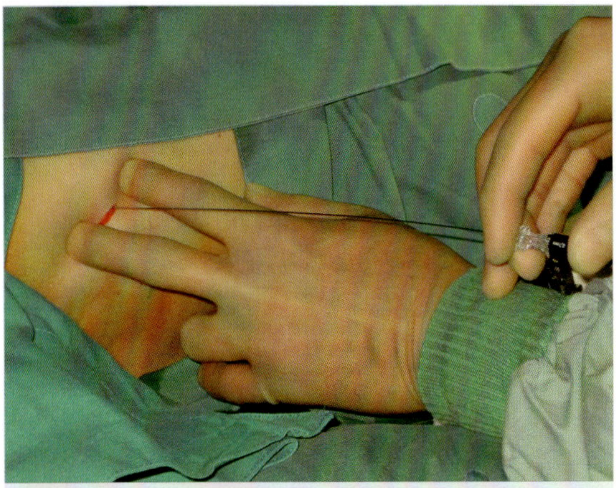

Fig. 20.4 A 0.7-mm Chiba needle is introduced blindly, without ultrasound guidance, along the superior border of the lower rib in the intercostal space.

Conventional Puncture of the Biliary Tree and Cholangiography

The biliary tree can be punctured in one or two steps using a single-needle or two-needle technique. The puncture needle is advanced into a peripheral bile duct under ultrasound guidance or 4 to 6 cm deep to the liver capsule using "blind" fluoroscopic technique. Bile aspiration is attempted with a syringe. Thereafter and during further needle withdrawal, contrast medium is injected to define the biliary tree (▶ Fig. 20.4).

Single-Needle Technique

An atraumatic 22-gauge (0.7-mm) Chiba needle is inserted into a peripheral bile duct in the sedated patient using freehand technique. An alternative is to use a larger-bore 18- or 20-gauge trocar system (1.1–1.3 mm; the 18-gauge needle will accommodate a 0.035-inch guidewire). As the needle is withdrawn after trocar removal, the escape of typical viscous biliary fluid will confirm correct placement. The bile is assessed for its color (turbidity), consistency, and odor, and a sample may be collected for microbiological analysis (Gram stain, culture, susceptibility testing). A small amount (0.5–2 mL) of contrast medium (e.g., Conray) can be injected to define the bile ducts (cholangiography). At this point a 5F (or 4F) sheath is introduced over a 0.018-inch guidewire to permit the insertion of a 0.035-inch wire.

Two-Needle Technique

This technique has become largely obsolete and is rarely practiced today. It involves two separate steps: primary puncture of the biliary tract with an atraumatic 22-gauge (0.7-mm) Chiba needle and contrast injection (cholangiography), followed by the insertion of a larger 18-gauge (1.3-mm) trocar system while the 22-gauge needle is still in place. The second needle is inserted parallel to the initial needle under fluoroscopic guidance.

We prefer a combination of sonographic and fluoroscopic guidance for the primary puncture of markedly distended intrahepatic bile ducts (> 5 mm) with an 18-gauge (1.3-mm) needle—or with a 20-gauge (1.1-mm) needle—followed by the fluoroscopically guided intervention. An ultrasound-guided puncture requires fewer needle passes than the conventional technique, so the primary use of a thicker needle poses no difficulty. In selected cases the entire procedure can be performed under ultrasound guidance alone, using a suitable ultrasound contrast agent (0.2 mL SonoVue [or less] in 10 mL of saline solution, swirled slowly). It should be noted that the needle tip echo may be displayed slightly distal to the actual tip position. As a rule, a 20-gauge needle is easier to see with ultrasound and is easier to control than needles with a smaller diameter.

There is still no demonstration of the superiority of one technique over another in terms of success rate, complication rate, or procedure time. Rotating the fluoroscopy unit (or repositioning the patient on the X-ray table) can provide three-dimensional orientation with respect to the opacified biliary tree.

Technique of Ultrasound-Guided PTCD

In ultrasound-guided PTCD, the initial puncture is performed under sonographic guidance (▶ Fig. 20.5, ▶ Fig. 20.6, ▶ Fig. 20.7).

In the "blind" puncture of peripheral bile ducts, major complications have been described in 2% of cholangiographies and in 10% of percutaneous interventions (e.g., sepsis, hemorrhage, abscess formation, peritonitis, hematobilia, especially in punctures close to the porta hepatis). On the other hand, complication rates depend significantly on patient comorbidity and operator experience. Ultrasound-guided PTCD has been described for dilated and nondilated bile ducts (e.g., postoperative bile leaks).[21,22] Several studies have shown a reduction of complication rates and particularly more rapid access to the bile ducts. Nevertheless, there is still no consensus on this score, and a preference for ultrasound-guided or unguided PTCD will depend on local priorities.[4,23–25]

Ultrasound can be used effectively at the start of the intervention to locate a bile duct that is ideally accessible. A trade-off must be made between the caliber of the bile duct and a needle path that is not too close to the main bile duct. In an ultrasound-guided puncture, the rates of complications and hemorrhage are less important considerations than stable positioning of the sheath. This is essential to ensure that the sheath is not displaced when the thin wire is exchanged for a thicker wire. For this reason, we target a relatively thin (peripheral) bile duct segment that runs at a 30° to 45° angle to the direction of needle insertion to facilitate puncture of the compliant

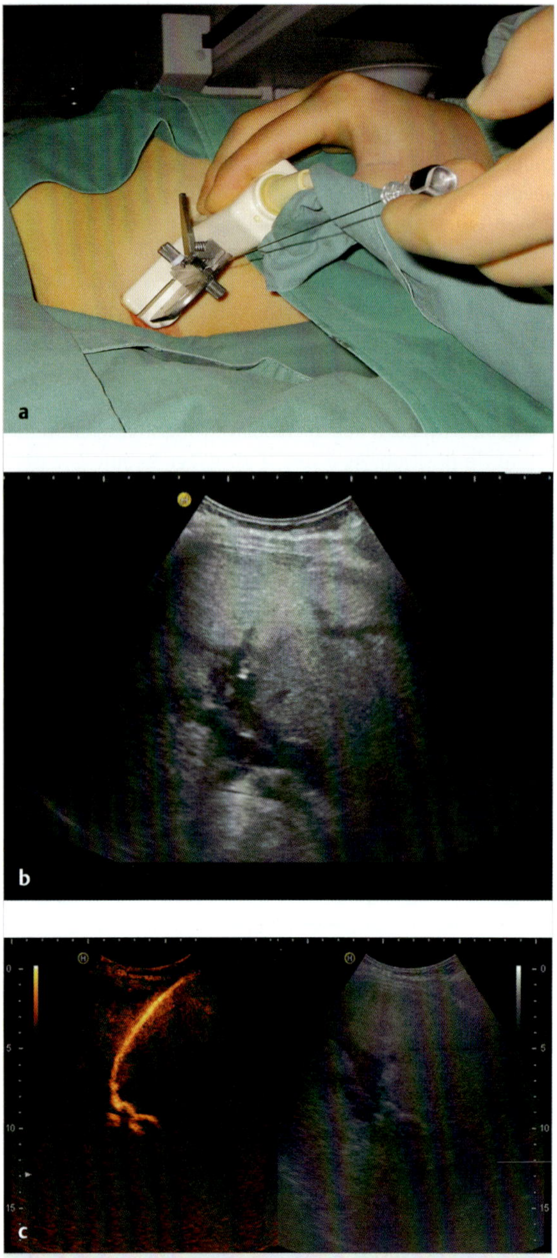

Fig. 20.5 The needle is introduced under ultrasound guidance, again at the superior border of the lower rib in the intercostal space.
a Puncture site.
b The needle is advanced to the targeted bile duct under sonographic guidance.
c Contrast administration (SonoVue) confirms correct placement in the bile duct.

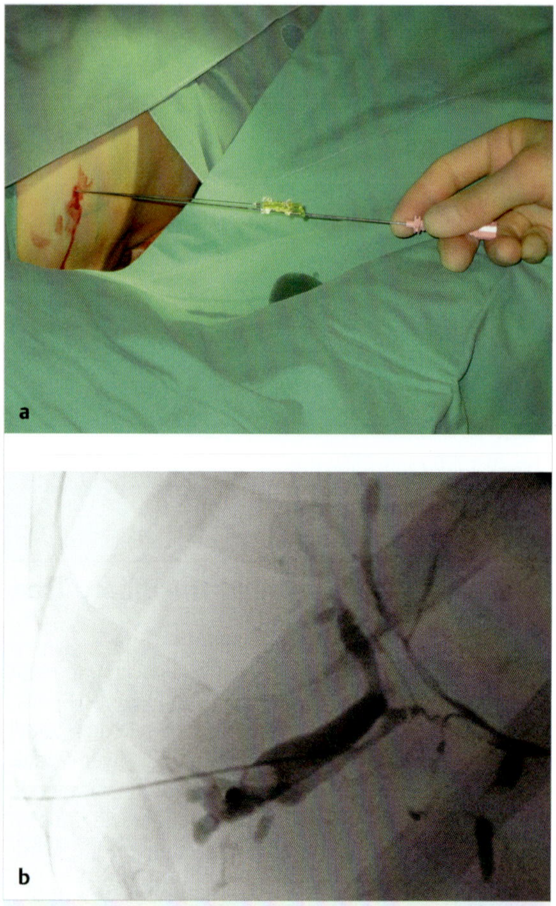

Fig. 20.6
a The trocar is removed. Escaping bile is inspected, and viscous bile of different coloration is collected for further analysis.
b Contrast medium opacifies the bile ducts for fluoroscopic documentation.

duct wall. The targeted duct should lie at a depth of 2 to 6 cm measured from the liver capsule.

Whether the needle is introduced through a biopsy transducer, through a needle guide, or freehand is a matter of operator preference. Ultrasound guidance makes it safe to use a thicker and more stable needle than the standard 22-gauge. Another advantage of the thicker needle is better ultrasound visualization. Ultrasound permits the primary use of an 18-gauge needle in a higher percentage of cases. This eliminates the need for an 0.018-inch wire, reducing costs and procedure times. Once the wire is in the biliary tract, the rest of the procedure is analogous to conventional technique.

Incorrect Needle Placement

If the initial needle placement is incorrect, as evidenced by parenchymography or contrast flow toward the periphery (arterial puncture) or toward the inferior vena cava (venous puncture), the needle can be slowly withdrawn with a contrast syringe attached while contrast medium is injected under fluoroscopic (or sonographic) guidance to confirm an intracanalicular position of the needle. If the needle cannot be maneuvered into a bile duct, it should be removed, the trocar reinserted, and the

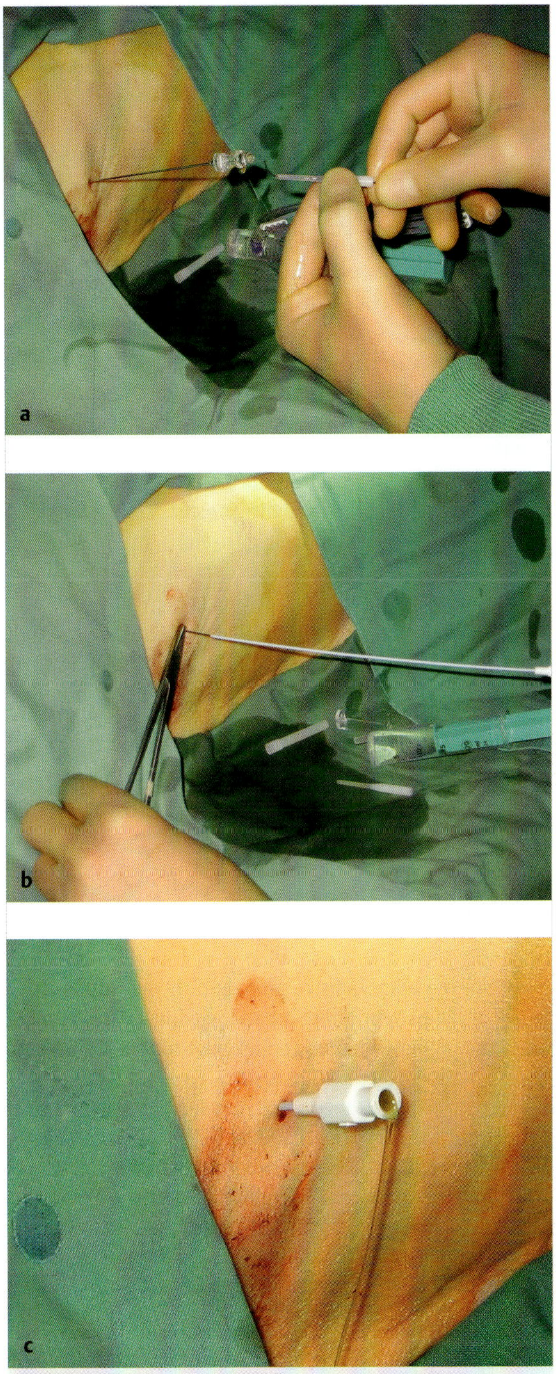

Fig. 20.7
a The guidewire is advanced into the bile ducts under sonographic or fluoroscopic guidance.
b The puncture needle is removed and the wire is secured at skin level (e.g., with a clamp). A lubricated 5F Teflon sheath is introduced over the wire into the bile ducts.
c Bile drips from the sheath, confirming correct placement.

puncture repeated while aiming the needle in a slightly different direction.

When frank cholangitis is present, biliary tract opacification should be done carefully and sparingly to avoid the risk of sepsis.

Confirming Correct Needle Placement and Planning the Procedure

When it has been confirmed that the needle is in the bile ducts, the next step in the standard technique is to introduce a lubricated 0.018-inch (0.46-mm) guidewire (e.g., OptiMed), followed by sheath insertion and exchange of the smaller wire for a 0.035-inch (0.89-mm) wire. This wire exchange does not require dilation of the access tract.

The wire is introduced primarily into the intrahepatic bile ducts and, in favorable cases, can be advanced through the stenosis and extrahepatic bile ducts and into the duodenum. This cannot always be done primarily, however. While the 0.035-inch guidewire is secured at skin level, and held in place with a clamp if necessary, a lubricated 5F Teflon sheath is introduced over the wire (generally without dilation) and is advanced distal to the stenosis if possible. The inner diameter of the 5F Teflon sheath will also accommodate the passage of 0.038-inch guidewires. This catheter may serve as an external drainage catheter for one or two nights, though it is not intended primarily for that purpose. Generally it is not durable enough for prolonged drainage. In principle, all further manipulations will be performed using the drainage catheter as an access sheath.

Some operators use special puncture sets in which a shorter catheter is premounted on a 40-cm-long Chiba needle. The advantage of this setup is that once the needle has entered the duct system, a catheter can be advanced immediately and atraumatically into the ducts and a 0.035-inch guidewire can be introduced for further dilation.

With a firm stenosis, it may be necessary to change to a steel wire (e.g., BardSelect from Bard Angiomed) or a stiff Teflon-coated guidewire (Lunderquist guidewire, Cook Medical). Wires with a flexible soft tip may be helpful in crossing tumor strictures. ERCP wires can be used in principle, but they are unwieldy due to their great length (260–400 cm) and are more expensive. The wires used for PTCD are usually 90 cm long and therefore cheaper. Another option is special wires with high stiffness and torque stability; these wires are not flexible enough for endoscopic use.

Contrast injection to define the biliary tree now permits an accurate assessment and selection of treatment mode: external drainage, combined external–internal drainage, or primary internal drainage alone. Primary internal drainage is preferred over external–internal drainage, which in turn is preferable to external drainage

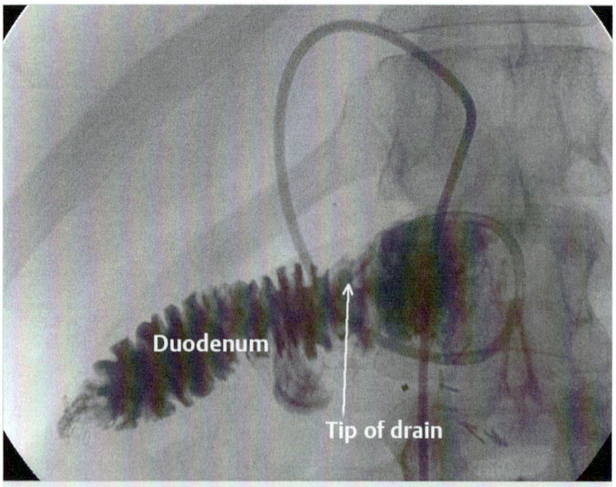

Fig. 20.8 The catheter is advanced over the wire toward the duodenum under fluoroscopic guidance. The dilated bile ducts proximal to the stenosis are no longer opacified.

alone, especially for the prevention of bile loss (▶ Fig. 20.8).

Dilation with Sheaths and Dilators (Seldinger Technique)

At this point the access tract is dilated over the guidewire (usually to a maximum of 10F in the first sitting). It should be dilated to a width around 2F less than the diameter of the drainage catheter. (Some operators dilate to the exact diameter of the drainage catheter.) Soft stenoses can be dilated with 5F to 10F Teflon sheaths. Dilators of the Nimura type (8F–16F, 60 cm long) have proven effective for hard strictures.

Yamakawa Drain, Munich Drain, Frimberger Drain, and Others

Polyethylene and polyurethane catheters can be used for biliary fluid drainage. Various models are available for external and internal–external drainage. A pigtail tip is generally used to prevent migration. Bile can be drained with catheter sizes from 8F to 16F. Drainage holes vary in their number and pattern, depending on the manufacturer.

The Yamakawa drain functions basically as an internal–external drain. Distinctive features are its very soft material, no pigtail, and low-profile skin plate, which can be capped off. This makes the drain easy to tolerate even while walking. In principle, the drain affords access for interventions while also providing internal biliary drainage to the bowel. An advanced design, called the Munich drain, is available in a range of lengths and calibers (8F to 16F). The disadvantage of this drain is that its very soft material requires adequate dilatation of the tract; otherwise the highly flexible material could not be advanced into the bile ducts. Some suppliers (Peter Pflugbeil) offer special stabilizing catheters that fit inside the drain.

Biliary Drainage Setup

We use the Munich-type drain, which was developed from the Yamakawa device (Peter Pflugbeil). The length of the catheter (primary length of 34 cm) can be modified by cutting off the catheter tip (at an angle) to suit anatomical requirements.

The lubricated drain, which preferably consists of a relatively soft material (polyethylene) for potential long-term drainage, is wire-guided with a slight twisting motion across the stenosis and advanced into the duodenum (or other small-bowel segment in postoperative patients) for external–internal drainage. Contrast injection is repeated at this time to confirm correct drain position.

If the guidewire cannot be advanced across the stenosis and into the intestine at the first sitting, a 6F or 7F pigtail catheter can be placed in the prestenotic segment. (A shortened Yamakawa or Munich drain is a possible alternative, although there is the problem of side holes extending into the channel in the liver with a potential for intraperitoneal or external bile leakage.) It should be noted that a more proximal drain placement carries a greater risk of migration. After the bile ducts have been decompressed and inflammatory processes have subsided (e.g., in 2–4 days), it is often possible to advance a guidewire into the duodenum and establish external–internal drainage (or internal drainage) across the stenosis (▶ Fig. 20.9).

Additional Treatment Options

Depending on the underlying disease, the level and nature of the biliary obstruction, and the age and comorbidity of the patient, there are many additional treatment options ranging from the rendezvous technique for continued drainage by a minimally invasive endoscopic technique to the percutaneous placement of a metal stent. Other percutaneous treatments are lithotripsy for cholelithiasis, the balloon dilation of stenoses, and procedures after liver transplantation (e.g., incremental dilation of a stenosis at intervals of several days from 8F to 14F, or occasionally to 16F to 18F) to establish an adequate percutaneous access tract. The placement of a Munich drain (usually 14F), sometimes for a relatively long period of several weeks or months, allows for appropriate therapy and consolidation of the affected area. The transhepatic approach to the biliary tract is also suitable for creating a sinus tract (biliary–cutaneous fistula) for percutaneous cholangioscopy (PTCS). This can provide access for selective biopsy, loop resection, electrocoagulation, laser therapy (mechanical, electrohydraulic, or laser), lithotripsy, or photodynamic therapy, and intraluminal brachytherapy or radiofrequency treatment. Generally this requires tract dilation to at least 18F.

In principle, endoscopic manipulation of the papilla is the most atraumatic procedure in cases where the papilla

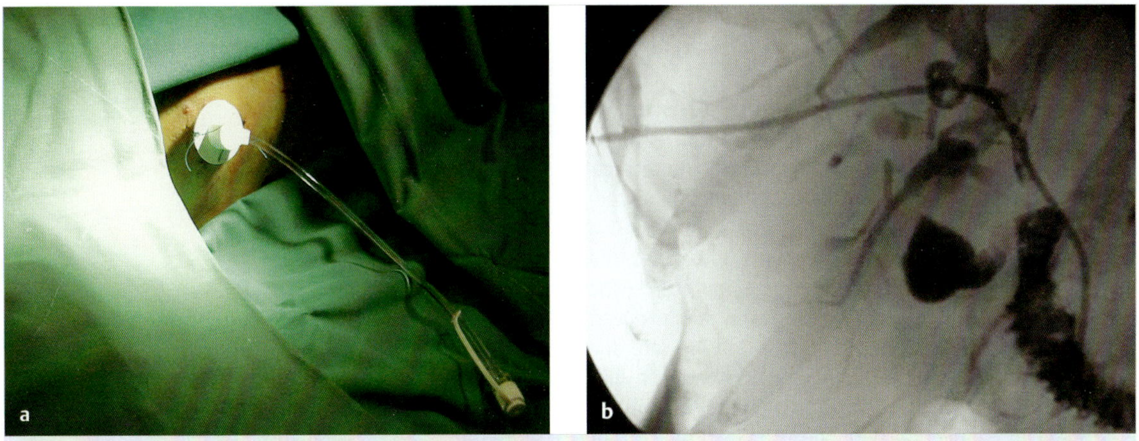

Fig. 20.9
a Placement of the biliary drain (8F Munich drain). The retention plate is secured to the skin with a suture.
b After the dressing is placed and the drainage bag connected, the result is documented by fluoroscopy.

is accessible. PTCD in itself does not generally provide sufficient access for papillotomy, stone extraction, or stent insertion. For this reason, a rendezvous technique with ERCP is usually the best option if the papilla is accessible to endoscopy. Patient positioning and sedation are the same as for ERCP. A 400-cm-long wire (Dreamwire, Jagwire) is advanced through the indwelling drain and into the duodenum. ERCP can then be performed. The wire is grasped in the duodenum using standard technique and is brought out through the duodenoscope. Devices (stent, papillotome) can then be advanced over the wire within the duodenum. Once access to the papilla has been secured, the operator can proceed with endoscopy in the usual manner.

Stent Placement

The stents available for ERCP can generally be used, but given the more traumatic approach compared with ERCP, metal stents are usually preferred because of their higher patency rates. The percutaneous transhepatic placement of metallic endoprostheses (8–10 mm diameter, 4–10 cm length) is particularly important for malignant strictures. Uncovered metal stents are best for stenoses close to the porta hepatis to avoid the occlusion of surrounding bile ducts, while covered metal stents (e.g., Wallflex, Boston Scientific) have proven effective for obstructions of the extrahepatic bile ducts close to the papilla. In principle, endoscopic material is possible but shorter delivery systems are more comfortable to handle and mostly more cost effective.

Attachment

The (external) retention plate, backed by a drain sponge, is sutured to the skin through at least two (or preferably three) opposing holes using No. 0 or No. 3 Mersilene suture material. A three-way stopcock is connected via an adapter; only then is a collection bag attached and the drain opened. This procedure reduces the risk of bacterial infection and sepsis while allowing the quantity and quality of the fluid output to be assessed. In the case of a Yamakawa or Munich drain, a clip-on cover that is exchangeable with a clip-on drain is provided

20.5.3 Procedure Time

The total procedure time is approximately 45 minutes for the physician and approximately 70 minutes for assisting personnel.[26]

20.6 Success Rate

PTC can be successfully performed in 95 to 98% of cases with dilated bile ducts and in 65 to 70% of patients with nondilated bile ducts ([27,28] and authors' data). Available data have been summarized by Dlugosch.[29]

20.6.1 Results with Plastic Endoprostheses

Hamlin reported a success rate of over 97% for external, internal, or combined percutaneous transhepatic cholangiodrainage in a series of 109 patients treated between 1979 and 1984.[30] Lammer described the successful deployment of plastic (Teflon, polyethylene, or polyurethane) endoprostheses in 100% of 162 patients.[31] Seitz (1994) published an equally high success rate for the insertion of a new-design Teflon stent.[32] Sommer (1987) reported the successful placement of an internal drain in 95% of cases using the combined rendezvous technique.[16]

20.6.2 Results with Metal Endoprostheses

Lammer described the initially successful placement of the Wallstent biliary endoprosthesis in all but 3 of 61 patients. The three failures related to problems in retracting the constraining membrane, but deployment was successful in a second attempt.[33] Huibregtse implanted a Wallstent endoprosthesis in 103 patients and achieved a technically correct primary placement in 97%.[34] The occlusion rates ranged from 10 to 50%, and the European Wallstent Study Group found that the occlusion rate due to biliary sludge was 5% at 175 days in 103 patients with malignant obstruction. One previously unknown problem was noted in connection with the plastic stents: tumor invasion of the stent lumen (in 7%).

Studies published on the Wallstent by Hoepffner, Schöfl, and Boguth with case numbers between 52 and 118 patients, all involving malignant obstructive jaundice, achieved a technically successful stent placement in 100% of cases.[35–37]

20.7 Complications

20.7.1 Incidence

Published data vary greatly regarding the number and severity of complications, but a general downward trend has been noted in recent years. PTCD has a significant morbidity rate of 2 to 5% and a mortality rate of 0.1 to 2%. The use of 0.7-mm needles is associated with a significantly lower complication rate than 1.3-mm needles.[38,39] Pleural and lung injuries and interposed colon (Chilaiditi syndrome) can be safely avoided or detected when ultrasound guidance is used.

Riemann (1984) analyzed complications in 2471 patients who underwent PTCD and found the frequency distribution shown in ▶ Table 20.2. This author made a distinction between major and minor complications.[40]

Table 20.2 Complications of PTCD

Complication	Incidence
Major complications of PTCD	**7.4%**
Bile leak, biliary peritonitis	2.0%
Sepsis	1.7%
Hematobilia	1.6%
Hemorrhage	1.6%
Retroperitoneal or subphrenic abscess	0.4%
Renal failure	0.1%
Minor complications of PTCD	**15.2%**
Catheter migration	6.6%
Cholangitis	5.9%
Fall in blood pressure	1.3%
Hyponatremia	1.0%
Pneumothorax	0.3%

Table 20.3 Early and late complications of biliary stenting

Complication	Incidence
Early complications	**5.5%**
Bile leak	3.5%
Intra-abdominal bleeding	1.8%
Pneumothorax	0.2%
Late complications	**13.4%**
Cholangitis with sepsis	5.7%
Perihepatic abscess	4.2%
Displacement	3.5%

Carrasco (1984) distinguished between early and late complications of percutaneous transhepatic stent drainage (random sample sizes of 455 and 462 patients)[41] (▶ Table 20.3).

20.7.2 Management of Complications

The incidence of complications and their severity depend mainly on the underlying disease, on the number of punctures required with associated trauma to the liver parenchyma and surrounding organs, vessels and ducts, and on the type, position, and caliber of the drainage catheter. Operator experience is also a factor.

Complications can be classified as early or late. Early complications are fever; cholangitis; bacteremia; sepsis; intrahepatic hematoma (bilioma); arterial, portal venous, or venous bleeding; leakage due to drain migration (respiratory excursions); (sero)pneumothorax; hemothorax; bile leakage from the puncture site (painful biliary peritonitis); hemobilia; and pancreatitis (in transpapillary biliary drainage). Late complications include the same complications and in addition drain obstruction, skin site infection, erosion of hepatic blood vessels, and pseudoaneurysm formation.

In the setting of PTCD-induced bleeding, hemostasis can be attempted by introducing a dilation balloon (often successful).

20.8 Aftercare

Vital signs should be checked every 30 minutes during the first 2 hours after the procedure then hourly for another 4 hours and should be documented on a monitoring chart. Particular attention should be given to signs of internal hemorrhage or sepsis. Additionally, hemoglobin and hematocrit may be checked 4 hours after the procedure (this is largely a traditional practice based on historical recommendations). Classic recommendations urge bed rest for 6 hours after the intervention and 12 hours of fasting; both recommendations are binding only in patients with postinterventional symptoms and corresponding follow-up plans. After a diagnostic PTC, it is

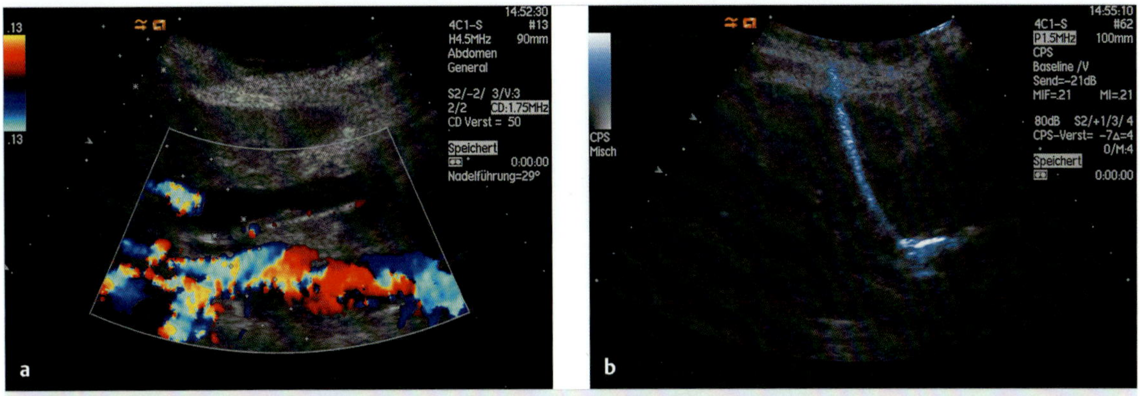

Fig. 20.10 In selected cases, contrast-enhanced ultrasound guidance (a) can also be used for the selective puncture (b) and drainage of central bile ducts.

wise to prescribe several days of minimal physical exertion. PTC can be performed on an outpatient basis when adequate surveillance is available after the procedure. Even PTCD can be done on an outpatient basis in selected tumor patients if the procedure is uneventful, good physician follow-up care is available, and no further interventions are planned.

External drainage is started immediately after placement in the case of obstructive symptomatic jaundice for a quick release of symptoms. After clinical relief, the drain can be clamped off to divert all drainage through the internal route. In the case of external drainage the volume of biliary drainage should be charted daily. A significant amount of blood-tinged drainage should be present only on the first day. Heavy bleeding should be investigated at once, generally by an abdominal ultrasound examination. A blood count may be considered based on the progression of vital signs and the volume of bloody drainage. The drain should be flushed 2 to 4 times daily with at least 10 mL of sterile saline to prevent clogging by blood clots or debris. Bile leakage from the puncture site is often a sign of ineffective drain placement or clogging. In this case the drain should be assessed by fluoroscopy and adjusted as needed. The duration of antibiotic therapy after successful PTCD depends on the individual clinical course. External–internal drains (e.g., of the Yamakawa type) should be changed every 2 to 3 months over a guidewire (initial fluoroscopy, guidewire insertion, drain exchange, reimaging, documentation).

20.9 Use of Intracavitary Ultrasound Contrast Agents

The intracavitary injection of ultrasound contrast agents is used for abscess visualization, for ultrasound-guided gastrostomy (Chapter 21), and for ultrasound-guided PTCD (contrast-enhanced PTCD, CEUS-PTCD).[42–44] Ultrasound contrast agent in a very high dilution (0.1–0.2 mL SonoVue per 20 mL physiologic saline solution) is injected into the bile ducts after the initial puncture to confirm intraductal placement or locate a possible stenosis. This technique has proven particularly helpful for difficult and occasional atypical punctures (▶ Fig. 20.10, ▶ Fig. 20.11, ▶ Fig. 20.12, ▶ Fig. 20.13, ▶ Fig. 20.14). Contrast solution can also be instilled into the small intestine after advancement of the sheath to visualize the

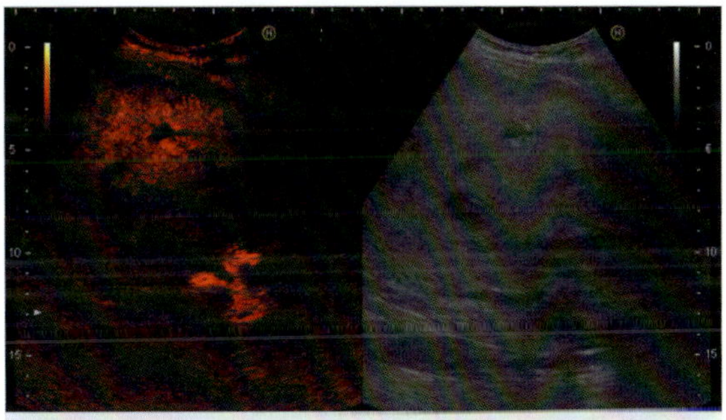

Fig. 20.11 Ultrasound contrast agent enters the small intestine in this woman with postsurgical anatomical changes in the biliodigestive tract.

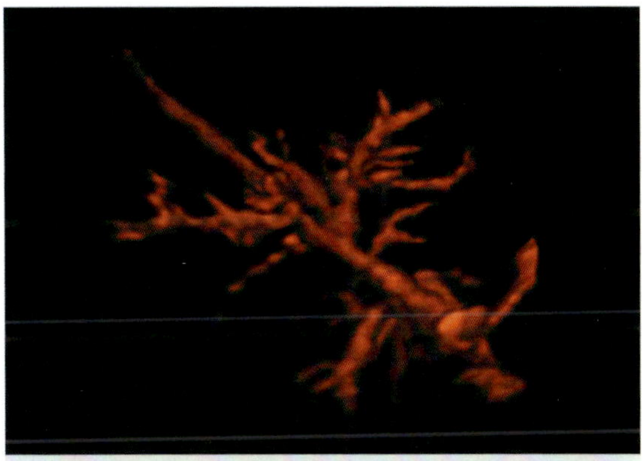

Fig. 20.12 Contrast agent-specific 3D image of internal–external drainage in a patient with advanced hepatocellular carcinoma. Biliary obstruction was caused by lymphadenopathy in the hepatoduodenal ligament.

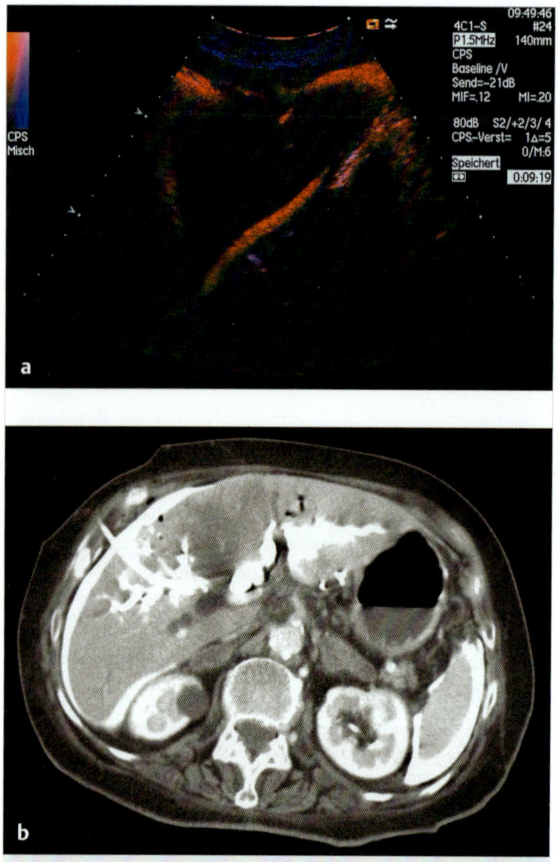

Fig. 20.13 Contrast agent visible around the left lobe of the liver.
a The extravasation site is visible at approximately the 1 o'clock position. A previous PTCD had been placed through this tract but it migrated. A new PTCD had to be inserted via a different route. When contrast agent was instilled through the new drain, it escaped through the old channel and defined the persistent leak.
b Corresponding axial CT view of perihepatic contrast agent.

small-bowel loops. A leak may be demonstrated in selected cases.[44] Other contrast applications have also been described.[45,46]

20.10 Analysis of the Literature

20.10.1 Present Authors' Data

Our own data from 69 patients with cholestatic jaundice, 31 women and 38 men with an average age of 63.5 years, were retrospectively analyzed. Percutaneous puncture of the bile ducts was successfully accomplished in 99% of cases. In the 29 patients who received an endoprosthetic stent, the device was successfully placed by the percutaneous route alone or by the rendezvous technique in 26 cases. Immediately life-threatening complications occurred in 3 of 69 patients (approximately 4%): biliary–venous fistula requiring intervention, sepsis, and an acute abdomen caused by stent perforation.[47]

20.10.2 Comparison of Endoprostheses

While only a few types of endoprosthesis were available in the late 1980s, today we can choose from of a variety of devices depending on the cause, type, length, and consistency of the stenosis. Two main types of device are available: plastic endoprostheses and metal stents. Wagner (1993) conducted a prospective, randomized trial comparing plastic endoprostheses (14F) with self-expanding metal stents (24F) in 20 patients with type II–IV hilar obstructions in the Bismuth classification.[48] Long-term stent failure occurred in 50% of the plastic group and in 18.2% of the metal stent (Wallstent) group (though the differences were not statistically significant). The main problem with the plastic endoprostheses was early occlusion with frequent associated cholangitis. Moreover, the reintervention rate was significantly lower in the metal stent group, so that the metal stents were more cost-effective than the plastic stents despite the higher initial cost of the metal stents. Knyrim (1993) obtained almost identical results in a long-term comparison of plastic versus metal stents in 85 inoperable patients with malignant biliary obstruction, except that the early complications (30 days after implantation) were similar in both groups.[49]

In reviewing the literature on metal stent designs arising from the evolution of vascular and urethral prosthetics, we find that the Gianturco stent, Wallstent, and Strecker stent have been the most widely used devices during the past decade. More recent developments include nitinol stents such as the self-expanding Zilver stent[50,51] and the Memotherm stent.[51,52] In the Mozart Study, a multicenter study of 241 patients with malignant biliary strictures, the endoscopically placed Zilver stent with a 10 mm diameter had occlusion rates similar to the Wallstent, also 10 mm in diameter (24% versus 21%). The 6-mm Zilver stent showed a significantly higher occlusion rate (40%).[53]

Gianturco Stent

The Gianturco stent (Cook Medical) consists of a self-expanding, nonflexible stainless steel wire mesh with an expanded diameter of approximately 12 mm and a length of approximately 3 cm. The constrained stent is delivered to the stricture in a 12F Teflon catheter by the percutaneous transhepatic route. Several stents are usually placed end-to-end due to their short individual lengths. Irving (1989) observed recurrent obstruction in 2 of 11 patients with benign strictures and in 7 of 13 patients with malignant strictures that had been treated with the stent. The failures in the malignant group were due to tumor ingrowth through the wire mesh of the Gianturco stent.[54] Mathieson (1994) reported a reocclusion rate of 35% in 26 patients with malignant obstructive jaundice after treatment with the Gianturco stent. The reocclusions

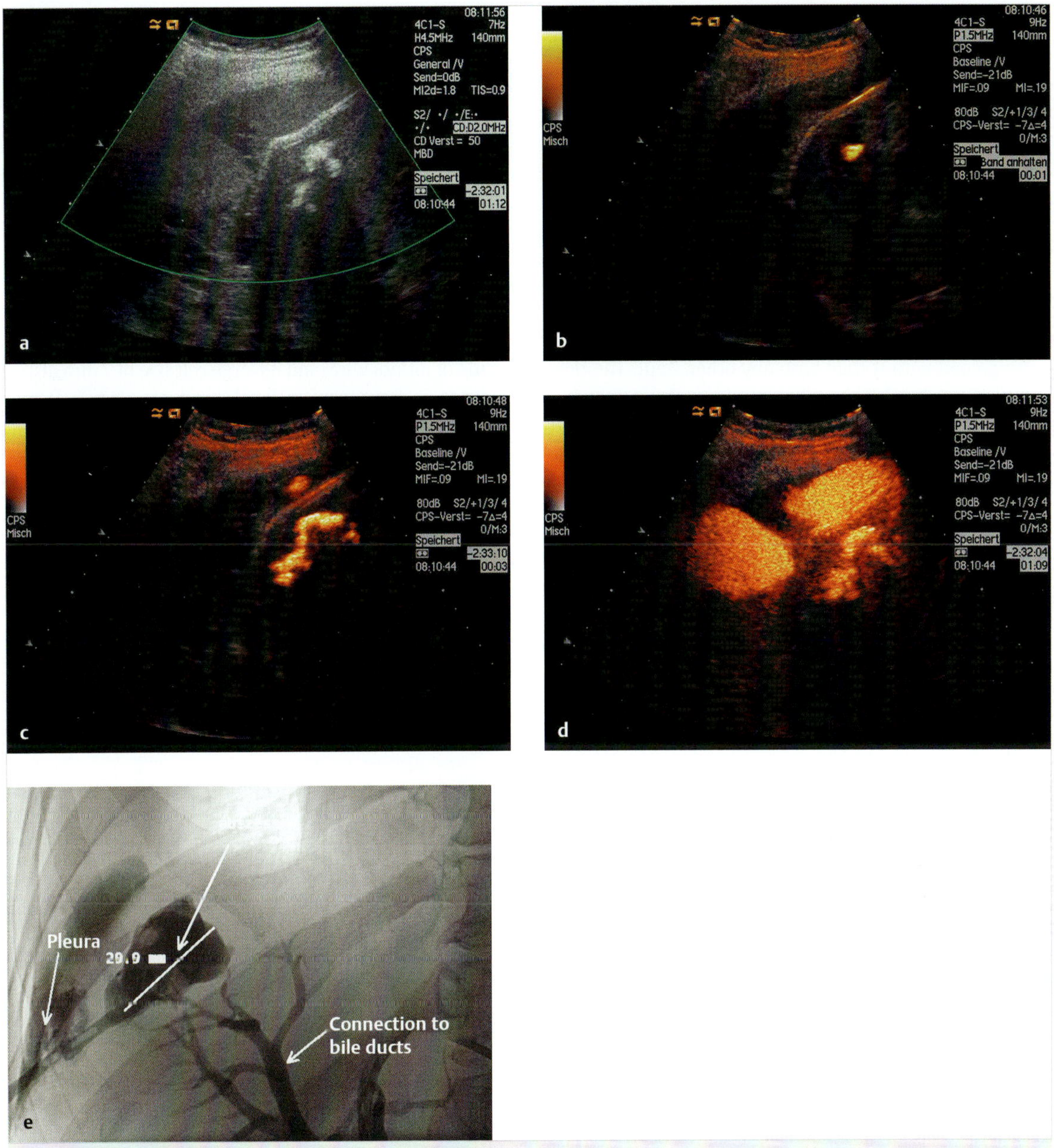

Fig. 20.14 Bile leakage from the abdomen into the chest, demonstrated by B-mode ultrasound (a), intracavitary SonoVue injection (b–d), and fluoroscopy (e).

were caused by tumor overgrowth at the edges of the device.[55]

Strecker Stent

The Strecker stent (Medi-Tech, Boston Scientific), with an original length of approximately 3.5 cm, is balloon-expanded to a maximum diameter of 8 mm after deployment. Neuhaus (1990) often placed several of these devices in series to prevent tumor overgrowth of the stent ends.[56] Today the Strecker stent is available in lengths up to 8 cm with larger diameters and is distinguished by its good radiopacity. Also, it undergoes minimal shortening when expanded. One disadvantage is the need to predilate the stenosis because the stent is released by two silastic sleeves that retract as the balloon is inflated.[57] Bethge (1992) reported problems with expansion of the Strecker stent during 6 (17%) of 34 insertions.[58] There were three additional cases of problems with balloon removal, and only part of the stent could be fully expanded in two patients. Successful deployment was achieved in all cases on the second or third attempt, however. It is also noteworthy that incomplete expansion occurred only after endoscopic placement, not after percutaneous placement. The authors attribute this to the longer working channel in the endoscopic retrograde approach compared with the percutaneous route, increasing the difficulty of pneumatic dilation.

Wallstent

Perhaps more has been written about the self-expanding Wallstent (formerly Medivent, Lausanne, Switzerland; now Boston Scientific) and more clinical experience has been gained with it than with any other stent. The flexible wire mesh tube has a lumen of approximately 1 cm when fully expanded by the retraction of a constraining plastic membrane. One advantage over rapid balloon expansion is that even rigid strictures can be dilated without pain.[59] The Wallstent is available in a range of lengths from approximately 3 to 10 cm. Several disadvantages have been described: poor radiographic visibility, the relatively sharp-edged ends, and shortening of the device on expansion.

Hoepffner (1994)[35] published the most comprehensive study to date based on 4 years' observation of 118 patients with malignant biliary strictures treated with a total of 127 self-expanding 10-mm Wallstents. Technical problems occurred in only 5 cases (4.2%). The constraining membrane could not be retracted in four patients, and stent expansion was incomplete in one patient. The Wallstent patency rates in patients who survived 1 year or longer were 86% at 6 months, 72% at 12 months, and 64% at 18 months. Stent occlusion occurred in 12% of patients after an average of 168 days. Hoepffner concluded from these results that patients surviving longer than 3 months after stent insertion were the ones most likely to benefit from this type of therapy.

ComVi

The ComVi stent is a covered metal stent consisting of a polytetrafluoroethylene membrane sandwiched between two wire stents. This creates a wire surface on both the inside and outside of the device. The individual layers are not attached to one another. This design allows for maximum flexibility during angulation. The radial force is higher than in the Wallstent. The high flexibility and minimal axial shortening on self-expansion are designed to prevent kinking and occlusion of the common bile duct.

A study was done in 47 patients with malignant distal biliary obstruction who had been treated with the ComVi stent.[60] The patients were matched with 47 patients who had been treated with a covered metal stent (Wallstent, Boston Scientific) at an earlier time. No significant differences were found in stent patency or patient survival. Stent occlusion occurred in 13 patients in the ComVi group and 10 patients in the Wallstent group. The incidence of stent migration was significantly lower with the ComVi.

Niti-S Stent

The Niti-S large-cell D-type biliary stent (Taewoong Medical)was developed to permit both unilateral and bilateral drainage of hilar biliary obstruction. Unlike traditional stents for bilateral placement, which have a low-density mesh in their central portion, the Niti-S stent provides contralateral drainage over its entire length with sufficient radial force for self-expansion owing to its greater wire thickness (0.178 versus 0.127 mm). The stent is made of nitinol wire, and its large cell size of 7 mm distinguishes it from conventional products (Niti-S D-type stent).[61] The stent was placed in 12 consecutive patients with unresectable Klatskin tumors. Five of the 12 patients (42%) had bilateral stent placement. The success rate was 100%. The mean duration of stent patency was 202 days.

References

[1] Misra S, Melton GB, Geschwind JF, Venbrux AC, Cameron JL, Lillemoe KD. Percutaneous management of bile duct strictures and injuries associated with laparoscopic cholecystectomy: a decade of experience. J Am Coll Surg 2004; 198: 218–226

[2] Jakobs R, Weickert U, Hartmann D, Riemann JF. [Interventional endoscopy for benign and malignant bile duct strictures]. Z Gastroenterol 2005; 43: 295–303

[3] Krömer MU, Maier M, Benz CA et al. Bile duct stenoses and leakage after cholecystectomy: endoscopic diagnosis, therapy and treatment outcome- [Article in German]. Z Gastroenterol 1996; 34: 167–172

[4] Takada T, Yasuda H, Hanyu F. Technique and management of percutaneous transhepatic cholangial drainage for treating an obstructive jaundice. Hepatogastroenterology 1995; 42: 317–322

[5] Ferrucci JT, Wittenberg J, Sarno RA, Dreyfuss JR. Fine needle transhepatic cholangiography: a new approach to obstructive jaundice. AJR Am J Roentgenol 1976; 127: 403–407

[6] Laufer U, Kirchner J, Kickuth R, Adams S, Jendreck M, Liermann D. A comparative study of CT fluoroscopy combined with fluoroscopy versus fluoroscopy alone for percutaneous transhepatic biliary drainage. Cardiovasc Intervent Radiol 2001; 24: 240–244

[7] Koito K, Namieno T, Nagakawa T, Morita K. Percutaneous transhepatic biliary drainage using color Doppler ultrasonography. J Ultrasound Med 1996; 15: 203–206

[8] Fölsch UR, Wurbs D, Classen M, Creutzfeldt W. [A comparison of percutaneous transhepatic cholangiography and endoscopic retrograde cholangiopancreatography (author's transl)]. Dtsch Med Wochenschr 1979; 104: 625–628

[9] Jander HP, Galbraith J, Aldrete JS. Percutaneous transhepatic cholangiography using the Chiba needle: comparison with retrograde pancreatocholecystography. South Med J 1980; 73: 415–421

[10] Albert JG, Ulrich F, Zeuzem S, Sarrazin C. [Endoscopic-retrograde cholangiopancreatography in patients with surgical modification of anatomy]. Z Gastroenterol 2010; 48: 839–849

[11] Tischendorf JJ, Meier PN, Schneider A, Manns MP, Krüger M. Transpapillary intraductal ultrasound in the evaluation of dominant bile duct stenoses in patients with primary sclerosing cholangitis. Scand J Gastroenterol 2007; 42: 1011–1017

[12] Tischendorf JJ, Krüger M, Trautwein C et al. Cholangioscopic characterization of dominant bile duct stenoses in patients with primary sclerosing cholangitis. Endoscopy 2006; 38: 665–669

[13] Nuernberg D, Ignee A, Dietrich CF. [Ultrasound in gastroenterology. Biliopancreatic system]. Med Klin (Munich) 2007; 102: 112–126

[14] Stanley J, Gobien RP, Cunningham J, Andriole J. Biliary decompression: an institutional comparison of percutaneous and endoscopic methods. Radiology 1986; 158: 195–197

[15] Pedersen FM. Endoscopic management of malignant biliary obstruction. Is stent size of 10 French gauge better than 7 French gauge? Scand J Gastroenterol 1993; 28: 185–189

[16] Sommer A, Burlefinger R, Bayerdörffer E, Ottenjann R. [Internal biliary drainage in the "rendezvous" procedure. Combined transhepatic endoscopic retrograde methods]. Dtsch Med Wochenschr 1987; 112: 747–751

[17] Shorvon PJ, Cotton PB, Mason RR, Siegel JH, Hatfield AR. Percutaneous transhepatic assistance for duodenoscopic sphincterotomy. Gut 1985; 26: 1373–1376

[18] Hauenstein KH, Wimmer B, Salm R, Farthmann EH. [Percutaneous diagnosis and therapy of the bile ducts and gallbladder. Feasibility and status]. Radiologe 1991; 31: 132–140

[19] Hauenstein KH, Salm R, Vineé P, Tribukait U. [Percutaneous interventions on the bile duct in obstructive jaundice. A meaningful or excruciating prolongation of life?]. Radiologe 1992; 32: 13–21

[20] Wenz W. [Percutaneous transhepatic cholangiography]. Radiologe 1973; 13: 41–46

[21] Cozzi G, Severini A, Civelli E et al. Percutaneous transhepatic biliary drainage in the management of postsurgical biliary leaks in patients with nondilated intrahepatic bile ducts. Cardiovasc Intervent Radiol 2006; 29: 380–388

[22] Lee W, Kim GC, Kim JY et al. Ultrasound and fluoroscopy guided percutaneous transhepatic biliary drainage in patients with nondilated bile ducts. Abdom Imaging 2008; 33: 555–559

[23] Makuuchi M, Yamazaki S, Hasegawa H, Bandai Y, Ito T, Watanabe G. Ultrasonically guided cholangiography and bile drainage. Ultrasound Med Biol 1984; 10: 617–623

[24] Sukigara M, Taguchi Y, Watanabe T, Koshizuka S, Koyama I, Omoto R. Percutaneous transhepatic biliary drainage guided by color Doppler echography. Abdom Imaging 1994; 19: 147–149

[25] Takada T, Hanyu F, Kobayashi S, Uchida Y. Percutaneous transhepatic cholangial drainage: direct approach under fluoroscopic control. J Surg Oncol 1976; 8: 83–97

[26] Phillip J, Sahl RJ, Ruus P, Rösch T, Classen M. [Time factors in endoscopic studies. A survey in West Germany]. Z Gastroenterol 1990; 28: 1–9

[27] Mueller PR, Harbin WP, Ferrucci JT, Wittenberg J, vanSonnenberg E. Fine-needle transhepatic cholangiography: reflections after 450 cases. AJR Am J Roentgenol 1981; 136: 85–90

[28] Mueller PR, van Sonnenberg E, Ferrucci JT. Percutaneous biliary drainage: technical and catheter-related problems in 200 procedures. AJR Am J Roentgenol 1982; 138: 17–23

[29] Dlugosch J. Die perkutane transhepatische Cholangiographie und Drainage im Verlauf von Gallenwegserkrankungen. Frankfurt am Main: Johann Wolfgang Goethe Universität; 1996

[30] Hamlin JA, Friedman M, Stein MG, Bray JF. Percutaneous biliary drainage: complications of 118 consecutive catheterizations. Radiology 1986; 158: 199–202

[31] Lammer J, Neumayer K. Biliary drainage endoprostheses: experience with 201 placements. Radiology 1986; 159: 625–629

[32] Seitz U, Vadeyar H, Soehendra N. Prolonged patency with a new-design Teflon biliary prosthesis. Endoscopy 1994; 26: 478–482

[33] Lammer J, Klein GE, Kleinert R, Hausegger K, Einspieler R. Obstructive jaundice: use of expandable metal endoprosthesis for biliary drainage. Work in progress. Radiology 1990; 177: 789–792

[34] Huibregtse K, Carr-Locke DL, Cremer M et al. Biliary stent occlusion—a problem solved with self-expanding metal stents? European Wallstent Study Group. Endoscopy 1992; 24: 391–394

[35] Hoepffner N, Foerster EC, Högemann B, Domschke W. Long-term experience in Wallstent therapy for malignant choledochal stenosis. Endoscopy 1994; 26: 597–602

[36] Schöfl R, Brownstone E, Reichel W et al. Malignant bile-duct obstruction: experience with self-expanding metal endoprostheses (Wallstents) in Austria. Endoscopy 1994; 26: 592–596

[37] Boguth L, Tatalovic S, Antonucci F, Heer M, Sulser H, Zollikofer CL. Malignant biliary obstruction: clinical and histopathologic correlation after treatment with self-expanding metal prostheses. Radiology 1994; 192: 669–674

[38] Harbin WP, Mueller PR, Ferrucci JT. Transhepatic cholangiography: complicatons and use patterns of the fine-needle technique: a multi-institutional survey. Radiology 1980; 135: 15–22

[39] Burke DR, Lewis CA, Cardella JF et al. Society of Cardiovascular and Interventional Radiology. Quality improvement guidelines for percutaneous transhepatic cholangiography and biliary drainage. J Vasc Interv Radiol 1997; 8: 677–681

[40] Riemann JF. Complications of percutaneous bile drainage. In: Classen M, Geenen J, Kawai U, eds. Nonsurgical Biliary Drainage. Berlin: Springer Verlag; 1984:29–35

[41] Carrasco CH, Zornoza J, Bechtel WJ. Malignant biliary obstruction: complications of percutaneous biliary drainage. Radiology 1984; 152: 343-346

[42] Dietrich CF. Comments and illustrations regarding the guidelines and good clinical practice recommendations for contrast-enhanced ultrasound (CEUS)—update 2008. Ultraschall Med 2008; 29 (Suppl 4): S188–S202

[43] Dietrich CF, Schreiber-Dietrich D, Schuessler G, Ignee A. [Contrast enhanced ultrasound of the liver—state of the art]. Dtsch Med Wochenschr 2007; 132: 1225–1231

[44] Ignee A, Baum U, Schuessler G, Dietrich CF. Contrast-enhanced ultrasound-guided percutaneous cholangiography and cholangiodrainage (CEUS-PTCD). Endoscopy 2009; 41: 725–726

[45] Zuber-Jerger I, Endlicher E, Schölmerich J, Klebl F. Endoscopic retrograde cholangiography with contrast ultrasonography. Endoscopy 2008; 40 (Suppl 2): E202

[46] Dietrich CF. Contrast-enhanced low mechanical index endoscopic ultrasound (CELMI-EUS). Endoscopy 2009; 41 (Suppl 2): E43–E44

[47] Dietrich CF, Dlugosch J, Wehrmann T, Hellstern A. PTC(D) im Verlauf von Gallenwegserkrankungen. Endosk Heute 1997; 10: 90

[48] Wagner HJ, Knyrim K, Vakil N, Klose KJ. Plastic endoprostheses versus metal stents in the palliative treatment of malignant hilar biliary obstruction. A prospective and randomized trial. Endoscopy 1993; 25: 213–218

[49] Knyrim K, Wagner HJ, Pausch J, Vakil N. A prospective, randomized, controlled trial of metal stents for malignant obstruction of the common bile duct. Endoscopy 1993; 25: 207–212

[50] Han YH, Kim MY, Kim SY et al. Percutaneous insertion of Zilver stent in malignant biliary obstruction. Abdom Imaging 2006; 31: 433–438

[51] Inal M, Akgül E, Aksungur E, Demiryürek H, Yağmur O. Percutaneous self-expandable uncovered metallic stents in malignant biliary obstruction. Complications, follow-up and reintervention in 154 patients. Acta Radiol 2003; 44: 139–146

[52] Chiou YY, Tseng HS, Chiang JH, Hwang JI, Chou YH, Chang CY. Percutaneous placement of metallic stents in the management of malignant biliary obstruction. J Formos Med Assoc 2005; 104: 738–743

[53] Loew BJ, Howell DA, Sanders MK et al. Comparative performance of uncoated, self-expanding metal biliary stents of different designs in 2 diameters: final results of an international multicenter, randomized, controlled trial. Gastrointest Endosc 2009; 70: 445–453

[54] Irving JD, Adam A, Dick R, Dondelinger RF, Lunderquist A, Roche A. Gianturco expandable metallic biliary stents: results of a European clinical trial. Radiology 1989; 172: 321–326

[55] Mathieson JR, McLoughlin RF, Cooperberg PL et al. Malignant obstruction of the common bile duct: long-term results of Gianturco-Rosch metal stents used as initial treatment. Radiology 1994; 192: 663–667

[56] Neuhaus H, Hagenmüller F, Classen M. [Self-expanding and expandable bile duct prostheses]. Z Gastroenterol 1991; 29: 306–310

[57] Strecker EP, Romaniuk P, Schneider B et al. [Percutaneously implantable balloon-inflatable vascular prostheses. Initial clinical results]. Dtsch Med Wochenschr 1988; 113: 538–542

[58] Bethge N, Wagner HJ, Knyrim K et al. Technical failure of biliary metal stent deployment in a series of 116 applications. Endoscopy 1992; 24: 395–400

[59] Jaschke W, Busch HP, Georgi M. [The treatment of bile duct stenoses using metal mesh endoprostheses (stents)]. Radiologe 1992; 32: 8–12

[60] Isayama H, Kawabe T, Nakai Y et al. Management of distal malignant biliary obstruction with the ComVi stent, a new covered metallic stent. Surg Endosc 2010; 24: 131–137

[61] Kogure H, Isayama H, Nakai Y et al. Newly designed large cell Niti-S stent for malignant hilar biliary obstruction: a pilot study. Surg Endosc 2011; 25: 463–467

[62] van der Gaag NA, Rauws EA, van Eijck CH et al. Preoperative biliary drainage for cancer of the head of the pancreas. N Engl J Med 2010; 362: 129–137

[63] Baron TH, Kozarek RA. Preoperative biliary stents in pancreatic cancer—proceed with caution. N Engl J Med 2010; 362: 170–172

[64] Kennedy EP, Rosato EL, Yeo CJ. Preoperative drainage in pancreatic cancer. N Engl J Med 2010; 362: 1344, author reply 1345

[65] Mönkemüller K. Preoperative drainage in pancreatic cancer. N Engl J Med 2010; 362: 1344, author reply 1345

[66] Tsujino T, Isayama H, Koike K. Preoperative drainage in pancreatic cancer. N Engl J Med 2010; 362: 1343–1344, author reply 1346

21 Percutaneous Gastrostomy

A. Ignee, G. Schuessler, C. F. Dietrich

A gastrostomy can be performed by surgical or nonsurgical means. Nonsurgical methods are broadly subdivided into endoscopic procedures and interventional radiology.

Endoscopic techniques are well established, and the "pull" method for percutaneous endoscopic gastrostomy tube delivery is the most commonly used. It is easily learned and has low complication rates.

Interventional radiology using fluoroscopy or ultrasound can eliminate the need for endoscopic access. The strength of imaging techniques is that they can safely avoid extraluminal structures such as the liver and transverse colon and prevent endoscopic access.

This chapter will examine the role of ultrasonography both as an adjunct and as a standalone guidance modality for percutaneous gastrostomy placement. The potential benefits of the method and its indications will be explored.

21.1 Indications

Percutaneous gastrostomy is generally done to provide intermediate- or long-term nutrition in patients who cannot take food orally. It follows the principle that, whenever possible, enteric feeding is preferable to parenteral nutrition. Thus the indications include patients on long-term ventilatory support and patients with acquired diseases or disturbances of deglutition, as in CNS diseases. A gastrostomy may also be placed to decompress the stomach contents when gastrointestinal continuity is disrupted due to a malignant bowel obstruction.

21.2 Contraindications

The only acute situation that would require an emergency gastrostomy is tube placement for gastric decompression because of bowel obstruction. This may be done for palliation in patients with, say, a malignant stricture distal to the stomach.

Feeding tube placement is contraindicated in unstable patients, who should be adequately managed by temporary parenteral nutrition.

In principle, a feeding gastrostomy is a palliative option in a terminally ill patient only if it would subjectively improve the patient's quality of life.

21.3 Materials and Equipment

Two standard systems used for percutaneous gastrostomy placement are the Wills–Oglesby gastrostomy sets (Cook Medical Europe), which are available in a conventional version and in the Mallinckrodt Institute modification. The retention mechanism in both versions is a locking pigtail loop. The conventional system measures 12F, while the modification has a 14F catheter. All initial drainages must be exchanged. We prefer the 12F system as its smaller diameter affords a certain degree of safety, especially at the start of the learning curve. It is supplied with a long Lunderquist wire together with 7F, 10F, and 12F dilators. The Mallinckrodt system is supplied with a 100-cm Amplatz wire and only two dilator sizes (12F and 14F). With both systems, the T-fasteners that are necessary for pulling the stomach wall against the abdominal wall must be ordered separately. The fasteners are available in a twin-pack. Similar systems are offered by other companies. These techniques require the use of very stiff, torque-stable guidewires. The Lunderquist wire is even stiffer than the Amplatz wire; both are made of coated stainless steel.

The Freka-Pexact gastrostomy tube (Fresenius Kabi) is an alternative set for the placement of a 15Ch (15F) balloon tube designed for insertion by an introducer. The manufacturer recommends the use of endoscopic guidance. Special features include placement with a special gastropexy system, which is described later in the chapter. Also, the abdominal wall is not punctured with a guidewire followed by dilators as in the traditional introducer technique. Instead, the puncture is performed directly with a 16F trocar covered with a sheath. The solid steel trocar is then removed, and the sheath provides access for placing the gastrostomy tube. The sheath is then peeled apart and removed.

21.4 Types of Gastrostomy

The following nonsurgical procedures are most widely practiced:

- Percutaneous endoscopic gastrostomy (PEG) using the pull method, the push method, or the introducer method
- Percutaneous radiologic gastrostomy (PRG)
- Percutaneous sonographic gastrostomy (PSG)

21.4.1 Percutaneous Endoscopic Gastrostomy

Pull Method

The "pull" method is the standard technique. First the puncture site is identified endoscopically by transillumination or digital indentation and a needle is passed through the abdominal wall into the stomach. A thread is passed through the needle, grasped with an endoscopic forceps, and brought out through the mouth with the endoscope. The feeding tube is attached to the thread. The percutaneous end of the thread is then pulled to draw the PEG tube down the esophagus and against the stomach and abdominal wall, where it is fixed with a retention system. The advantage of this method is that sturdy, stable retention plates can be delivered through a normally patent esophagus.

Push Method

This method is rarely if ever used today. The technique is analogous to the pull method, except that the PEG tube is pushed into the stomach over the guidewire.

Introducer Method

In the conventional introducer method, a needle is passed into the stomach at a point identified by transillumination and/or indentation. Then a guidewire is introduced and placed in the gastric fundus. Most but not all authors perform a gastropexy. The tract is then dilated over the wire to allow the placement of an approximately 12F gastrostomy catheter. This tube must have a retaining device that can "collapse" during the insertion process and allow the tube to enter the stomach. Balloon retention catheters are most often used for this purpose. Other alternatives are locking pigtails or retention baskets.

Direct puncture systems are available in which a peel-away plastic sheath is introduced over a trocar, creating access for the placement of a 15Ch (15F) balloon catheter (Freka Pexact, Fresenius Kabi).

Percutaneous Radiologic Gastrostomy

The stomach is distended with 500 to 1500 mL of air via stomach tube and is punctured at a site located by transillumination. Some authors perform a contrast enema to opacify the transverse colon. Then a guidewire is passed into the gastric fundus. Many authors recommend performing a gastropexy. But there is no consensus on the number and positioning of gastropexy devices. Then the tract is enlarged with serial dilators, and a gastrostomy catheter is placed as in the introducer method.

21.4.2 Percutaneous Sonographic Gastrostomy

The technique is described below in the section on Ultrasound-Assisted PEG.

21.5 Advantages and Disadvantages of Different Methods

The advantages and disadvantages of the various gastrostomy methods are outlined in ▶ Table 21.1.

Table 21.1 Advantages and disadvantages of gastrostomy methods

Method	Advantages	Disadvantages
Endoscopy	The luminal view permits accurate placement of a stable retention plate and allows safe gastric distention.	Interposed liver or colon cannot be seen. The endoscope itself may cause complications in some cases. Most patients require sedation.
Fluoroscopy	Clear visualization; the entire stomach can be seen. The colon can be visualized.	In most cases the colon requires opacification by contrast enema. The liver is poorly visualized. Radiation exposure.
Ultrasonography	Needle insertion can be monitored in real time while also visualizing the transverse colon and liver.	Ultrasound does not give a clear view of the stomach.

21.6 Success Rates of Different Gastrostomy Techniques

It is difficult to compare the success rates of different gastrostomy techniques because published patient cohorts have been heterogeneous with a range of underlying diseases. Success rates and complication rates vary widely in neurologic patients, patients with head and neck tumors, and patients with upper gastrointestinal tumors.

Endoscopic placement is frequently preferred. Nevertheless, local practices and preferences—in short, local expertise—will often dictate the selection of a particular gastrostomy method. If it is unsuccessful, an alternative procedure will be used. Thus there is a preselection of critical patients or patients with a complicated anatomy for the "second choice" method. Accordingly, local expertise will have a significant impact on complications and success rates.

The success rates stated in the literature are probably too high, and no randomized comparative studies are available. Reported success rates are generally in the range of 92 to 100% for PEG, 99 to 100% for PEG using the introducer technique, 95 to 100% for PRG, and 98 to 100% for PSG in the few studies that have been published on ultrasound-guided placement. With few exceptions, all the studies on PSG published to date have been feasibility studies.

21.7 Complication Rates of Different Gastrostomy Techniques

Complications can be classified as follows:

- Endoscopy-related complications (perforation, etc.)

Table 21.2 Complication rates of different gastrostomy methods as reported in the literature

	Major	Minor	Mortality	Source (reference no.)
PSG with a stomach tube	0%	0%	0%	7
PSG without a stomach tube	0–3%	0–14%	0–2%	7,10
US-assisted PEG	7%	14%	0%	5
PRG	0–16%	6–56%	0–8%	2,3,11–16
PEG by pull method	0.5–16%	3–45%	0–6%	2,11,12,15–20
PEG by introducer method	0.70%	11%	0%	21

Abbreviations: PEG, percutaneous endoscopic gastrostomy; PRG, percutaneous radiologic gastrostomy; PSG, percutaneous sonographic gastrostomy; US, ultrasound.

- Sedation-related complications (allergies, respiratory arrest, etc.)
- Puncture-related complications (perforation, hemorrhage, etc.)
- Later complications (dislodgment, infection, peritonitis, etc.)

As far as sedation is concerned, we note that procedural sedation (brief general anesthesia) is used in most PEG studies while some radiologic studies use local anesthesia alone. Upper gastrointestinal endoscopy does not require sedation in itself, and the same is true for the abdominal intervention. Issues of comorbidity and compliance are more important factors in determining whether sedation should be used in any given case (uncooperative patients, children).

Moreover, no reliable data have been published on the incidence of complications. The reasons for this were mentioned in the preceding section. It is also difficult to distinguish between major and minor complications, as the underlying data are not presented in all studies.

The complication rates stated in the literature are summarized in ▶ Table 21.2.

An important observation is that the complication rates of endoscopic gastrostomy, especially using the pull method, are higher in patients with head and neck tumors. Alternative or supportive techniques are particularly recommended in this subset of patients. It should be possible to cross the stenosis with the thinnest available gastroscope and then place the tube percutaneously using Seldinger technique. Sonographic guidance for the puncture can provide additional safety.

In a series of 79 patients with head and neck carcinoma, Tucker and colleagues found that the pull method ($n = 50$) and introducer method ($n = 29$) had the same success rates but that the pull method was associated with a significantly higher complication rate.[1]

In one study of 177 gastrostomies placed endoscopically and 193 placed fluoroscopically, no significant differences were found in the success rates or complication rates.[2]

The studies that have been published on ultrasound-assisted gastrostomies probably do not report valid complication rates due to small case numbers and a presumed selection bias, which will be discussed later in this chapter.

21.8 Role of Ultrasonography

21.8.1 General

The methods described above should be viewed not as separate procedures but as techniques that can be combined when necessary to achieve the therapeutic goal.

We feel that fluoroscopic guidance is helpful only for operators who desire constant confirmation of an intragastric wire position. Fluoroscopy offers no additional advantages over sonographic guidance. The argument that fluoroscopy is necessary to define the transverse colon[3,4] is no longer tenable when high-resolution ultrasound scanners are used. Generally the transverse colon is easily identified sonographically as a second gas containing structure below the abdominal wall in craniocaudal orientation that is separate from the stomach (▶ Fig. 21.1).

Not infrequently, optimum transillumination cannot be obtained in patients with prior upper abdominal surgery. Ultrasound can be used in these cases to define a safe needle path. In patients with esophageal patency, we place a PEG tube by the pull method as this allows for a sturdier retention plate that is more resistant to dislodgment.[5,6] Schlottmann et al reported negative transillumination in 28 of 753 PEG placements (4%).[5] This is fairly consistent with our own experience.

It is necessary to withhold endoscopy only in rare cases. Endoscopes are available with a 5.5 mm outer diameter, and this should be small enough to cross even tight esophageal strictures. If the endoscope cannot find the correct path, the stenosis can be crossed initially with a soft-tip guidewire. When fluoroscopy has confirmed that the wire is in the stomach, the endoscope can be carefully advanced down the esophagus. If the endoscope still cannot be passed into the stomach, a slender tube can at least be advanced into the stomach by Seldinger technique. When tube placement has been checked by administration of a radiologic or ultrasound contrast

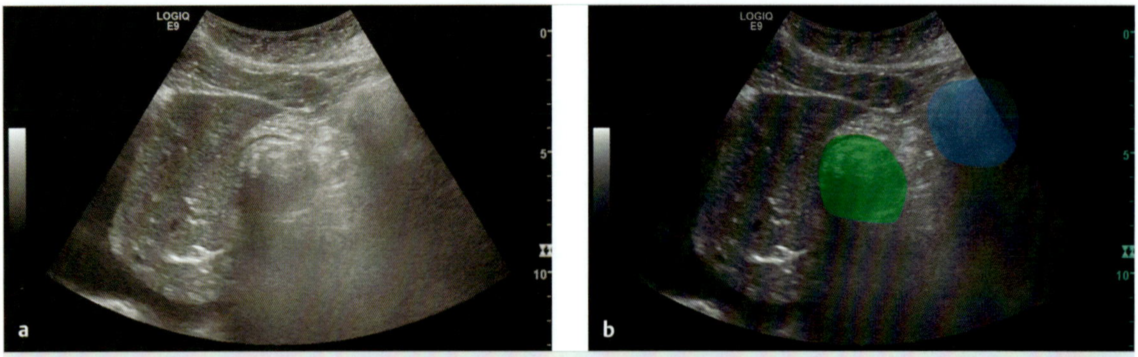

Fig. 21.1
a Local anatomy is clearly displayed in an upper abdominal longitudinal ultrasound scan just to the right of the midline.
b The gastric antrum (shaded green) is visible just below the liver. The transverse colon (shaded blue) appears in cross-section caudal to the stomach.

agent, it can be used to distend the stomach and the percutaneous gastrostomy can be continued under sonographic guidance, for example.

Practice

Tube placement can be assessed sonographically by instilling a highly diluted SonoVue solution (0.1 mL in 20–50 mL of saline solution) through the tube.

The strength of ultrasonography lies in its flexibility, low costs, and lack of side effects. It can be used at any time, the only requirement being enough space to accommodate the ultrasound machine. A sterile cover for the ultrasound probe may incur additional costs (less than 10 EUR, < 13.30 USD). We use a curved-array transducer and freehand technique. The stomach is usually imaged in a sagittal plane, as this will display the liver and transverse colon just cranial and caudal to the stomach and show their relationship to the stomach and antrum.

Practice

The stomach should be scanned with ultrasound before it is fully distended with air. The following anatomical landmarks can be identified along the midline in the craniocaudal direction:

- Left lobe of the liver
- Stomach in cross section
- Pancreas and splenic vein
- Transverse colon

The skin area is prepped and draped to expose an area large enough for needle and transducer contact. Local anesthesia is then administered. For orientation, the needle is introduced at an approximately 90° angle to the body surface while maintaining safe clearance from the left lobe of the liver and transverse colon.

The needle is usually introduced just to the right of the midline using freehand technique.

21.8.2 Ultrasound-Assisted PEG

The standard needle from the PEG set is generally used for ultrasound-assisted PEG (US-PEG). The diameter of this needle permits clear ultrasound visualization. In principle, the passage of the needle through the abdominal wall cannot always be clearly tracked with ultrasound. This step can be aided by reducing the gain setting for a sufficiently high dynamic range (> 75 dB) so that the needle will appear as a string of bright echoes against a dark background. The difference from a purely ultrasound-guided gastrostomy is that the stomach is air-distended through the endoscope and is not filled with water. The stomach is distended through the endoscope under sonographic control, then the needle is advanced through a small skin incision (4 mm) also under sonographic guidance. Generally the entry of the needle into the air-filled stomach is indicated by a conspicuous echo at the needle tip (► Fig. 21.2).

Practice

When the needle comes into contact with the stomach wall, it will produce a visible indentation. At that point the sonographer should advance the needle with a fast jabbing motion to penetrate the stomach wall. Needle entry into the stomach is marked by a high-amplitude artifact behind the air artifact from the stomach.

Now the needle has entered the stomach and air can be aspirated. The needle is simultaneously visible in the endoscopic view. The steel needle is removed, leaving the plastic sheath in the stomach. A thread can now be introduced through the sheath and grasped with the endoscopic forceps.

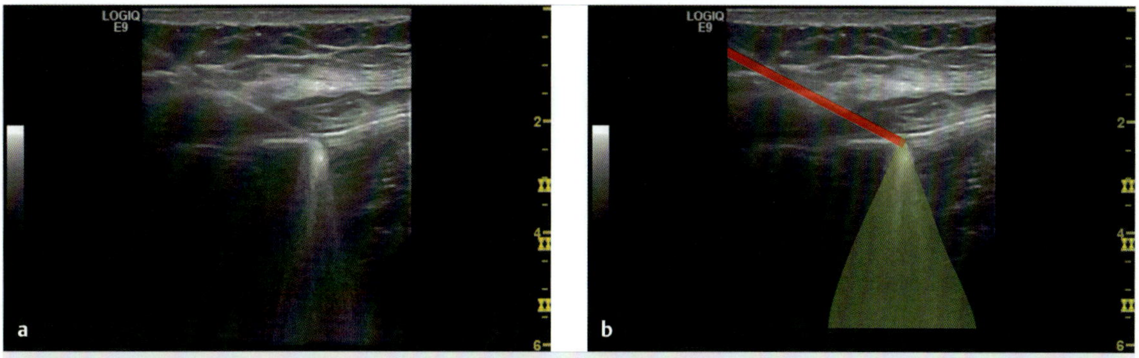

Fig. 21.2 Entry of the needle into the stomach.
a A high-amplitude artifact marks the intragastric position of the needle tip.
b In this scan the needle is highlighted in red and the artifact is shaded green. In the case shown here, the angle of needle insertion is too oblique. Ideally the needle track should be perpendicular to the abdominal wall.

Practice

The stomach is much easier to puncture when fully distended than in a lax condition. On the other hand, sonographic orientation is obtained more easily when the stomach is not fully distended.

When the thread has been grasped, the sonographic phase is complete and the procedure is continued as in a standard PEG tube placement. Thus the endoscope is withdrawn, bringing the forceps-held suture out through the mouth, and the PEG tube is attached to the suture and pulled back through to the stomach wall while the free hand of the nonendoscopic investigator stabilizes the plastic sheath in the abdominal wall. When the gastrostomy tube engages against the sheath, the sheath and the tube are both withdrawn from the stoma tract until resistance is felt, indicating that the retention plate is abutting the stomach wall. Then the thread is cut from the gastrostomy tube and the external retention system is connected to the tube.

21.8.3 Technique of Percutaneous Sonographic Gastrostomy

When performing a gastrostomy with sonographic guidance alone (PSG), we use an 18-gauge 10-cm needle for the initial puncture. This needle is sufficiently large and has a tip that is clearly visible at ultrasound. Two operators should carry out the intervention.

If a stomach tube can be passed, we distend the stomach with physiologic saline solution (500–1000 mL). Correspondingly smaller volumes are used in children. The fluid-distended stomach is clearly visible. Bleck and colleagues instill enough fluid to distend the antrum to > 5 cm.[7]

Now the first gastropexy T-anchor (T-fastener) is introduced through the puncture needle (▶ Fig. 21.3). This device is used to fasten the stomach to the abdominal wall and promote epithelialization of the stoma tract. For this purpose the metal T-anchor with attached suture is inserted into the needle and pushed into the stomach

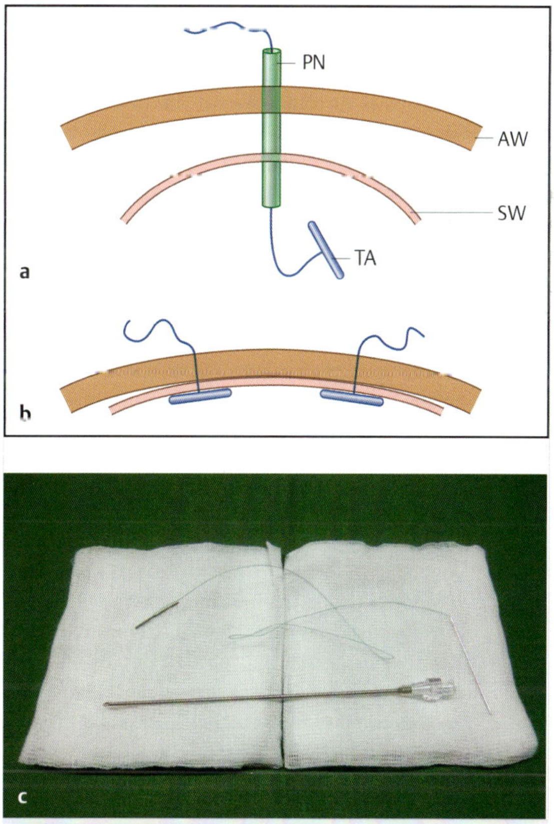

Fig. 21.3 Gastropexy with T-anchors. Usually two anchors are placed 2 cm apart, and the gastrostomy site is positioned midway between them. (AW, abdominal wall; SW, stomach wall; TA, T-anchor; PN, puncture needle.)
a, b Diagrammatic representations.
c View of the anchor on a suture with a cannula. A needle is attached to the other end of the suture.

with a wire. The wire is 0.035 inches in diameter and has a soft tip. The wire may remain in place while gentle tension is applied to test the fixation of the T-anchor. Then the needle is removed and reinserted approximately 2 cm from the first puncture site (usually at a more caudal level), advancing the needle into the stomach under vision. The second T-anchor is now placed using the same technique as before.

If a stomach tube cannot be passed, the stomach is distended with 500 to 1000 mL of physiologic saline solution instilled through the needle tract before the first T-anchor is placed. Bleck and colleagues also recommend the use of an infusion pump.[7] This technique has a higher complication rate than the conventional procedure. An infusion system is connected to the Luer lock fitting of the needle, and the stomach is distended. Manual pressure on a plastic infusion bottle aids the fluid instillation. One ampule of butylscopolamine can be administered by IV injection (barring contraindications) to inhibit gastric emptying.

An alternative is a gastropexy system offered by Fresenius Kabi, which was originally developed for endoscopic placement (introducer technique). In this system, described briefly above in the section Types of Gastrostomy, two needles are introduced through a parallel needle guide (▶ Fig. 21.4a). One needle is used to insert a wire loop, which is directed toward the other needle. A suture is then passed through the second needle, and the wire loop is withdrawn, snaring the suture and pulling it against the needle tip. This creates a resistance to further withdrawal of the wire loop (confirms snaring). Now the system is withdrawn and the suture ends are tied together to complete the gastropexy (▶ Fig. 21.4b). Number 2 nonabsorbable monofilament suture material is used.

Next a 7F or 8F dilator is advanced over a thick, stiff guidewire. The gastropexy sutures should exert some traction on the stomach wall at this time. We now dilate the tract to 10F and then 12F. Next a 12F catheter with a locking pigtail is introduced (▶ Fig. 21.5). A balloon-retained catheter may be used as an alternative.

Practice

We check the position of the tube by injecting a low dose of an ultrasound contrast agent in a standard dilution that we use for intracavitary applications: 0.1 mL in 20 mL of saline solution is sufficient to enhance a volume > 0.5 L. By comparison, note that 1.2 to 2.4 mL (up to 4.8 mL) is sufficient to obtain good enhancement of the blood compartment (5–7 L). An alternative is to inject radiographic contrast agents when fluoroscopic guidance is used.

As a rule, the initial catheter should be replaced after development and epithelialization of the stoma tract (in approximately 2 weeks) due to the manufacturer's recommendations.

The instillation of diluted ultrasound contrast solution provides a rapid and clear overview, will not clog the tube, and can be dispersed by high-energy ultrasound pulses if troublesome contrast residues remain. Contrast instillation is effective in detecting complications. In ▶ Fig. 21.6, heavy granulations in the gastrostomy tract led to incorrect measurement of the tract length for a button system, resulting in the placement of a catheter that was too short. Pain occurred during balloon inflation. Contrast-enhanced ultrasound confirmed the intragastric position of the catheter tip, while contrast injection into the balloon demonstrated that the balloon was within the stomach wall.

In ▶ Fig. 21.7, contrast injection through the tube after placement shows the extragastric position of the tube. Presumably one of the anchors was dislodged after tract dilation.

21.9 Questions Relevant to Percutaneous Sonographic Gastrostomy

21.9.1 Use of a Spasmolytic Agent

Various authors describe the use of a spasmolytic agent such as glucagon (0.1 mg) or *N*-butylscopolamine (20 mg). The efficacy of this measure has not yet been evaluated.

21.9.2 Prophylactic Antibiotics

A meta-analysis of 10 PEG studies in a total of 1059 patients was conducted in 2007 to determine the efficacy of antibiotic prophylaxis.[8] It was found that antibiotic prophylaxis led to an absolute risk reduction of 15% with a "number needed to treat" of 8. Penicillin-based regimens were superior to cephalosporin-based regimens. There is no evidence that results would be different in ultrasound-guided gastrostomy tube placements. This means that antibiotic prophylaxis is appropriate for PRG and PSG.

21.9.3 Use of a Guidewire

The use of a guidewire is recommended. The wire is placed in the gastric corpus or fundus, followed by tract dilation or direct insertion by the trocar technique.

21.9.4 Need for Gastropexy

The gastropexy described above fixes the stomach wall to the abdominal wall, making it possible to dilate the tense stomach wall without the dilator pushing the stomach wall aside. A gastropexy is consistently performed even though it is not mandatory. It is used in the PEG introducer method as well as in PRG and PSG. The conventional

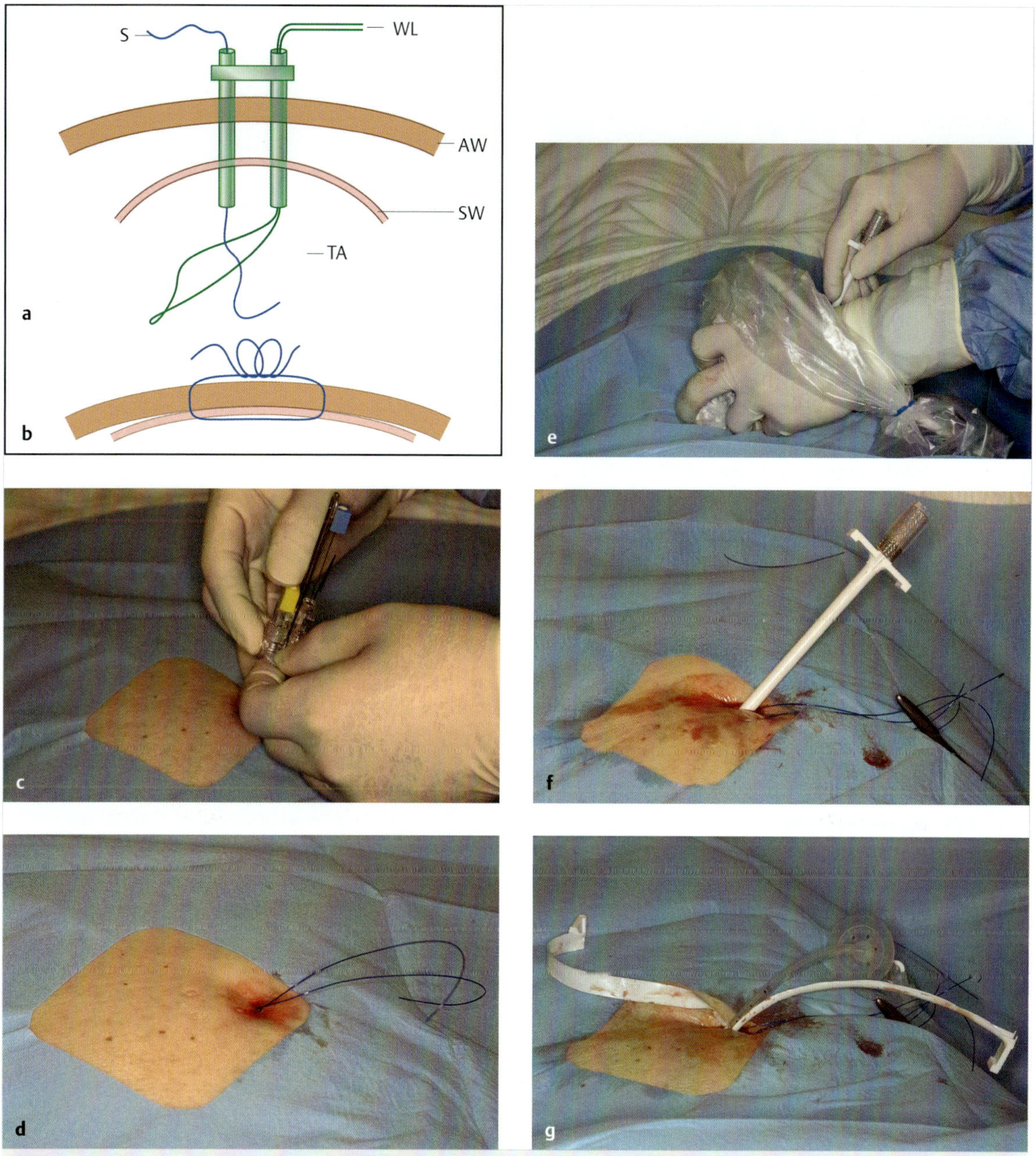

Fig. 21.4 Use of a gastropexy system.
a, b Diagram of the principle. S, suture; WL, wire loop; TA, T-anchor; SW, stomach wall; AW; abdominal wall.
c–g Intraoperative photographs document the further steps. The abdominal and stomach walls are pierced, and the gastropexy is performed. Next the trocar is introduced into the stomach lumen, and the gastrostomy tube is placed through the sheath, which is peeled apart.

technique employs 1, 2, or 3 percutaneous T-anchors (T-fasteners). This device consists of a short metal sleeve attached to a suture. It is pushed with a wire through the needle and into the gastric lumen. When out of the needle, the sleeve will move automatically into a position when drawn back where it holds back the stomach wall, and is then sutured into place. An alternative is the automated gastropexy system described above. It is unclear how long the gastropexy must be kept in place. Generally this period is described as lasting until a stoma tract is formed, i.e., approximately 7 to 21 days.

21.9.5 Type of Drainage

Performing a gastropexy without endoscopy requires the use of a collapsible retention system that can be passed

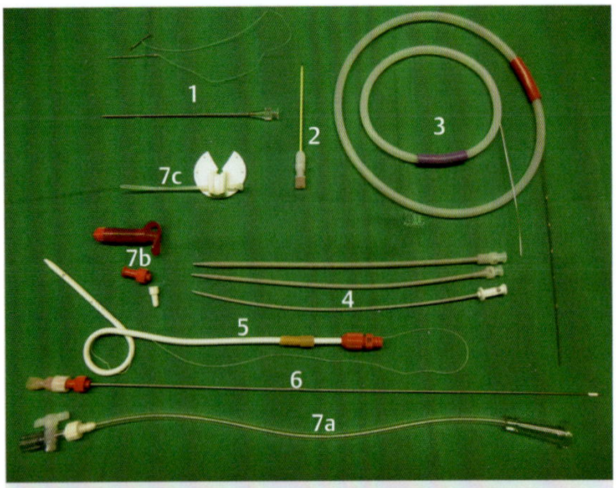

Fig. 21.5 Materials for the percutaneous placement of an ultrasound-guided gastrostomy, illustrated for a 12F drain with a retention pigtail. **1**, T-anchor; **2**, introducer sheath; **3**, guidewires; **4**, dilators (7F, 10F, 12F); **5**, 12F gastrostomy tube; **6**, introducer–stiffener needle (blunt); **7a,b,c**, distention and fixation materials.

with the tube through the tract and then deployed inside the stomach. As well as a locking pigtail, balloon catheters are most commonly used. Balloon retention carries a risk of rupture or fluid loss. Basket retention devices are very rarely used today.

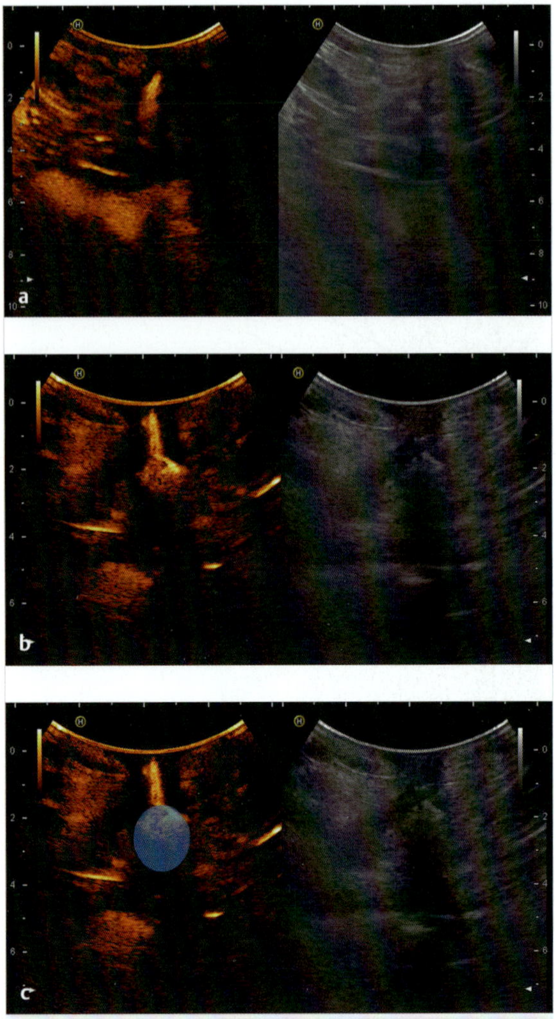

Fig. 21.6 Contrast instillation for detecting complications.
a Contrast injection after changing a gastrostomy button system retained by a balloon. Tract length was measured and a new button system was placed, but balloon inflation elicited pain. The injection of 0.1 mL SonoVue in 20 mL saline solution showed the button partially introduced into the stomach.
b Injecting the same SonoVue concentration into the balloon shows that the balloon is within the stomach wall.
c The balloon is shown in purple; the persistent contrast pool in the stomach is shown in yellow.

21.10 Summary

In principle, PEG placement by the "pull" method is ideal because it allows the use of a stable retention plate that prevents dislodgment. Endoscopy allows for safe placement of the tube. The needle tract is not visualized, however. This is not a problem in the great majority of cases. The introducer technique can be used to avoid trauma to the esophagus in the presence of stenosis and/or a tumor, especially in squamous cell carcinoma due to tumor implantation into the abdominal or gastric wall.

PRG is an established and reliable procedure whose complication rate is usually overestimated because (except at specialized centers) PRG is frequently used as a second-line option performed after PEG failure. Consequently, the cohorts for PEG and PRG often cannot be meaningfully compared with each other. Unfortunately, the gastrostomy catheters initially used in the nonendoscopic procedures have a limited diameter compared with PEG tubes, which increases their susceptibility to clogging.

Every endoscopy department should have the capability of assisting a PEG placement by image guidance in cases where obstacles or difficulties are encountered. Ultrasonography is an ideal modality in experienced hands, owing to its modest logistical requirements compared with fluoroscopy (no need for radiation protection, no special room) and the ability to positively identify the stomach and perigastric structures.

Ultrasound-assisted PEG offers the highest degree of patient safety. Given the advantages of conventional PEG, however, ultrasound guidance should be reserved for exceptional cases (obesity, abdominal surgery or other obstacles to transillumination).

When we consider the simple capabilities of percutaneous ultrasound guidance, we do not feel that guidance by endosonography is a reasonable option.[9]

PSG without endoscopic support is reserved for cases in which the stomach is not accessible to endoscopy.

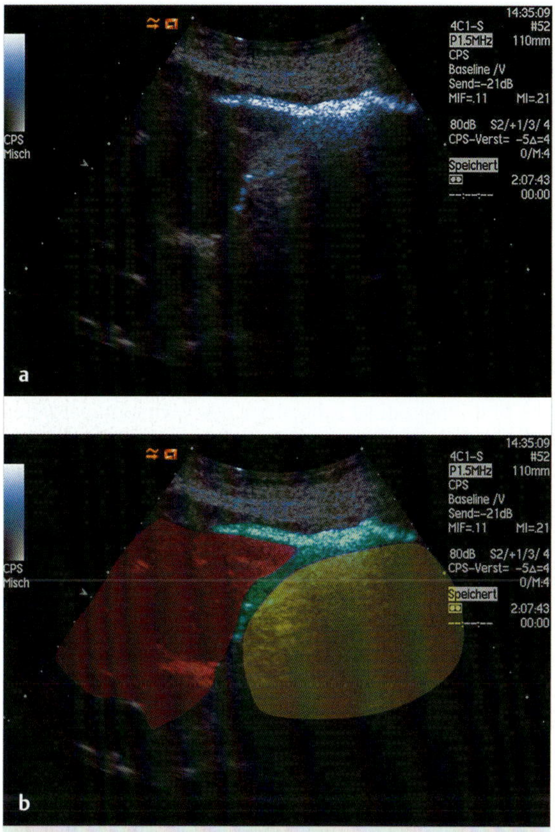

Fig. 21.7 Percutaneous sonographically guided gastrostomy (PSG) without esophageal intubation, done for palliation in a woman with anaplastic stenosing thyroid carcinoma. The ultrasound images are sagittal scans.
a Tract dilation led to dislodgment of the gastrostomy tube. The injection of ultrasound contrast agent shows perihepatic enhancement.
b For anatomical orientation, the left lobe of the liver is shown in red, the stomach in yellow, and the perigastric/perihepatic contrast pool in green.

The approach used at our institution can be outlined as follows:

- **Standard procedure:** PEG by the pull method.
- **Problems and strategies for solution:**
  - Head and neck tumors, stenosing esophageal tumors, bleeding risk, and tumor seeding (especially with squamous cell carcinoma): introducer PEG with an automated gastropexy system and trocar technique, generally with sonographic assistance.
  - Failure of transillumination, especially in previously operated or very obese patients, or after gastrectomy: ultrasound-assisted PEG (puncture under sonographic control; sonography phase ends when the endoscopic forceps grasps the intragastric suture).
  - Esophageal stricture impassable by an endoscope: placement of a feeding tube with endoscopy and X-ray assisted Seldinger technique if possible, followed by PSG.

References

[1] Tucker AT, Gourin CG, Ghegan MD, Porubsky ES, Martindale RG, Terris DJ. 'Push' versus 'pull' percutaneous endoscopic gastrostomy tube placement in patients with advanced head and neck cancer. Laryngoscope 2003; 113: 1898–1902

[2] Silas AM, Pearce LF, Lestina LS et al. Percutaneous radiologic gastrostomy versus percutaneous endoscopic gastrostomy: a comparison of indications, complications and outcomes in 370 patients. Eur J Radiol 2005; 56: 84–90

[3] Cory DA, Fitzgerald JF, Cohen MD. Percutaneous nonendoscopic gastrostomy in children. AJR Am J Roentgenol 1988; 151: 995–997

[4] Stehr W, Farrell MK, Lucky AW, Johnson ND, Racadio JM, Azizkhan RG. Nonendoscopic percutaneous gastrostomy placement in children with recessive dystrophic epidermolysis bullosa. Pediatr Surg Int 2008; 24: 349–354

[5] Schlottmann K, Klebl F, Wiest R et al. Ultrasound-guided percutaneous endoscopic gastrostomy in patients with negative diaphanoscopy. Endoscopy 2007; 39: 686–691

[6] Höroldt BS, Lee FK, Gleeson D, McAlindon ME, Sanders DS. Ultrasound guidance in the placement of a percutaneous endoscopic gastrostomy (PEG): an adjuvant technique in patients with abdominal wall varices? Dig Liver Dis 2005; 37: 709–712

[7] Bleck JS, Reiss B, Gebel M et al. Percutaneous sonographic gastrostomy: method, indications, and problems. Am J Gastroenterol 1998; 93: 941–945

[8] Jafri NS, Mahid SS, Minor KS, Idstein SR, Hornung CA, Galandiuk S. Meta-analysis: antibiotic prophylaxis to prevent peristomal infection following percutaneous endoscopic gastrostomy. Aliment Pharmacol Ther 2007; 25: 647–656

[9] Chaves DM, Kumar A, Lera ME et al. EUS-guided percutaneous endoscopic gastrostomy for enteral feeding tube placement. Gastrointest Endosc 2008; 68: 1168–1172

[10] Lorentzen T, Nolsøe CP, Adamsen S. Percutaneous radiologic gastrostomy with a simplified gastropexy technique under ultrasonographic and fluoroscopic guidance: experience in 154 patients. Acta Radiol 2007; 48: 13–19

[11] Chishty IA, Haider Z, Khan D, Pasha S, Rafiq Z, Akhter W. Percutaneous radiologic gastrostomy: results and complications. J Ayub Med Coll Abbottabad 2006; 18: 36–39

[12] Schrag SP, Sharma R, Jaik NP et al. Complications related to percutaneous endoscopic gastrostomy (PEG) tubes. A comprehensive clinical review. J Gastrointestin Liver Dis 2007; 16: 407–418

[13] Park JH, Kang SW. Percutaneous radiologic gastrostomy in patients with amyotrophic lateral sclerosis on noninvasive ventilation. Arch Phys Med Rehabil 2009; 90: 1026–1029

[14] Quadri A, Umapathy N, Orme R. Percutaneous gastrostomy in patients with complete obstruction of the upper digestive tract. Eur J Radiol 2005; 56: 74–77

[15] Wollman B, D'Agostino HB, Walus-Wigle JR, Easter DW, Beale A. Radiologic, endoscopic, and surgical gastrostomy: an institutional evaluation and meta-analysis of the literature. Radiology 1995; 197: 699–704

[16] Grant DG, Bradley PT, Pothier DD et al. Complications following gastrostomy tube insertion in patients with head and neck cancer: a prospective multi-institution study, systematic review and meta-analysis. Clin Otolaryngol 2009; 34: 103–112

[17] Ljungdahl M, Sundbom M. Complication rate lower after percutaneous endoscopic gastrostomy than after surgical gastrostomy: a prospective, randomized trial. Surg Endosc 2006; 20: 1248–1251

[18] Lockett MA, Templeton ML, Byrne TK, Norcross ED. Percutaneous endoscopic gastrostomy complications in a tertiary-care center. Am Surg 2002; 68: 117–120

[19] Blum CA, Selander C, Ruddy JM, Leon S. The incidence and clinical significance of pneumoperitoneum after percutaneous endoscopic gastrostomy: a review of 722 cases. Am Surg 2009; 75: 39–43

[20] Larson DE, Burton DD, Schroeder KW, DiMagno EP. Percutaneous endoscopic gastrostomy. Indications, success, complications, and mortality in 314 consecutive patients. Gastroenterology 1987; 93: 48–52

[21] Foster JM, Filocamo P, Nava H et al. The introducer technique is the optimal method for placing percutaneous endoscopic gastrostomy tubes in head and neck cancer patients. Surg Endosc 2007; 21: 897–901

22 Interventional Endosonography

C. F. Dietrich, M. Hocke, C. Jenssen

Diagnostic and therapeutic endoscopic ultrasound (EUS) has established itself as the interdisciplinary "royal discipline" of interventional endoscopy.[1] The combination of ultrasound and endoscopy permits the use of high-frequency ultrasound scanning and supplemental ultrasound techniques in anatomical regions that are poorly accessible or inaccessible to transabdominal or transthoracic ultrasound. A familiarity with conventional ultrasonography combined with the extraordinary capabilities of side-viewing endoscopy are essential prerequisites for successful therapeutic endosonography.

The capabilities of EUS-guided biopsy techniques have increased the importance of EUS as a diagnostic tool. The advantage of these EUS-guided techniques is that they can accurately direct a needle under vision into a previously inaccessible target lesion located deep in the mediastinum, retroperitoneum, or pelvis.

Endosonography can play an important role in interdisciplinary planning and in the treatment of pancreatic pseudocysts, (peri)pancreatic abscesses and necrosis, pancreatic duct obstructions, biliary strictures, pancreatic duct stones, and many other minimally invasive applications while providing a remarkably low complication rate.[2,3]

22.1 Cost–Benefit Analysis

Today endosonography is and in the future will remain on a competitive footing with other interventional guidance modalities such as CT and MRI (based on cost–benefit analysis of personnel costs, training costs [personal experience], and equipment and operating costs [endoscope, ultrasound scanner]). Thus, because EUS requires a high degree of practical experience and the equipment entails additional investment costs (although modest relative to those for CT and MRI), it can be particularly effective in interdisciplinary settings, despite the fact that multidisciplinary frameworks are not available at every institution.

22.2 Historical Introduction

The development of endosonography began in the early 1980s, coinciding with the advent of mechanical radial ultrasound scanners and electronic linear scanners.[4–6] Olympus offered the first commercially available radial echoendoscope in 1983, equipped with a motor-driven rotating sector scanner. At the same time, companies such as Siemens, Acmi, and Toshiba/Machida developed rotating sector scanners in addition to longitudinal echoendoscopes equipped with linear array transducers.[7,8] In 1990, T. Rösch and colleagues published the first report on the successful use of miniaturized radial transducers passed through the working channel of an endoscope ("miniprobe").[9]

Despite the appealing image quality, endosonography initially met with limited acceptance. It became widely practiced only after the introduction of EUS-guided interventions, which in a first step consisted mainly of fine needle biopsies. These procedures became possible when Picker, working with Pentax in the early 1990s, developed the first longitudinal echoendoscope with a miniaturized curved-array transducer and a working channel.[10] Initial results of EUS-guided fine needle aspiration biopsies were published in 1993.[11,12] Other milestones in the development of endoscopic ultrasound were the introduction of electronic radial scanners by Olympus/Aloka and Hitachi/Pentax in the early 2000s and the introduction of real-time endosonographic elastography and contrast-enhanced endosonography.[13–16]

The era of therapeutic endosonography was launched by Maurits Wiersema in 1996 with the first reports on endosonographic celiac plexus neurolysis and EUS-guided drainage of pseudocysts.[17,18] Reports published in 2002 and 2003 described initial experience with EUS-guided biliary drainage[19] and pancreatic duct drainage.[20]

Meanwhile, EUS-guided fine needle aspiration biopsy (EUS-FNA) has had a crucial impact on therapeutic decision-making by providing a definitive diagnosis for lesions demonstrated by endoscopic ultrasound. In Germany, an average of 15% of endosonographic procedures include fine needle biopsy, and the biopsy rates at some centers are considerably higher (up to 30%). EUS-guided therapeutic interventions enrich the spectrum of interventional endoscopy, although they are mostly limited to centers that possess the necessary expertise. Approximately 3% of endosonographies performed in Germany are therapeutic procedures. The most common procedure is the drainage of pancreatic fluid collections and necrosis (60%), followed by biliary and pancreatic duct drainage (23%), celiac plexus neurolysis or blockade (8%), and the drainage of nonpancreatic fluid collections (9%) (www.eus-degum.de).

22.3 Materials and Equipment

22.3.1 Requirements of the Endoscopy Unit

The EUS procedure room should meet the general requirements of an interventionally equipped endoscopy unit and must also have the necessary sonographic and endosonographic equipment. The following are required:

- Fluoroscopy unit (fixed or portable C arm)
- Video processor, cold light source
- Monitors (endoscopy, fluoroscopy)
- Imaging documentation systems (PACS, etc.)
- Electrosurgical unit
- Surveillance monitor (including continuous measurement of oxygen saturation, pulse rate, ECG leads, and blood pressure monitoring)
- Oxygen port, continuous oxygen delivery
- Additional suction equipment

Other necessary gear includes lead aprons, thyroid shields, and radiation dosimeters for operators and assistants. Every endoscopy unit should have an emergency kit with essential drugs as well as equipment for intubation and bag ventilation.

Optional accessories include the following:

- Video duodenoscope, therapeutic forward-viewing upper GI endoscope ("gastroscope")
- Assorted guidewires (0.035-inch, 4 m)
- Radiographic contrast medium (in sterile bottle or dish; e.g., Ultravist 370, Bayer HealthCare Pharmaceuticals [L-lysine amidotrizoate])
- Fixed-diameter dilators (5F–9F)
- Balloon dilators (6–20 mm)
- Self-expanding metal stents (metal biliary stents)
- 0.9% NaCl (in sterile bottle or dish)
- Sterile 10-mL syringes
- Sterile gauze pads
- Polyp retriever
- Dormia basket
- Polyp retrieval net, polyp retrieval basket (rotatable)
- Miscellaneous polypectomy snares (rotatable)

▶ **Documentation.** Written documentation should cover the indication for the procedure, the scope of informed consent, premedication, the endoscopes and materials used, the course of the procedure, treatment results, aftercare recommendations, as well as endoscopic (and possibly radiologic) image documentation. Radiologic documentation includes the fluoroscopy time and radiation dose product. Nursing documentation includes patient identification data, course of the procedure, procedure time, monitoring parameters, and nursing care recommendations after the intervention.

22.3.2 Which Endosonography Systems Have Become Established?

Concurrently with the development of radial EUS techniques (not suitable for interventional use), initial experience was published on the use of electronic linear-array scanners, which initially could not be used for interventions (ACMI, Machida, Siemens, Toshiba). The first longitudinal echoendoscope (the FG 32-UA) was marketed in 1991, making it possible to direct a needle to a targeted site under endosonographic guidance (Picker/Hitachi-Pentax).[10,11] Since then, longitudinal endosonography has become an established tool, owing especially to its usefulness for therapeutic interventions. The working channel should have an inner diameter > 3 mm, preferably 3.7 to 3.8 mm (Pentax-Hitachi, Olympus, Fujinon).

A detailed analysis of available systems and their technical characteristics (electronic or mechanical, working channel, instrument length, tip, field of view, transducer frequency, Doppler capabilities, elastography) was recently published by Janssen[21] and by Sudholt and Vilman.[22] Details may be found in descriptions of individual interventional techniques.

▶ **Our own experience.** Today a top-level endoscopy facility should combine optimal sonographic techniques with endoscopes that have high maneuverability and interventional stability. Desirable sonographic capabilities include color Doppler scanning, contrast-enhanced imaging, and elastography.

Typical EUS instruments are illustrated in ▶ Fig. 22.1, ▶ Fig. 22.2, ▶ Fig. 22.3, and ▶ Fig. 22.4.

22.3.3 Which Biopsy Needles and Techniques Have Become Established?

Biopsy devices were developed in the early 1990s by Peter Vilman and Soeren Hancke in cooperation with the German endoscopic accessories manufacturer Medi-Globe Ltd. (formerly GIP Medizintechnik).

Most present day needle systems are based on the designs introduced at that time. The first needle systems were homemade devices used as prototypes, and their successors are now available commercially from companies such as Cook Medical (wide selection of 25- to 19-gauge EchoTip aspiration needles and histology needles

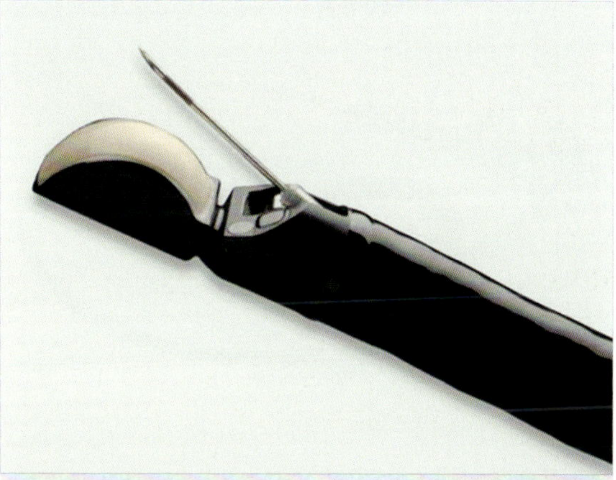

Fig. 22.1 Longitudinal echoendoscope EG 3870 UTK (Hitachi/Pentax) with fine needle deployed through a 3.8-mm working channel.

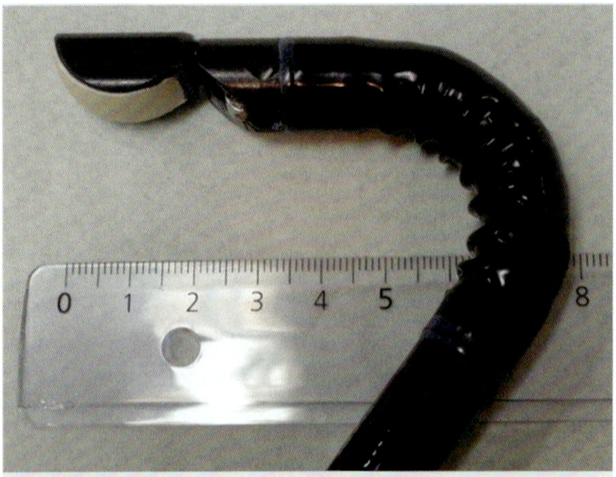

Fig. 22.2 Longitudinal echoendoscope EG 3830 UT (Hitachi/Pentax) has an approximately 45-mm-long rigid introducer section (diameter 12.8 mm) with a micro-convex probe (approximate length 20 mm, 120° scan angle, 5–10 MHz), side-viewing endoscopic lens (120°), and a 3.8-mm working channel with an Albarran lever.

[Quick-Core 19G, EUSN-19-QC; ProCore 25G, 22G and 19G, Echo-HD-25/22/19C]); Boston Scientific (Expect 25G, 22G, 19G; Expect 19 Flex); Medi-Globe (ProControl aspiration needles 25G to 19G); Olympus (EZ shot 2 aspiration needles 25G to 19G); Beacon Endoscopic/Covidien (bnx system 25G, 22G, 19G). The first successful needle design widely used in studies was a metal needle system with a metal stylet (GIP, 170 cm length, 0.8 mm diameter = 22 gauge), which mounts on the instrument channel of the endoscope by a Luer lock connector. Current aspiration needle designs are characterized by a plastic coil, metal stylet, and Luer lock fitting. Trucut core needle systems are offered by Cook Medical (Quick-Core) but have not become widely implemented as first- and second-generation systems.[23]

In a recent innovation, developed in the United States, a 19-gauge "access needle" uses the stylet as a needle rather than a needle-protector as in conventional assemblies (EUS-19 Access, Cook Medical). When thin-lumen biopsy needles are used in echoendoscopes with a large working channel (3.7 mm), it is sometimes difficult to center the needle tip in the channel. This led Medi-Globe to introduce 25-gauge and 22-gauge needles covered by a distal sheath to help stabilize the needle tip. Beacon Endoscopic has developed the bnx needle exchange system facilitating the passage of multiple needles of various diameters (25, 22, and 19 gauge) through a single delivery system, which is kept in place during the fine needle intervention (distribution: Covidien). So far the bnx system is the only one with a needle stick prevention device.

Needles with 19-gauge diameter can be used in all longitudinal echoendoscopes even without a therapeutic working channel, although the use of a diagnostic endoscope limits interventional capabilities (e.g., stent placement is not possible without changing the scope). 19G Nitinol-needles (Boston Scientific; Beacon Endoscopic/Covidien) have higher flexibility, allowing EUS-guided biopsy and interventional procedures also in bent scope positions. Various biopsy techniques have been described, although large comparative studies have not yet been published.

On the basis of the current literature the following observation can be made:

- Biopsy and cytology needles should have the smallest possible effective diameter.
- Any tissue particles that are retrieved should be immersed in formalin for histologic processing.
- The thin needles used to date cannot consistently retrieve histologic specimens, despite the very promising results published by some authors.

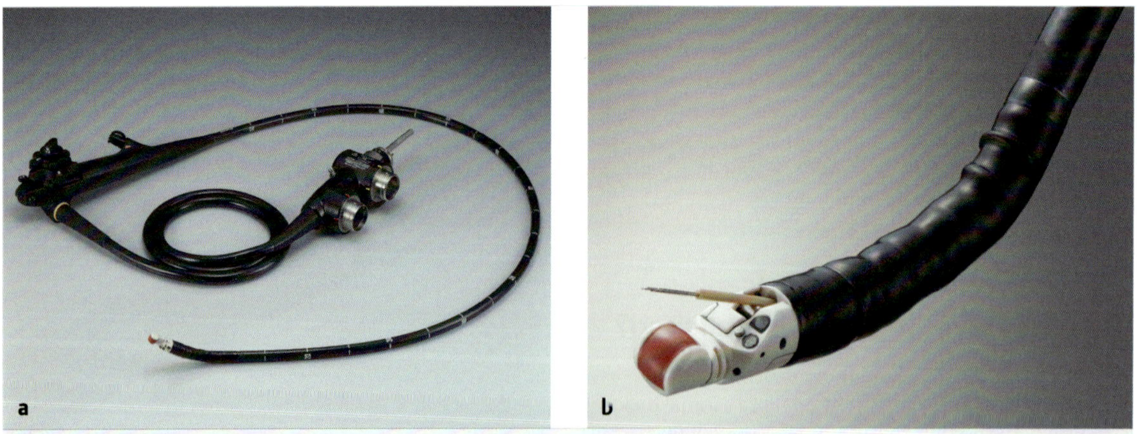

Fig. 22.3 Olympus GF-UCT180 therapeutic ultrasound gastroscope with CHE capability and 180° longitudinal scan. (Source: Reproduced with kind permission of Olympus Deutschland GmbH, Hamburg, Germany.)
a General view.
b Distal end.

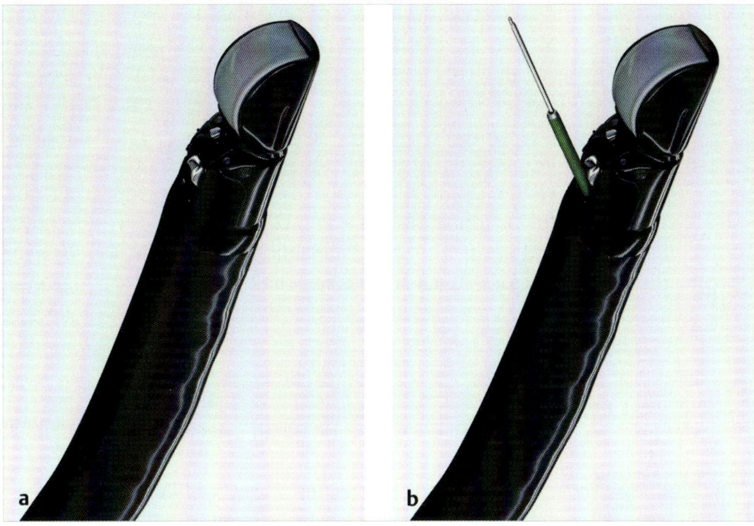

Fig. 22.4 Fujinon EG 530 UT therapeutic ultrasound gastroscope.
a Without needle system.
b With needle system.

- The cell block technique, based on the cytocentrifugation of aspirated material, can duplicate the advantages of histologic tissue sampling.
- Cell block cytology yields tissuelike cell aggregates that can be embedded in paraffin for both histologic and immunocytologic study.[24]
- Conventional rigid needle systems for histologic tissue sampling (19-gauge) do not (yet) have the versatile guidance needed for critical biopsy applications, especially in the pancreatic head, and are in need of further refinement.

▶ **Our own experience.** We have found the 22-gauge needle to be excellent for aspiration cytology. It is uncertain whether 25-gauge needles, with their presumed lower complication rate and simplified use (biopsy of hard tissues), would be advantageous for this application. For interventional endosonography we use 19-gauge needles (Cook Medical, Olympus, Boston Scientific, Beacon Endoscopic/Covidien), which can accommodate a 0.035-inch guidewire. It should be noted that the 19-gauge needles supplied by Medi-Globe, with their slightly smaller inner lumen, cannot accommodate a 0.035-inch wire, only wires with a maximum diameter of 0.030 inch.

Typical EUS aspiration needles are illustrated in ▶ Fig. 22.5 and ▶ Fig. 22.6.

22.3.4 Guidewires

Today a great variety of guidewires are available commercially. Their suitability depends on the specific indication. Radiopaque wires in lengths of 260 to 450 cm are usually flexible at the tip (made of Teflon or PVC), have a nitinol core for stability, and may have high torque stability. A hydrophilic coating facilitates wire insertion, and various color markers or centimeter scales allow for wire placement without continuous fluoroscopic guidance. The two preferred guidewires in current use are the Jagwire (Boston Scientific) and the Metro (Cook Medical) (▶ Fig. 22.7). The Terumo wire, designed for angiologic use, should be well wetted before insertion and is useful for wayfinding, especially when dealing with Klatskin tumors (HS^+, FS^-). The hybrid wire has a tip that is similar to the Terumo wire (continuous flush) but not quite as soft. The hybrid wire is useful after the precut and for delivering metal stents into the duodenum (the wire is 40 cm longer).

Our preferred access wires are the Jagwire and the Super Stiff wire. Both have a flexible tip that reduces the risk of perforation after insertion into the cyst lumen. In the atraumatic access technique (dilation), we have found that the Jagwire is often too unstable to provide effective guidance for a dilator. The Super Stiff wire has proven useful in this situation; it keeps the dilator in line with the dilation axis, creating an optimum vector for force transfer. One disadvantage of the conventional Super Stiff wire is the steel core of the fixed shaft; as a result the wire is not kink-resistant and must be used with caution. An improvement is the super-stiff cyst access wire developed by the firm MTW Endoskopie. This wire resists kinking, but its short length prevents the use of certain accessory devices (e.g., colon dilation balloon). Also, the wire is not insulated so it is not suitable for electrosurgical access with a cystotome or diathermy ring, for example. Medi-Globe offers a similar stiff steel wire (length 400 cm) with a flexible tip, but this wire is uncoated too, and therefore is not suitable for diathermy use.

Both the Jagwire and Metro wire are suitable for access with electrosurgical cutting instruments such as a needle-knife papillotome or the newly developed diathermy ring with circular cutting edge. The tissue can be cut with very little force application, and the wire coating is compatible with a diathermy current.

One disadvantage of coated wires is that difficult placement maneuvers (e.g., EUS-guided biliary drainage) or attempts to adjust the wire position may shear off the

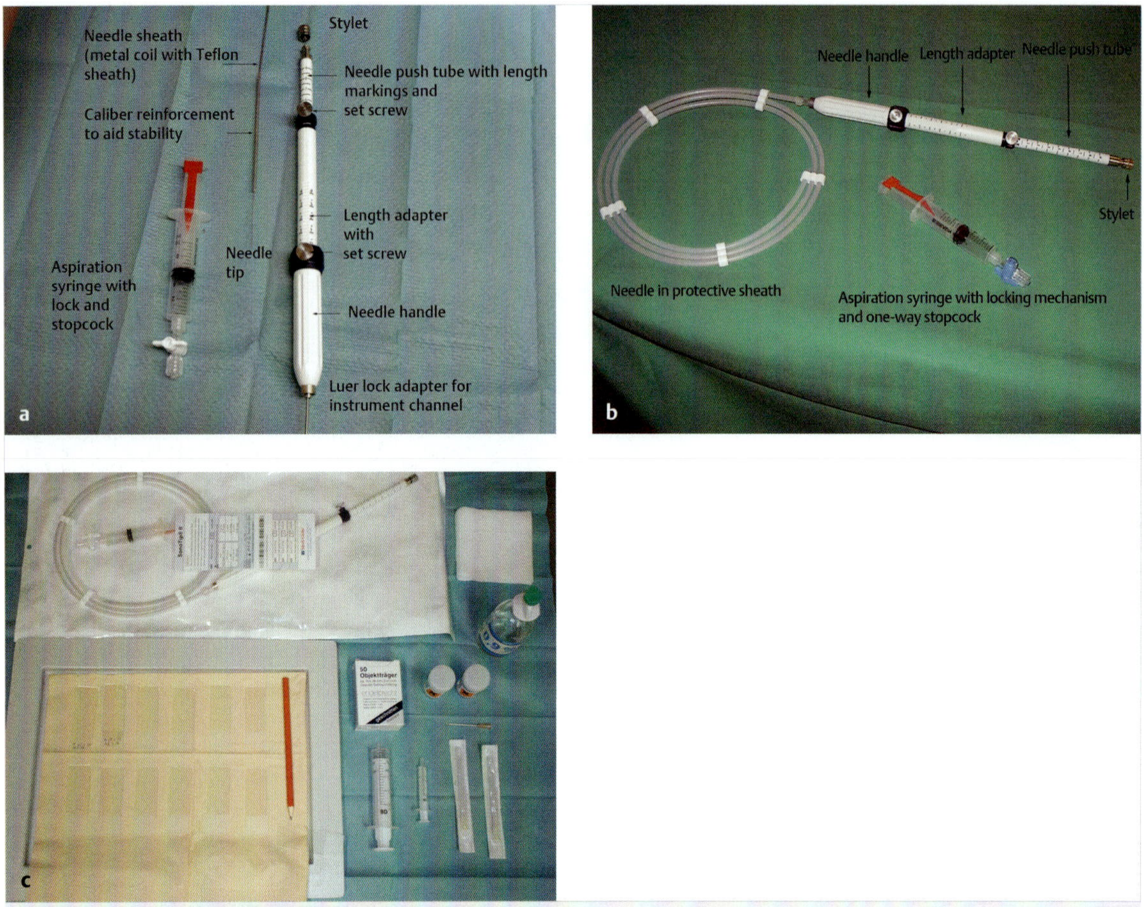

Fig. 22.5 The 22-gauge SonoTip II EUS aspiration needle (Medi-Globe). The system components are labeled (**a**, **b**) and a table setup is shown (**c**).

Terumo tip or the Teflon sheath at the sharp needle tip, which would jeopardize the success of the intervention and may lead to complications (▶ Fig. 22.8).

A special 19-gauge intervention needle assembly (EchoTip Access, Cook Medical) with a blunt hollow needle and pointed stylet has recently been developed to minimize this risk (▶ Fig. 22.9).

As an alternative to a 19-gauge needle, diathermy devices (diathermy rings, cystotomes, needle knives) can be used to establish primary access to pancreatic and nonpancreatic fluid collections. Various manufacturers offer these devices, as well as fixed-diameter and balloon dilators of various diameters for enlarging a wire-secured access tract. The specific device will depend on the targeted lesion and the characteristics of the access route.

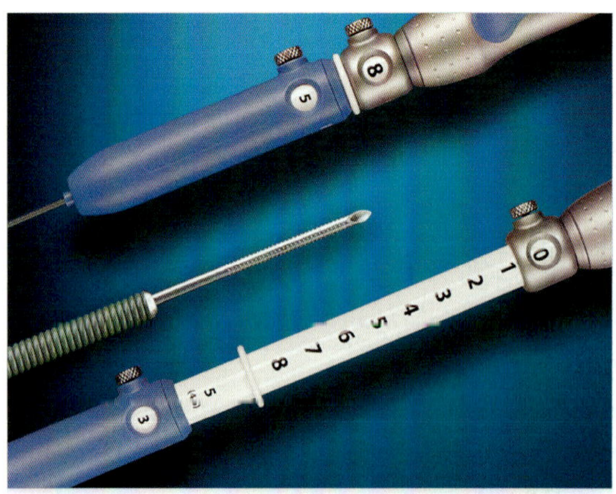

Fig. 22.6 The 19-gauge EchoTip Ultra EUS aspiration needle (Cook Medical), the standard needle for EUS-guided interventions.

22.3.5 Fixed-Diameter Dilators

Tissue dilators ranging from 5F to 9F (▶ Fig. 22.10) can provide atraumatic access following needle insertion and wire placement. As a rule, the transgastric access route established by the guidewire is initially enlarged with a

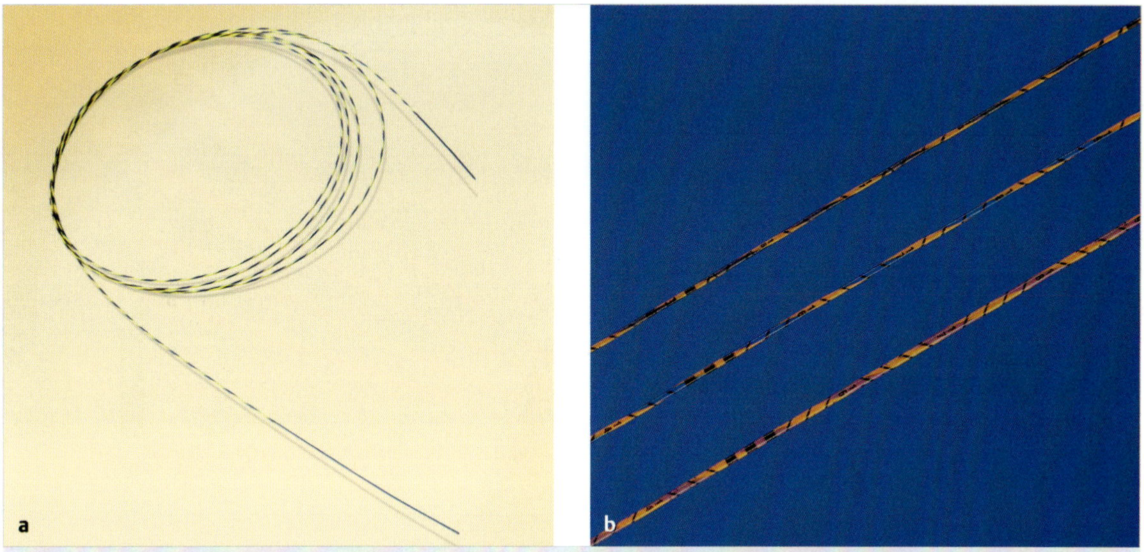

Fig. 22.7 Guidewires. The Hydra Jagwire (Boston Scientific) (**a**) and Metro Wire (Cook Medical) (**b**) are shown.

6F biliary dilator. Because the 5F and 6F dilators have identical tips, the greater stability of the 6F dilator is better for tract enlargement. Successful dilation to 6F is followed by a second dilation with a 7F dilator, which will establish sufficient access for inserting a balloon dilator. We have also had good experience with graduated dilators such as the Cotton dilator (5–7–8.5F, 5–7–10F; Cook Medical).

22.3.6 Balloon Dilators

The most suitable access balloon for cyst drainage is a multidiameter balloon such as the CRE balloon dilator (Boston Scientific). This type of device differs from single-diameter biliary balloon dilators (▶ Fig. 22.11, ▶ Fig. 22.12).

Cook Medical now offers a similar device (Quantum TTC). The balloons are introduced in a very low-profile configuration on the delivery system permitting easy access after initial dilation to 7F or initial cutting with a needle-knife papillotome or diathermy ring. Because no waisting occurs at the center of the balloon, care should be taken on initial access that the balloon is centered in the stomach wall and does not slip into the cyst lumen or displace outward. If this occurs, we recommend deflating and repositioning the device, which is often made easier by creating an artificial waist in the balloon. The Titan

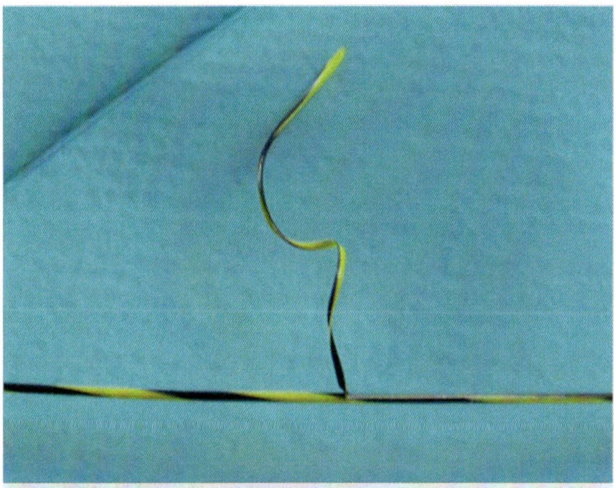

Fig. 22.8 Endoglide coating has been sheared off the guidewire by the sharp tip of a 19-gauge needle during the transgastric EUS-guided placement of a biliary drain.

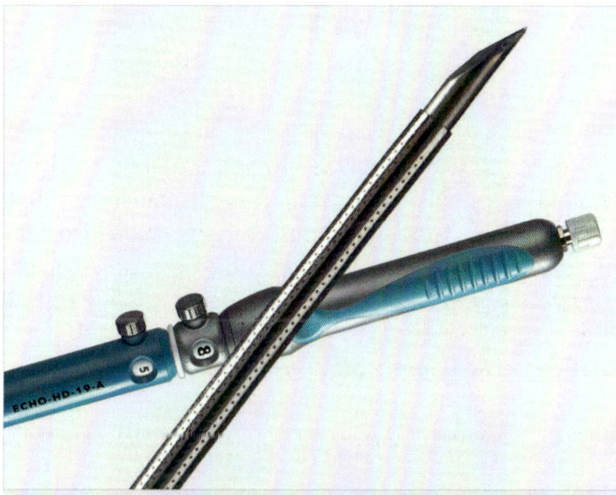

Fig. 22.9 Access needle (Cook Medical). This 19-gauge access needle uses the stylet as a needle (rather than protecting the needle with the stylet as in traditional designs).

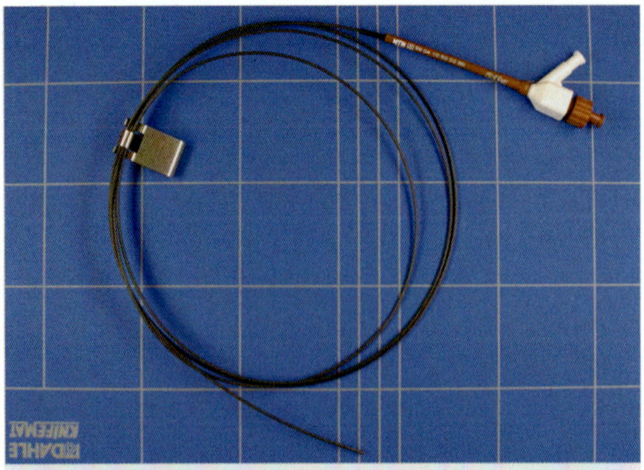

Fig. 22.10 Dilator (MTW Endoskopie).

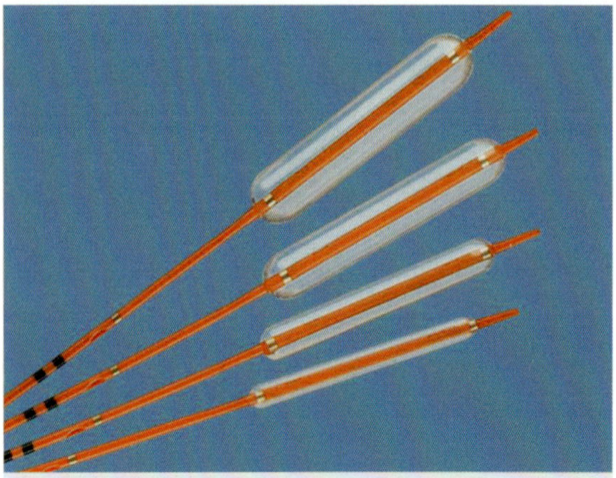

Fig. 22.12 Titan balloon dilators (Cook Medical).

balloon dilators (Cook Medical) inflate uniformly from the proximal and distal ends through a multiport system, making it less likely that the balloon will slip if not optimally centered.

The necessary balloon size depends on the proposed intervention. For example, a 6-mm biliary balloon dilator is usually adequate for cholangiodrainage. A 6–7–8-mm multidiameter balloon dilator can provide good initial access for a simple cyst drainage or planned cystoscopy. On the other hand, an emergency situation requiring immediate intervention and endoscopic débridement may require dilation to at least 12 mm, if not to 15 or 20 mm. Redilations or extensive interventions may require up to 35 mm for sufficient access. Since there are no balloons designed specifically for that purpose, an achalasia balloon dilator must be used.

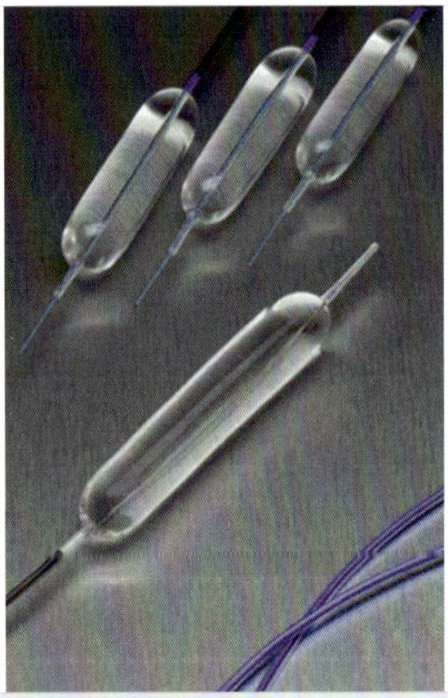

Fig. 22.11 CRE balloon dilators (Boston Scientific).

The CRE wire-guided balloon dilation catheter can produce three distinct pressure-controlled diameters. Balloon sizes are printed on each package and labeled hub. The CRE balloon dilation catheter is designed to fit through the working channel of an endoscope and can accommodate a 0.035-inch guidewire. This catheter is supplied with a preloaded 0.035-inch flexible-tip guidewire in its guidewire lumen. The guidewire is 25 cm longer than the balloon catheter, with excess length protruding from the catheter hub. For safety, balloons should not be reinflated or tested before use.

22.3.7 Plastic Stents (Pigtail)

Two main plastic stent designs are used: double-pigtail stents with a loop at both ends and straight stents with or without side holes (▶ Fig. 22.13). Both types have advantages and disadvantages for cyst drainage as described below. Single-pigtail stents do not have a role in endosonographic interventions. Straight stents have better drainage properties because the absence of a curve makes the lumen less susceptible to clogging. Drains with side holes (Amsterdam stents) have the best drainage properties but poorer site stability because they generally require an inner and outer barb for retention. To solve this problem, "Tannenbaum" (Christmas tree) stents were developed that have four barbs at each end for more stable retention.

We generally use 8F double-pigtail stents, as we have found that the actual drainage efficiency of the stent is of minor importance for cyst drainage or even necrosectomy. The drainage effect depends on the size of the access tract that has been created, and so the function of the stent is basically reduced to maintaining tract patency. Double-pigtail stents have the best retention properties because they are atraumatic on the cyst side and the pigtail provides a good anchoring effect in the cyst and in the stomach.

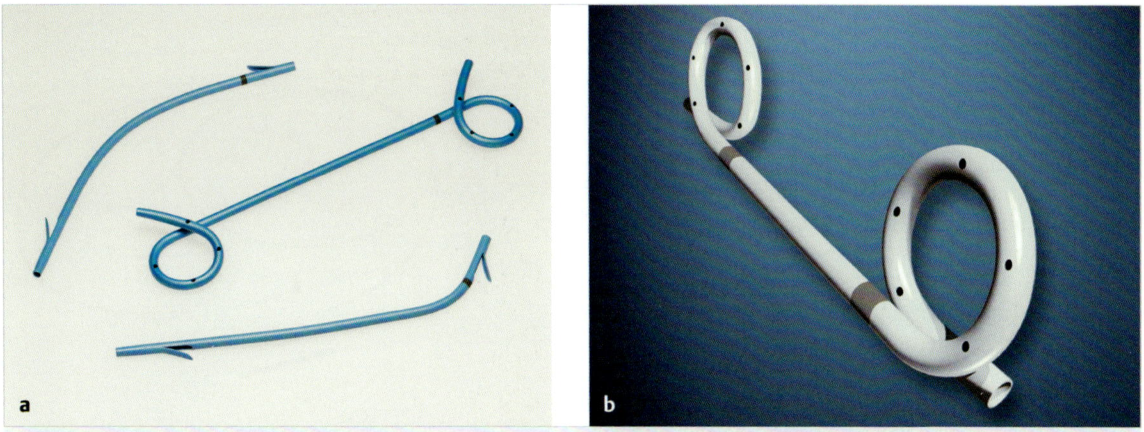

Fig. 22.13 Innovative plastic stents. The photograph illustrates a double-pigtail plastic stent along with conventional straight and angled designs (Advanix, Boston Scientific) (**a**). The double-pigtail stent (Solos, Cook Medical) in (**b**) has two radiopaque markers; it is available in 10F with the Solus introducer set for one-step placement. The set includes the radiopaque 10F stent, 10F/165-cm delivery catheter, and 5F/210-cm guide catheter. A 0.035-inch guidewire is recommended.

It is best to use a stent with center and edge markers because following deflation of the balloon, the draining cyst fluid will obscure vision of the puncture site and increase the risk of advancing the stent too far into the fluid collection.

22.3.8 Metal Stents

Traditional biliary stents (Amsterdam stents) can be used for EUS-guided biliary and pancreatic duct drainage. The stent sizes most often used for these applications are 7F or 10F. It is important to have an adequate stent length in the liver or stomach, as movements of the stomach are apt to cause stent migration. The use of covered metal stents has recently been advocated (▶ Fig. 22.14, ▶ Fig. 22.15). These devices have the advantage of a large lumen and lower occlusion rates.

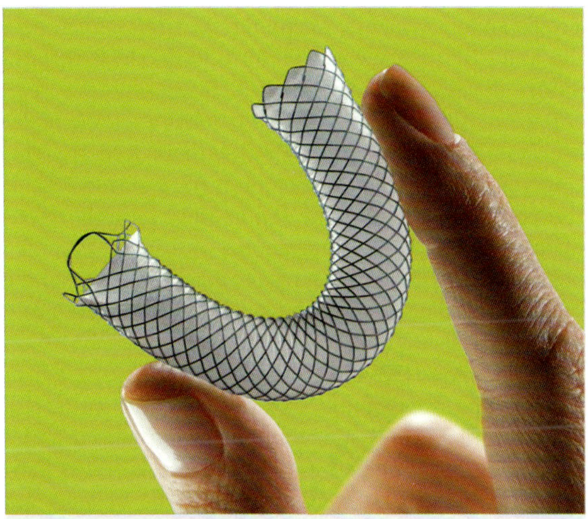

Fig. 22.14 WallFlex metal stent.

Biliary metal stents are available in many designs, either with or without covering. Most stents are made of nitinol because of its outstanding properties but differ in their weave and wire gauge; these differences cause differences in X-ray visibility. Some stents are cut from nitinol in a way that prevents shortening during deployment. Metal stents with a thin wire weave usually carry additional radiopaque markers to ensure adequate visibility. For transgastric, transduodenal, or transjejunal EUS-guided biliary drainage, only covered stents should be used, however, in order to avoid bile leakage. Metal stents

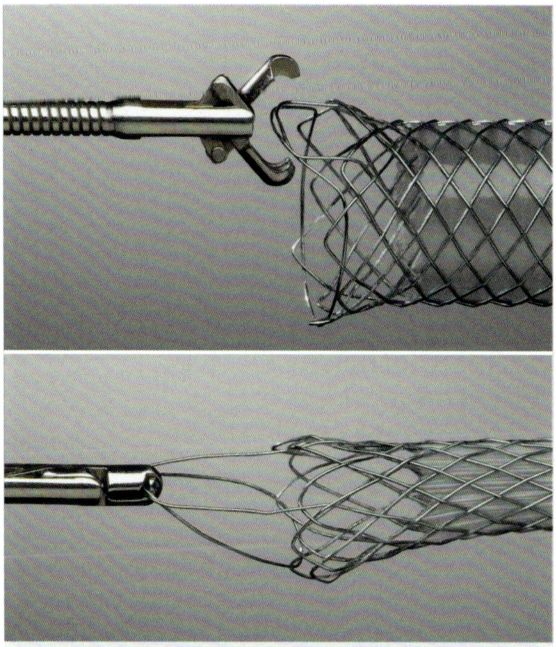

Fig. 22.15 WallFlex metal stent with forceps retrieval option.

should also have some reserve length in the liver or stomach to prevent migration.

Some authors are currently testing the use of large-bore metal stents to maintain access for pseudocyst drainage or necrosectomy. This can be done with short esophageal metal stents (Ultraflex 18 mm, length 7 cm [Boston Scientific], Aixstent Esophagus 102–20–060, length 60 mm [Leufen Medical]), or specially developed pseudocyst access stents (e.g. Aixstent Pseudocyst, diameter 10 and 14 mm, nitinol, length 20 mm, fully covered [Leufen Medical]). Initial reports confirm better access for necrosectomy. The stent is only temporary, however, and must be retrievable at the end of the procedure. K. Binmoeller and his group have developed two innovative devices for endosonographic drainage: a needle- and balloon-assisted access system that employs two guidewires (Navix); and a short, covered apposition stent (Axios), also available as a combined system from Xlumena, Inc.

The unique Platinol wire construction of the WallFlex RX biliary stent system (▶ Fig. 22.14, ▶ Fig. 22.15) is setting new standards with its characteristics:

- Flexibility to aid placement in tortuous anatomies and maintain luminal patency
- Full-length radiopacity to improve visibility during stent placement
- Radial force to maximize the stent diameter
- Yellow marker on the end of the stent
- Reconstrainability of the stent up to 80% of deployment to aid in repositioning
- Multiple markers to increase placement accuracy
- Ability to remove fully or partially covered stents to meet acute requirements
- Platinol wire construction

Other features include:

- Integrated retrieval loop (fully or partially covered)
- Rounded and flared stent ends to resist migration
- Closed-cell design and coating options
- Permalume covering
- Biliary RX delivery system
- Four fluoroscopy markers
- Yellow transition zone on the catheter
- Repositioning limit marker on the handle

22.3.9 Diathermy Devices, Cystotome

Occasionally, wire-guided access to a pseudocyst, necrotic area, or duct cannot be achieved with dilators. In this case various diathermy devices, known mostly from their use in endoscopic retrograde cholangiopancreatography (ERCP), can be used following needle-assisted wire placement (▶ Fig. 22.16, ▶ Fig. 22.17a). These devices consist of monopolar needle knives delivered over a guidewire (this is essential; otherwise access to the cyst would be lost after the cut), circular metal rings or cones mounted at the tip of a wire-guided catheter (cystotome or diathermy ring), and a device that combines a central cutting wire with a larger-diameter cutting ring. Generally these instruments are powered by a software-controlled high-frequency current (Endocut). Access to a fluid collection or obstructed duct is achieved through a combination of electrosurgical tissue destruction and a mechanical pushing force.

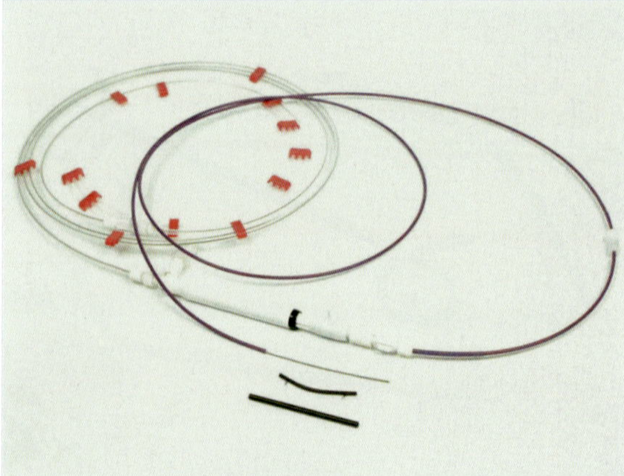

Fig. 22.16 Giovannini set (Cook Medical).

Wire guidance is necessary to ensure that the cutting device does not stray from the intended target.

Caution

Note that the gas generated by electrosurgical tissue destruction may cause significant artifacts, which are particularly troublesome in EUS-guided cholangiodrainage.

Suitable instruments are double- or triple-lumen needle-knife papillotomes (Huibregste HPC-3 Triple Lumen Needle Knife [Cook Medical], KD-V 441 M triple-lumen needle knife [Olympus]; Microknife XL triple-lumen needle knife [Boston Scientific]; BII GSP 34 20 020 wire-guided papillotome [Medi-Globe]), diathermy rings (e.g., MTW Endoskopie), and other BII papillotomes. We prefer the Cysto-Gastro Set (Endo-Flex) without a central cutting wire, available in diameters of 6F, 8.5F and 10F, or the cutting ring cystotome (Endo-Flex) recently developed by U. Will. One disadvantage of using multilumen needle-knife or BII papillotomes is the space between the guidewire and needle, which may make it difficult to gain entry into the cyst in some circumstances.

A cystotome (CST-10, Cook Medical, ▶ Fig. 22.17) or needle-knife papillotome can also be used primarily, without prior needle insertion, when introduced under endosonographic guidance. Needle-based access is definitely safer, however, because the needle knife is not kink-resistant and may skid off the firm cyst wall after passing through the intestinal wall.

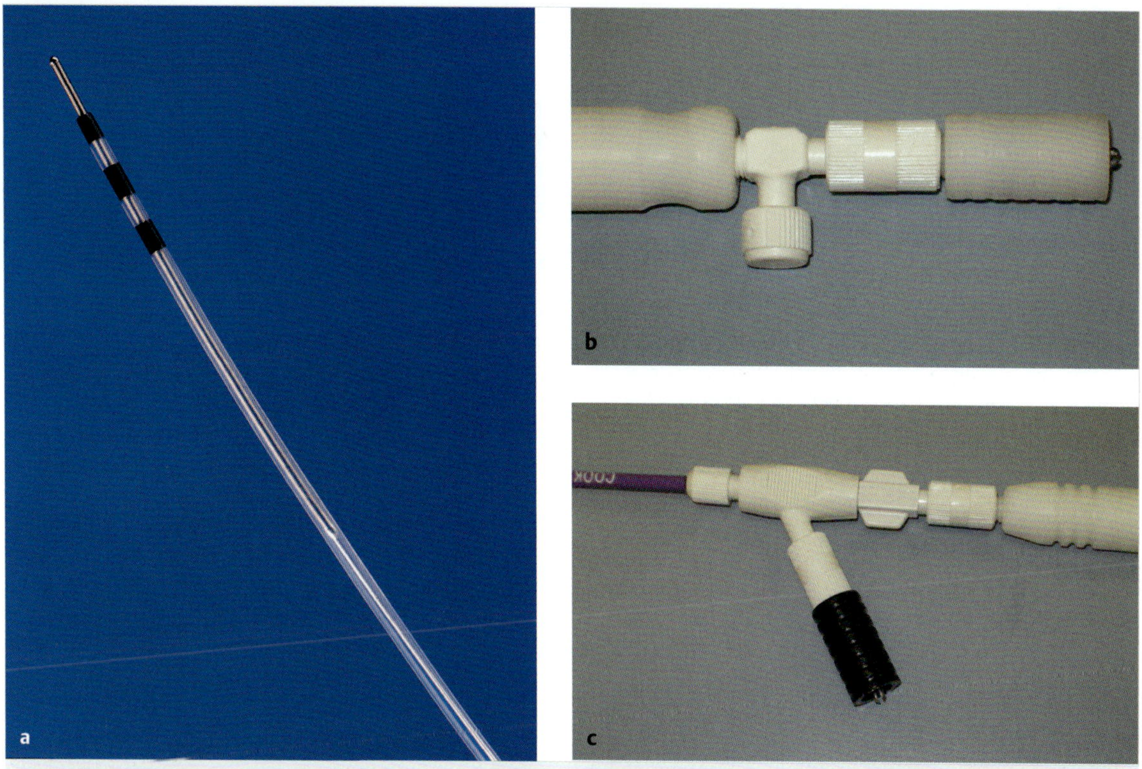

Fig. 22.17 a–c Cystotome. CST-10 cystotome (Cook Medical) for electrosurgical transgastric or transduodenal cystoenterostomy of a pancreatic pseudocyst visibly bulging into the gastrointestinal tract. The system has a minimum working channel 3.7 mm in diameter, a 10F/165-cm outer catheter, a 5F/190-cm inner catheter, and a 10F diathermy ring. The manufacturer recommends the Tracer Metro Direct guidewire (0.035-inch). The handle has two separate HF ports in contrasting colors (step one: white port; step two: black port for the 10F diathermy ring).

Cook Medical developed an all-in-one system in which a cutting wire is used to create initial access followed by the placement of a dilator and an 8.5F stent ("Giovannini set," ▶ Fig. 22.16).

A very similar cyst drainage set was designed by Dr. C. Grotjahn (MTW Endoskopie). Once the diathermy needle has entered the cyst lumen, however, it must be replaced by a flexible wire before the preloaded straight 8.5F stent can be delivered. Unfortunately, the access obtainable with this system is no larger than the stent diameter, so that no further interventions can be carried out. Another disadvantage is the relatively high risk of primary or secondary migration of the relatively short, straight plastic stents.

A new development is the diathermy ring produced by MTW Endoskopie. This is a cutting knife with a circular (tapered cylindrical) cutting edge that surrounds the guidewire. The wire keeps the ring centered on the target and creates access comparable to a 6F dilator, facilitating further interventions.

Despite a lack of supportive data, the main difference between atraumatic dilation and diathermy access lies in the potential for hemorrhage. In theory, the dilator compresses the vessels in the stomach wall to minimize bleeding risk, while a cutting process may increase the risk of vascular disruption.

Cystotomes (fistulotomes) are available from Cook Medical (CST-10 10F cystotome [necessary working channel 3.7 mm], the Endoflex 2-stage fistulotome model XS 99900000340 [10F] and XS 99900000341 [8.5F]), and the diathermy ring cystotome designed by Uwe Will is available from MTW Endoskopie.

The triple-lumen needle knife (Olympus) has separate channels for a guidewire, cutting wire, and contrast instillation. Other features are a radiopaque tip and a needle knife 5 mm long and 0.2 mm in diameter.

22.3.10 Retrievers

Stent retrievers are wire-guided flexible metal coils that have a threaded conical tip (▶ Fig. 22.18). The tip is "screwed" into the distal end of a straight plastic stent by rotating the instrument shaft clockwise. This allows plastic stents to be removed through the working channel while the endoscope and guidewire remain in place. Combined with a stiff guidewire, this instrument can also be used in EUS-PD and pseudocyst drainage to mechanically enlarge a primary needle tract through fibrotic pancreatic tissue or a tough pseudocyst capsule.

The Soehendra stent retriever (SSR-x, Cook Medical) is available in diameters of 5, 7, 8.5, 10 and 11.5F. It is

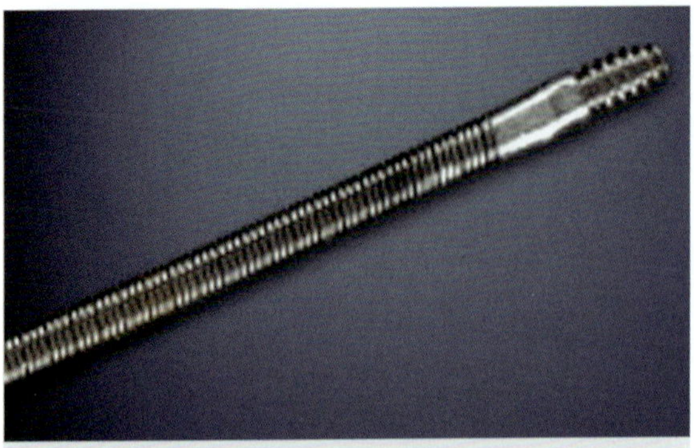

Fig. 22.18 Soehendra retriever (Cook Medical).

designed primarily for engaging and removing biliary and pancreatic duct stents with the guidewire *still in place.* It is particularly useful for pancreatic duct drainage performed during an EUS-guided intervention. The minimum working channel matches the corresponding French size (▶ Fig. 22.18).

22.3.11 Supplementary Techniques in EUS-guided Biopsy

The success of an intervention depends critically on the personal experience of the operator in ultrasonography and endoscopy (which includes institution-specific features), the puncture technique including specimen collection (number of needle passes), and specimen processing in cooperation with the cytologist (cellularity) or pathologist (formalin fixation, correct identification of tissue fragments versus blood clots). Supplies should include an adequate number of glass slides (> 5) with a frosted end for labeling, formalin solution for tissue fixation, isotonic (0.9%) saline solutions, and special media.

Special tests are applied selectively, such as immunocytochemical tests and FISH in lymphoma diagnosis, PCR and culture for detection of tuberculosis, and tumor marker assays (especially CEA but also CA19–9, AFP, CA15–3) in fluid samples from, say, cystic pancreatic lesions for clinical and chemical evaluation (cell differentiation, tumor markers, microbiology, etc.). Attention should be given to various cytologic methods. Wet fixation for cytologic analysis is necessary only if Papanicolaou staining is to be done. But many cytologists now use the simpler May–Grünwald–Giemsa stain, which requires simple air dried slides. It should be noted that immunocytology also requires air-dried slides because a wet-fixed specimen will not take additional staining. Detailed clinical information is necessary for a discriminating analysis (genetic analysis, proliferation indices). Accurate lymphoma classification requires the examination of a whole lymph node because some lymphomas can be correctly classified only by their infiltration pattern in specific lymph node regions.

22.4 Procedure

The patient is generally placed in a left lateral decubitus position that is turned slightly toward the table to reduce aspiration risk. The patient may be positioned prone for papillary lesions or, less commonly (also due to aspiration risk) supine for pancreatic drainage.

22.4.1 Sedation

The goal of sedation is to immobilize the patient so that the technically challenging intervention can be carried out. Sedation is induced by the fractionated administration of Disoprivan (Propofol in initial dose of 40–60 mg), which may be supplemented if necessary by midazolam (e.g., Dormicum [Roche Pharma] 1–2.5 mg). Pulse oximetry, ECG, and blood pressure monitoring should be supervised by a physician experienced in critical care medicine (Chapter 11). Peri-interventional oxygen supplementation is standard at our facility. Generally there is no need to add topical oropharyngeal anesthetics (e.g., Xylocaine [lidocaine] spray [AstraZeneca]) or analgesics such as pethidine hydrochloride (Dolantin, Sanofi).[1,25]

22.4.2 Other Medications

The administration of *N*-butylscopolamine (Buscopan, Boehringer Ingelheim Pharma) or atropine is necessary only in exceptional, justified cases. Antibiotic prophylaxis follows published recommendations and is mandatory in the puncture of cystic lesions. Suitable antibiotics are aminopenicillins (e.g., amoxicillin IV or oral, 3 × 1 g), cephalosporins (e.g., ceftriaxone 2 g IV, single shot), and fluoroquinolones (ciprofloxacin or levofloxacin, 400 mg IV, 500 mg or oral twice, but only on the intervention day).

22.4.3 Orientation

The patient's neck should be slightly hyperextended during insertion of the echoendoscope (due to the relatively stiff instrument tip). The procedural protocol and orientation are not standardized. We have found it helpful to advance the scope under combined endoscopic and endosonographic guidance. Possible complications have been described in detail and should be avoided.[26,27] Mural lesions may be approached under endoscopic vision, though this is not mandatory. Whenever possible, we rely more on endosonographic than endoscopic orientation. Generally it is unnecessary to distend the stomach with water, and we do not use balloon distention.

22.4.4 General Rules for Needle Insertion

EUS-guided drainage generally employs an echoendoscope with a large-bore working channel (3.7 mm or

3.8 mm, depending on the manufacturer) and an Albarran lever. When an echoendoscope with a small working channel is used, the initial puncture must be made with a 22-gauge needle. After insertion of a 0.025-inch guidewire, the initial scope is then exchanged for a therapeutic duodenoscope or gastroscope so that further therapeutic steps can be carried out. A 22-gauge needle is generally adequate for EUS-guided injection therapy. The ultrasound platform should permit color duplex scanning to ensure a high degree of procedural safety.

22.4.5 Biopsy Technique

After the targeted lesion has been identified, the ultrasound probe is brought to bear on the lesion and placed in a stable position (artifact-free endoscope coupling with no troublesome air echoes). Because the access angle is relatively flat, it is helpful to adjust the control wheel to position the lesion at the top of the image before the needle is introduced. Color duplex scan can exclude interposed blood vessels. The metal coil or Teflon sheath (together with the retracted needle) is then introduced into the biopsy channel. The needle should be fixed at this point to avoid damage to the EUS probe. The coil is introduced completely, and the handle is firmly connected to the endoscope by the Luer lock mechanism. With adjustable-length needles, the length should be adjusted so that the metal coil or Teflon sheath of the needle is just visible sonographically and/or endoscopically. If a needle with Teflon sheath is advanced too far, it may accidentally perforate the sheath (▶ Fig. 22.19). In this case a wire can no longer be passed when the needle is withdrawn. The working channel may also be damaged during needle removal.[26]

To perform the biopsy, the blunt stylet inside the fixed needle is withdrawn by about 10 mm so that the sharp point can be advanced by 6 to 8 cm (or farther in some cases). In needles with a pointed stylet, it is unnecessary to withdraw the stylet. On reaching the target lesion, some authors recommend readvancing the stylet to reduce contamination of the aspirate by mural epithelial cells. Other authors reject this technique on hygienic grounds, since advancing any object from the needle constitutes contamination. When the needle tip has reached the target lesion, the stylet is removed and suction is applied to the needle with the 10-mL Luer lock syringe. At this point the needle is repeatedly moved back and forth in the lesion under constant EUS vision to aspirate cells and tissue. Any suction that is applied should be discontinued before the needle is removed to avoid aspirating nonlesional tissue and luminal fluid. Other authors do not use a stylet or suction at all (proving that even this technique can yield acceptable results). After the biopsy is completed, the needle is first retracted into the sleeve and then removed from the working channel together with the sleeve and handle.

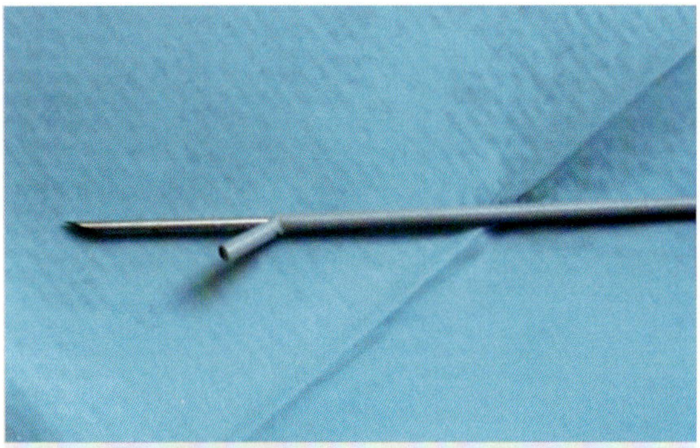

Fig. 22.19 The Teflon sheath of this 19-gauge EchoTip aspiration needle (Cook Medical) was perforated by the sharp steel needle during the aspiration biopsy of a pseudocyst.

To sample a different site in a presumably malignant lesion, the needle should be changed. If blood residues are sampled, the needle should be flushed between passes with sterile saline solution and then "blown out" with an air-filled syringe to avoid fluid-induced artifacts due to cellular swelling.

22.4.6 Suction

Aspiration techniques (with or without suction) vary greatly in clinical practice. Biopsy without suction is based on the experience published by Wallace et al that applying suction during the EUS-FNA of lymph nodes increases the blood contamination of smears and therefore does not improve the diagnostic yield despite the greater cellularity.[20] On comparing intermittent and continuous suction as well as aspiration syringes of different volumes, Bhutani et al found that continuous suction with smaller syringe volumes (5–10 mL) provided an optimum cell yield.[29] It may be that aspiration at higher suction can improve the recovery of material suitable for histologic evaluation.[30,31]

22.4.7 Specimen Processing

The stylet is slowly advanced within the needle to expel cells and any tissue fragments onto a tilted glass slide held beneath the needle tip. The material is then smeared, air-dried, and processed further for cytologic examination. Small tissue cores or formed clots are placed in formalin solution for histologic evaluation (▶ Fig. 22.20, ▶ Fig. 22.21, ▶ Fig. 22.22, and ▶ Fig. 22.23). Procedural details and problems relating to blood in the aspirate and specimen processing are described elsewhere[26,32] (see Chapter 6).

All specimens should be clearly labeled and the indication stated. For some clinical indications (gastrointestinal stromal tumors [GIST], lymphoma, etc.) the cytologist should be contacted directly for special test requests (e.g., proliferation indices, CD34, c-kit analysis).

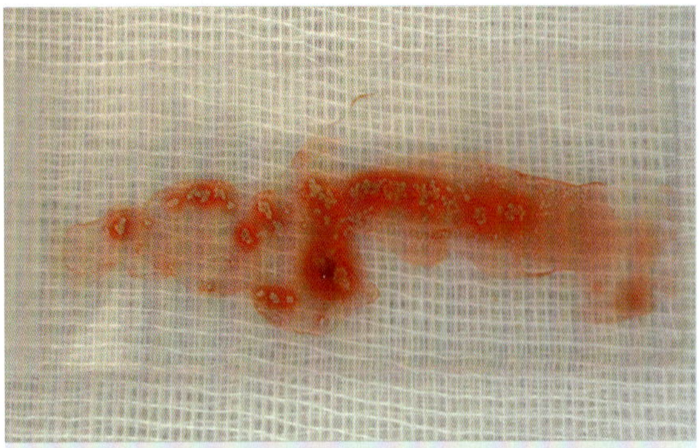

Fig. 22.20 Fine, light tissue fragments with slight admixture of serosanguinous fluid, well suited for preparing a cytologic smear. The specimen should be smeared quickly to avoid drying.

Factors that may affect diagnostic yield are outlined in ▶ Table 22.1. Lesions that can be sampled by EUS-FNA are listed in order of difficulty in ▶ Table 22.2.

22.5 Diagnostic Interventions

Biopsies should be performed with the smallest possible needle diameter that is still effective. The yield from a 25-gauge needle (Cook Medical or Medi-Globe) is generally adequate for the benign/malignant differentiation of lesions. A 22-gauge or 19-gauge needle (Cook Medical; Medi-Globe; Olympus; MTW Endoskopie; Boston Scientific) is more likely to harvest material that can be evaluated histologically. The same applies to desired immunocytochemical tests (lymphoma classification, GIST), which consistently require the use of a 19-gauge needle.[26]

The operator and the cytologist (pathologist) are both critical for a high cytologic and histologic accuracy rate, which should range from 70% (pancreas) to approximately 100% (lymph nodes, adrenal gland) depending on the targeted area.[33] On-site cytology is particularly helpful for beginners as it provides immediate feedback on diagnostic yield.

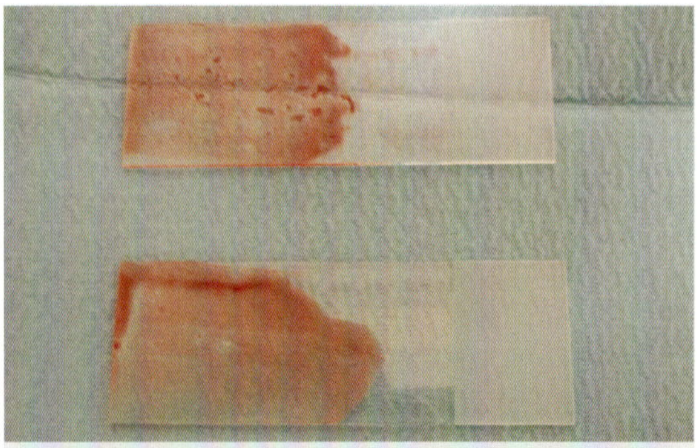

Fig. 22.22 Completed smears. The frosted end of the slide should be clearly labeled.

22.5.1 Indications

EUS-FNA has proven its ability to supply a tissue diagnosis for lesions and lymph nodes in the mediastinum, hepatobiliary system, and retroperitoneum; for stage-adapted tumor therapy (multimodal therapies, especially neoadjuvant treatment strategies); and for the identification of inflammatory conditions (tuberculosis, sarcoidosis).[26] The importance of EUS-FNA for the classification of intramural tumors in the gastrointestinal tract is controversial.[34] Indications for EUS-FNA in the gastrointestinal tract are as follows:

- N-staging of tumors of the upper and lower gastrointestinal tract and lung (also the M-staging of certain tumors [left lobe of the liver, porta hepatis])
- Investigation of subepithelial (submucous) tumors in the esophagus, stomach, duodenum, rectum, and colon
- Investigation of abscesses and fluid collections in the chest, abdomen, and pelvis
- Investigation of mediastinal and retroperitoneal lymphadenopathy
- Investigation of small liver lesions (left lobe of the liver, porta hepatis)
- Investigation of lesions in the left adrenal gland

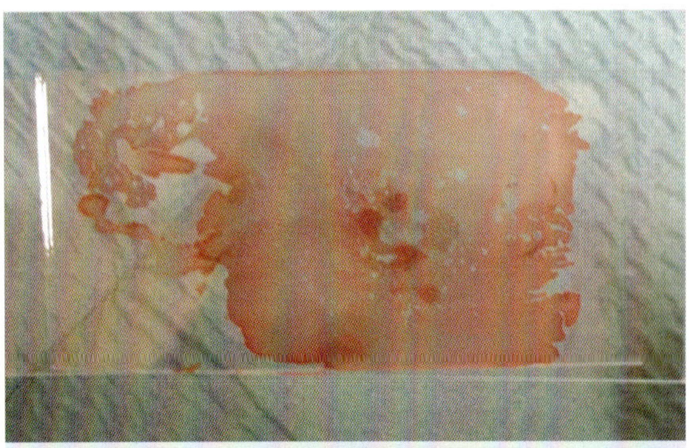

Fig. 22.21 The specimen is smeared between two glass slides, which are slid in opposite directions while gentle pressure is applied.

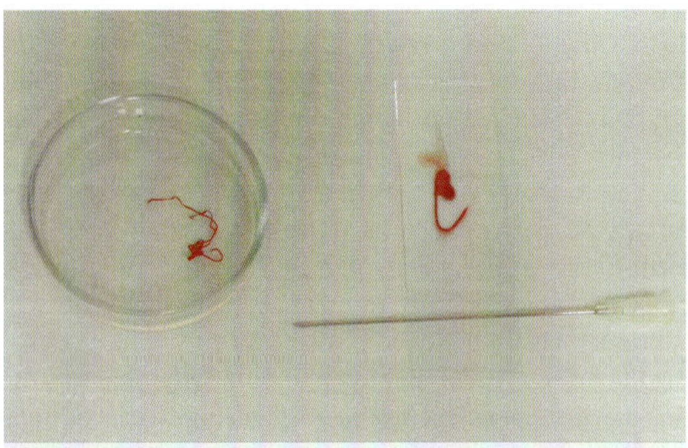

Fig. 22.23 Small tissue cores or clots should be picked up from the slide with a hypodermic needle and placed in formalin solution.

Table 22.1 Factors that may affect diagnostic yield

Factors	Relevance	Problems
Target organ or tissue		
Location	+	Problems with specimen collection: genu of the pancreas, head of the pancreas, especially the uncinate process starting from the descending part of the duodenum; gastrointestinal wall lesions; interposed blood vessels
Benign/malignant differentiation	+	Less than optimum diagnostic yield: benign lesions, well-differentiated adenocarcinoma of the pancreas
Tumor type	++	Problems with specimen collection: subepithelial tumors, pancreatic carcinoma, cystic neoplasms
Vascularity	+	Contamination of smears with blood
Size of lesion	+	Problems with specimen collection: very small lymph nodes and tumors, very large tumors (necrosis)
Technical variables		
Needle diameter, needle type	+	Affects specimen yield for cytology and histology; also affects the technical difficulty of the biopsy
Applied suction	+	Affects cellularity, histologic specimen yield, and blood contamination
Number of needle passes	++	Necessary number of needle passes depends on the target organ and tumor type
Organizational and structural variables		
Clinical-pathologic interaction	+	On-site cytology can increase diagnostic yield by 10–15%
Experience and training (endosonographer, cytopathologist)	++	Distinct learning curve
Different cytopathologic techniques	+	Can improve diagnostic yield in certain cases
Standard quality management	+	Can reduce diagnostic errors
Other factors		
Contamination by tissue from the needle tract or pancreatic acinar cells	+	May hamper smear interpretation, raise problems of differential diagnosis
Significant blood contamination	+	Hampers smear interpretation

Source: reference[32].

- Investigation of lesions in the spleen
- Investigation of lesions in the prostate and seminal vesicles
- Confirmation of inoperable pancreatic cancer and differential diagnosis of atypical pancreatic masses

22.5.2 Risk of Complications

The risk of complications in diagnostic and even more in therapeutic EUS-guided interventions is significantly higher than in diagnostic EUS but is still considered to be low.[27] The following risks should be disclosed during informed consent:

- Bleeding
- Infection (especially in interventions on cystic lesions)
- Tumor seeding
- Pancreatitis (in pancreatic interventions)

Mild, self-limiting intraluminal and extraluminal bleeding may occur. The risk of intralesional hemorrhage is higher in the biopsy of cystic lesions. Strategies for preventing or reducing potential risks include noting the individual benefit and comorbidity of the patient and creating optimum conditions for the planned endosonographic intervention. Endoscopy prior to EUS, using a forward-viewing gastroscope, should precede side-viewing EUS to exclude a stenosis. The complication risk of endosonographic procedures was recently reviewed by Jenssen et al.[27]

Table 22.2 Degree of difficulty of EUS-FNA

Degree of difficulty by lesion (increasing from 1 to 9)	Lesion/site
9	Stomach wall (subepithelial lesions)
8	Pancreatic head lesions
7	Peripancreatic lymph nodes
6	Lesions of pancreatic body and tail
5	Gastric lymph nodes
4	Adrenal glands
3	Liver lesions
2	Mediastinal lymph nodes
1	Large mediastinal tumors

Source: reference[22].

Table 22.3 Overview of EUS-guided therapeutic procedures and their current role

Goal	Procedure	Current role
Symptomatic	**Pain management:**	
	EUS-guided celiac plexus block/neurolysis	Clinical practice
	EUS-guided pancreatic duct drainage	Clinical studies, experts procedure
	Biliary decompression:	
	EUS-guided biliary drainage	Clinical studies, expert procedure
Palliative	**EUS anastomosis:**	
	EUS gastrojenunostomy	Animal studies
	Endosonographic tumor intervention:	
	Ethanol injection	Clinical studies
	Gene therapy	Clinical studies
	Brachytherapy	Animal studies
	Radiofrequency ablation	Clinical studies
Curative	**Endosonographic treatment of pseudocysts, necrosis, abscesses**	Clinical practice
	Endosonographic vascular intervention:	
	Obliteration of perforator veins, varices, ulcer vessels, tumor vessels; (transjugular) intrahepatic portosystemic stent shunt	Animal studies, clinical studies

22.5.3 Contraindications

Contraindications include lack of informed consent, questionable diagnostic and therapeutic benefit, poor patient performance status (ECOG > 2, Karnofsky index < 70%), other prognostically relevant comorbidity, significant coagulopathy (INR > 1.5–2, platelets < 40–50 × 10^9/L), and significant prolongation of bleeding time (depending on the indication). If doubt exists, bleeding time should be the deciding factor. Blood vessels in the needle path and nonvisualization of the puncture needle should also be noted.

22.6 Therapeutic Interventions, General Aspects

22.6.1 Therapeutic EUS-Guided Interventions

Therapeutic EUS-guided interventions have permanently enriched available treatment options in recent years.[35] The foremost therapeutic procedures are the drainage of (peri)pancreatic fluid collections, mediastinal, retro- and extraperitoneal abscesses (including perirectal lesions), celiac plexus neurolysis, and EUS-guided cholangiopancreatic drainage techniques. Some treatments are still experimental and are in clinical trials, such as EUS-guided injection therapies for malignant neoplasms using chemotherapeutic agents or immunomodulators as well as EUS-guided radiofrequency thermoablation and other tumor ablation techniques (laser techniques, photodynamic therapies).

Other proposed techniques are of dubious benefit, such as the EUS-guided treatment of peri-intestinal varices and EUS-guided botulinum toxin injection for achalasia (▸ Table 22.3).

22.6.2 Endoscopes and Needle Types

For most interventions we use a 19-gauge needle (Cook Medical; Olympus; Boston Scientific), which can accommodate a high-performance 0.035-inch guidewire, combined with the Hitachi Preirus platform and Pentax EG 3830 UT echoendoscope with a 3.8-mm working channel adequate for all essential techniques. Another option is the Aloka Olympus GF-UCT 140 unit, which lacks only the elastography feature. The puncture site should be identified by both endosonographic and optical viewing criteria to ensure that clear visualization is maintained when the tip of the scope is moved away so that subsequent steps can be completed. We know from experience that the access site is often close to the cardia, where the maneuverability of the endoscope may be greatly limited. The 19-gauge needle should be straightened for insertion into the echoendoscope. The evaluation of needle position outside the echoendoscope relies on visual endoscopic control. An optimum position is reached when the needle sheath protrudes approximately 5 mm past the Albarran lever.

The target lesion is visualized and, with the stylet retracted, the needle is introduced at the targeted site as described above, making sure to avoid interposed vessels. The Albarran lever helps to avoid needle insertion at an angle that is too tangential. Another technique is to anchor the needle tip in the wall and advance the echoendoscope slightly to increase the insertion angle.

22.6.3 General Rules for Needle and Wire Handling

Some helpful technical tips:

- Position the echoendoscope without tension (to minimize the risk of wire dislodgment).
- Do not advance the wire after removing the needle.
- Avoid looping the wire (risk of dislodgment).
- Place controlled traction on the wire when advancing a stent, fixed dilator or balloon dilator (increases the delivery force).
- Seal the endoscope channel with the rubber cap (to prevent air escape).

22.6.4 Indications

The indications are listed and explained in the sections below.

22.6.5 Contraindications

The main contraindications are as follows:

- Lack of informed consent
- Poor patient performance status (ECOG > 2, Karnofsky index < 70%)
- Coagulation disorder (Quick value < 40–50%; platelets < 50×10^9/nL).

22.7 Drainage of Peripancreatic Fluid Collections

22.7.1 History

The first endoscopic transmural cyst drainage was described by Rogers in 1975. Percutaneous gastrocystic (internal) drainage, developed by Hancke and Henriksen[36] and Bernadino,[37] broadened the spectrum of available techniques. Combined ultrasound-guided percutaneous endoscopic transgastric cyst drainage completes the published techniques.[38] The history of the drainage of peripancreatic fluid collections was recently reviewed[39] and was the subject of a recent multicenter study.[40]

22.7.2 Basic Anatomical Considerations

For endoscopic therapy to be effective, the retroperitoneal area that requires drainage must be fully accessible from the stomach (or duodenum), whether by transmural puncture or by the transpapillary route through the pancreatic duct. The drainage procedure should never establish an open connection with the peritoneal cavity. The retroperitoneal position of the pancreas determines both the spread and the boundaries of pancreatogenic fluid collections. The pancreas is separated from the stomach anteriorly by the omental bursa (a space between the peritoneal layers). The omental bursa predisposes to a peripancreatic fluid collection that could drain into the free abdominal cavity through a patent epiploic foramen. The occlusion of this connection by inflammatory scarring (adhesions) must occur to permit the low-risk drainage of fluid collections arising from the pancreas. These collections, frequently necrotic and infected, generally spread parallel to the pancreas (along the transverse body axis) and may track into the porta hepatis, splenic hilum, and pleural space (with or without bronchial involvement), anteriorly along the paravertebral muscles, and into the retroperitoneal pelvis. Remarkably, despite their complex configuration, these fluid collections can often be effectively drained from a single point, allowing the inflammatory tracts arising from the pancreas to dry up and resolve.

A feared complication is an oozing venous hemorrhage due to portal hypertension or a collateral circulation that often develops in response to splenic vein thrombosis. Another feared complication is arterial bleeding from the splenic or gastroduodenal artery or branches of the hepatic artery (listed by frequency of pseudoaneurysm formation).

22.7.3 Pathophysiologic Considerations

Many classification systems for peripancreatic fluid collections have been published, some based on the 1992 Atlanta Classification or ductal changes,[41,42] and need not be described here. Abnormal cavities about the pancreas can be classified by a variety of features, noting that the features from one category (e.g., "size") do not always correlate with those in another category (e.g., "prognosis"). The pathophysiology of pancreatic interventions is explored more fully by Seifert and Dietrich.[39]

22.7.4 Diagnostic Workup

Transabdominal ultrasound scans, contrast-enhanced CT, and acceptable coagulation parameters are absolute prerequisites for EUS-guided drainage. MRI (MRCP) has also proven helpful for the evaluation of complex cystic lesions in selected cases. ERCP is not considered mandatory before drainage, as it has been found that the therapeutic procedure should not depend on the presence or absence of fistulous duct connections. Criteria to be evaluated are technical feasibility, wall thickness, interposed blood vessels, and distance from the gastric (or duodenal) wall.

22.7.5 Indications

Indications for the interventional treatment of fluid collections are an infected cyst or necrosis, septic complications (fever, elevated CRP), and clinical manifestations. The most frequent indication for a therapeutic intervention for pseudocysts is severe pain, followed by nausea and vomiting (compression of the gastric or intestinal lumen), weight loss, and jaundice. Intralesional hemorrhage is a less common indication.

Relative indications are bacterial contamination (positive aspirate in the absence of symptoms), bloating, anorexia, weight loss, oligosymptomatic (pseudo)cysts with persistence (> 6 weeks) or enlargement of a necrotic area or of cystic lesions.

If less urgent indications for interventional treatment are not present (including the patient's desire for treatment after detailed disclosure), we follow the patient for 2 to 6 weeks. Prophylactic antibiotic therapy will reduce septic complications, at least in patients with extensive necrosis, even if signs of bacterial infection are absent. The choice of antibiotics and the duration of therapy are not standardized (e.g., levofloxacin 500 mg daily for 3 weeks).

22.7.6 Timing of the EUS Intervention

Pseudocysts and peripancreatic necrosis with septic complications are always indications for therapeutic intervention. The situation is usually less clear in clinical practice, however, so it is important to be familiar with the spontaneous course. The anticipated spontaneous course of a pancreatic pseudocyst depends on the timing of the observation. If a cystic mass develops during the acute phase of pancreatitis, it most likely represents peripancreatic edema with a good chance of spontaneous resolution. Even in some cases of extensive necrosis, we have successfully adopted a wait-and-see approach until the lesion finally consolidated. This approach requires patience and carries a risk of septic complications. Hemorrhage, rupture, and infection are possible complications that may arise in untreated cases. There are no reliable data on the best timing for an intervention, although it would be logical to schedule the less invasive endoscopic intervention at an earlier time than a surgical procedure.

The timing of the EUS intervention depends on the severity of complaints, the acuteness of the disease, the degree of cyst maturity (ideally 3–6 weeks), patient age and comorbidity (and also operator experience). Acute necrotizing pancreatitis is treated interventionally when secondary infection supervenes. The treatment of pseudocysts is indicated only if clinical symptoms are present or complications (abscess, fistula, hemorrhage) arise. Cystic pancreatic neoplasms should be excluded before the intervention. The diagnostic workup should at least include evaluation of the cyst wall and septa and a fluid analysis (CEA, cytology).[43–45]

22.7.7 Selection of Procedure

In principle, the best interventional procedure is the one with the lowest morbidity and mortality. Interdisciplinary management of these complex diseases by a gastroenterologist and surgeon and an awareness of surgical options are essential.

22.7.8 Technique

The endoscopic treatment of intra- or peripancreatic fluid collections can be done by the transpapillary route or by transmural puncture and drainage. The transmural approach always requires endosonographic guidance so that bleeding complications can be avoided and even complex anatomical relationships can be appreciated. Although this distinction does not have support from any published comparative study, any experienced operator with access to EUS can act upon it the given practical circumstances.

Drainage may be performed in one or two steps. *One-step* drainage employs a suitable EUS scope with a working channel of 3.7 to 3.8 mm with the ability to deliver 8.5F stents. *Two-step* drainage involves exchanging the diagnostic EUS scope for a therapeutic gastroscope with a working channel of 3.7 to 4.2 mm that can deliver 10F stents. The scopes are exchanged by simultaneously (and carefully) advancing the guidewire while withdrawing the EUS scope. The therapeutic endoscope is introduced over a guidewire threaded into the working channel with a catheter. The endoscope is positioned as close to the puncture site as possible and under as little tension as possible.

22.7.9 One-Step Systems

The first hand-made, one-step system described in the literature was successful, although it did not conform to aseptic requirements.[46,47] The custom-made stent is inserted directly over a stainless steel puncture needle and stylet, aided by a pusher connected to the stent with a suture. Stent position can be adjusted by movements of the needle. Removal of the stylet releases the suture, detaching the stent from the pusher and endoscope and leaving it in the correct drainage position.

Later the Cook Medical Giovannini needle system, which was popular for a time, had an electrosurgical needle knife at the tip that allowed for one-step puncture and dissection under vision. This system has poor guidance stability, however, and has largely been abandoned.

General Rules for Needle and Wire Handling

Several basic rules should be followed:

- Position the echoendoscope without tension (to minimize the risk of wire dislodgment).

- Do not advance the wire after removing the needle.
- Avoid looping the wire (risk of dislodgment).
- If possible, do not withdraw the wire while the sharp puncture needle is still in place (risk of shearing off the wire covering).
- Place controlled traction on the wire when advancing a stent, fixed dilator, or balloon dilator (to increase the delivery force).
- After needle removal: Seal the instrument channel with a rubber cap (to avoid vision loss due to escaping air).

The needle should pass through hypovascular wall-adherent structures (often hypoechoic) and should not perforate into the peritoneal cavity. The posterior wall of the gastric body and the proximal portions of the antrum have proven to be favorable access sites. If possible, the gastric fundus (difficult further dissection) and antral pyloric region (wall thickness) should be avoided. After the stylet is removed, 10 mL of cyst contents is collected for visual assessment (criteria are color, consistency, and odor [described as serous, mucinous, pus, blood]), laboratory testing (CEA, if necessary CA19–9 and lipase), microbiologic testing, and cytologic analysis. Then a 0.035-inch guidewire with a soft tip (e.g., Jagwire) is introduced. Placing two or three coils of wire inside the cyst should reduce the risk of wire dislodgment. Fluoroscopic control, with or without contrast administration, is helpful but not mandatory.

Wire Application

The puncture needle is now withdrawn, leaving the wire in place (preferably with two or three coils in the cyst but none in the stomach).

Further dissection (fenestration) can now be performed bluntly with a dilator or balloon or sharply with a cystotome (or needle knife). Blunt dissection is more advantageous as it can minimize bleeding. Access cannot always be accomplished with a push-type dilator, especially with a firm cyst wall or long pathway to the cyst. Access with an electrosurgical system is preferred in these cases.

Dissection with a Dilator and Balloon

We perform initial dilation (transmural fenestration) of the tract with a 6F biliary balloon dilator (e.g., Max-Force, Boston Scientific) followed by through-the-scope balloon dilation (10–14 mm or 14–20 mm, depending on wall hardness) with a CRE esophageal balloon dilator (Boston Scientific), which is consistently successful. Dilation in septic patients with a relatively soft gastrointestinal wall is usually done in one step to 16 mm (or to 20 mm in selected cases), whereas chronically ill patients with a scarred wall may require incremental dilation over a period of several days. Biliary tract dilators from 5F to 9F can also provide atraumatic access following needle insertion and drain placement.

Dissection with the Cystotome or Diathermy Ring

The cystotome or diathermy ring (7F, 8.5F, 10F) is introduced over the wire (and through the rubber cap), and the tip of the needle knife is extended approximately 1 to 2 mm under endoscopic vision. A blended current (cutting + coagulation) is applied to penetrate the stomach wall, preferably under fluoroscopic control (to maintain guidance through mobile tissue planes), while slight traction is placed on the wire to stabilize its position.

Dissection with the Needle Knife

The needle knife carries a risk of vascular injury and is of limited effectiveness in thick walls. It has proven helpful in selected cases where the duodenal route is used. The use of other papillotome designs for wall incisions has a higher bleeding risk and should be avoided.

Stent Placement

The rest of the procedure depends on the diagnosis. Symptomatic pancreatic pseudocysts can be drained with a 8.5F (or 10F) pigtail-retained stent with a 4- to 6-cm straight segment (e.g., Boston Scientific, Cook Medical, Olympus, [double pigtail]) placed through a therapeutic endoscopic with a working channel of 3.7 to 4.2 mm. Several suppliers offer pigtail stents with color and radiopaque markers at the center of the straight segment to aid accurate positioning and prevent primary migration (Medi-Globe). Straight stents (e.g., the Tannenbaum stent) should be avoided as they are prone to migration. We use a standard pusher such as the Endoflex (Olympus). The placement of covered self-expanding metal stents (for intestinal use) has also been described and has the advantage of creating stable, large-bore access for repeated endoscopic débridement.

The steps in the endosonographic drainage of (peripancreatic) fluid collections are summarized in ▶ Fig. 22.24.

Special Issues Relating to Abscesses and Infected Necrosis

Abscesses and infected necrosis can often be atraumatically (bluntly) dilated to 14 to 20 mm by contrast-controlled balloon dilation, continuing until the balloon waist disappears as pus or necrotic fluid is drained. There is a potential for major fluid influx into the stomach with risk of aspiration, so an adequate suction system should be provided. The placement of one to three 8.5F or 10F pigtails stents is helpful for securing the access tract (gastrocystomy) as described above (▶ Fig. 22.25). If the clinical situation permits, it is best to wait at least one day so that a maximum amount of fluid can be drained. Visualization of the necrotic area or abscess cavity should be significantly improved by the next day (or several days later).

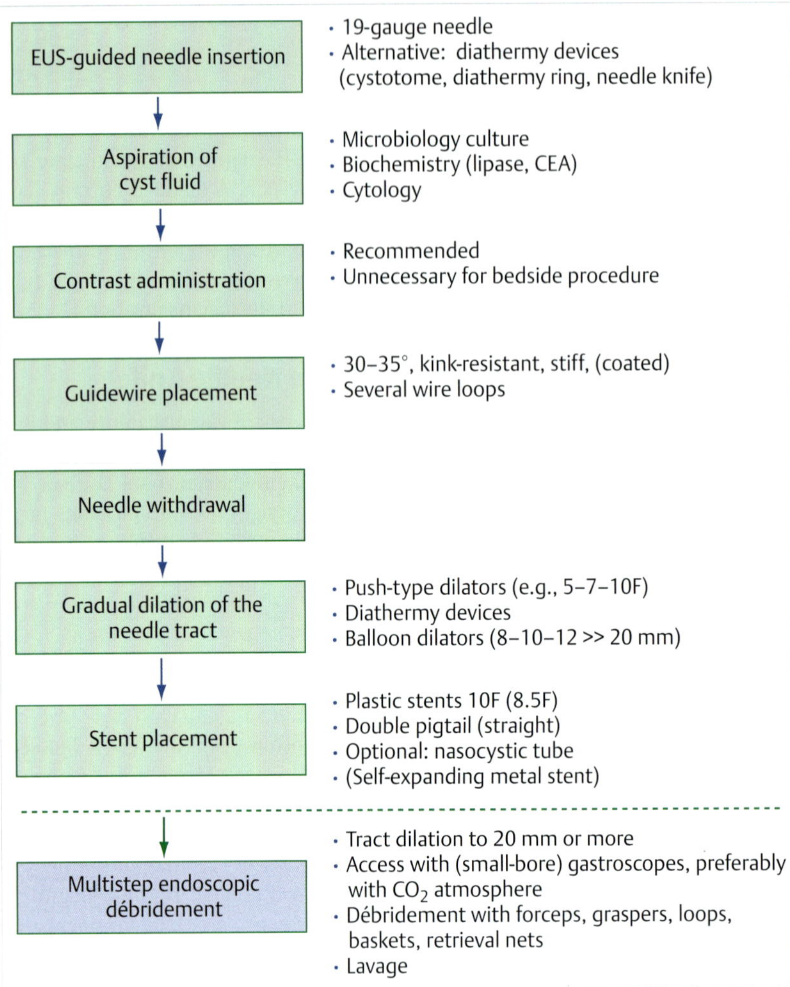

Fig. 22.24 Steps in the endosonographic drainage of (peripancreatic) fluid collections.

The immediate evacuation of necrotic areas is not strictly necessary and even harbors risks. Feared complications are venous oozing, which is very difficult to localize, and erosive arterial hemorrhage (e.g., from the splenic artery), which may be fatal within minutes. The placement of a nasocystic irrigation tube may be helpful despite patient discomfort. Irrigation with 500 to 1000 mL of 0.9% NaCl or Ringer solution is repeated two or three times daily. Combined endoscopic-percutaneous drainage and irrigation is a controversial measure to speed the healing of abscesses and infected necrosis. The more rapid evacuation and better irrigation must be weighed against the risks of a "blind" percutaneous puncture with greater risk of injury to unseen arterial and venous vessels. The percutaneous drain should have an adequate caliber (12F–18F). Irrigation may be done continuously (at 100–200 mL/h) or every 2 to 4 hours until the necrotic cavity is clean. Necrotic areas (which may show a remarkable capacity for reabsorption) can then be débrided endoscopically once the fluid has been adequately drained.

After the acute treatment phase, three 8.5F to 10F pigtail drains can be placed and removed at 1 to 6 months. It should be noted that the drainage pathway along the stents is more important than drainage through the stents, so the placement of multiple stents has proven effective.

It is important to recognize dependent portions of the pancreas that can be treated endoscopically by transpapillary stent placement, for example, and reconstructed by stenting with a plastic prosthesis (with or without additional transmural drainage of associated fluid collections). Any proximal stenoses should be dilated and pancreatic calculi removed.

22.7.10 Treatment of Nonpancreatic Fluid Collections

The EUS-guided drainage technique described above may also be successfully applied to other fluid collections that require treatment and are located in close proximity to

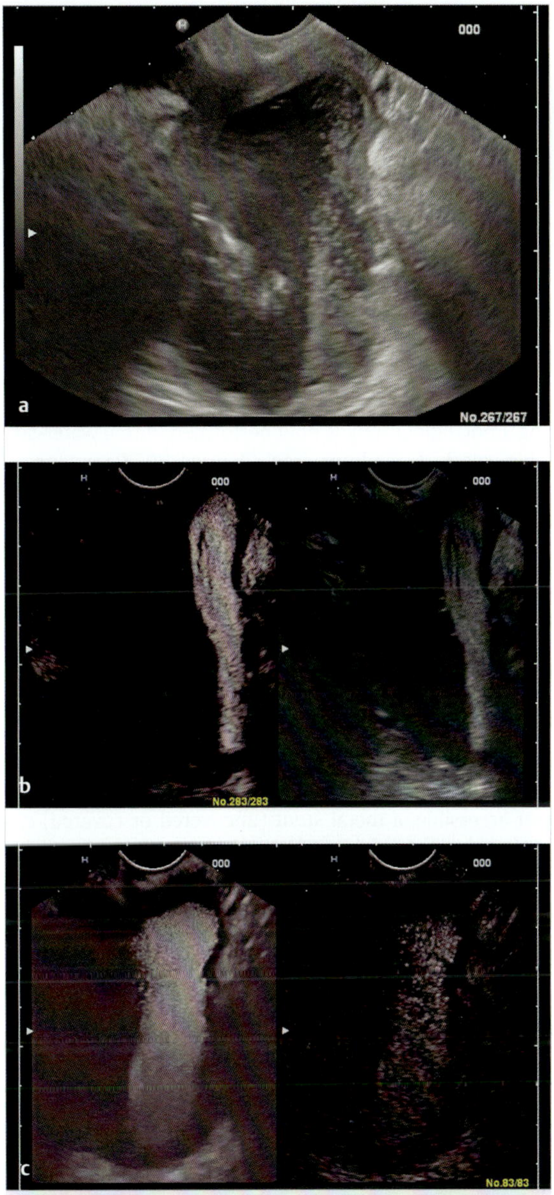

Fig. 22.25 a–c Pancreatic abscess, demonstrated by EUS-guided puncture and intralesional injection of SonoVue. (Source: www.efsumb.org.)

the gastrointestinal tract. EUS-guided drainage has been described for biliomas, for example, as well as (postoperative) subphrenic, retroperitoneal, mediastinal, and perirectal abscesses and abscesses in the left lobe of the liver.

Assessing the Result, Postinterventional Care, Complications

The drainage of pus or pseudocystic fluid, and the very rapid clinical improvement that usually follows, are the main criteria for evaluating the success of interventional drainage. Percutaneous ultrasound follow-ups will document shrinkage of the fluid collection, correct drain placement, and air echoes inside the lesion. Possible severe complications besides bleeding include free perforation and stent migration leading to peritonitis and secondary infection due to stent malfunction. The postinterventional sonographic or radiographic detection of free intraperitoneal air is common and may be interpreted as a perforation only within the context of clinical findings.

Percutaneous Drainage

The percutaneous drainage of uncomplicated pancreatic pseudocysts is a low-risk procedure when proper sonographic technique is followed and can yield good results, at least in the short term.[35,48] The drainage may be evaluated by CT or ultrasonography. The percutaneous débridement of pancreatic necrosis using special catheters has also been reported. Very long procedure and fluoroscopy times are required.

22.7.11 Surgical Options

The goal of surgical treatment has been well defined for decades: to prevent complications by removing necrotic and infected material, then draining and irrigating the resulting cavities. There is disagreement as to the best surgical technique, which may be a question of individual anatomy and operator experience. Some surgeons favor longitudinal incision and anastomosis of the pancreatic duct (Partington–Rochelle pancreaticojejunostomy). While this operation does establish drainage, like the endoscopic techniques, it may not eliminate chronic inflammatory foci that are often present in the pancreatic head. Also, the basic problem of pancreatogenic distal biliary stenosis remains untreated. Even specialists do not agree on whether a duodenum-preserving pancreatic head resection or a modified Whipple operation with pancreaticoduodenectomy (pylorus-preserving or not) is preferred.[49]

We will dispense with further image sequences at this point and refer the reader to a current textbook of endosonography.[39]

22.8 EUS-Guided Cholangiodrainage

22.8.1 Introduction

EUS-guided cholangiodrainage (EUS-CD) was first published by Eike Burmester and has been developed and advanced individually by other interventionalists. Meanwhile, at least six different access routes and procedures have been employed. The access or drainage route may be transgastric using a rendezvous technique, or obstructed intrahepatic bile ducts can be drained into the stomach (hepaticogastrostomy). Other approaches are a rendezvous maneuver or direct drainage from the duodenal bulb or (in postoperative cases) from the jejunum to the porta hepatis (hepaticoduodenostomy, hepaticojejunostomy) or periampullary drainage (choledochoduodenostomy).

22.8.2 Indications and Treatment Goals

The palliative indication for EUS-guided cholangiodrainage includes the symptomatic treatment of patients with obstructive lesions for which internal drainage cannot be established by simpler, lower-risk methods such as endoscopic retrograde cholangio(pancreato)graphy (ERC[P]) or percutaneous transhepatic cholangiodrainage (PTCD) due to an impassable papillary stenosis, complete biliary stricture, pyloric stenosis, or duodenal stenosis. EUS-CD can be performed as a rendezvous procedure in patients with an accessible but impassable papilla or as primary transmural EUS-CD following gastrectomy, a Kausch–Whipple procedure, hepaticojejunostomy, or other conditions that make the papilla inaccessible. Factors that would argue against external PTC drainage (and in favor of EUS-CD) are the loss of bile and quality-of-life issues raised by external drainage tubes.

The primary goal of EUS-CD is to restore papillary drainage by passing a needle into the intrahepatic (or extrahepatic) bile ducts, advancing a guidewire across the papilla, and placing a drain such as a metal stent. If this is unsuccessful, the obstructed bile ducts can still be drained directly into the stomach, duodenum, or jejunum through an endosonographically placed plastic stent or covered metal stent.

22.8.3 Equipment

The intervention room must be equipped with EUS and standard endoscopic equipment, monitoring unit (as described above), and fluoroscopy unit.

22.8.4 Preparatory Measures

Preparations include antibiotic prophylaxis with ceftriaxone (Rocephin [Roche Pharma AG], 2 g IV), for example. Alternatives are amoxicillin or gyrase inhibitors as described above. The site and topography of the stenosis should be determined by transabdominal ultrasonography (and MRCP if necessary).

22.8.5 Technique

The patient is placed in a prone or left lateral decubitus position. Access for a rendezvous maneuver can be obtained through the left lobe of the liver, duodenal bulb, or even the gallbladder. The problem with puncturing the duodenal bulb is that the wire must be passed upward to establish drainage for a complete distal obstruction. In areas without any layered wall structure (especially after surgery), adhesions are generally present that will allow safe access without breaching the peritoneal cavity. The EUS-guided puncture of dilated intrahepatic bile ducts is usually done at a relatively far peripheral site in the left lobe of the liver, directing the needle toward the porta hepatis. This is done both to provide a good force vector for advancing the guidewire and to create an access tract stable enough for dilation. The peripheral (tangentially directed) puncture of the bile ducts facilitates subsequent dilation of the "liver tract." Following successful needle insertion, the stylet is removed and approximately 10 mL of bile is aspirated and collected for microbiological testing. Cholangiography is now performed with a water-soluble contrast medium (see Chapter 20, Percutaneous Transhepatic Cholangiodrainage) to evaluate the stenosis.

A 0.035-inch guidewire such as the Jagwire (Boston Scientific) with a soft tip, or a noninsulated, noncutting stiff wire (GGW-08-30-400 from Medi-Globe), is inserted tangentially into a peripheral bile duct, aiming toward the porta hepatis. Non-kink-resistant wires should be avoided since necessary wire manipulations will tend to kink and strip the coating. The goal is to advance the wire across the stenosis and bring it out in the papilla so that a stent can be placed with a duodenoscope using the rendezvous technique. If the papilla is not accessible, a metal stent (uncovered or covered) can be delivered across the stenosis from the antegrade side (also crossing the papilla if necessary). If the wire cannot cross the stenosis, a stable wire position with adequate wire length should be established in the bile duct to allow for serial dilation (from 6F to 10F) and transmural placement of a covered metal stent or plastic stent. "Burn-in" with a cystotome is rarely necessary.

The tract is dilated over the guidewire with a conventional 6F biliary dilator (e.g., Cook Medical or MTW Edoskopie) or a 6F balloon dilator (e.g., Boston Scientific). Care is taken to avoid wire dislodgment during device exchanges. Good results have been obtained by using a covered biliary metal stent, (4 to) 6 cm long with an uncovered portion of 10 mm length (e.g., Boston Scientific). As a rule, 6 cm is sufficient to bridge the distance from the lumen to the bile duct. Shorter stents tend to migrate, while the covered portion of longer stents may compress the bile ducts or indent (and even perforate) the stomach or bowel wall. The stent covering should be clearly visible on the luminal side (> 10 mm) to prevent bile leakage. Clips have been recommended for keeping the stent in place. When plastic stents are used, we prefer the straight design over double-pigtail stents as they can be exchanged over a guidewire with a Soehendra stent retriever (Cook Medical) (▶ Fig. 22.26).

A "mini-rendezvous" version of the same method can be used in patients with an impassable papilla. This technique utilizes the close proximity of the common

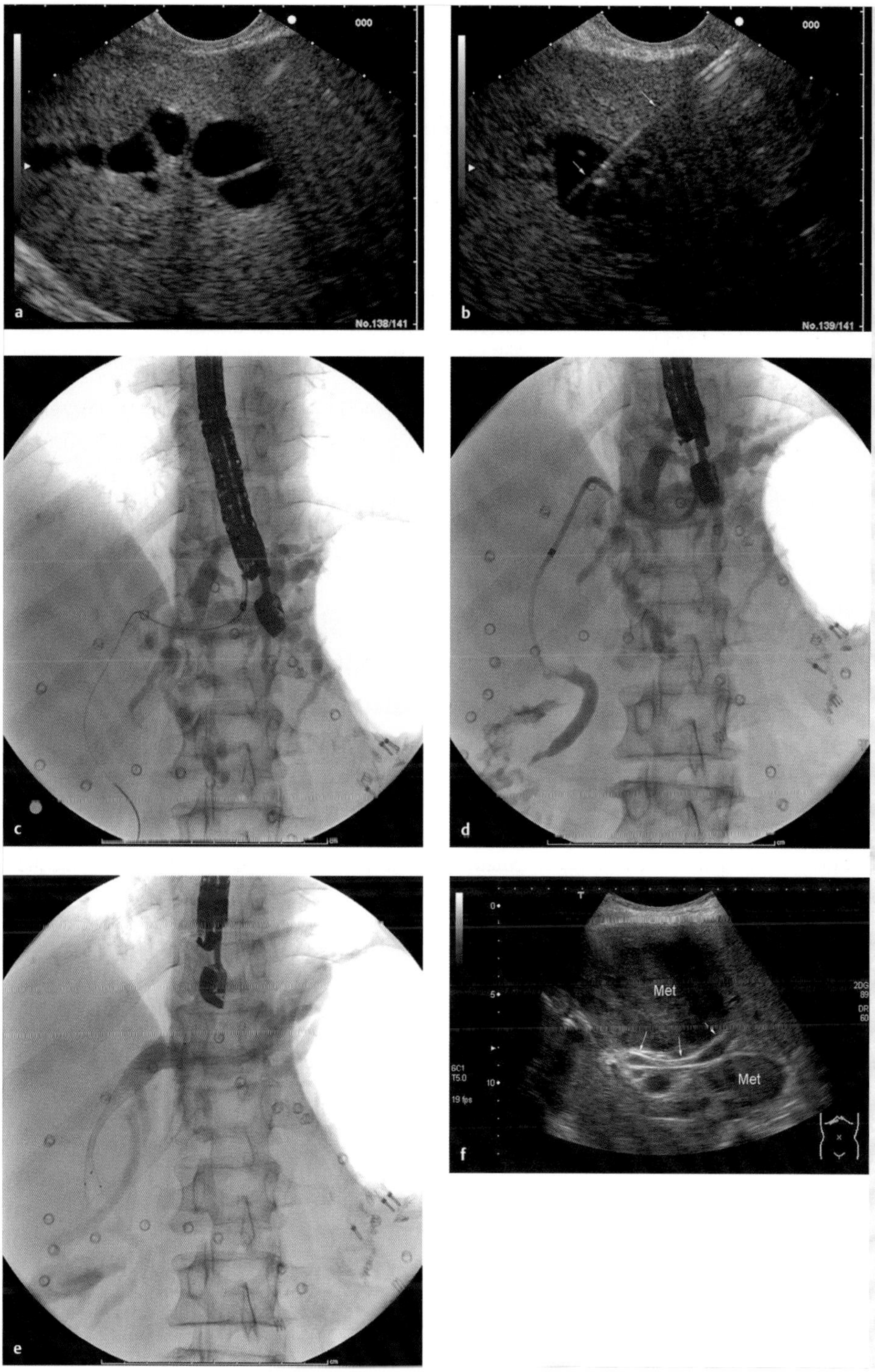

Fig. 22.26 Cholangiodrainage. Antegrade EUS-guided drainage of a perihilar biliary stenosis using an uncovered metal stent.
a Dilated intrahepatic bile ducts in the left lobe of the liver, imaged from the stomach by endosonography.
b EUS-guided puncture with a 19-gauge needle.
c Placement of a guidewire.
d Opacified bile ducts with guidewire brought out through the papilla.
e Placement of the metal stent system.
f Expanded metal stent, sonographic result (Met, metastases; arrows indicate the expanded metal stent). (Source: taken from references [2] and [54].)

bile duct to the duodenal wall to enable a simple, uncomplicated puncture. Because the needle is directed toward the papilla (with the scope in the duodenal bulb or descending duodenum), a guidewire passed through the needle can be brought out through the papilla in the great majority of cases. The wire can then be picked up with a side-viewing scope and used to perform the papillotomy that was previously unsuccessful. After the papillotomy the wire is removed and the ERCP is continued in a conventional way.

This technique spares affected patients the need to undergo a percutaneous (PTC-based) rendezvous procedure, which has a considerably higher risk of complications.

22.8.6 Assessing the Result, Postinterventional Care, Complications

The drainage of bile and contrast medium and the presence of air in the bile ducts document successful internal drainage. Percutaneous ultrasonography is essential for evaluating the result. The most serious complications are stent migration with the development of biliary peritonitis, large bilioma formation, and cholangitis due to stent malfunction.

22.9 EUS-Guided Pancreatic Duct Drainage

22.9.1 Indications and Treatment Goals

The indications for endosonographically guided drainage of the pancreatic duct (EUS-PD) are symptom relief and pain management in patients with nonneoplastic obstructive pancreatic duct disease (chronic obstructive pancreatitis) and patients with pancreatic duct fistulas where internal drainage cannot be established by simpler, lower-risk methods (ERC[P]).

EUS-PD can be performed by a rendezvous technique in patients with an accessible but impassable papilla or as primary transmural EUS-PD following gastrectomy, a Kausch–Whipple procedure, hepaticojejunostomy, or other conditions that make the papilla inaccessible.

22.9.2 Technique

The preparations and technique are analogous to EUS-CD. The intervention is performed in the prone or left lateral decubitus position. The needle is passed into the obstructed pancreatic duct at a tangential angle under EUS guidance, directing it toward the papilla if a rendezvous technique is planned. In consideration of scarring and calcifications in the pancreatic parenchyma, the "pancreatic tract" from the wall to the pancreatic duct should be as short as possible.

After the needle has been placed, the stylet is removed and pancreatic juice is aspirated for laboratory testing (carcinoembryonic antigen [CEA], if necessary CA 19–9, lipase), cytologic analysis, and possible microbiologic testing. The viscosity is assessed and documented. A CEA value > 200 ng/mL is considered evidence of a mucinous neoplasm. Pancreatography is now performed to characterize the stenosis and aid further wire maneuvers.

A 0.035-inch guidewire (e.g., Jagwire) is inserted toward the papilla. Often the pancreatic parenchyma is too firm for duct dilation with fixed-diameter or balloon dilators, and this can be facilitated with a Soehendra stent retriever (7F or 10F, Cook Medical) or diathermy ring cystotome (MTW Endoskopie). The problems described for EUS-CD apply equally to EUS-PD. In particular, the use of (stiff) wires without a Terumo tip should be avoided. The goal is to advance the wire across the stenosis and bring it out through the (minor) papilla so that a stent can be placed with a duodenoscope using rendezvous technique. Brush cytology is advised in selected cases and can be done prior to stent placement. If the wire cannot cross the stenosis, a stable wire position with adequate wire length should be established in the pancreatic duct to allow for the transmural placement of a plastic stent or covered metal stent (*caution:* an uncovered metal stent will allow leakage of pancreatic juice into the omental bursa).

The risk of dislodgment of the 19-gauge puncture needle and wire is greater in EUS-PD than in EUS-CD. It is also more difficult to dilate the access tract through the fibrotic pancreatic parenchyma, requiring the use of very stable guidewires and possibly the use of a Soehendra stent retriever to open up the duct.

22.9.3 Assessing the Result, Postinterventional Care, Complications

The drainage of pancreatic secretions and contrast medium plus air in the pancreatic duct document successful internal drainage. Percutaneous ultrasonography is essential for evaluating the result. The most important potential complications are hemorrhage and severe pancreatitis.

We will dispense with further image sequences and refer the reader to a current textbook of endosonography.[48]

22.10 Celiac Plexus Neurolysis and Celiac Plexus Blockade

22.10.1 Indications and Treatment Goals

Irreversible celiac plexus neurolysis (CPN) induced by the injection of a long-acting local anesthetic (20 mL bupivacaine) and concentrated alcohol (96%, 20 mL) has proven helpful in patients with tumor infiltrating the corresponding ganglia and nerve fibers (especially ductal adenocarcinoma of the pancreas) (▶ Fig. 22.27). Reversible celiac plexus blockade (CPB) is favored in patients with chronic pancreatitis, for example, although the results are poorer and ultimately disappointing due in part to the higher complication rate.

Patient selection is based on the following criteria: WHO recommendations on pain management have been exhausted, and continuous care is no longer available, as in countries with a limited infrastructure (developing countries).

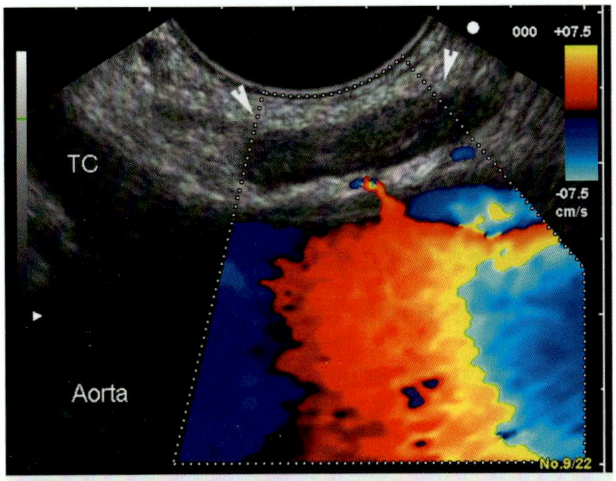

Fig. 22.27 Endosonographic visualization of the ganglia of the celiac plexus (arrowheads) cranial to the origin of the celiac trunk (TC). The ganglia can be positively distinguished from lymph nodes by noting the typical architectural features of lymph nodes in inflammatory liver disease[55–57] and by evaluating the course of the disease.[58]

Two key questions should be answered in assessing the need for treatment:

- Is tumor infiltration present?
- Has tumor infiltrated the nerve pathways that would be blocked by CPN?

In selected patients with ductal adenocarcinoma of the pancreas, it may be possible to perform locoregional staging, fine needle aspiration cytology, and celiac plexus neurolysis in one sitting.

Celiac plexus blockade by the injection of a long-acting local anesthetic (20 mL bupivacaine) and a corticosteroid (20–200 mg triamcinolone) has been proposed in patients with chronic pancreatitis and inflammatory infiltration of the peripancreatic nerve pathways. The complication rate of this therapy is higher than in neoplastic conditions, however, and the efficacy is much lower.

Celiac plexus neurolysis through a posterior approach under CT guidance is no longer recommended due to problems with needle placement and the imprecise approach.

22.10.2 Materials

We use a standard 19-gauge needle. A 20-gauge needle with side holes is also available (EUSN-20 CPN). Neurolysis is induced by bupivacaine (0.25%, 5–30 mL) plus 96% alcohol ("absolute alcohol") or 80 of mg triamcinolone. On the basis of published experience, we use only 5 mL of bupivacaine to avoid overdiluting the alcohol concentration (20 mL is used for EUS-CPB).

22.10.3 Technique

The celiac trunk is visualized to the left of the midline approximately 44 cm (33–44–55 rule) from the dental arch. There is disagreement whether the celiac ganglia can be identified by endosonography, and the ganglia may be confused with lymph nodes, at least in some cases (▶ Fig. 22.27). Once the target area has been visualized, the 19-gauge needle is advanced into the area and an aspiration test done to exclude intravascular placement of the needle tip. Endosonography is sufficient for needle guidance; we do not use fluoroscopic guidance with radiopaque contrast medium. From 10 to 30 mL of bupivacaine is injected just above the origin of the celiac trunk. An additional 10 mL can be injected on the left side. The needle is repositioned by withdrawing it slightly and directing it away from the aorta, as the injection often produces tiny air echoes (acoustic artifacts) that obscure the field. As little air as possible should be injected with the solution. Another technique avoids repositioning the needle by injecting up to 40 mL of long-acting local anesthetic at one site only. The bupivacaine injection is followed by the injection of at least 20 mL of 96% alcohol with the needle in the same position (▶ Fig. 22.28). A technique has been described in which the celiac ganglia are identified by endosonography, allowing direct injection into the ganglia.[50]

The initial puncture can also be done with a saline-filled (air-free) lumen without a stylet. An aspiration test is done before the injection to confirm extravascular needle placement. The large 19-gauge needle diameter has proven better than smaller diameters for safely excluding intravascular (aorta, celiac trunk) needle placement.

22.10.4 Assessing the Result, Postinterventional Care, Complications

Possible side effects are (often transient) diarrhea and hypotension, so peri-interventional circulatory monitoring and intravenous volume replacement are indicated. Acute pain exacerbations correlate with long-term success of CPN but should be managed with analgesics. Septic and ischemic complications are more serious but rare. (Endo)Sonographic assessment of blood flow in the celiac trunk and its branches is mandatory following injection therapy.

22.11 Tumor Ablation with Alcohol

While EUS-guided tumor ablation by the injection of an agent such as absolute alcohol (96%) is not a widely established procedure, it was described in an insulinoma patient,[51] for example, and has since been performed for a variety of indications (especially in patients with functioning neuroendocrine tumors and neoplastic pancreatic cysts). Possible indications are patient age, comorbidity, and patient refusal of surgical treatment. The volume of the targeted tumor should equal the injected volume of

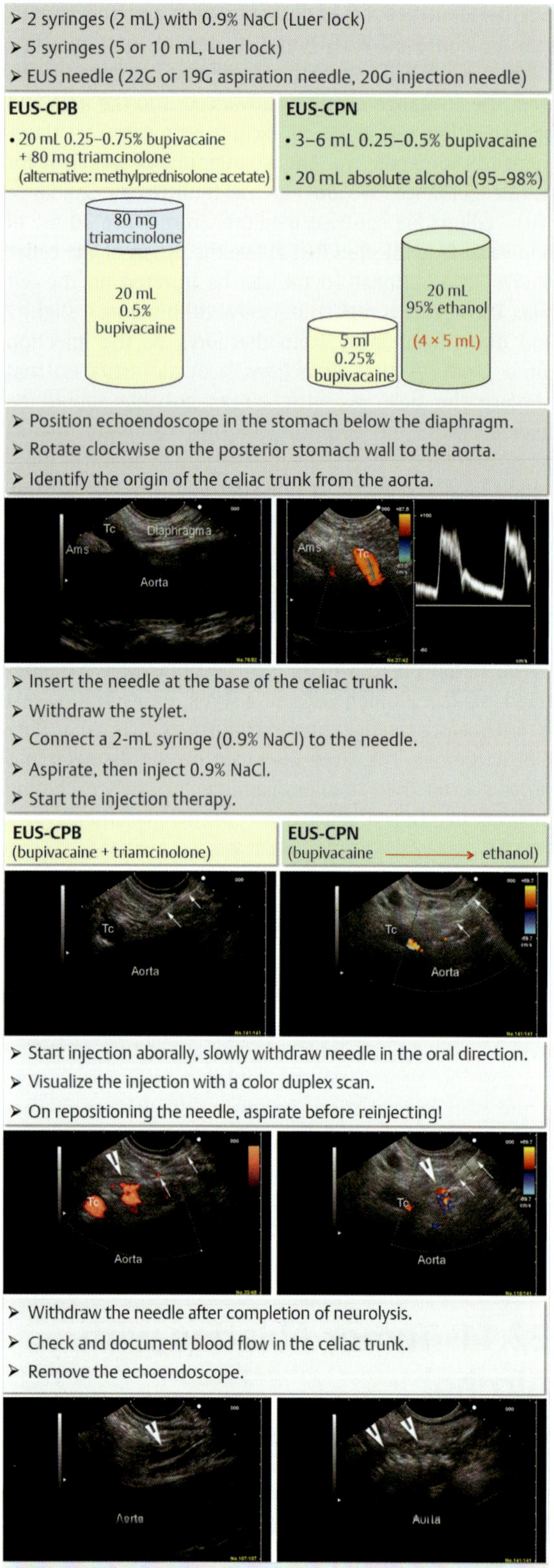

Fig. 22.28 Sequence of steps in the EUS-guided neurolysis and blockade of the celiac plexus. (Source: reference[2].)

absolute alcohol, at least for the initial treatment. Complications due to alcohol-induced necrosis of healthy adjacent tissue have been described. The alcohol ablation of neoplastic pancreatic cysts is unable to eradicate all the neoplastic epithelium in most cases, leading us to question its value.

22.12 EUS-Guided Vascular Interventions

22.12.1 Indications and Treatment Goals

EUS-guided angiography and the associated EUS-guided creation of a portocaval shunt have so far been evaluated only in animal studies. EUS-guided techniques of hemostasis may assume practical importance when endoscopic methods fail. This applies to refractory ulcer bleeding, bleeding from subepithelial tumors or visceral pseudoaneurysms, and bleeding varices.[52]

22.12.2 Materials

EUS-guided vascular therapy is performed with 22-gauge and 19-gauge aspiration needles. Various hemostatic agents may be administered, depending on the nature of the bleeding lesion: epinephrine solution, 96% alcohol, human thrombin solution, fibrin glue, cyanoacrylate, or coils.

22.12.3 Technique

The successful delivery of embolization coils used in angiography (MWCE-18S-8/4 Embolization Microcoil, Cook Medical) through a 22-gauge aspiration needle to control bleeding from anastomotic varices after pancreaticojejunostomy has been described. The needle was guided into the varix by endosonography, and the coil was introduced through the needle lumen with a stylet. Several authors have described the EUS-guided sclerotherapy of perforator veins for recurrent variceal bleeding. There are also isolated case reports of immediate thrombosis induced by the injection of 96% alcohol or human thrombin solution into visceral pseudoaneurysms. Bleeding ulcer vessels (e.g., in patients with a Dieulafoy ulcer or pseudoxanthoma elasticum) and tumor vessels (e.g., in GISTs) can be selectively obliterated with epinephrine solution, sclerosants, cyanoacrylate, or thrombin solution under endosonographic guidance.[53]

22.12.4 Assessing the Result, Postinterventional Care, Complications

The efficacy of treatment is usually assessed at once by endoscopy and endosonography. Postinterventional care is the same as that following the endoscopic treatment of gastrointestinal bleeding. The efficacy of treatment for visceral pseudoaneurysms is also assessed by transabdominal ultrasound. No serious complications have been described to date. There is a conceivable risk of severe ischemic complications or even exacerbation of bleeding due to ineffective EUS-guided angiotherapy.

22.13 Complications

The complication rates of EUS-guided therapeutic interventions depend strongly on the type of intervention and the underlying disease. The principal complications are bleeding, perforation leading to peritonitis, and infection (pseudocyst infection, cholangitis) (▶ Table 22.4).

New EUS-guided procedures should be performed only at high-volume centers that deal with large case numbers and have a high degree of expertise in the procedures.

Two recent papers reviewed the complications of endosonography and explored risk evaluation and prevention.[26,27] They found that diagnostic endosonography without EUS-FNA is a safe procedure with complication rates very close to those of diagnostic endoscopy of the upper digestive tract. The most frequent complications are perforations of the esophagus and duodenum, which may relate to specific mechanical and optical characteristics of the echoendoscopes. Operators can minimize the perforation risk by becoming familiar with the technical characteristics of their echoendoscopes and knowing specific anatomical details in their patients (e.g., esophageal stricture, esophageal and duodenal diverticula). Esophageal dilation to enable the passage of an echoendoscope for staging esophageal cancer should be avoided in the presence of very tight strictures and in all cases where the EUS locoregional staging result would be very unlikely to affect treatment planning.

Most complications of endosonography occur during fine needle aspiration biopsy, Trucut biopsy, and therapeutic interventions. The total complication rate of EUS-FNA appears to be 0.3 to 2.2%, depending especially on the indication and the way in which complications are identified. The mortality rate is close to zero, and deaths have occurred in only a very few isolated cases. The main complications are bleeding, acute pancreatitis, and infectious complications. The risk of infectious complications and bleeding is higher with cystic lesions than with solid lesions. It appears, however, that the infection of pancreatic cysts after EUS-FNA can be almost completely prevented by peri-interventional antibiotic prophylaxis.

Table 22.4 Success rates and complications of EUS-guided therapeutic interventions (supplemented by current data from references [59] and [64])

EUS-guided intervention	Success rates	Complications
EUS-guided pseudocyst drainage	Several case series (> 500 patients) Technical success: 84–100% Long-term clinical success: 80–97%	0–18% (hemorrhage, stent migration, stent occlusion, pseudocyst infection, pneumoperitoneum, perforation and peritonitis)
EUS-guided transmural necrosectomy and drainage of pancreatic abscesses	Several case series (> 250 patients) Technical success: 77–100% Long-term clinical success: 80–93%	0–31% (hemorrhage, stent migration, stent occlusion, pseudocyst infection, pneumoperitoneum, gallbladder puncture, perforation and peritonitis, air embolism)
EUS-CPN/CPB	Several case series, retrospective and prospective (controlled) studies. Clinical success: 1. EUS-CPN: 80.1% (n = 283, 8 studies)[a] 72.5% (n = 119, 5 studies)[b] 2. EUS-CPB: 59.5% (n = 376, 9 studies)[a] 51.5% (n = 221, 6 studies)[b]	1.6% (major: 0.55%)[c] to 8.2% (major: 0.6%)[a] (self-limiting hypotension and diarrhea, retroperitoneal abscess, self-limiting postinterventional pain, retroperitoneal hemorrhage, two isolated case reports: ischemia in territory of celiac trunk). The risk of major complications seems to be higher in EUS-CPB (0.6%) than in EUS-CPN (0.2%) (data from 20 series comprising 1,162 patients).
EUS-CD	Several case series (approximately 150 patients) Technical success: 75–100% Long-term clinical success: 67–100%	0–20% (stent migration, stent occlusion, cholecystitis, intraluminal bleeding/hemobilia, pneumoperitoneum, plastic stent ileus, pancreatitis) Mortality: up to 4%[35]
EUS-PD	Five case series (92 patients) Technical success: 25–92% Long-term clinical success: 69–78%	14–25% (pancreatitis, hemorrhage, infection, pneumoperitoneum, pseudocyst formation, perforation)
EUS-guided ablation of cystic pancreatic lesion	Three case series (64 patients) Complete cyst resolution (imaging): 35–79%	3.4% (pancreatitis)[60]

[a] Meta-analysis by Puli et al, 8 studies with 283 patients CPN, 9 studies with 376 patients CPB.[61]
[b] Meta-analysis by Kaufman et al, 5 studies with 119 patients CPN, 6 studies with 221 patients CPB.[62]
[c] Pooled complication rates in 6 studies (n = 170).[63]
[d] Complication rates in the prospective study by O'Toole and Schmulewitz (2009), n = 189.[63]

Table 22.5 Complication rates of EUS-FNA (summary of the literature)

First author, year[a]	Study design, number of EUS-FNAs (*n*)	Complication rate (%)
Williams et al 1999	Single-center, prospective, *n* = 333	0.3
Mortensen et al 2005	Single-center, prospective, *n* = 670	0.3
Bournet et al 2006	Single-center, prospective, *n* = 224	2.2
Al-Haddad et al 2008	Single-center, prospective, *n* = 483	1.4
Eloubeidi and Tamhane 2008	Single-center, prospective, *n* = 656	1.1
O'Toole et al 2001	Single-center, retrospective, *n* = 322	1.6
Carrara et al 2009	Single-center, prospective, *n* = 1034 pancreas	1.2
Wiersema et al 1997	Multicenter (4), prospective, *n* = 457	1.1
Buscarini et al 2006	Multicenter (6), retrospective, *n* = 787	0.88
Jenssen et al 2008	Multicenter (67), retrospective, *n* = 13,223	0.29
Wang et al 2011	Meta-analysis (51 studies), *n* = 10,941	0.98

[a] References (in order of citation):
Williams DB, Sahai AV, Aabakken L et al. Endoscopic ultrasound guided fine needle aspiration biopsy: a large single centre experience. Gut 1999;44:720–726
Mortensen MB, Fristrup C, Holm FS et al. Prospective evaluation of patient tolerability, satisfaction with patient information, and complications in endoscopic ultrasonography. Endoscopy 2005;37:146–153
Bournet B, Migueres I, Delacroix M et al. Early morbidity of endoscopic ultrasound: 13 years' experience at a referral center. Endoscopy 2006;38:349–354
Al-Haddad M, Wallace MB, Woodward TA et al. The safety of fine-needle aspiration guided by endoscopic ultrasound: a prospective study. Endoscopy 2008;40:204–208
Eloubeidi MA, Tamhane A. Prospective assessment of diagnostic utility and complications of endoscopic ultrasound guided fine needle aspiration. Results from a newly developed academic endoscopic ultrasound program. Dig Dis 2008;26:356–363
O'Toole D, Palazzo L, Arotcarena R et al. Assessment of complications of EUS-guided fine-needle aspiration. Gastrointest Endosc 2001;53:470–474
Carrara S, Arcidiacono PG, Mezzi G et al. Pancreatic endoscopic ultrasound-guided fine needle aspiration: complication rate and clinical course in a single centre. Dig Liver Dis 2010;42:520–523
Wiersema MJ, Vilmann P, Giovannini M et al. Endosonography-guided fine-needle aspiration biopsy: diagnostic accuracy and complication assessment. Gastroenterology 1997;112:1087–1095
Buscarini E, De Angelis C, Arcidiacono PG et al. Multicentre retrospective study on endoscopic ultrasound complications. Dig Liver Dis 2006;38:762–767
Jenssen C, Faiss S, Nürnberg D. [Complications of endoscopic ultrasound and endoscopic ultrasound-guided interventions – results of a survey among German centers]. Z Gastroenterol 2008;46:1177–1184
Wang KX, Ben QW, Jin ZD et al. Assessment of morbidity and mortality associated with EUS-guided FNA: a systematic review. Gastrointest Endosc 2011;73:283–290

The risk of bleeding after EUS-FNA is not increased by NSAID or aspirin therapy but may possibly be increased by low-molecular weight heparins, even when taken in a prophylactic dose. For this reason, low-molecular weight heparins should be promptly discontinued in patients scheduled for EUS-FNA. Antiplatelet drugs other than aspirin should also be discontinued whenever possible. The EUS-FNA of benign pancreatic lesions appears to have a higher complication rate than the FNA of pancreatic malignancies. To date, there have been only isolated case reports of needle-tract or peritoneal seeding of tumor cells by EUS-FNA.

Every endoscopy department should keep a prospective record of the complications of endosonography and EUS-guided biopsies and therapeutic procedures. An adequate training program that includes practical workshops in EUS and EUS-FNA is the key to reducing the risks and increasing the benefits of endosonographic examinations and procedures. Limiting EUS-FNA to cases in which the cytologic or histologic result will very likely influence treatment planning is the most effective way to prevent complications.[27] The literature on EUS-FNA complication rates is reviewed in ▶ Table 22.5, and complications and predisposing factors in EUS-guided interventions are summarized in ▶ Table 22.6.

22.14 Postinterventional Care

Although severe complications in EUS-guided procedures are very rare, postinterventional care is still an important concern and is geared toward the type of sedation used and the interventional technique. Inpatient care is recommended after biopsies and therapeutic procedures and has contributed greatly to the low published complication rates.

The administration of proton pump inhibitors is controversial because the rise in gastric pH may promote infection.

Table 22.6 Complications and predisposing factors in endosonographic interventions (data from reference [27])

Complication	Predisposing factors
Perforation	Diagnostic EUS: approximately 0.03% (cervical esophagus, duodenum)
	Therapeutic interventions: significantly higher complication rate
	Distal rigidity of the echoendoscope
	Pathologic changes in wall and tissue structures
	Water distention of the esophagus and stomach Poor elevation of the upper body
Aspiration	Bacteremia rate up to 2%, usually resolves without sequelae
	Febrile episodes up to 1%
	Severe infection: cystic lesions, necrotic tumors or lymph nodes
	Needle penetration from an area colonized by microbes to a sterile extraintestinal site
	Spread of infectious material from abscesses or infected necrotic tissues
Bacteremia and septic complications	Penetration or perforation of the obstructed bile duct without drainage
Biliary peritonitis and cholangitis	Approximately 2% of pancreatic punctures
	Benign pancreatic diseases
	Puncture of the pancreatic duct
Acute pancreatitis	Up to 4%, clinically insignificant in most cases
	Puncture of hypervascular lesions and of cysts
	Vessels in the needle path
	Portal hypertension
	Antiplatelet therapy with clopidogrel
	INR > 1.5, therapeutic heparinization, anticoagulants started too soon
Hemorrhage	Very rare (7 published cases)
	Improper handling of the needle
Tumor seeding	Excessive air insufflation
	"Microperforation" by the needle
	Long procedure times
Abdominal or chest pain	

References

[1] Dietrich CF. Evidenzbasierter Einsatz der Endosonographie in der gastroenterologischen Diagnostik. Up2Date 2007; Themenheft Gastroenterologie

[2] Dietrich CF, Hocke M, Jenssen C. Interventional endosonography [Article in German]. Ultraschall Med 2011; 32: 8–22, quiz 23–25

[3] Dietrich CF, Jenssen C. Evidence based endoscopic ultrasound [Article in German]. Z Gastroenterol 2011; 49: 599–621

[4] DiMagno EP, Buxton JL, Regan PT et al. Ultrasonic endoscope. Lancet 1980; 1: 629–631

[5] Strohm WD, Phillip J, Hagenmüller F, Classen M. Ultrasonic tomography by means of an ultrasonic fiberendoscope. Endoscopy 1980; 12: 241–244

[6] Dimagno EP, Regan PT, Clain JE, James EM, Buxton JL. Human endoscopic ultrasonography. Gastroenterology 1982; 83: 824–829

[7] Heyder N, Lutz H, Lux G. [Ultrasound diagnosis via the gastroscope]. Ultraschall Med 1983; 4: 85–91

[8] Asaki S, Ota K, Kanazawa N, Ohara S, Onodera H, Goto Y. Ultrasonic endoscopy. Tohoku J Exp Med 1983; 141: 9–12

[9] Rösch T, Classen M. A new ultrasonic probe for endosonographic imaging of the upper GI-tract. Preliminary observations. Endoscopy 1990; 22: 41–46

[10] Vilmann P, Khattar S, Hancke S. Endoscopic ultrasound examination of the upper gastrointestinal tract using a curved-array transducer. A preliminary report. Surg Endosc 1991; 5: 79–82

[11] Vilmann P, Hancke S, Henriksen FW, Jacobsen GK. Endosonographically-guided fine needle aspiration biopsy of malignant lesions in the upper gastrointestinal tract. Endoscopy 1993; 25: 523–527

[12] Giovannini M, Seitz JF, Monges G, Perrier H, Castellani P. [Guided puncture-cytology under electronic sectorial ultrasound endoscopy. Results in 26 patients]. Gastroenterol Clin Biol 1993; 17: 465–470

[13] Dietrich CF. Echtzeit-Gewebeelastographie. Anwendungsmöglichkeiten nicht nur im Gastrointestinaltrakt. Endosk Heute 2010; 23: 177–212

[14] Giovannini M, Hookey LC, Bories E, Pesenti C, Monges G, Delpero JR. Endoscopic ultrasound elastography: the first step towards virtual biopsy? Preliminary results in 49 patients. Endoscopy 2006; 38: 344–348

[15] Dietrich CF, Ignee A, Frey H. Contrast-enhanced endoscopic ultrasound with low mechanical index: a new technique. Z Gastroenterol 2005; 43: 1219–1223

[16] Dietrich CF. Contrast-enhanced low mechanical index endoscopic ultrasound (CELMI-EUS). Endoscopy 2009; 41 (Suppl 2): E43–E44

[17] Wiersema MJ. Endosonography-guided cystoduodenostomy with a therapeutic ultrasound endoscope. Gastrointest Endosc 1996; 44: 614–617

[18] Wiersema MJ, Wiersema LM. Endosonography-guided celiac plexus neurolysis. Gastrointest Endosc 1996; 44: 656–662

[19] Burmester E, Niehaus J, Leineweber T, Huetteroth T. EUS-cholangio-drainage of the bile duct: report of 4 cases. Gastrointest Endosc 2003; 57: 246–251

[20] Bataille L, Deprez P. A new application for therapeutic EUS: main pancreatic duct drainage with a "pancreatic rendezvous technique". Gastrointest Endosc 2002; 55: 740–743

[21] Janssen J, Dietrich CF. Radial-, Longitudinal- oder Minisonden-Endosonographie: Wie viele Systeme braucht eine Endoskopieabteilung? In: Dietrich CF, ed. Endosonographie. Stuttgart, New York: Thieme; 2008:39–46

[22] Sudholt HW, Vilmann P. Die endosonographisch gesteuerte diagnostische Feinnadelpunktion – Ausrüstung und Technik. In: Dietrich CF, ed. Endosonographie. Stuttgart, New York: Thieme; 2008:76–86

[23] Gerke H, Rizk MK, Vanderheyden AD, Jensen CS. Randomized study comparing endoscopic ultrasound-guided Trucut biopsy and fine needle aspiration with high suction. Cytopathology 2010; 21: 44–51

[24] Ardengh JC, Lopes CV, de Lima LF et al. Cell block technique and cytological smears for the differential diagnosis of pancreatic neoplasms after endosonography-guided fine-needle aspiration. Acta Gastroenterol Latinoam 2008; 38: 246–251

[25] Riphaus A, Wehrmann T, Weber B et alSektion Enoskopie im Auftrag der Deutschen Gesellschaft für Verdauungs- und Stoffwechselerkrankungen e.V. (DGVS). Bundesverband Niedergelassener Gastroenterologen Deuschlands e. V. (Bng). Chirurgische Arbeitsgemeinschaft für Endoskopie und Sonographie der Deutschen Gesellschaft für Allgemein- und Viszeralchirurgie (DGAV). Deutsche Morbus Crohn/Colitis ulcerosa Vereinigung e. V. (DCCV). Deutsche Gesellschaft für Endoskopie-Assistenzpersonal (DEGEA). Deutsche Gesellschaft für Anästhesie und Intensivmedizin (DGAI). Gesellschaft für Recht und Politik im Gesundheitswesen (GPRG). [S3-guidelines—sedation in gastrointestinal endoscopy]. Z Gastroenterol 2008; 46: 1298–1330

[26] Jenssen C, Dietrich CF. Endoscopic ultrasound-guided fine-needle aspiration biopsy and trucut biopsy in gastroenterology – an overview. Best Pract Res Clin Gastroenterol 2009; 23: 743–759

[27] Jenssen C, Alvarez-Sánchez MV, Napoléon B, Faiss S. Diagnostic endoscopic ultrasonography: assessment of safety and prevention of complications. World J Gastroenterol 2012; 18: 4659–4676

[28] Wallace MB, Kennedy T, Durkalski V et al. Randomized controlled trial of EUS-guided fine needle aspiration techniques for the detection of malignant lymphadenopathy. Gastrointest Endosc 2001; 54: 441–447

[29] Bhutani MS, Suryaprasad S, Moezzi J, Seabrook D. Improved technique for performing endoscopic ultrasound guided fine needle aspiration of lymph nodes. Endoscopy 1999; 31: 550–553

[30] Voss M, Hammel P, Molas G et al. Value of endoscopic ultrasound guided fine needle aspiration biopsy in the diagnosis of solid pancreatic masses. Gut 2000; 46: 244–249

[31] Larghi A, Noffsinger A, Dye CE, Hart J, Waxman I. EUS-guided fine needle tissue acquisition by using high negative pressure suction for the evaluation of solid masses: a pilot study. Gastrointest Endosc 2005; 62: 768–774

[32] Jenssen C, Möller K, Wagner S, Sarbia M. [Endoscopic ultrasound-guided biopsy: diagnostic yield, pitfalls, quality management part 1: optimizing specimen collection and diagnostic efficiency]. Z Gastroenterol 2008; 46: 590–600

[33] Jenssen C, Dietrich CF. [Ultrasound and endoscopic ultrasound of the adrenal glands]. Ultraschall Med 2010; 31: 228–247, quiz 248–250

[34] Jenssen C, Dietrich CF. Endoscopic ultrasound of gastrointestinal subepithelial lesions. Ultraschall Med 2008; 29: 236–256, quiz 257–264

[35] Will U. [Therapeutic endosonography]. Z Gastroenterol 2008; 46: 555–563

[36] Hancke S, Henriksen FW. Percutaneous pancreatic cystogastrostomy guided by ultrasound scanning and gastroscopy. Br J Surg 1985; 72: 916–917

[37] Bernardino ME, Amerson JR. Percutaneous gastrocystostomy: a new approach to pancreatic pseudocyst drainage. AJR Am J Roentgenol 1984; 143: 1096–1097

[38] Dunkin BJ, Ponsky JL, Hale JC. Ultrasound-directed percutaneous endoscopic cyst-gastrostomy for the treatment of a pancreatic pseudocyst. Surg Endosc 1998; 12: 1426–1429

[39] Seifert H, Dietrich CF. Pancreatic interventions. In: Dietrich CF, ed. Endoscopic Ultrasound, an Introductory Manual and Atlas. Stuttgart, New York: Thieme; 2011: 366–386

[40] Seifert H, Biermer M, Schmitt W et al. Transluminal endoscopic necrosectomy after acute pancreatitis: a multicentre study with long-term follow-up (the GEPARD Study). Gut 2009; 58: 1260–1266

[41] Nealon WH, Walser E. Main pancreatic ductal anatomy can direct choice of modality for treating pancreatic pseudocysts (surgery versus percutaneous drainage). Ann Surg 2002; 235: 751–758

[42] Jenssen C, Dietrich CF. [Endoscopic ultrasound in chronic pancreatitis]. Z Gastroenterol 2005; 43: 737–749

[43] Dietrich CF, Jenssen C, Allescher HD, Hocke M, Barreiros AP, Ignee A. [Differential diagnosis of pancreatic lesions using endoscopic ultrasound]. Z Gastroenterol 2008; 46: 601–617

[44] Dietrich CF, Ignee A, Braden B, Barreiros AP, Ott M, Hocke M. Improved differentiation of pancreatic tumors using contrast-enhanced endoscopic ultrasound. Clin Gastroenterol Hepatol 2008; 6: 590–597, e1

[45] Beyer-Enke SA, Hocke M, Ignee A, Braden B, Dietrich CF. Contrast enhanced transabdominal ultrasound in the characterisation of pancreatic lesions with cystic appearance. JOP 2010; 11: 427–433

[46] Seifert H, Dietrich C, Schmitt T, Caspary W, Wehrmann T. Endoscopic ultrasound-guided one-step transmural drainage of cystic abdominal lesions with a large-channel echo endoscope. Endoscopy 2000; 32: 255–259

[47] Seifert H, Faust D, Schmitt T, Dietrich C, Caspary W, Wehrmann T. Transmural drainage of cystic peripancreatic lesions with a new large-channel echo endoscope. Endoscopy 2001; 33: 1022–1026

[48] Will U. Forcierte Interventionelle Endosonographie – Praktische Tipps und Tricks. In: Dietrich CF, ed. Endosonographie. Stuttgart, New York: Thieme Verlag; 2008: 463–475

[49] Besselink MG, de Bruijn MT, Rutten JP, Boermeester MA, Hofker HS, Gooszen HG. Dutch Acute Pancreatitis Study Group. Surgical intervention in patients with necrotizing pancreatitis. Br J Surg 2006; 93: 593–599

[50] Levy MJ, Topazian MD, Wiersema MJ et al. Initial evaluation of the efficacy and safety of endoscopic ultrasound-guided direct ganglia neurolysis and block. Am J Gastroenterol 2008; 103: 98–103

[51] Jürgensen C, Schuppan D, Neser F, Ernstberger J, Junghans U, Stölzel U. EUS-guided alcohol ablation of an insulinoma. Gastrointest Endosc 2006; 63: 1059–1062

[52] Levy MJ, Wong Kee Song LM, Farnell MB, Misra S, Sarr MG, Gostout CJ. Endoscopic ultrasound (EUS)-guided angiotherapy of refractory gastrointestinal bleeding. Am J Gastroenterol 2008; 103: 352–359

[53] Levy MJ, Chak A. EUS 2008 Working Group. EUS 2008 Working Group document: evaluation of EUS-guided vascular therapy. Gastrointest Endosc 2009; 69 (Suppl): S37–S42

[54] Jenssen C. Diagnostische Endosonographie – State of the Art 2009. Endosk Heute 2009; 22: 89–104

[55] Dietrich CF, Leuschner MS, Zeuzem S et al. Peri-hepatic lymphadenopathy in primary biliary cirrhosis reflects progression of the disease. Eur J Gastroenterol Hepatol 1999; 11: 747–753

[56] Dietrich CF, Lee JH, Herrmann G et al. Enlargement of perihepatic lymph nodes in relation to liver histology and viremia in patients with chronic hepatitis C. Hepatology 1997; 26: 467–472

[57] Hirche TO, Russler J, Braden B et al. Sonographic detection of perihepatic lymphadenopathy is an indicator for primary sclerosing cholangitis in patients with inflammatory bowel disease. Int J Colorectal Dis 2004; 19: 586–594

[58] Dietrich CF, Stryjek-Kaminska D, Teuber G, Lee JH, Caspary WF, Zeuzem S. Perihepatic lymph nodes as a marker of antiviral response in patients with chronic hepatitis C infection. AJR Am J Roentgenol 2000; 174: 699–704

[59] Jenssen C, Dietrich CF. Endoscopic ultrasound in chronic pancreatitis. In: Dietrich CD, ed. Endoscopic Ultrasound, an Introductory Manual and Atlas. Stuttgart, New York: Thieme; 2011: 284–322

[60] Ho KY, Brugge WR. EUS 2008 Working Group. EUS 2008 Working Group document: evaluation of EUS-guided pancreatic-cyst ablation. Gastrointest Endosc 2009; 69 (Suppl): S22–S27

[61] Puli SR, Reddy JB, Bechtold ML, Antillon MR, Brugge WR. EUS-guided celiac plexus neurolysis for pain due to chronic pancreatitis or pancreatic cancer pain: a meta-analysis and systematic review. Dig Dis Sci 2009; 54: 2330–2337

[62] Kaufman M, Singh G, Das S et al. Efficacy of endoscopic ultrasound-guided celiac plexus block and celiac plexus neurolysis for managing abdominal pain associated with chronic pancreatitis and pancreatic cancer. J Clin Gastroenterol 2010; 44: 127–134

[63] O'Toole TM, Schmulewitz N. Complication rates of EUS-guided celiac plexus blockade and neurolysis: results of a large case series. Endoscopy 2009; 41: 593–597

[64] Alvarez-Sánchez MV, Jenssen C, Faiss S et al. Interventional endoscopic ultrasonography: an overview of safety and complications. Surg Endosc 2014; 28: 712–734

23 Special Issues Regarding Interventions in the Spleen

C. F. Dietrich

Interventional procedures in the spleen are relatively rare. This is due to a lack of "hard indications" for splenic biopsy but also to the (culturally instilled) attitude of many operators that it is too dangerous to puncture the spleen because of the risk of hemorrhage. This reluctance stems in part from a lack of awareness of necessary indications (benefits) and the risks relating to the proximity of the pleura (risk of a two-cavity procedure) and bowel (risk of injury).[1] The technique of percutaneous splenic biopsy and drainage is basically the same as that described for liver biopsies and abscess drainage and need not be detailed here.

23.1 Diffuse Splenic Changes

The differential diagnosis of diffuse splenic changes includes portal hypertension, acute and chronic infectious diseases, tumors, and hemato-oncologic conditions. Potential systemic or malignant causes are diffusely infiltrating lymphomas and myeloproliferative syndromes. Right heart failure, portal vein thrombosis, splenic vein thrombosis, metabolic and storage diseases, and amyloidosis should also be considered. Splenomegaly may have numerous other causes:

- Portal hypertension
- Myeloproliferative syndrome (chronic myeloid leukemia, polycythemia vera)
- Osteomyelosclerosis
- Hairy cell leukemia
- Storage diseases especially Gaucher disease)
- Chronic infections such as kala-azar (leishmaniasis)
- Form of anemia with severe hemolysis
- Infections, acute
- Infections, chronic
- Congestive heart failure
- Anemia due to hemolysis
- Hemato-oncologic disease (except for myeloproliferative syndromes)
- Acute and chronic lymphocytic leukemia
- Acute myeloid leukemia
- Hodgkin and non-Hodgkin lymphoma
- Portal vein thrombosis, splenic vein thrombosis
- Autoimmune diseases
- Storage diseases (except for Gaucher disease)

The spleen usually has a homogeneous structure when imaged by ultrasound. Tuberculosis, candidiasis, or syphilis may produce scattered foci or decreased or greatly increased echogenicity.

Ultrasound contrast agents have proven helpful for the exclusion of tiny, circumscribed splenic changes that may indicate malignant or inflammatory infiltration with microabscess formation in the setting of *Candida* sepsis or other bacterial infections.[1–7] It should be emphasized that plain B-mode imaging with a high-resolution transducer (7–17 MHz) can yield equally good results.[8] Similar voids may be found in hemophagocytic syndrome (personal data, previously unpublished).

Diffuse splenic changes in themselves are not an indication for splenic biopsy, which would be absolutely contraindicated in patients with portal hypertension, for example.

Possible complications of splenomegaly:

- Splenic infarction (splenic abscess)
- Splenic capsule rupture with hemorrhage
- Splenic fibrosis
- Pulmonary ventilation disorders

Note

Diffuse splenic changes are not an indication for splenic biopsy.

23.2 Specific Disorders

23.2.1 Splenic Rupture

Splenic rupture is a threatening condition because it may lead to hemorrhagic shock culminating in death. Splenic injuries usually appear as hypoechoic foci that may be hyperechoic in the acute stage. Splenic rupture may have a traumatic etiology or may occur spontaneously in patients with underlying splenic pathology. Splenic injuries are discussed further in Chapter 31.

Intraparenchymal injury is distinguished from subcapsular hematoma formation and injury to the splenic capsule. In doubtful cases with unexplained ascites and a suspected splenic rupture, ultrasound-guided fluid aspiration can be performed to confirm the hemorrhage. Abscess formation is observed in rare cases (for treatment see Chapter 15).

23.2.2 Splenic Infarction

Splenic infarctions usually resolve completely without sequelae or by scarring of the infarcted area. They most often occur in association with endocarditis, myeloproliferative syndromes, and septic diseases and generally do not require an ultrasound-guided intervention.[1]

23.2.3 Focal Splenic Changes

Cystic Masses

Dysontogenetic cysts appear echo-free with smooth margins, may contain internal septa, and display typical cystic features such as an entry echo and distal acoustic enhancement. Echogenic splenic cysts are more common than in the liver and require interventional investigation only in selected cases. Solitary echinococcal cysts are very rare; their management is discussed under PAIR treatment (puncture, aspiration, injection, reaspiration) for hydatid liver cysts in Chapter 17.[9]

Primary Splenic Tumors

Benign tumors of the spleen are relatively rare. As in the liver, the most common entities are capillary hemangiomas, which are usually echogenic; cavernous hemangiomas, which are hypoechoic or show variable echogenicity; and splenomas. Hemangiomas require differentiation from other mesenchymal tumors and littoral cell angioma. Only histology can furnish a definitive diagnosis. Benign/malignant differentiation in most cases relies on the progression of sonographic (imaging) findings. Primary malignant tumors of the spleen are extremely rare; most are mesenchymal tumors (angiosarcoma, leiomyofibrosarcoma).

Secondary Focal Splenic Changes

These changes are usually due to secondary infiltration by lymphoma, which may determine the individual prognosis (stage I or II [with primary mediastinal involvement] versus stage IV with splenic involvement). Lymphomatous infiltrates usually appear as hyperechoic, circumscribed lesions of variable size and with variable margins. They are distinguishable from a number of other changes (bacterial and fungal abscesses) only by histologic examination. Indolent non-Hodgkin lymphomas tend to show a diffuse or micronodular pattern of involvement, while more aggressive lymphomas may form conglomerate masses of variable size with mixed echogenicity and scalloped margins.

Splenic Abscesses

A distinction is made between macroabscesses and microabscesses (< 10 mm). Splenic abscesses usually exhibit low or mixed echogenicity and are rarely echo-free. An echogenic perifocal reaction may be seen, depending on host immune status. Macroabscesses in the spleen most commonly result from the secondary infection of an infarcted area, the spread of pancreatitis, or hematogenous spread. The early stages of an abscess (pyogenic inflammation) may show increased vascularity. Microabscesses are typical of *Candida* infection. Multiple small focal lesions are found in immunosuppressed patients or patients who have had neutropenic fever. Hepatosplenic candidiasis is not manifested during neutropenic fever, and imaging findings appear only after recovery of the granulocyte count. For this reason, ultrasound is of little help in excluding HLC during the cytopenic phase.

Abscess regression in response to antimycotic therapy can be monitored sonographically. The differential diagnosis is broad and includes bacterial and fungal abscess, parasitic diseases, granulomatous inflammations, as well as lymphoma and hemophagocytic syndrome.

Isolated microabscesses < 10 mm may determine the prognosis in any given case and are confirmed histologically (recommended needle diameter: 0.95 mm or 1.2 mm). Abscesses up to 50 (or 70) mm in size can be drained by percutaneous needle aspiration, while larger abscesses require catheter drainage as described in Chapter 15.

Splenic Metastases

Splenic metastases at the end stage of an aggressive cancer illness are more common than is generally assumed but rarely determine the prognosis. Splenic metastases are often hypoechoic, but some have a cystic appearance with echogenic elements while others show complex and variable echogenicity. Hypervascular metastases are found in association with neuroendocrine tumors and renal cell carcinoma, while relatively hypovascular metastases are more characteristic of gastrointestinal cancers.

23.3 Procedures

23.3.1 Clinical Scenarios

Splenic changes are often found in the setting of other organ manifestations. Splenomegaly seldom occurs in isolation (portal hypertension, infections, and hemato-oncologic diseases). Circumscribed splenic changes in otherwise healthy, asymptomatic patients generally have a benign etiology and require only follow-up.

Diagnostic and therapeutic interventions (drainage) are performed under primary sonographic guidance owing to the advantages described earlier. The indications and procedures are not standardized (ultrasound-guided splenic biopsy, laparoscopy, [exploratory] laparotomy [splenectomy], or wait and see). The indication for fine needle aspiration biopsy (FNAB) should be carefully considered in terms of the risk of hemorrhage and the alternatives of diagnostic and perhaps therapeutic splenectomy. The diagnostic accuracy of FNAB is high, however, and the postinterventional complication rate is low.

23.3.2 Anatomical Considerations in Splenic Interventions

The anatomical relationships of the spleen should be considered prior to splenic interventions. The spleen is intraperitoneal, occupying a subdiaphragmatic and subcostal location in the left upper quadrant of the abdomen. The upper pole of the spleen is closely related to the gastric fundus, aorta, pancreatic tail, adrenal gland, and left lobe of the liver. It is relevant to interventions that, with deep inspiration, the spleen may be covered by air in the costophrenic angle. The lower pole of the spleen is anterolateral to the left kidney and borders on the left colic flexure. The splenic artery runs cranial to the pancreatic body and along the pancreatic tail to the splenic hilum. The spleen can be identified in an initial flank scan above the left kidney, and an intercostal scan aimed at the splenic hilum should then demonstrate the spleen without artifacts (the patient's left arm is raised to open up the intercostal space). The splenic vein and pancreatic tail should also be visible. The beam is directed anteromedially to display the stomach and inferolaterally to display the left kidney.

23.3.3 Procedures for Specific Applications

We prefer a fine needle aspiration (needle diameter 0.095 mm) for the investigation of splenic metastases and a cutting needle biopsy (needle diameter 1.2 mm) for the characterization of splenic tumors. This is because, as in the liver, thinner needles are assumed to be less useful for tumor characterization (especially benign tumors and lymphomas) while larger needles increase the risk of hemorrhage.

23.4 Abscess Drainage

Abscess drainage follows the rules covered in Chapter 15 (▶ Fig. 23.1).[10]

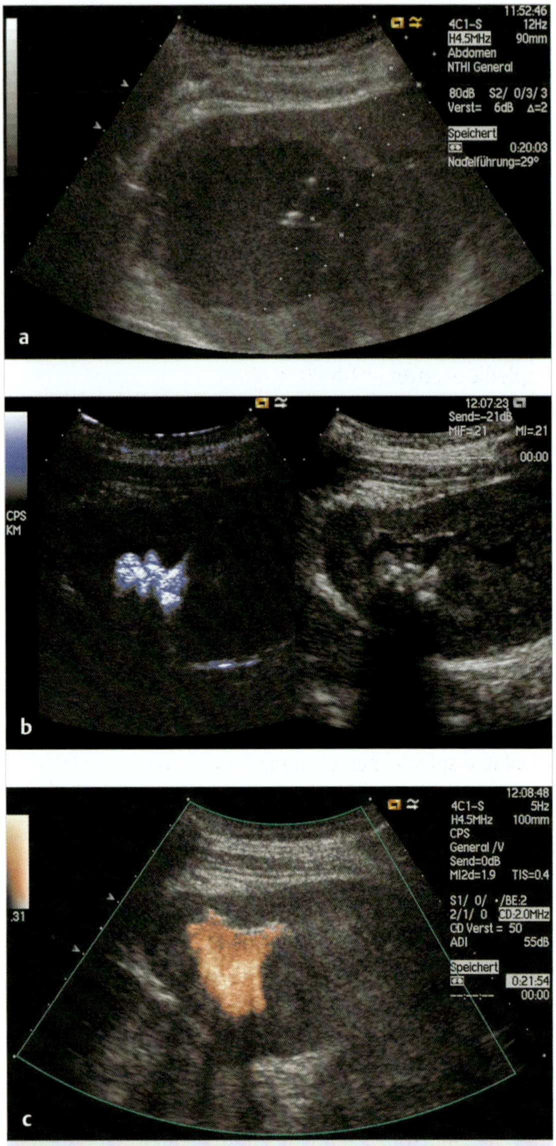

Fig. 23.1 a–c Splenic abscess drainage. The abscess is punctured with a needle (**a**). After contrast agent is injected via the drainage, the structure of the abscess cavity is demonstrated, and there is no communication between abscess and surrounding structures (**b, c**).

23.5 Indications

Splenic biopsy or drainage is appropriate in all cases where the clinical benefit is well defined and is expected to alter diagnostic and/or therapeutic management or is considered necessary to make a prognosis.[3,11,12] Thus we cannot offer any simple, general rules, although we can present cases that illustrate the range of indications.

23.6 Contraindications

Besides the contraindications noted in the chapters on the liver and abscess drainage, a splenic intervention should be withheld if the clinical benefit is not clearly defined and the procedure will not alter diagnostic and/or therapeutic management or is unnecessary for making a prognosis.

Patients with known amyloidosis have a relatively high risk of spontaneous intrasplenic hemorrhage. As a general rule, splenic biopsy is unsuitable for the diagnosis of amyloidosis.[13]

23.7 Indications for Splenic Biopsy Drawn from Case Data

We can cite specific indications for splenic biopsy based on an analysis of more than 100 splenic interventions performed at our center. Illustrative case reports and a limited number of literature citations are available for the list of indications that can be definitively diagnosed by splenic biopsy. We do not consider the list to be complete, and we invite interested readers to submit their own indications and experience (e.g., on the "Case of the

Month" page at the website of the European Federation of Societies for Ultrasound in Medicine and Biology, www.efsumb.org). Our indications are as follows:

- Localized mediastinal lymphadenopathy associated with a circumscribed splenic change that would influence the diagnosis and treatment of Hodgkin and non-Hodgkin lymphoma. For example, the exclusion of splenic involvement by a suspected benign mesenchymal neoplasm (e.g., splenic hemangioma, splenoma, other tumors) could affect treatment options.[3]
- Systemic lupus erythematosus in patients on immunosuppressant therapy with isolated small, circumscribed splenic changes (< 10–20 mm).
- Splenic biopsy to detect or exclude a secondary lymphoma with manifestations confined to the spleen, a fungal infection, or a hemophagocytic syndrome.
- Differential diagnosis of fungal infection during treatment of systemic hematologic disease.
- Bone marrow suppression with isolated circumscribed splenic changes to detect or exclude extramedullary hematopoiesis versus infiltration by lymphoma.[14]
- Postpancreatic pseudocyst infiltration versus cystic pancreatic tumor[15] versus primary splenic tumor (for optimum control of drainage therapy for a pancreatic abscess or infected pancreatic pseudocyst, for example).
- Isolated splenic masses in sarcoidosis to differentiate granulomatous infiltration of the spleen from other neoplastic infiltration.[8]
- Scarring of the spleen and splenic infarction associated with a lymphoma at a different site, e.g., isolated pancreatic lymphoma in HIV infection.[14,16,17]
- Isolated splenic tuberculosis (rare).[18–21]
- Echinococcosis of the spleen.[9,22,23]
- Isolated splenic metastases from melanoma, ovarian carcinoma, poorly differentiated small-cell lung cancer,[24] etc. (*Comment:* Splenectomy without a prior biopsy may be a better option.)
- Isolated organ manifestation of aggressive T-cell lymphoma.[7]
- Inflammatory pseudotumor of the spleen.[25–27]
- Littoral cell angioma.[28–31]
- Pancreatic carcinoma infiltrating the spleen primarily and presenting as a splenic tumor.[32]
- Atypical accessory spleen.[33] (*Comment:* In almost every case, an accessory spleen can be accurately diagnosed by contrast-enhanced ultrasonography.[34])
- Primary sarcomas of the spleen.[35–38] (*Comment:* In everyday oncology practice, splenectomy without a prior biopsy is recommended for a suspected primary sarcoma of the spleen.)

23.8 Postinterventional Care

Postinterventional care follows the same rules as for percutaneous liver biopsy and abscess drainage. If symptoms arise, ultrasound scans should be performed to detect or exclude free fluid and intrasplenic hemorrhage. An ultrasound follow-up should be scheduled for the day after the intervention.

23.9 Complications

Complications of splenic biopsies are rarely reported.[1,39–43] In 20 years of follow-up in more than 100 splenic interventions, we have recorded 3 cases of minor postinterventional bleeding but have had no complications requiring surgical treatment or transfusion. Civardi et al observed less than a 1% incidence of major complications in 398 fine needle biopsies of the spleen.[41]

23.10 Preinterventional Vaccinations

Because loss of the spleen (whether surgical, traumatic or functional) weakens host defenses against polysaccharide encapsulated bacteria, patients should be vaccinated against the following organisms prior to the intervention:

- Meningococci
- Pneumococci
- *Haemophilus influenzae* type B

▸ **Timing of the vaccination.** Necessary vaccines should be administered at least 10 days before an elective splenectomy. With an unplanned splenectomy, vaccination should be initiated after the patient has recuperated but before hospital discharge. Immunosuppressed patients should be vaccinated as soon as possible; some patients may require antibiotic coverage until that time.

References

[1] Nuernberg D, Ignee A, Dietrich CF. Ultrasound in gastroenterology—liver and spleen [Article in German]. Z Gastroenterol 2006; 44: 991–1000

[2] Görg C, Faoro C, Bert T, Tebbe J, Neesse A, Wilhelm C. Contrast enhanced ultrasound of splenic lymphoma involvement. Eur J Radiol 2011; 80: 169–174

[3] von Herbay A, Barreiros AP, Ignee A et al. Contrast-enhanced ultrasonography with SonoVue: differentiation between benign and malignant lesions of the spleen. J Ultrasound Med 2009; 28: 421–434

[4] Görg C. The forgotten organ: contrast enhanced sonography of the spleen. Eur J Radiol 2007; 64: 189–201

[5] Görg C, Bert T. Second-generation sonographic contrast agent for differential diagnosis of perisplenic lesions. AJR Am J Roentgenol 2006; 186: 621–626

[6] Görg C, Bert T. Contrast enhanced sonography of focal splenic lesions with a second-generation contrast agent. Ultraschall Med 2005; 26: 470–477

[7] Dietrich CF. 3D real time contrast enhanced ultrasonography,a new technique [Article in German]. Rofo 2002; 174: 160–163

[8] Dietrich CF, Ignee A, Trojan J, Fellbaum C, Schuessler G. Improved characterisation of histologically proven liver tumours by contrast enhanced ultrasonography during the portal venous and specific late phase of SHU 508A. Gut 2004; 53: 401–405

[9] Dietrich CF, Mueller G, Beyer-Enke S. Cysts in the cyst pattern. Z Gastroenterol 2009; 47: 1203–1207

[10] Schwerk WB, Görg C, Görg K, Richter G, Beckh K. Percutaneous drainage of liver and splenic abscess [Article in German]. Z Gastroenterol 1991; 29: 146–152
[11] Bert T, Tebbe J, Görg C. What should be done with echoic splenic tumors incidentally found by ultrasound? Z Gastroenterol 2010; 48: 465–471
[12] Görg C, Hoffmann A. Metastases to the Spleen in 59 cancer patients: a 14-year clinicosonographic study [Article in German]. Ultraschall Med 2008; 29: 173–178
[13] Barreiros AP, Otto G, Ignee A, Galle P, Dietrich CF. Sonographic signs of amyloidosis. Z Gastroenterol 2009; 47: 731–739
[14] Huynh MQ, Barth P, Sohlbach K, Neubauer A, Görg C. B-mode ultrasound and contrast-enhanced ultrasound pattern of focal extramedullary hematopoiesis of the spleen in a patient with myeloproliferative disease. Ultraschall Med 2009; 30: 297–299
[15] Beyer-Enke SA, Hocke M, Ignee A, Braden B, Dietrich CF. Contrast enhanced transabdominal ultrasound in the characterisation of pancreatic lesions with cystic appearance. JOP 2010; 11: 427–433
[16] Görg C, Seifart U, Görg K. Acute, complete splenic infarction in cancer patient is associated with a fatal outcome. Abdom Imaging 2004; 29: 224–227
[17] Görg C, Zugmaier G. Chronic recurring infarction of the spleen: sonographic patterns and complications. Ultraschall Med 2003; 24: 245–249
[18] Dixit R, Arya MK, Panjabi M, Gupta A, Paramez AR. Clinical profile of patients having splenic involvement in tuberculosis. Indian J Tuberc 2010; 57: 25–30
[19] Udgaonkar U, Kulkarni S, Shah S, Bhave S. Asymptomatic, isolated tubercular splenic abscess, in an immunocompetent person. Indian J Med Microbiol 2010; 28: 172–173
[20] Barreiros AP, Braden B, Schieferstein-Knauer C, Ignee A, Dietrich CF. Characteristics of intestinal tuberculosis in ultrasonographic techniques. Scand J Gastroenterol 2008; 43: 1224–1231
[21] Mahi M, Chaouir S, Amil T, Hanine A, Benameur M. [Isolated tuberculosis of the spleen. Report of a case]. J Radiol 2002; 83: 479–481
[22] Culafić DM, Kerkez MD, Mijac DD et al. Spleen cystic echinococcosis: clinical manifestations and treatment. Scand J Gastroenterol 2010; 45: 186–190
[23] Yuksel M, Demirpolat G, Sever A, Bakaris S, Bulbuloglu E, Elmas N. Hydatid disease involving some rare locations in the body: a pictorial essay. Korean J Radiol 2007; 8: 531–540
[24] Busić Z, Cupurdija K, Kolovrat M et al. Isolated splenic metastasis from colon cancer—case report and literature review. Coll Antropol 2010; 34 (Suppl 1): 287–290
[25] Chen WH, Liu TP, Liu CL, Tzen CY. Inflammatory pseudotumor of the spleen. J Chin Med Assoc 2004; 67: 533–536
[26] Oz Puyan F, Bilgi S, Unlu E et al. Inflammatory pseudotumor of the spleen with EBV positivity: report of a case. Eur J Haematol 2004; 72: 285–291
[27] Yesildag E, Sarimurat N, Ince U, Numan F, Buyukunal C. Nonsurgical diagnosis and management of an inflammatory pseudotumor of the spleen in a child. J Clin Ultrasound 2003; 31: 335–338
[28] Wang YJ, Li F, Cao F, Sun JB, Liu JF, Wang YH. Littoral cell angioma of the spleen. Asian J Surg 2009; 32: 167–171
[29] Tee M, Vos P, Zetler P, Wiseman SM. Incidental littoral cell angioma of the spleen. World J Surg Oncol 2008; 6: 87
[30] Qu ZB, Liu LX, Wu LF, Zhao S, Jiang HC. Multiple littoral cell angioma of the spleen: a case report and review of the literature. Onkologie 2007; 30: 256–258
[31] Görg C, Barth P, Backhus J, Boecker J, Neubauer A. Sonographic patterns of littoral cell angioma: case report and review of the literature [Article in German]. Ultraschall Med 2001; 22: 191–194
[32] Wang HJ, Zhao ZW, Luo HF, Wang ZY. Malignant nonfunctioning islet cell tumor of the pancreas with intrasplenic growth: a case report. Hepatobiliary Pancreat Dis Int 2006; 5: 471–473
[33] Kanazawa H, Kamiya J, Nagino M et al. Epidermoid cyst in an intrapancreatic accessory spleen: a case report. J Hepatobiliary Pancreat Surg 2004; 11: 61–63
[34] von Herbay A, Vogt C, Häussinger D. The ultrasound contrast agent levovist helps with the differentiation between accessory spleen and lymph nodes in the splenic hilum: a pilot study [Article in German]. Z Gastroenterol 2004; 42: 1109–1115
[35] Trojan J, Hammerstingl R, Engels K, Schneider AR, Zeuzem S, Dietrich CF. Contrast-enhanced ultrasound in the diagnosis of malignant mesenchymal liver tumors. J Clin Ultrasound 2010; 38: 227–231
[36] Chen WL, Hsu YJ, Tsai WC, Tsao YT. An unusual case of febrile neutropenia: acute myeloid leukemia presenting as myeloid sarcoma of the spleen. J Natl Med Assoc 2008; 100: 957–959
[37] Hsu JT, Ueng SH, Hwang TL, Chen HM, Jan YY, Chen MF. Primary angiosarcoma of the spleen in a child with long-term survival. Pediatr Surg Int 2007; 23: 807–810
[38] Thompson WM, Levy AD, Aguilera NS, Gorospe L, Abbott RM. Angiosarcoma of the spleen: imaging characteristics in 12 patients. Radiology 2005; 235: 106–115
[39] Kang M, Kalra N, Gulati M, Lal A, Kochhar R, Rajwanshi A. Image guided percutaneous splenic interventions. Eur J Radiol 2007; 64: 140–146
[40] Zerem E, Bergsland J. Ultrasound guided percutaneous treatment for splenic abscesses: the significance in treatment of critically ill patients. World J Gastroenterol 2006; 12: 7341–7345
[41] Civardi G, Vallisa D, Bertè R et al. Ultrasound-guided fine needle biopsy of the spleen: high clinical efficacy and low risk in a multicenter Italian study. Am J Hematol 2001; 67: 93–99
[42] Zeppa P, Picardi M, Marino G et al. Fine-needle aspiration biopsy and flow cytometry immunophenotyping of lymphoid and myeloproliferative disorders of the spleen. Cancer 2003; 99: 118–127
[43] López JI, Del Cura JL, De Larrinoa AF, Gorriño O, Zabala R, Bilbao FJ. Role of ultrasound-guided core biopsy in the evaluation of spleen pathology. APMIS 2006; 114: 492–499

Thorax

24 Thoracic Interventions . . . 260

24 Thoracic Interventions

W. Blank, A. Heinzmann

The chest wall, including the thoracic inlet and axillae, can be defined in exquisite detail with small, lightweight, high-resolution ultrasound transducers and modern ultrasound technology (▶ Fig. 24.1).

Pulmonary lesions can be visualized if they are in contact with the visceral pleura or are accessible to ultrasound scans through a sound-conducting medium (pleural effusion, atelectasis).[1–4]

Approximately 75% of clinically significant mediastinal masses in adults are located in the anterior and middle mediastinum and can be imaged sonographically from a suprasternal or parasternal site (left and right lateral decubitus).[5]

Only a few thoracic masses can be accurately classified etiologically on the basis of typical sonographic findings. Often a definitive diagnosis will require additional biochemical, microbiologic, cytologic, or histologic evaluation. The specimens necessary for these studies can be acquired by various means:

- Percutaneous aspiration or core biopsy (ultrasound- or CT-guided)
- Endoluminal access (bronchoscopy, endoluminal ultrasound)
- Surgical access (mediastinoscopy, mediastinoscopic ultrasound, thoracoscopy, or open exposure)

24.1 Advantages of Ultrasound-Guided Interventions

Masses that are detectable by ultrasound are usually accessible to percutaneous biopsy unless the targeted lesion or needle path cannot be clearly visualized.

In the chest as elsewhere, an ultrasound-guided intervention offers definite advantages over CT guidance in suitably selected cases[6,7]:

- The procedure can be performed quickly and at bedside.
- There is no radiation exposure to the patient, physician, or staff.
- The needle can be introduced in any direction and its path can be observed continuously.
- Ultrasound guidance can protect blood vessels (color Doppler), nerves (nerve plexuses at the thoracic inlet, ▶ Fig. 24.1), and aerated lung from injury (low incidence of pneumothorax) (▶ Fig. 24.2).
- Active tumor elements (color Doppler, contrast agents) can be selectively targeted and sampled with a high success rate (▶ Fig. 24.3).

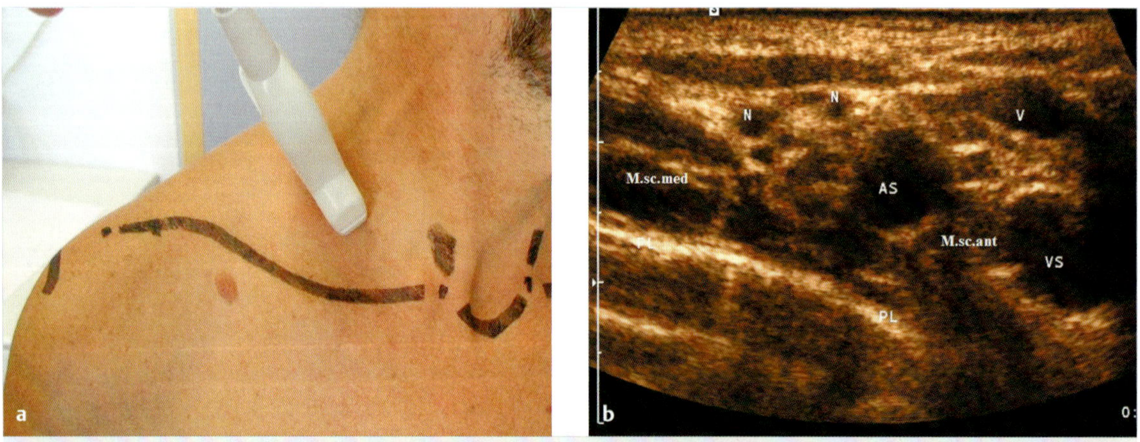

Fig. 24.1
a The thoracic inlet is examined sonographically in sagittal, axial, coronal, and lesion-adapted planes. Small high-resolution ultrasound probes, preferably with a sector image format (on a system with variable electronic formatting), are advantageous for displaying the complex anatomy about the thoracic inlet. The scan plane shown in the figure can display the brachial plexus and subclavian artery in the anterior scalene interval.
b Ultrasound image of the region scanned in panel **a**. The structures between the middle scalene muscle (M.s.c. med.) and anterior scalene muscle (M.s.c. ant.) are the subclavian artery (AS) anteriorly and a cross section of the hypoechoic nerve fascicles of the brachial plexus (N) posteriorly. It is important to preserve these neurovascular structures during the percutaneous biopsy of lymph nodes, apical lung tumors, etc., calling for a skilled biopsy technique. VS, subclavian vein; PL, summation echo from the parietal pleura, visceral pleura, and lung surface.

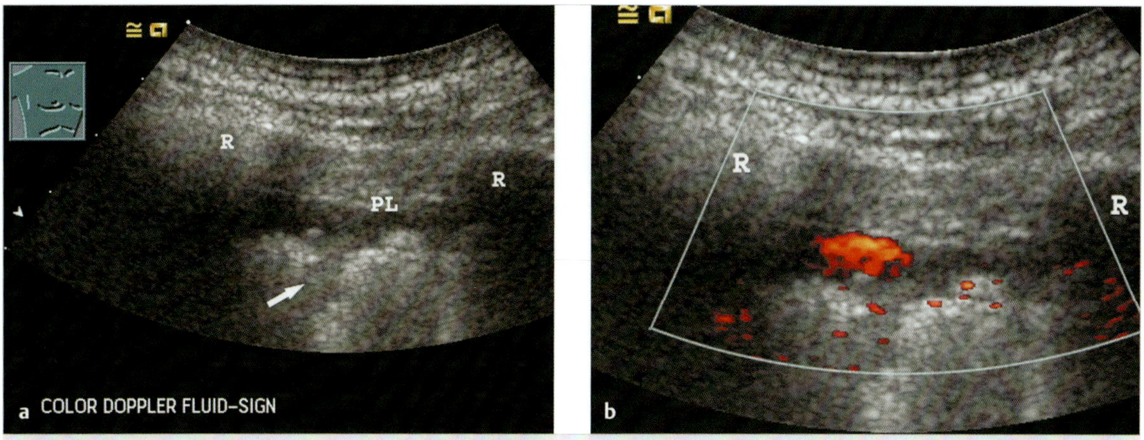

Fig. 24.2
a The parietal pleura (PL) appears as a slightly echogenic line. Subpleural deposits are visible along the irregular lung surface (arrow). A hypoechoic band appears between the lung surface and parietal pleura. Even the moving image (deep respiratory excursions) could not positively distinguish between a small effusion or a solid mass. R, rib.
b Power Doppler image during a deep respiratory excursion demonstrates the typical color Doppler fluid sign. This "motion artifact" is caused by moving fluid (low pulse repetition frequency, sensitive machine setting). Even tiny pleural effusions can be detected, and lesions can be precisely targeted to avoid unproductive biopsies.

- Peripheral lung tumors can be distinguished from pneumonic or atelectatic lung areas by color Doppler and contrast-enhanced ultrasound (less production of motion artifacts).[8,9]

24.2 Indications

Although any sonographically visible mass can be biopsied in principle, an ultrasound-guided percutaneous biopsy is indicated only if it will have therapeutic implications (e.g., chemotherapy or radiation) or is expected to yield important prognostic information. When a peripheral tumor suspicious for malignancy is detected in an operable patient, it should not be biopsied but should undergo primary resection. There is no point in confirming an already established or plausible diagnosis. Biopsy should also be withheld if the same information can be obtained by less invasive means.[10–13]

The following indications are recognized for percutaneous biopsy or drainage procedures in the chest:

1. The investigation of fluid collections in the pleural space (benign/malignant effusion, empyema). Very small effusions can be distinguished from solid pleural thickening at once by the "fluid color sign" on color Doppler imaging (▶ Fig. 24.2); this avoids unproductive needle aspirations.[9] Individual chambers in loculated pleural effusions can be selectively aspirated if empyema is suspected.
2. Paracentesis and pleural drainage for malignant and bloody pleural effusions. Early diagnostic confirmation and treatment of pleural empyema can prevent significant formation of septa. If septa have already formed, they can be lysed by the instillation of urokinase.[3]
3. Chest wall masses (tumors, hematomas, abscesses) including masses and destructive lesions of the ribs and sternum
4. Pleural masses
5. Peripheral lung changes in contact with the chest wall (lung tumor, pneumonia, lung abscess)
6. Mediastinal lesions, especially when located in the anterior or superior mediastinum

24.3 Contraindications

A severe coagulation disorder with INR > 2 and platelet count < 50×10^9/L is an absolute contraindication to a thoracic intervention.

Relative contraindications: bullous pulmonary emphysema and pulmonary hypertension. Severe respiratory compromise and poor blood gas values would contraindicate percutaneous drainage unless the intervention can improve the patient's status.[14]

Percutaneous biopsy or drainage should be withheld if the intended target cannot be visualized or a safe needle path cannot be confirmed.[15]

24.4 Selection of Materials

24.4.1 Ultrasound Technology

High-frequency transducers (7.5 to 12 MHz) have excellent near-field resolution for detailed visualization of the chest wall. A small transducer footprint (4–6 cm) facilitates acoustic coupling and the biopsy procedure itself. Trapezoid imaging with an expandable field of view improves visualization of the intercostal space and of

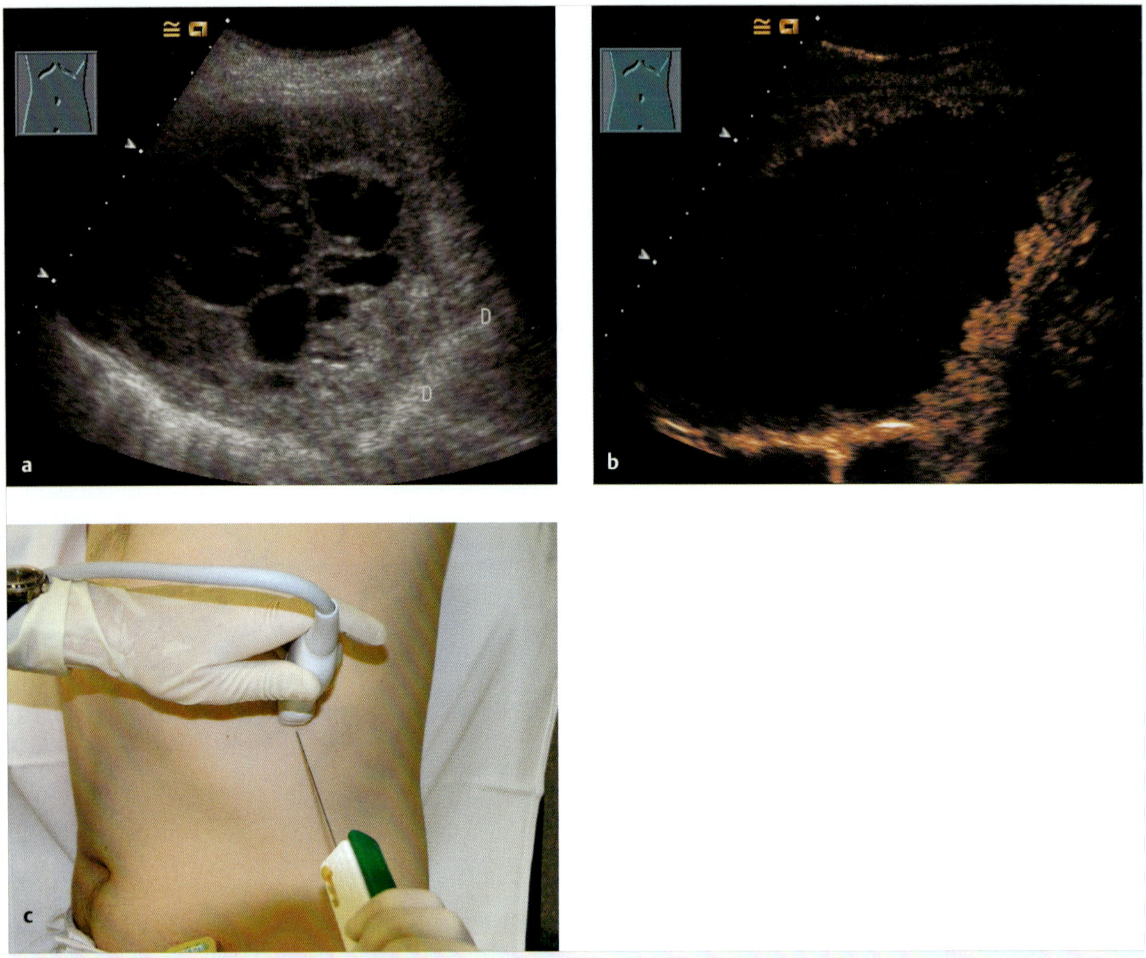

Fig. 24.3
a Where radiographs showed opacity in the left lower lung zone, B-mode ultrasound shows a solid-appearing mass with central cystic components. Color Doppler showed no definite blood flow even at a very sensitive setting. D, diaphragm.
b Contrast-enhanced ultrasound with a low mechanical index (low MI) shows enhancement confined to the peripheral portions of the mass.
c The areas that enhanced (with SonoVue [Bracco]) were selectively biopsied with a BioPince needle (Peter Pflugbeil). Histology revealed adenocarcinoma.

pleural areas bordering the ribs. Sector-type probes with a small footprint are advantageous for scanning pulmonary lesions.

Active tumor sites can be detected more sensitively by color Doppler and contrast-enhanced ultrasound, enabling the sites to be biopsied with greater precision and a higher success rate (▶ Fig. 24.3).[16] These techniques can also be used to assess the efficacy of treatment, such as the palliative radiofrequency thermal ablation (RFTA) of chest wall tumors (e.g., metastatic hepatocellular carcinoma [HCC]).

Color Doppler ultrasound can identify the mammary arteries and other blood vessels that must be spared in percutaneous needle procedures.[5]

24.4.2 Biopsy Devices

Economically priced needles without a stylet are satisfactory for aspiration cytology. No. 1 needles with an outer diameter of 0.9 mm (20-gauge) like those used for drawing blood have good echogenicity and produce a high-amplitude double echo at the needle tip. These needles can also be used for the aspiration of fluid collections (Sterican, Braun Melsungen).

Cutting biopsy needles can harvest tissue cores for histologic examination.

Coordinated manipulations of the ultrasound probe and needle tip are most easily accomplished with a "one person–one hand" technique. It is easier to maneuver the instruments in three dimensions, and needle tip adjustments can be made more quickly.[7]

Automated one-hand needle systems, or biopsy guns, are particularly suitable for thoracic lesions. They facilitate targeting, shorten the procedure time, and the fast needle stroke tends to penetrate rather than deflect the lung tissue. This leads to better biopsy results and lower complication rates, including a lower incidence of pneumothorax.

Several biopsy needles, all substantially equivalent, are available on the market, but it is best for an operator to become familiar with one needle type.

Currently we prefer the BioPince principle (BioPince Full Core Biopsy Instrument, Peter Pflugbeil) in which a special retention clip traps the tissue core inside the needle. Larger tissue cores can be harvested with this needle and retrieved safely.

A needle diameter of 1.2 mm provides a significantly better yield for histologic evaluation than a fine needle diameter (< 1 mm), with only a minimal increase in complication rate.

The Trucut principle captures the tissue core in a specimen notch so that it cannot be lost (Trucut Needle, Bard). Disadvantages are that the tissue cores are short and thin relative to the needle diameter, and the system is relatively difficult to handle.

The Autovac single-use biopsy system (Surecut principle) by Bard (formerly Angiomed) is more favorably priced than the BioPince needle. The tissue core is excised by a rapid forward thrust of the needle. When the needle is withdrawn, the tissue core is retained in the needle by suction. In contrast to the BioPince needle, the specimen may be lost if the suction mechanism fails (with risk of tumor seeding in the needle track!) (▶ Fig. 24.4).

It is rarely necessary to use needle diameters larger than 1.2 mm. Simple aspiration needles are used for highly viscous fluids. A large-volume Trucut needle can be used for histologic differentiation, especially of benign chest wall lesions and occasionally of interstitial lung changes.

The diameter of a **drainage catheter** depends on the viscosity of the fluid collection. In principle, the drain can be placed by the trocar or Seldinger technique. The trocar technique is most commonly used in the chest (▶ Fig. 24.5).

Available Devices

- Sterican single-use injection needle, No. 1 (G 20/ 0.9 × 40/80 mm). B. Braun Melsungen AG, D-34209 Melsungen, Germany.
- Sonocan single-use set for ultrasound-guided full-core biopsy (G 20/0.9 × 100/150 mm), B. Braun Melsungen. Supplier: Nicolai GmbH & Co. Ostpassage 7, D-30853 Langenhagen, Germany.
- BioPince single-use full-core biopsy gun (G 18/ 1.2 × 100/150 mm), InterV-MDTech, Gainesville, Florida, USA. Supplier: Pflugbeil-Amedic.

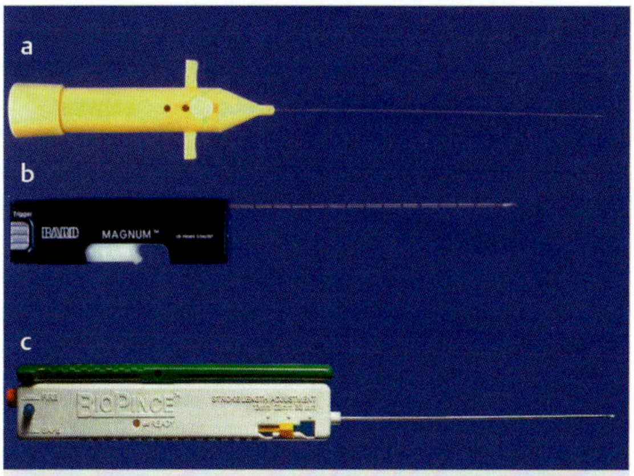

Fig. 24.4 This photograph illustrates three types of biopsy guns. The desired biopsy depth (measured sonographically) can be set on each device.
a Autovac single-use biopsy system (Bard, formerly Angiomed). The tissue core is excised by a rapid forward movement of the needle and is retained by suction.
b Reusable biopsy gun with Trucut needle inserted (Bard). The Trucut needle captures the tissue sample in a specimen notch so that it cannot be lost when the needle is withdrawn. This device yields only a half-diameter core, however, and is somewhat cumbersome to use.
c BioPince biopsy gun (Pflugbeil-Amedic). A retention clip traps the full core inside the needle so that it cannot be lost.
Source: Reprinted from Chest Sonography, 3rd ed. (ed. Gebhard Mathis), 2011 with kind permission of Springer Science and Business Media.

- Max-Core disposable core biopsy instrument (G 20–16/ 0.9–1.2 × 100/160 mm). Bard GmbH, Wachhausstrasse 6, D-76227 Karlsruhe, Germany.
- Magnum reusable core biopsy instrument, Bard.
- Magnum disposable needles (G 20–16/0.9–1.2 × 100/ 160 mm), Bard.
- Navarre Universal Drainage Catheter with nitinol (6–12 F × 30 cm), Bard. Universal adapter with Luer lock, Bard.
- Argyle trocar catheter (12F–17F/4–6 mm). Sherwood Medical, Tullamore, Ireland. EC rep: Gosport, PO 13 OAS, UK.
- Argyle Sentinel Seal Chest Drainage Unit. Tyco Healthcare, Tullamore, Ireland.

24.5 Preparations

The basic equipment for percutaneous biopsy or drainage procedures includes syringes, cannulas, biopsy needles, gloves, local anesthesia, and sterile draping material. As in any intervention, the patient must be duly informed about the steps in the procedure and its risks.

Coagulation status should be assessed (except for chest wall biopsies). Antiplatelet drugs are discontinued 4 to 5 days before an elective procedure. For urgent procedures (e.g., abscess, symptomatic pleural effusion), the risk should be determined on a case-by-case basis.

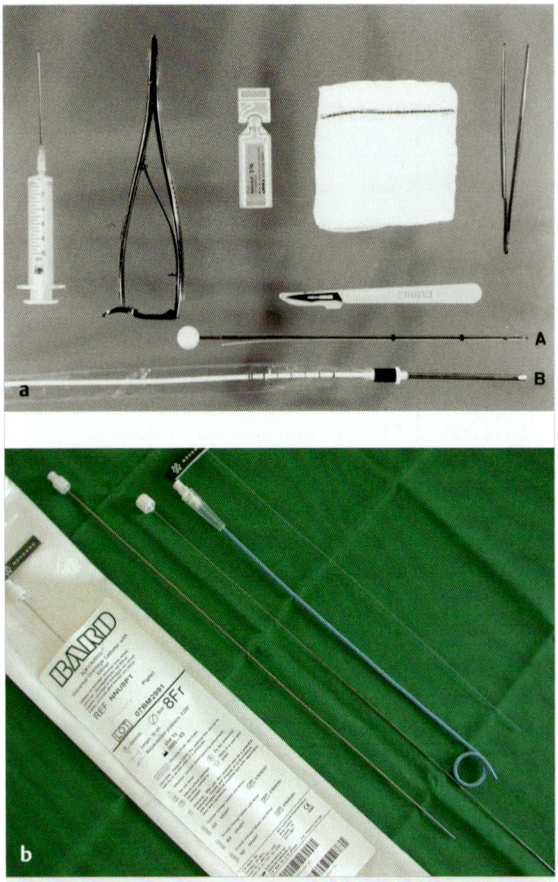

Fig. 24.5
a Pleural drainage set (trocar technique). **A:** classic trocar catheter (Argyle); small- and large-bore catheters are available. **B:** small-bore Pneumocat catheter (12F, Intra).
b Navarre universal drainage catheter (Bard-Angiomed, 8–12F). This is our favorite catheter at present. It has many advantages: it can be introduced directly through a small stab incision; it is easily inserted without prior dilatation; it is kink-resistant; it rarely clogs; and it has pigtail retention.
Source: Reprinted from Chest Sonography, 3rd ed. (ed. Gebhard Mathis), 2011 with kind permission of Springer Science and Business Media.

The initial diagnostic work-up consists of thoracic ultrasonography and may include a chest radiograph or CT examination. Next, four determinations are made: the intended target, the puncture site, the direction of needle insertion, and the needle path.

Blood vessels and nerves (e.g., plexuses) should be visualized and identified to prevent neurovascular injury (▶ Fig. 24.1).

Nonsterile ultrasound gel is removed. Percutaneous biopsy requires sterile gloves and a local antiseptic spray (not tolerated by all ultrasound probes; check with the manufacturer) or sterile catheter gel (which costs less than sterile ultrasound gel).

Local anesthesia is necessary only for multiple punctures or large-bore needles, although many patients desire it.

The patient is positioned—sitting, supine, lateral, or prone—to facilitate lesion imaging and interventional access. The patient should perform a short breath-hold when the needle is introduced.

24.6 Technique

24.6.1 Chest Wall Lesions

Most chest wall tumors can be clearly visualized with ultrasound. Whenever possible, the biopsy needle should be directed parallel to the lung surface (▶ Fig. 24.6). This should result in a very echogenic needle with minimal risk of pneumothorax. Even large-caliber needles (1.2–2 mm), which are particularly useful in the differentiation of benign lesions, can be used with this technique.[3,17–19]

Fluid collections are usually treated by a single percutaneous aspiration or, if necessary, by repeated aspirations. If these attempts are unsuccessful, a drain should be placed.

Rib metastases usually produce defects in the cortical bone. These lesions can be clearly defined sonographically, along with the surrounding soft tissue reaction, and biopsied under sonographic guidance.[20]

Fine needle aspiration biopsy (FNAB) is adequate for differentiating inflammation from malignancy, providing a success rate of 88 to 100%. If a plasmacytoma is suspected, FNAB is always preferable to core needle biopsy because the lesion is easier to diagnose in a smear (▶ Fig. 24.7). Core biopsy may sometimes be necessary for determining the histologic type of a malignant tumor.

24.6.2 Pleural Space

Thoracentesis

With large-volume effusions, ultrasound can be used to define the extent of the effusion and mark the puncture site in the optimum intercostal space. The procedure is then performed on the ward (▶ Fig. 24.8a). With complicated effusions (small, loculated, encapsulated, difficult site), it is safer to perform thoracentesis under continuous ultrasound guidance (▶ Fig. 24.8b). This will significantly reduce the incidence of pneumothorax (< 1%). The success rate is 97%. Unproductive thoracentesis can be avoided by noting the "fluid color sign" on color Doppler imaging (▶ Fig. 24.2). Plastic indwelling cannulas are preferred for thoracentesis due to the risk of lung injury from metal cannulas.[21]

▶ **Technique in brief.** Following local anesthesia, the plastic cannula with stylet (e.g., Abbocath [Hospira]) is advanced to the pleura along the superior rib border in the selected intercostal space. A slight increase in resistance is felt when the needle enters the pleura. The stylet is then removed. Special pleural drainage sets allow for manual aspiration within a closed drainage system.

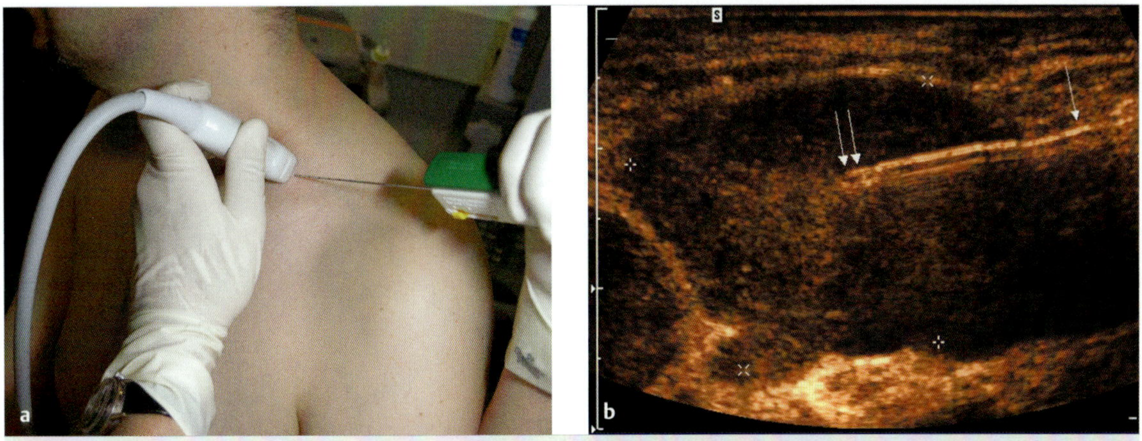

Fig. 24.6 For biopsy of a hypoechoic lymph node (+ – +) at the thoracic inlet, the needle is introduced at a small angle, almost parallel to the skin surface (a), to improve needle visualization and protect deeper structures. The needle is clearly visible as an echogenic double line (b). Needle tip (↓ ↓); needle shaft (↓) (BioPince needle 1.2 mm diameter). This technique can also be used with larger-caliber needles (1.2–2 mm), which may be necessary for subtyping lymphomas or differentiating benign chest wall lesions.
Source: Reprinted from Chest Sonography, 3rd ed. (ed. Gebhard Mathis), 2011 with kind permission of Springer Science and Business Media.

Uncomplicated pleural effusions in the setting of heart failure and even small pneumothoraces after needle biopsy can be treated by thoracentesis. Malignant pleural effusions and collections of pus or blood should be treated by catheter drainage due to the risk of septation (▶ Fig. 24.9).

The success rate of cytology for malignant effusions is only 50 to 75%. Pathogen detection in tuberculous effusions is successful in only 20 to 40% of cases. Because classic blind pleural biopsy using the Abrams or Ramell technique has a success rate of only 50% in malignant effusions, video-assisted thoracoscopy is increasingly used. Ultrasound-guided pleural biopsy is a possible alternative, achieving an accuracy rate of 83% in the small case numbers reported to date. If video-assisted thoracoscopy is unavailable or cannot be done in patients requiring intensive care, for example, an ultrasound-guided forceps biopsy of the pleura can be performed as an alternative (▶ Fig. 24.10).[22] The FNAB of pleural thickenings is of no value and should be limited to the investigation of focal changes.[7]

Percutaneous Pleural Drainage

Malignant, bloody, and inflammatory pleural effusions can be treated by ultrasound-guided percutaneous pleural drainage in suitably selected cases. Small-bore catheters (7–12F, such as Pleurocath [Prodimed]) are adequate for malignant effusions. The drain is usually placed by the trocar technique, positioning the catheter at the lowest point in the pleural space. Correct catheter placement can be documented sonographically by the instillation of NaCl solution (10 mL). Sensitivity can be increased by adding one drop of ultrasound contrast agent (SonoVue, Bracco) to the solution, provided suitable equipment is available. Catheter malposition or displacement can be detected with high sensitivity. Septations with associated poor drainage can be recognized by failure of the contrast agent to spread throughout the pleural space.[23,24]

Pleurodesis for Malignant Pleural Effusions

Multiple percutaneous aspirations of malignant pleural effusions should be avoided whenever possible due to the very rapid septation that occurs. Pleurodesis is performed by first draining all fluid from the pleural space and then instilling a sclerosing agent (cytostatic agent, acidic tetracycline, fibrin glue). Residual effusions, with or without septations, will significantly lower the success rate and should be aspirated prior to sclerotherapy.

Pleural Empyema

The prompt diagnostic confirmation of pleural empyema is important because percutaneous therapy is likely to be successful (success rate 72 to 88%) only in the acute phase during weeks 1 to 4. When septa have already formed, the results of drainage therapy can be significantly improved by the instillation of urokinase (50,000 to 100,000 IU per treatment).

24.6.3 Subpleural Lung Lesions

Peripheral lung lesions can be visualized and biopsied under ultrasound guidance when they are in contact with the pleura or when poststenotic atelectasis or pneumonia provides an acoustic window. The least accessible regions are the mediastinum, diaphragm, and areas behind the ribs and scapula.

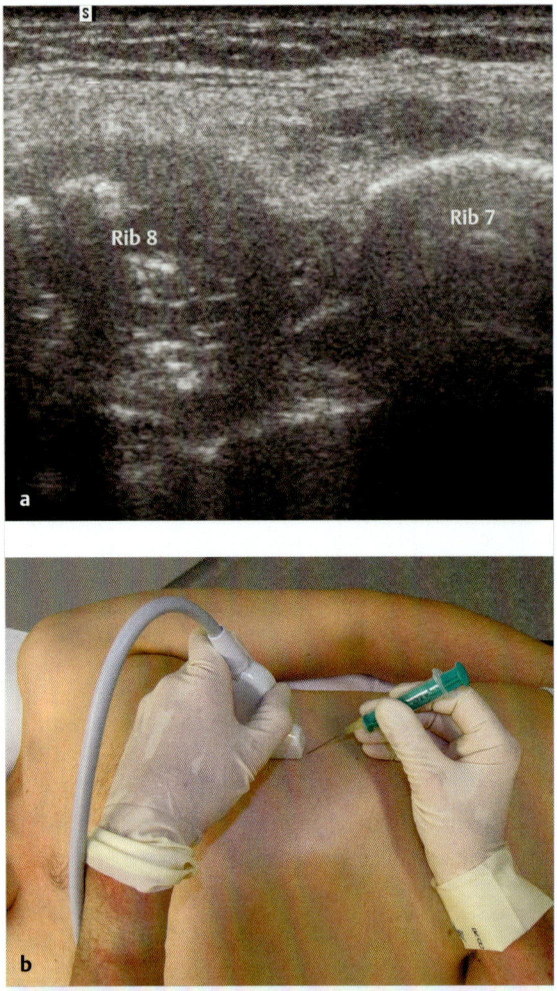

Fig. 24.7
a The normal seventh rib produces a curved, high-amplitude echo with a posterior acoustic shadow that obscures pleuropulmonary structures deep to the rib. The eighth rib shows destructive changes with disruption of the cortical surface echo, and the pleura beneath the rib is partially visible. The area around the altered rib shows a hypoechoic rim consistent with a perifocal soft tissue reaction. Usually a rib with destructive changes of this kind is easily biopsied.
b The biopsy procedure is shown. Fine needle aspiration biopsy is usually adequate for differentiating inflammation from malignancy and is preferred over cutting needle biopsy for diagnosing plasmacytoma.

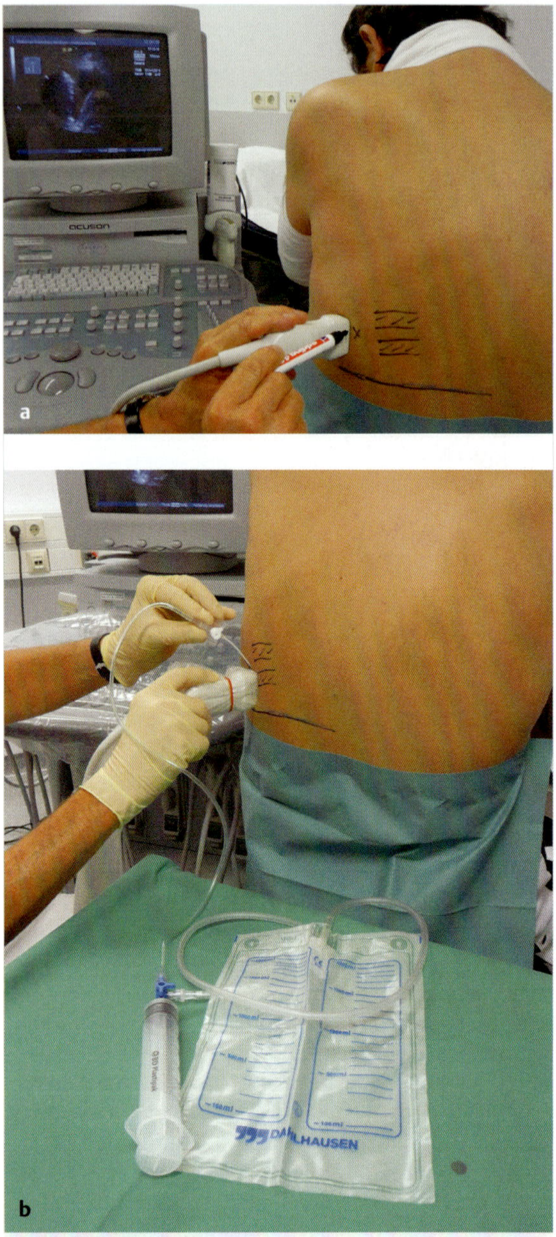

Fig. 24.8
a With a larger pleural effusion, the puncture site is marked in the optimum intercostal space, preferably with the patient in a sitting position. Thoracentesis can then be performed on the ward.
b Complicated pleural effusions should be drained under sonographic guidance. The plastic cannula is introduced at the superior border of the rib. Special pleural drainage sets allow the fluid to be aspirated manually within a closed system.

Approximately two-thirds of lung cancers are no longer curable at the time of diagnosis. Histology should be established before palliative treatment (chemotherapy, radiation) is begun. Peripheral tumors > 3 cm should be investigated by fine needle core biopsy for histologic evaluation (▶ Fig. 24.11b). This procedure has a 70–90% success rate.[25] Peripheral lung lesions < 3 cm should be investigated by fine needle aspiration cytology[25] (▶ Fig. 24.11a).

Fine needle biopsy is often inadequate for the differentiation of benign tumors (success rate only about 70%), and it is better to proceed with a thoracoscopic wedge resection.[14]

Larger tumors can be biopsied under continuous sonographic guidance using classic technique as in a thyroid biopsy (see Chapter 27). The needle is positioned in the

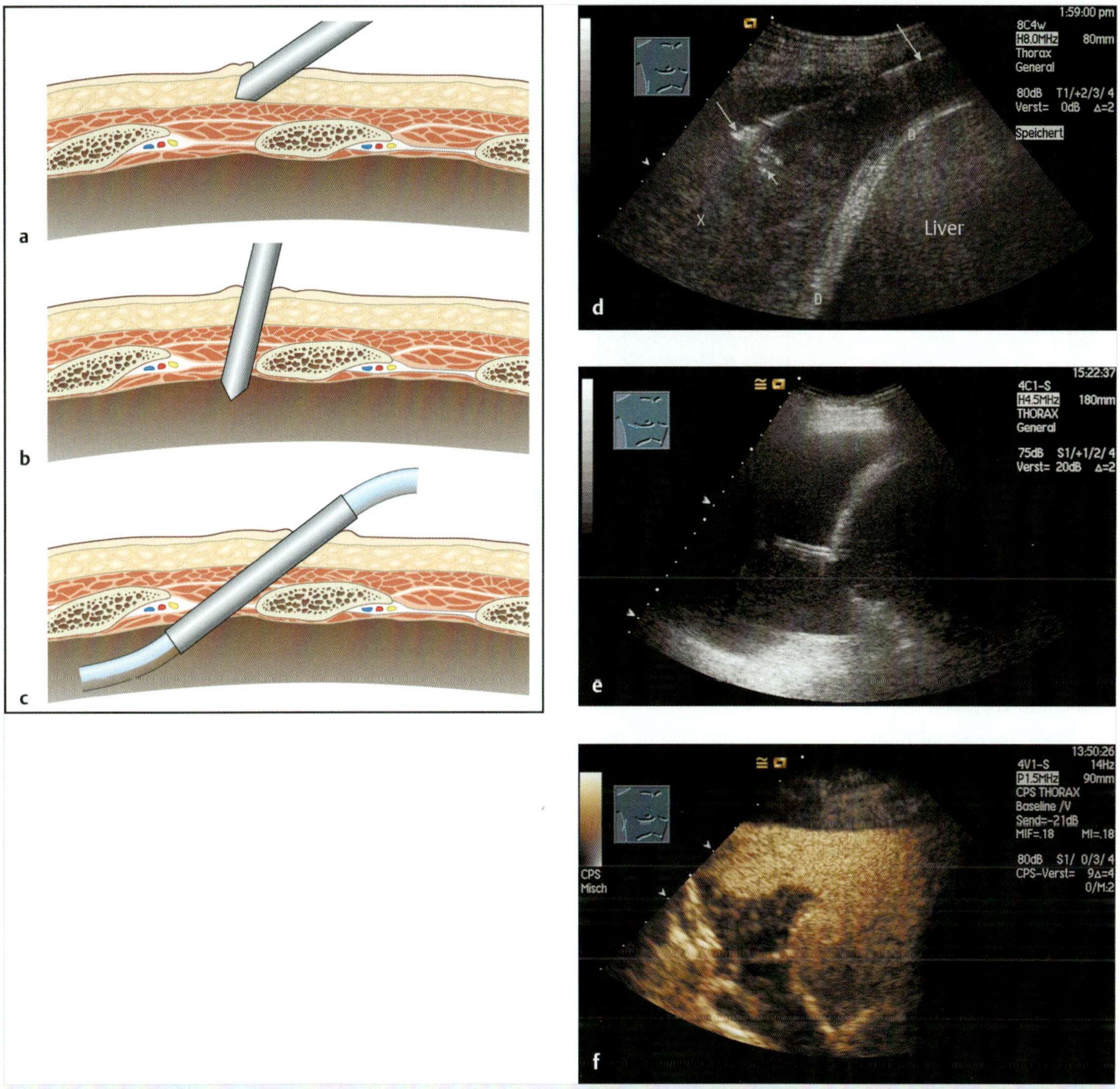

Fig. 24.9 Pleural drainage.
a–c Diagrammatic representation of the thoracentesis technique. Following a stab incision (under local anesthesia), the drainage catheter (Navarre) is advanced obliquely upward into the pleural space along the superior border of the rib, preferably under sonographic guidance, appearing as a smooth, high-amplitude linear echo.
d When saline solution is instilled, an echogenic cloud is visible at the catheter tip (→ ←).
e After removal of the stylet, fluid drainage appears as an echogenic double line. This feature may be difficult to see in complicated effusions.
f After instillation of saline solution with a small amount of contrast agent added (one drop of SonoVue), the agent spreads throughout the pleural effusion. This confirms correct drain placement and is predictive of a good result.

same plane as the transducer. The needle tip is advanced to the parietal pleura, the peripheral lung lesion is identified, and when the biopsy gun is favorably aligned with the target, it is activated for rapid sample acquisition. The biopsy depth is measured beforehand, and the stroke length is adjustable on most automated biopsy guns. This protects healthy lung tissue and minimizes the risk of pneumothorax.

Even small peripheral lung lesions can be biopsied by experienced operators. The technique must be modified somewhat, however, as the classic biopsy technique usually cannot be employed. As with small thyroid lesions, an "atypical" biopsy is performed (Chapter 27). The needle is introduced almost perpendicular to the skin a slight distance from the center of the probe, which is fanned in a "radarlike" pattern to detect the needle tip. This biopsy technique is more difficult to learn.

Another option for small lesions is to mark the puncture site with the tip of a ballpoint pen, for example (making an annular impression in the skin), and then

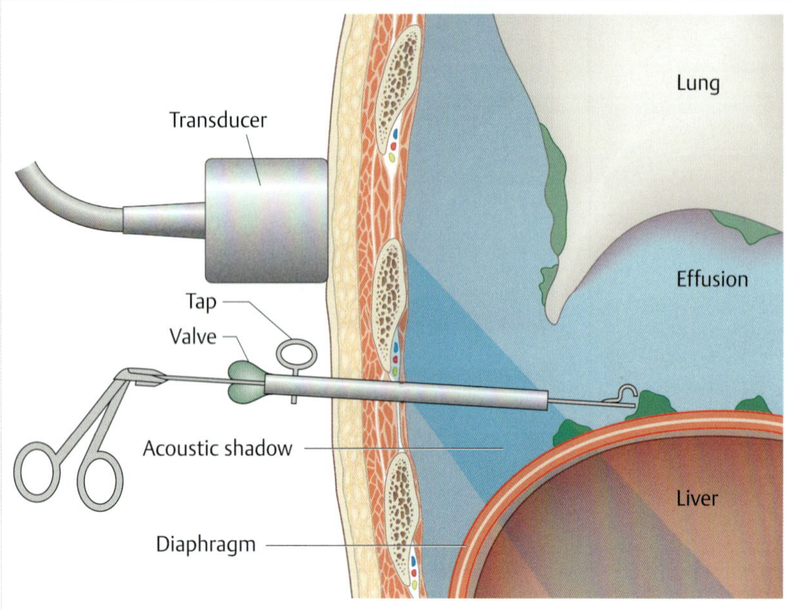

Fig. 24.10 Diagrammatic representation of a pleural forceps biopsy by the Seitz technique, using a Seitz pleural biopsy forceps (Karl Storz).

performing the biopsy "by memory." In experienced hands the results are not inferior to those of continuous ultrasound guidance.

A small, perforated biopsy transducer can also be used if available (needle-guide technique).[10]

24.6.4 Pulmonary Abscesses

Lung abscesses are rarely an indication for a percutaneous intervention. Small abscesses can be defined much more clearly than on chest radiographs. Small abscesses can be detected with even greater sensitivity by contrast-enhanced ultrasound. If an abscess does not respond to primary antibiotic therapy (e.g., in immunosuppressed patients), ultrasound-guided aspiration of the abscess can isolate the causative organism in two-thirds of cases (▶ Fig. 24.12). Rarely, ultrasound-guided drainage is necessary after other therapies have failed. The risk of fistula formation can be reduced by finding the shortest access route and approaching the lesion through solid, homogeneous, infiltrated or atelectatic tissue whenever possible.[8]

24.6.5 Mediastinum

Only a few mediastinal masses (retrosternal goiter, aneurysm, cyst, thrombosis) permit an accurate etiologic classification based on typical sonographic findings.

Atraumatic tissue sampling without creating a significant tissue defect is particularly important in the workup of surgically removable masses, and this goal can be achieved more easily by percutaneous biopsy than by excisional biopsy.

The majority of masses are located in the anterior mediastinum and can usually be biopsied percutaneously

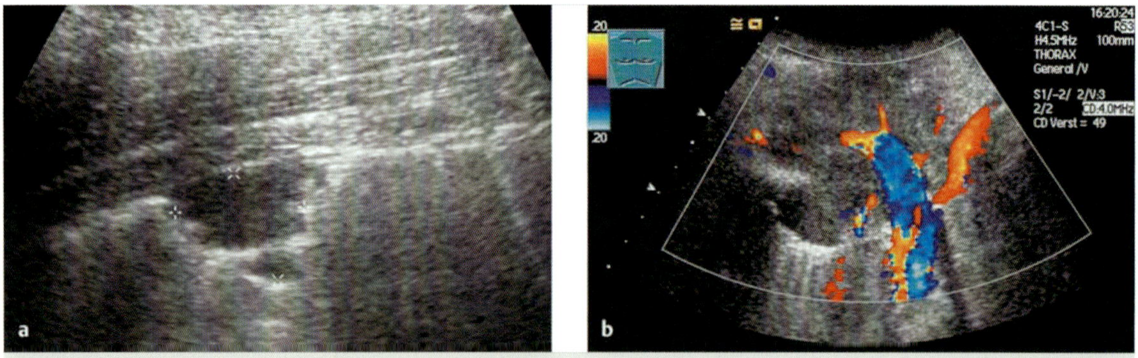

Fig. 24.11
a Multiple small (15 mm), peripheral lung nodules suspicious for metastases. Fine needle aspiration biopsy showed that the lesions were metastatic to follicular thyroid carcinoma.
b Vascular encasement by a Pancoast tumor. The diagnosis was confirmed by cutting needle biopsy (1.2-mm BioPince needle). Histology: squamous cell carcinoma.

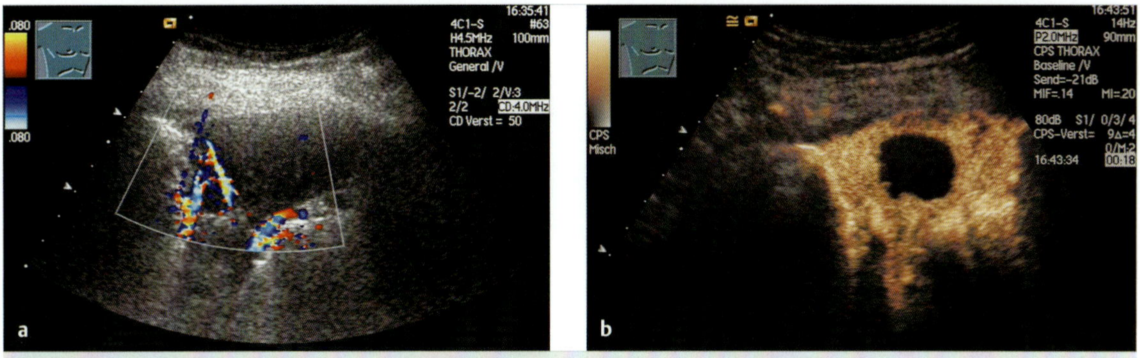

Fig. 24.12

a Refractory pneumonia. B-mode ultrasound shows no evidence of an abscess. Color Doppler scan shows a partial "absence" of vascularity.

b Contrast-enhanced ultrasound shows a punched-out defect from which pus could be aspirated for culturing.

from a suprasternal or parasternal approach (right or left lateral decubitus) under sonographic guidance[7,26] (▶ Fig. 24.13).

Because most superficial mediastinal masses are thymomas or lymphomas, the differentiation of these lesions requires larger tissue samples. The BioPince needle that we use (1.2 mm diameter) will usually retrieve samples adequate for tissue differentiation. Larger needle diameters are needed only in exceptional cases.

Lesions of the posterior and inferior mediastinum are usually not accessible to ultrasound-guided percutaneous biopsy. In some cases these lesions can be biopsied by the endosonographic transesophageal technique.[19,27–30]

24.7 Steps in the Procedure

24.7.1 Preparations

The following steps should be carried out, and the following questions answered, in preparing for the interventional procedure:

- Review previous findings (chest radiograph, CT, bronchoscopy).
- Determine thoracic ultrasound status.
- Is there an indication for percutaneous biopsy?
- Is an ultrasound-guided biopsy technically feasible?
- Are there contraindications to percutaneous biopsy?
- Obtain written informed consent from the patient.
- Fine needle aspiration cytology or core biopsy?
- Select the appropriate equipment (needle, drain).

24.7.2 Technique

The steps in the procedure are as follows:

1. Position the patient (sitting, supine, lateral, or prone).
2. Determine the puncture site and access route to the lesion.
3. Remove nonsterile ultrasound gel.
4. Administer local anesthesia if required.
5. Introduce the needle during a breath-hold.
6. For aspiration cytology: prepare and evaluate a smear.
7. With core biopsy: evaluate the tissue core.
8. Repeat if necessary.

24.7.3 Postprocedure Care

The patient should be positioned with the biopsied side down. Postprocedure ultrasonography should be performed if complaints arise, or routinely at 3 to 4 hours. The images are read and the results documented in a brief written report that is discussed with the patient. Barring complications, the patient may be given a follow-up appointment if necessary and discharged home.

24.8 Problems and Complications

Ultrasound-guided percutaneous biopsies have a very low complication rate when done by a technically proficient operator in suitably selected patients.[31]

24.8.1 Postbiopsy Pneumothorax

If a lesion is no longer visible after percutaneous biopsy, a pneumothorax should be suspected. When pneumothorax is present, the normally moving lung surface ("pleural" sliding sign with respirations) is no longer seen. Reverberations (artifacts) posterior to the lung surface visible by B-mode ultrasound can be displayed as corresponding color artifacts by color Doppler imaging. The color Doppler energy mode (CDE, power mode) can demonstrate the respiration-dependent sliding sign with excellent clarity and can document it even in an upright image. This color artifact ("motion artifact") is no longer demonstrated when pneumothorax is present (▶ Fig. 24.14).

Ultrasonography has high sensitivity (90–95%) in the detection of pneumothorax. It cannot quantify the free

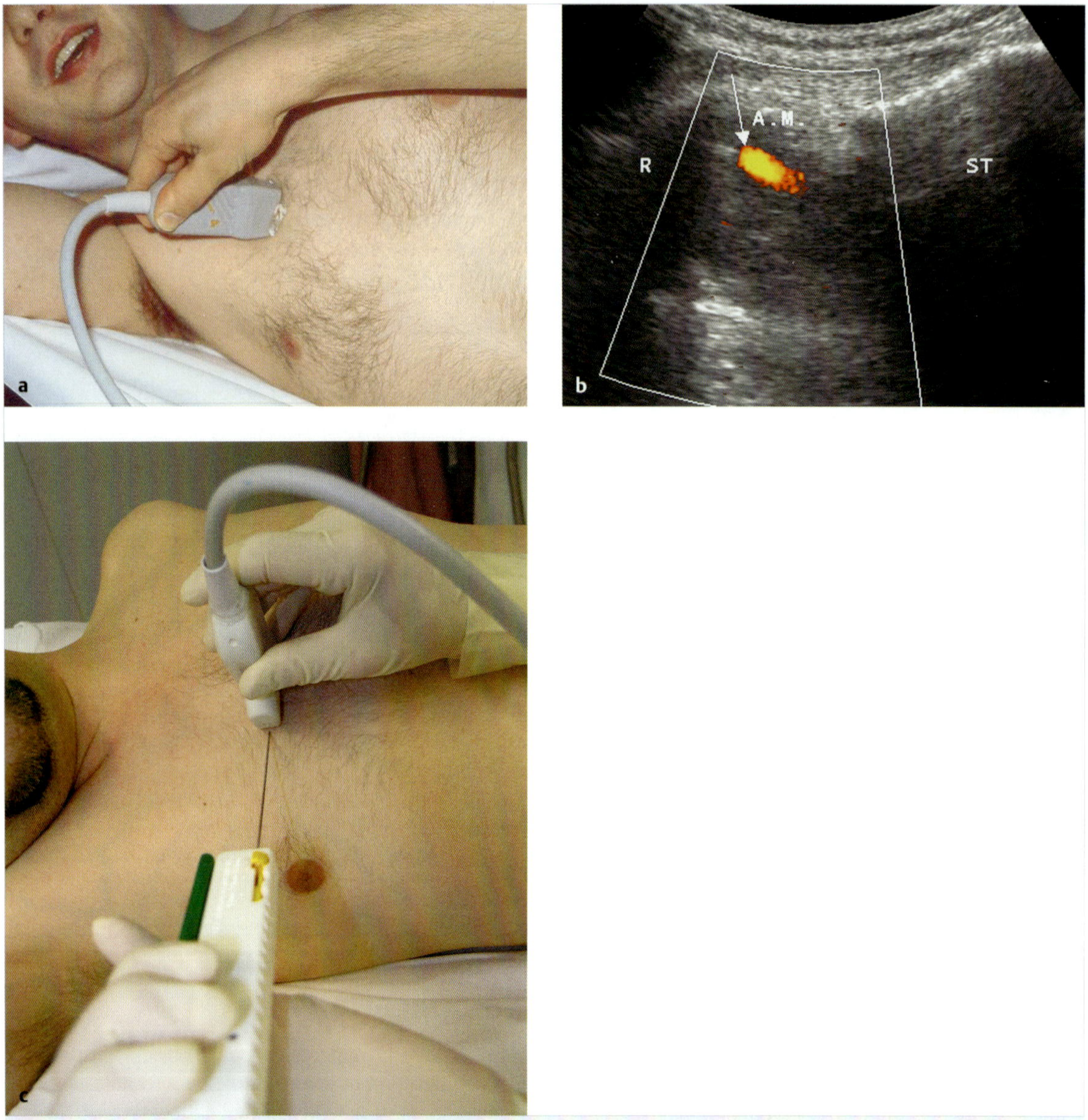

Fig. 24.13
a Parasternal ultrasound scan in right lateral decubitus displays portions of the anterior and middle mediastinum. The ultrasound probe is placed in the intercostal spaces lateral to the sternum to perform transverse and sagittal scans in angled planes.
b The parasternal scan in right lateral decubitus shows a hypoechoic mass in the anterior mediastinum. The parasternal mammary vessels are imaged with color Doppler (here using CDE or power mode) to avoid injury during core needle biopsy.
c The biopsy procedure using classic technique (BioPince needle in the transducer plane).

air volume, however, and a chest radiograph should be obtained if the sliding sign is absent.[2]

Other complications such as hemorrhage or hemoptysis are rarely observed (0–2%). To date there have been no reports of air embolism or deaths.

Seeding of the needle tract with tumor cells (inoculation metastasis) is very rare (less than 0.003%) and usually is not clinically significant. Tumor seeding is more commonly observed in patients with malignant pleural mesothelioma.[32]

24.9 Postprocedure Care and Follow-Up

A pneumothorax will generally reach its maximum size in 3 hours, so ultrasound scans should be obtained at least 3 hours after the interventional procedure, even if the patient is free of complaints. A routine chest radiograph is unnecessary after an ultrasound-guided percutaneous biopsy. If a pneumothorax is diagnosed

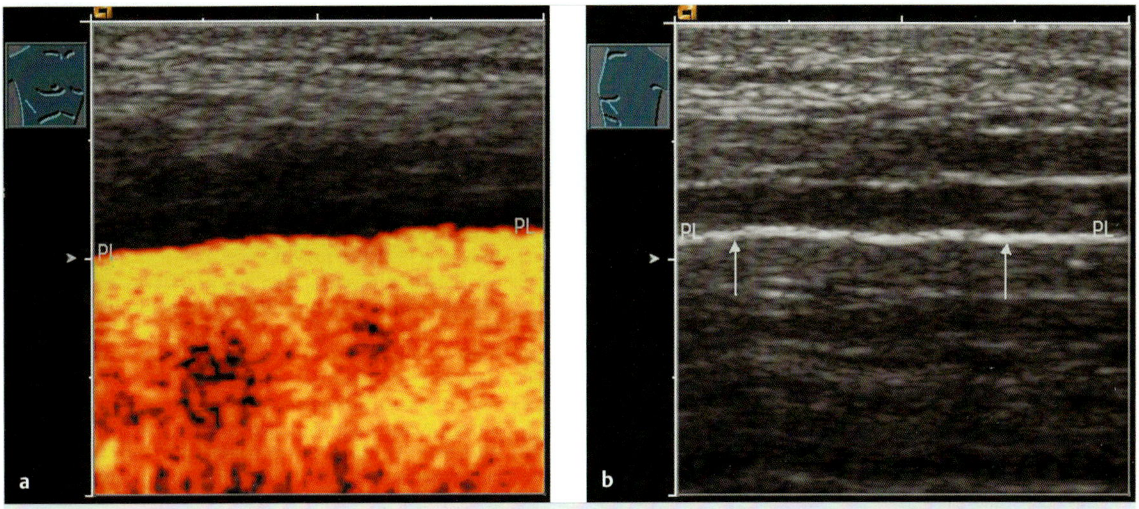

Fig. 24.14
a Lung mobility during respirations can be sensitively tracked in a dynamic examination (deep respiratory excursions), even with B-mode ultrasound. This sliding sign is vividly depicted by color Doppler (preferably using CDE or power mode) and can be clearly documented even in a standing image.
b When pneumothorax is present, the air in the pleural space displaces the lung surface so that the pleural sliding sign is no longer present. The color artifacts ("motion artifacts") are no longer visible. Quantification of the air volume in the pleural space to evaluate the extent of the pneumothorax cannot be done sonographically and requires a chest radiograph.

(absence of the lung sliding sign), a chest radiograph is taken to quantify the free air volume. If the patient is symptomatic or a large air volume is found, it should be treated by primary thoracentesis. Analogous to the percutaneous aspiration of effusions (Chapter 8), a plastic cannula with stylet (e.g., Abbocath [Hospira]; Angiocath [Becton Dickinson]) is introduced along the superior border of the rib and advanced to the pleura. A slight increase in resistance is felt as the needle penetrates the pleura. In obese patients, the skin-to-pleura distance can be determined sonographically. Next the stylet is removed and the plastic cannula is preferably connected to a special pleural drainage set to allow for manual aspiration of the air within a closed system. If all "free" pleural air can be removed, the lung sliding sign will reappear. The success rate during the first 10 hours is 90%. If a recurrence of lung collapse is seen, a percutaneous drain should be placed.

If postprocedure ultrasound does not show a pneumothorax or hemorrhage, patients are discharged with instructions to return at once if they experience shortness of breath, pain, fever, pallor, or dizziness. Finally, the patients are told when and how they will be informed of the biopsy result.

References

[1] Chandrasekhar AJ, Reynes CJ, Churchill RJ. Ultrasonically guided percutaneous biopsy of peripheral pulmonary masses. Chest 1976; 70: 627–630

[2] Mathis G, ed. Bildatlas der Lungen- und Pleurasonographie. 3rd ed. Berlin Heidelberg New York: Springer-Verlag; 2010

[3] Sistrom CL, Wallace KK, Gay SB. Thoracic sonography for diagnosis and intervention. Curr Probl Diagn Radiol 1997; 26: 1–49

[4] Wang HC, Doelken P. Ultrasound guided drainage procedures and biopsies. In: Bolliger CT, Herth FJF, Mayo PH, Miyazawa T, Beamis JF, eds. Clinical Chest Ultrasound. From the ICU to the Bronchoscopy Suite. Basel: JF Karger-Verlag: 2009. Progress in Respiratory Research; Vol 37

[5] Blank W, Schuler A, Wild K, Braun B. Transthoracic sonography of the mediastinum. Eur J Ultrasound 1996; 3: 179–190

[6] Heilo A. US-guided transthoracic biopsy. Eur J Ultrasound 1996; 3: 141–151

[7] Ikezoe J, Morimoto S, Arisawa J, Takashima S, Kozuka T, Nakahara K. Percutaneous biopsy of thoracic lesions: value of sonography for needle guidance. AJR Am J Roentgenol 1990; 154: 1181–1185

[8] vanSonnenberg E, D'Agostino HB, Casola G, Wittich GR, Varney RR, Harker C. Lung abscess: CT-guided drainage. Radiology 1991; 178: 347–351

[9] Wu RG, Yang PC, Kuo SH, Luh KT. "Fluid color" sign: a useful indicator for discrimination between pleural thickening and pleural effusion. J Ultrasound Med 1995; 14: 767–769

[10] Blank W. Sonographisch gesteuerte Punktionen und Drainagen. In: Braun B, Günther R, Schwerk WB, eds. Ultraschalldiagnostik. Lehrbuch und Atlas. Landsberg/Lech: Ecomed; 1994;III-11.1:1–79

[11] Koegelenberg CF, Bolliger CT, Plekker D et al. Diagnostic yield and safety of ultrasound-assisted biopsies in superior vena cava syndrome. Eur Respir J 2009; 33: 1389–1395

[12] Mathis G, Bitschnau R, Gehmacher O, Dirschmid K. Ultrasound-guided transthoracic puncture [Article in German]. Ultraschall Med 1999; 20: 226–235

[13] Pedersen OM, Aasen TB, Gulsvik A. Fine needle aspiration biopsy of mediastinal and peripheral pulmonary masses guided by real-time sonography. Chest 1986; 89: 504–508

[14] Beckh S, Bölcskei PL. Biopsy of thoracic space-occupying lesions—from computerized tomography to ultrasound-controlled puncture [Article in German]. Ultraschall Med 1997; 18: 220–225

[15] Yang PC, Chang DB, Yu CJ et al. Ultrasound-guided core biopsy of thoracic tumors. Am Rev Respir Dis 1992; 146: 763–767

[16] Zimmermann C, Werle A, Schuler A, Reuss J, Gemacher O, Blank W. Echosignalverstärker in der sonographischen Diagnostik des Thorax. Ultraschall Med 2003; 24: 31

[17] Bradley MJ, Metreweli C. Ultrasound in the diagnosis of the juxta-pleural lesion. Br J Radiol 1991; 64: 330–333

[18] Diacon AH, Theron J, Schubert PT et al. Ultrasound-assisted transthoracic biopsy: fine-needle aspiration or cutting-needle biopsy? Eur Respir J 2007; 29: 357–362

[19] Gleeson F, Lomas DJ, Flower CDR, Stewart S. Powered cutting needle biopsy of the pleura and chest wall. Clin Radiol 1990; 41: 199–200

[20] Civardi G, Livraghi T, Colombo P, Fornari F, Cavanna L, Buscarini L. Lytic bone lesions suspected for metastasis: ultrasonically guided fine-needle aspiration biopsy. J Clin Ultrasound 1994; 22: 307–311

[21] Reuss J. Sonographic imaging of the pleura: nearly 30 years experience. Eur J Ultrasound 1996; 3: 125–139

[22] Seitz K, Pfeffer A, Littmann M, Seitz G. Ultrasound guided forceps biopsy of the pleura [Article in German]. Ultraschall Med 1999; 20: 60–65

[23] Heinzmann A, Müller T, Leitlein J, Braun B, Kubicka S, Blank W. Endocavitary contrast enhanced ultrasound (CEUS)—work in progress. Ultraschall Med 2012; 33: 76–84

[24] Weiss H, Weiss A. Therapeutic interventional sonography [Article in German]. Ultraschall Med 1994; 15: 152–158

[25] Hsu WH, Chiang CD, Hsu JY, Kwan PC, Chen CL, Chen CY. Ultrasound-guided fine-needle aspiration biopsy of lung cancers. J Clin Ultrasound 1996; 24: 225–233

[26] Heilo A. Tumors in the mediastinum: US-guided histologic core-needle biopsy. Radiology 1993; 189: 143–146

[27] Gupta S, Gulati M, Rajwanshi A, Gupta D, Suri S. Sonographically guided fine-needle aspiration biopsy of superior mediastinal lesions by the suprasternal route. AJR Am J Roentgenol 1998; 171: 1303–1306

[28] Rubens DJ, Strang JG, Fultz PJ, Gottlieb RH. Sonographic guidance of mediastinal biopsy: an effective alternative to CT guidance. AJR Am J Roentgenol 1997; 169: 1605–1610

[29] Schlotterbeck K, Schmid J, Klein F, Alber G. Transesophageal ultrasound for staging lung tumors [Article in German]. Ultraschall Med 1997; 18: 153–157

[30] Schuler A, Blank W, Braun B. Sonographisch-Interventionelle Diagnostik bei Thymomen. Ultraschall Med 1995; 16: 62

[31] Weiss H, Düntsch U. Complications of fine needle puncture. DEGUM survey II [Article in German]. Ultraschall Med 1996; 17: 118–130

[32] Wang HC, Yu CJ, Chang DB et al. Transthoracic needle biopsy of thoracic tumours by a colour Doppler ultrasound puncture guiding device. Thorax 1995; 50: 1258–1263

Urogenital System

25 Percutaneous Renal Biopsy . . . 274

26 Interventional Urology . . . 280

25 Percutaneous Renal Biopsy

U. Goettmann, B. K. Kraemer

Percutaneous renal biopsy has become the gold standard for the diagnosis of renal diseases. The combined evaluation of biopsy specimens by light microscopy, immunohistology, and electron microscopy has made it possible to establish a uniform terminology, especially for the many different types of glomerular disease. Renal biopsy has also become an indispensable tool in renal transplantation. Besides the time-zero biopsy (intraoperative tissue sampling), protocol biopsies are again being used increasingly to monitor organ function. The results of renal biopsy should always be interpreted within the context of the clinical presentation and laboratory findings.

25.1 Indications

Currently there is no standard protocol used in selecting patients for renal biopsy. The overall frequency of renal biopsies ranges from 75 to 250 per 1 million population, depending on the selection criteria used by the treating nephrologist. The decision for renal biopsy is made largely by weighing therapeutic benefit against potential complications. After the exclusion of pre- and postrenal causes, unexplained acute renal failure with rapid deterioration of renal function is considered an absolute indication for biopsy, especially if there is coexisting nephritic urinary sediment with suspicion of rapidly progressive glomerulonephritis.[1]

In nephrotic syndrome, defined as the presence of proteinuria greater than 3.5 g/24 h/1.73 m^2, renal biopsy is generally advocated in adults due to the broad differential diagnosis and the value of biopsy findings in directing appropriate immunosuppressant therapy.[2] Renal biopsy is usually withheld in children under age 6 years with initial manifestations of nephrotic syndrome due to the fact that minimal-change glomerulonephritis exists in more than 90% of these patients.

In transplantation medicine, renal biopsy is used both in the acute postoperative period (to distinguish acute renal failure from acute rejection) and in patients with chronic allograft dysfunction.

The principal indications for renal biopsy are listed below:

- Acute renal failure with rapid deterioration of function after exclusion of pre- and postrenal causes, especially if rapidly progressive glomerulonephritis is suspected
- Nephrotic syndrome (proteinuria > 3.5 g/24 h/1.73 m^2), decide case-by-case in patients with suspected diabetic nephropathy
- Glomerular hematuria and associated proteinuria > 1 g/day
- Renal involvement by systemic disease, especially in lupus erythematosus, vasculitis, and amyloidosis
- The need to assess disease activity in response to immunosuppressant therapy
- Acute and chronic loss of renal function after renal transplantation
- Severe acute renal failure during pregnancy (except preeclampsia)

Isolated microhematuria is not an indication for renal biopsy. If microhematuria is associated with persistent proteinuria > 1 g/day, histologic evaluation is recommended at most centers. In patients with advanced chronic renal failure (glomerular filtration rate < 30 mL/min, kidney size < 9 cm), renal biopsy is generally withheld due to the lack of therapeutic implications and higher complication rate (bleeding risk). Selected references may be consulted for further considerations on renal biopsy indications.[1–5]

25.2 Contraindications

Absolute prerequisites for an elective renal biopsy are a cooperative patient and an intact hemostasis system with a normal prothrombin time and partial thromboplastin time and a normal platelet count. Platelet function should be tested in patients with a prior history of bleeding episodes and may be tested in patients who have been taking antiplatelet drugs or NSAIDs. Platelet function can be assessed by the determination of bleeding time or by performing a platelet function assay (PFA).[6] The PFA-100 analyzer provides better sensitivity and specificity than in vivo bleeding time.[7] Contradictory data have been published on the significance of a prolonged bleeding time or abnormal PFA in predicting bleeding complications after renal biopsy.[8–11] More recent studies have shown, however, that even aspirin use does not increase the risk of severe complications after ultrasound-guided percutaneous renal biopsy.[12,13]

On the other hand, we believe that antiplatelet drugs and NSAIDs should be stopped whenever possible prior to an elective renal biopsy. In some cases a prolonged bleeding time can be corrected by treatment with fast-acting desmopressin (0.3 µg/kg IV).[14]

Relative contraindications are hydronephrosis, pyelonephritis, renal abscess, uncontrolled hypertension (upper limit 150 mm Hg systolic and 95 diastolic), anomalies of renal shape and position (horseshoe kidney), large renal tumors, and small kidneys (increased bleeding risk). A single kidney does not contraindicate renal biopsy in carefully selected patients.[2,14]

25.3 Materials and Equipment

Special biopsy transducers (linear-array transducers) with an integrated biopsy channel as well as curved arrays with a side-mounted adjustable needle guide have proven effective for ultrasound-guided renal biopsies. Linear-array transducers provide high near-field resolution and stable contact with the skin, allowing for more accurate needle guidance. Both the transducer and needle guide are sterilized before each use.

The sector transducer has a smaller footprint and a more variable scan angle, which may be helpful in dealing with rib shadows or overlying bowel, for example. It also provides the cost-effective ability to convert an existing 3.5-MHz probe to a biopsy transducer by adding a biopsy attachment (▸ Fig. 25.1 and ▸ Fig. 25.2).

Most ultrasound manufacturers offer adjustable needle guides for their transducer systems. We use a sterile, disposable procedure kit that includes a needle guide and inserts for 14-gauge to 18-gauge needles, sterile ultrasound gel, and a sterile transducer cover (▸ Fig. 25.3).

A core biopsy technique using special 14- to 18-gauge Trucut needles (length 16 or 20 cm) has become widely practiced for percutaneous renal biopsies. Larger needles yield a greater number of glomeruli per core. Recent prospective randomized studies have shown no difference in the rate of bleeding complications with 14-gauge or 16-gauge needles in native kidneys or with 14-, 16-, or 18-gauge needles in renal allografts.[9,15] We generally use a 16-gauge needle for biopsies of native and transplanted kidneys (or an 18-gauge needle in selected cases).

Various suppliers offer both sterile disposable biopsy systems and sterilizable biopsy guns with sterile biopsy needles available separately.

25.4 Preparations

Informed consent should cover all the steps in the procedure, possible complications, and postbiopsy patient instructions. For forensic reasons, informed consent should be obtained on the day before the procedure and should be documented in writing. For a native kidney we generally biopsy the lower pole of the left or right kidney through a posterior approach in the prone patient. Most modern ultrasound systems have special biopsy programs that can superimpose the needle path on the screen. The patient should be fasted for 6 hours before the procedure but is allowed to drink liquids. Morning medications, especially for blood pressure, should be taken as usual. A prolonged cessation of fluid intake should be avoided in freshly transplanted patients. Laboratory values should include current coagulation status, simple blood count, creatinine, urea, and urinary status. Intravenous access should always be established. Body hair should be shaved over a wide area around the puncture site.

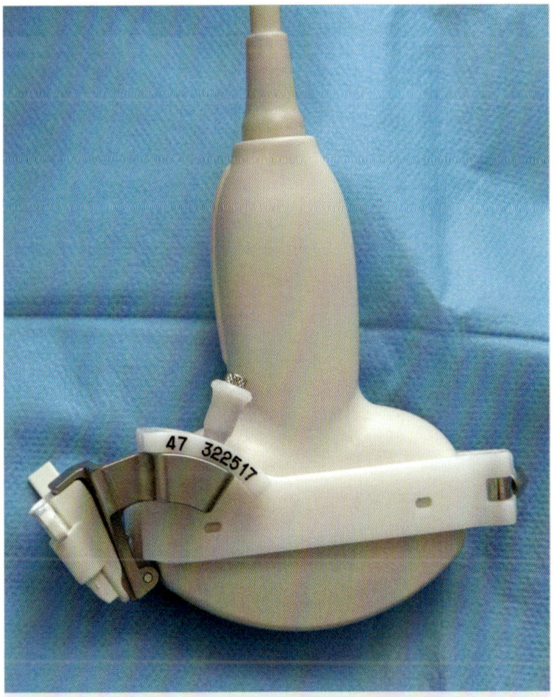

Fig. 25.1 Curved-array transducer with an adjustable needle guide.

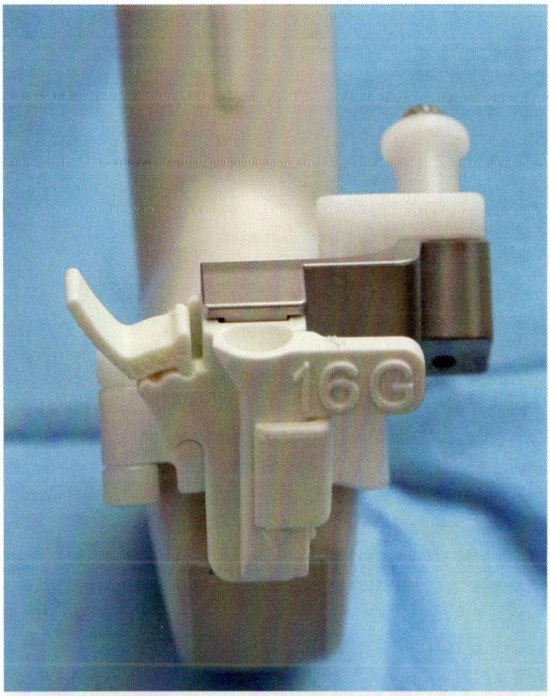

Fig. 25.2 Curved-array transducer with an adjustable needle guide, close-up view.

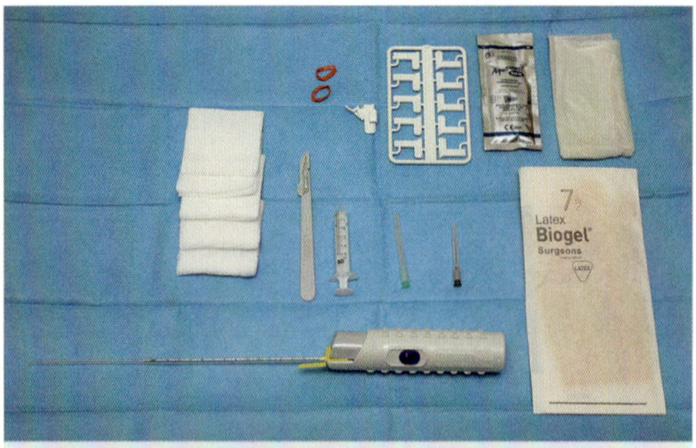

Fig. 25.3 Sterile, disposable procedure kit with needle guide and inserts, ultrasound gel packet, and a sterile disposable transducer cover (Ultra-Pro II needle guide [Civco]). A Max-Core automated sterile disposable biopsy device (Bard) and other materials are also shown.

25.5 Procedure

25.5.1 Native Renal Biopsy

After all necessary instruments have been laid out on a sterile table, the patient is positioned prone for biopsy of the native kidney. A foam roll is placed beneath the abdomen at the level of the umbilicus. With the patient in this position, the kidney should again be imaged sonographically prior to sterile draping and a suitable entry site marked on the skin with a permanent felt marker. At full inspiration the entry site should be as close to the lower renal pole as possible with adequate clearance from the lower ribs. Biopsy through the intercostal space should be avoided due to the risk of pneumothorax. If access is obstructed by ribs or bowel, the procedure should be switched to the contralateral kidney. The distance from the renal capsule to the skin should be determined to make sure that the biopsy needle, which has a centimeter scale, is not advanced too deeply.

Renal biopsy should always be performed under aseptic conditions. First the skin site is prepped with an antiseptic spray and covered with sterile drapes, leaving a wide area about the biopsy site undraped. After performing a surgical hand scrub, the operator should don sterile gloves and a surgical mask (plus a sterile gown if the patient is at high risk for infection). At this stage an assistant holds the transducer and maintains the renal image on the screen. It is sufficient for the assistant to wear a mask and sterile gloves.

When a conventional 3.5-MHz abdominal transducer is used, it is fitted with a needle guide attachment and then covered with a sterile disposable transducer cover. Previous to this a generous amount of ultrasound gel is placed in the base of the cover to improve mechanical coupling. Now the sterile needle guide with suitable biopsy insert is fastened to the side holder on the needle guide attachment (▶ Fig. 25.1 and ▶ Fig. 25.2). When a sterile linear biopsy transducer is used, the appropriate needle guide is mounted in the needle aperture of the transducer.

Topical anesthesia begins by raising a visible wheal in the skin with 2% mepivacaine, for example. A longitudinal stab incision is made with a pointed scalpel to help penetrate the epidermis. For infiltration of deeper tissues, a 21-gauge hypodermic needle is advanced through the needle guide and down to the renal capsule under ultrasound guidance, and a sufficient volume of local anesthetic is infiltrated along the needle tract. Careful deep infiltration will allow the biopsy to be performed with very little pain.

For the biopsy itself, the biopsy needle is inserted into the biopsy gun. The spring mechanism is cocked and the safety catch is released. Following another application of antiseptic spray, the biopsy needle is slowly advanced through the needle guide on the transducer under continuous ultrasound guidance, directing the needle as perpendicularly to the renal capsule as possible. The assistant maintains an optimum view of the ultrasound screen as the needle is advanced to the renal capsule (▶ Fig. 25.4).

A palpable resistance is usually felt when the needle reaches the capsule. If the needle tip echo is not clearly visible on the screen, the transducer can be angled slightly to one side. When the needle tip is in contact with the renal capsule at full inspiration, the patient is instructed to breath-hold and the biopsy gun is fired (▶ Fig. 25.5).

The needle appears as a bright echo as it advances into the renal parenchyma. Before the mechanism is fired, care should be taken that the needle has not already penetrated the renal capsule. That would result in a too-deep biopsy that would sample medullary tissue and increase

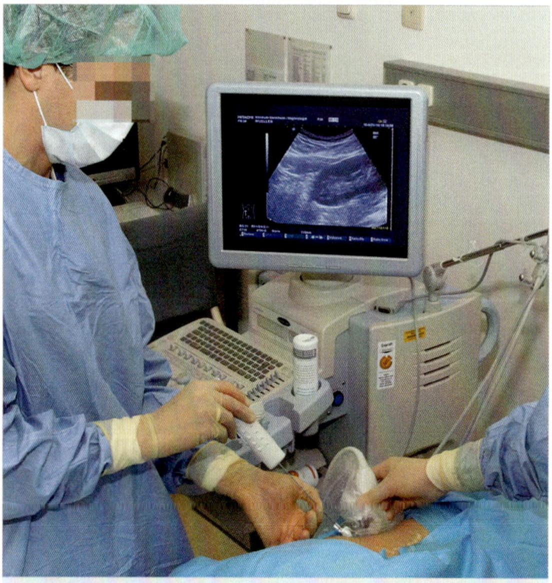

Fig. 25.4 The needle is carefully advanced to the left kidney under sonographic guidance.

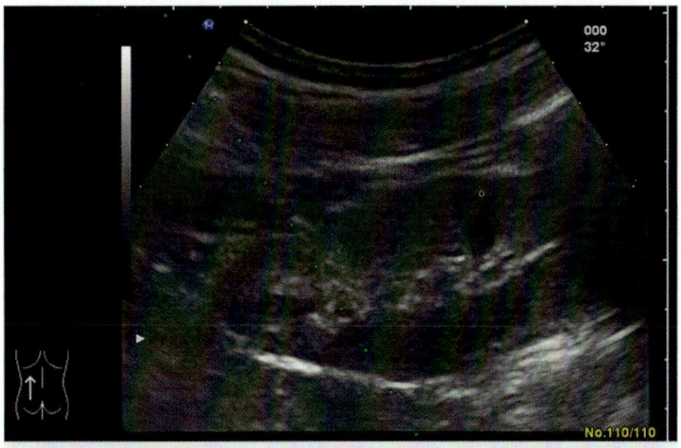

Fig. 25.5 Biopsy of the left kidney. The needle is clearly visible as a hyperechoic line.

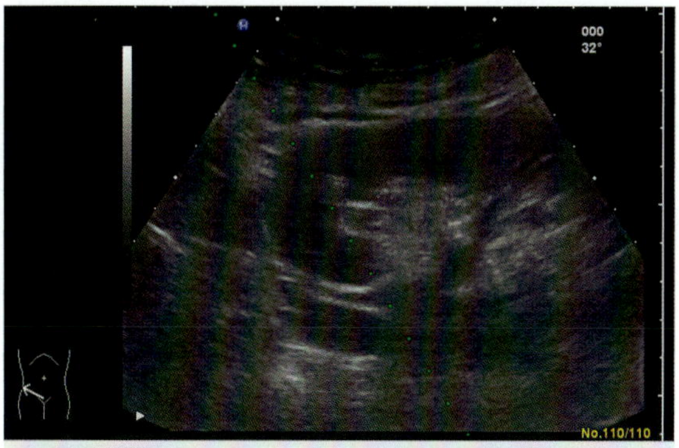

Fig. 25.6 Ultrasound image of a renal allograft in the lower right abdomen with an adjustable-angle needle guide (set here to 32°).

the bleeding risk. The needle should be fired during a breath-hold to avoid lacerating the kidney surface.

The harvested tissue core is carefully fixed in a prepared vessel with 4% buffered formalin and its quality is assessed. A specimen of acceptable quality is immediately sent to the pathologist. A detailed pathology report will require a tissue core at least 1 cm long and approximately 1.2 mm in diameter. The core should contain at least 10 to 12 glomeruli. If the adequacy of the specimen is uncertain, its glomerular content can be determined by examining the core under a light microscope at 6 × magnification. To increase the diagnostic yield, it is recommended that two tissue cores be obtained.

Immediately after the biopsy, the biopsied region is closely examined sonographically to check for bleeding complications. Local compression is applied to the area for 5 minutes, and the patient is positioned on a sandbag (native kidney) or a sandbag is placed over the biopsy site (renal allograft).

25.5.2 Review of the Procedure Steps

1. Sterile instruments are prepared, venous access is established, blood pressure is checked, and the patient is positioned prone on a foam roll.
2. The needle path is visualized on the ultrasound screen.
3. The most favorable needle path is determined at full inspiration with ultrasound visualization of the right or left renal lower pole, and the entry site is marked on the skin.
4. The field is draped.
5. The needle guide is attached to the transducer, and the biopsy site is rechecked sonographically under sterile conditions.
6. The skin site is infiltrated with local anesthetic, and a small stab incision is made with a scalpel. Deeper tissues are infiltrated down to the renal capsule with a 21-gauge needle under sonographic guidance.
7. The Trucut needle is mounted in the biopsy gun, the spring mechanism is cocked and the safety released.
8. The biopsy needle is introduced through the biopsy channel and carefully advanced to the renal capsule at the lower pole under ultrasound guidance.
9. The biopsy gun is fired during a breath-hold.
10. The harvested tissue core is carefully fixed in 4% formalin and assessed for acceptable quality.
11. The biopsy region is examined sonographically, the needle tract is compressed for 5 minutes, and the patient is positioned on a sandbag for 8 hours.

25.5.3 Biopsy of a Renal Allograft

A transplanted renal allograft (▶ Fig. 25.6) is usually biopsied at its upper pole in the supine patient owing to the superficial, extraperitoneal location of the graft in the iliac fossa. It is important to check for overlying bowel, especially after a combined renal and pancreatic transplantation (intraperitoneal placement of the renal allograft). If the lower pole must be biopsied for anatomical reasons, the anastomotic vessels and donor ureter close to the biopsy site can be identified by color duplex sonography. A superficial skin wheal should provide adequate anesthesia. The rest of the procedure is analogous to that for a native renal biopsy.

25.6 Complications

The primary complication of renal biopsy is bleeding. It may occur at any of three locations:

- The urinary outflow tract, resulting in micro- or macrohematuria
- Beneath the renal capsule, resulting in self-tamponade due to pressure and manifested by pain
- Bleeding into the perirenal space with the formation of a large hematoma and a marked fall in hemoglobin

Since the advent of ultrasound-guided biopsies and fully automated biopsy guns, however, severe bleeding complications of renal biopsy have become rare. Transient microhematuria occurs in almost all patients, and macrohematuria has a reported incidence of 0.8 to 7.5%, with 0.3 to 5% of affected patients requiring a transfusion.[9,11,16–18] Macrohematuria with bladder tamponade has become a rarity.[19] The most common bleeding complications are perirenal hematomas, which are usually asymptomatic. While postbiopsy CT studies have revealed the presence of small hematomas in over 50% of biopsies,[5] the incidence of clinically significant hematomas (flank pain, > 20 g/L fall in Hb) is only 1.5 to 2.5%.[9,16,20] Hematomas requiring operative treatment are extremely rare, and significant bleeding is usually managed by coiling the affected segmental artery of the biopsied kidney during angiography (up to 1.2% of cases).[11,16,17,19–21] Deaths after renal biopsy are rare, with several studies reporting a mortality rate of 0.02 to 0.1%.[5,18,20] Indeed, there are many highly specialized nephrology centers where renal biopsies have been practiced by experienced operators for decades with no deaths. Since the introduction of color duplex ultrasound, arteriovenous fistulas have been detected more frequently after renal biopsies as incidental sonographic findings. The incidence is higher for renal allografts (16.9%) than native kidneys (4.4%).[14] With a spontaneous healing rate of over 95%, these fistulas are of minor clinical importance. Performing renal biopsy as an outpatient procedure generally does not increase the procedural risk when an 8-hour observation period is enforced after the procedure.[5,22] Reports indicate that 67% of complications occur during the first 8 hours after a native renal biopsy and 90% within the first 12 hours,[18] while 87.5% of complications after an allograft biopsy occur within the first 8 hours.[23] Consequently, ambulatory renal biopsy still has a certain residual risk and we do not recommend it.

25.7 Postbiopsy Care

Following the biopsy, the patient should lie in the supine position and a total of 24 hours' bed rest should be maintained. A sandbag is placed beneath the biopsy site for 8 hours to prevent postbiopsy bleeding. We check pulse and blood pressure every 30 minutes for the first 2 hours, then hourly for another 4 hours and finally every 2 hours. A blood count and ultrasound examination are routinely performed the next morning. The blood count is also checked every 6 to 8 hours at our institution. A high fluid intake is maintained (approximately 3 L/24 h), and the urine is checked for hematuria. The patient is allowed to eat after the first normal blood count. The patient should be instructed to avoid heavy lifting and carrying, avoid strenuous exercise, and if possible avoid taking antiplatelet drugs for two weeks after the biopsy. Full anticoagulation should be withheld for at least one week after the biopsy if possible. Patients should be observed for at least 8 hours following an ambulatory biopsy.[5] Patients at our hospital are kept for overnight observation after a native or allograft biopsy and are released the following morning.

25.8 List of Materials and Equipment

- Linear or conventional 3.5-MHz curved-array transducer
- Adjustable-angle needle guide for a linear biopsy transducer, adjustable needle guide for curved arrays (e.g., EZU PA 7C1 [Hitachi]) (▶ Fig. 25.1, ▶ Fig. 25.2, ▶ Fig. 25.3)
- Sterile disposable procedure kit with needle guide, sterile ultrasound gel, and sterile disposable transducer cover (Ultra-Pro II needle guide [Civco])
- Needle for deeper infiltration anesthesia (e.g., 21-gauge, length 50 mm)
- 16- or 18-gauge Trucut biopsy needle (e.g., Magnum biopsy needle, length 20 cm, 1.7-mm sample notch)
- Biopsy gun (e.g., Bard Magnum or Max-Core sterile automated disposable biopsy system [Bard]; ▶ Fig. 25.3)

References

[1] Andreucci VE, Fuiano G, Stanziale P, Andreucci M. Role of renal biopsy in the diagnosis and prognosis of acute renal failure. Kidney Int Suppl 1998; 66: S91–S95

[2] Fuiano G, Mazza G, Comi N et al. Current indications for renal biopsy: a questionnaire-based survey. Am J Kidney Dis 2000; 35: 448–457

[3] Feneberg R, Schaefer F, Zieger B, Waldherr R, Mehls O, Schärer K. Percutaneous renal biopsy in children: a 27-year experience. Nephron 1998; 79: 438–446

[4] Gerth J, Wolf G. Nierenbiopsie: Indikation und Durchführung. Nephrologie 2008; 3: 169–177

[5] Korbet SM. Percutaneous renal biopsy. Semin Nephrol 2002; 22: 254–267

[6] Harrison P. Assessment of platelet function in the laboratory. Hamostaseologie 2009; 29: 25–31

[7] Favaloro EJ. Clinical utility of the PFA-100. Semin Thromb Hemost 2008; 34: 709–733

[8] Islam N, Fulop T, Zsom L et al. Do platelet function analyzer-100 testing results correlate with bleeding events after percutaneous renal biopsy? Clin Nephrol 2010; 73: 229–237

[9] Manno C, Strippoli GF, Arnesano L et al. Predictors of bleeding complications in percutaneous ultrasound-guided renal biopsy. Kidney Int 2004; 66: 1570–1577

[10] van den Hoogen MW, Verbruggen BW, Polenewen R, Hilbrands LB, Nováková IR. Use of the platelet function analyzer to minimize bleeding complications after renal biopsy. Thromb Res 2009; 123: 515–522

[11] Waldo B, Korbet SM, Freimanis MG, Lewis EJ. The value of postbiopsy ultrasound in predicting complications after percutaneous renal biopsy of native kidneys. Nephrol Dial Transplant 2009; 24: 2433–2439

[12] Atwell TD, Smith RL, Hesley GK et al. Incidence of bleeding after 15,181 percutaneous biopsies and the role of aspirin. AJR Am J Roentgenol 2010; 194: 784–789

[13] Mackinnon B, Fraser E, Simpson K, Fox JG, Geddes C. Is it necessary to stop antiplatelet agents before a native renal biopsy? Nephrol Dial Transplant 2008; 23: 3566–3570

[14] Stiles KP, Yuan CM, Chung EM, Lyon RD, Lane JD, Abbott KC. Renal biopsy in high-risk patients with medical diseases of the kidney. Am J Kidney Dis 2000; 36: 419–433

[15] Nicholson ML, Wheatley TJ, Doughman TM et al. A prospective randomized trial of three different sizes of core-cutting needle for renal transplant biopsy. Kidney Int 2000; 58: 390–395

[16] Hergesell O, Felten H, Andrassy K, Kühn K, Ritz E. Safety of ultrasound-guided percutaneous renal biopsy-retrospective analysis of 1090 consecutive cases. Nephrol Dial Transplant 1998; 13: 975–977

[17] Meola M, Barsotti G, Cupisti A, Buoncristiani E, Giovannetti S. Free-hand ultrasound-guided renal biopsy: report of 650 consecutive cases. Nephron 1994; 67: 425–430

[18] Whittier WL, Korbet SM. Timing of complications in percutaneous renal biopsy. J Am Soc Nephrol 2004; 15: 142–147

[19] Bach D, Wirth C, Klein B, Hollenbeck M, Grabensee B. Perkutane Nierenbiopsie. Nieren und Hochdruckkr 1998; 27: 355–360

[20] Mendelssohn DC, Cole EH. Outcomes of percutaneous kidney biopsy, including those of solitary native kidneys. Am J Kidney Dis 1995; 26: 580–585

[21] Riehl J, Maigatter S, Kierdorf H, Schmitt H, Maurin N, Sieberth HG. Percutaneous renal biopsy: comparison of manual and automated puncture techniques with native and transplanted kidneys. Nephrol Dial Transplant 1994; 9: 1568–1574

[22] Fraser IR, Fairley KF. Renal biopsy as an outpatient procedure. Am J Kidney Dis 1995; 25: 876–878

[23] Yablon Z, Recupero P, McKenna J, Vella J, Parker MG. Kidney allograft biopsy: timing to complications. Clin Nephrol 2010; 74: 39–45

26 Interventional Urology

D. Brix, A. Ignee, C. F. Dietrich

The first report on an interventional urologic procedure performed under continuous sonographic guidance was published in 1979. The procedure was successfully accomplished under dynamic ultrasound guidance without radiation exposure to the patient or staff.

Since our readers may be less familiar with urologic interventions than with other procedures described in this book, our discussions of interventional urology will include a review of some basic principles.[1]

26.1 Transrectal Ultrasonography of the Prostate

26.1.1 Introduction

Transrectal ultrasonography of the prostate (TRUS) has become an established diagnostic and therapeutic tool in urology. The close proximity of the rectum to the prostate permits the use of high-frequency transducers in the 6- to 10-MHz range, resulting in higher spatial resolution of the imaged structures.

Histologic studies of the prostate[2] have identified the presence of three glandular zones (peripheral, central, and transitional) and one stromal zone (anterior segment). This subdivision can also be appreciated on ultrasound images.[3]

26.1.2 Equipment Requirements

TRUS should be performed with a high-frequency transducer (6–10 MHz) in at least two standard planes. Also, the transducer should have a biopsy channel or needle guide to allow for ultrasound-guided biopsy, antibiotic injection, abscess drainage, or interstitial brachytherapy. Most modern ultrasound scanners have color Doppler and duplex capabilities, and some systems allow for contrast agent-specific imaging and elastography.

26.2 Diseases of the Prostate

26.2.1 Prostate Cancer

Etiology and Incidence

Prostate cancer is the most common visceral cancer affecting males in the Western population. The incidence in the United States is 241,740 new cases per year.[4]

A variety of etiologic factors have been discussed: ethnographic (incidence is 30 times higher in African Americans than in Japanese); dietary (high-fat, low-fiber foods increase the cancer risk, soy consumption reduces it); genetic (positive family history is linked to higher risk); environmental (occupational cadmium exposure); and hormonal (androgenic stimulation).

Diagnosis

The diagnosis of prostate cancer is based on digital rectal examination, serum PSA (prostate specific antigen) level, and TRUS of the prostate. Most prostate cancers develop in the peripheral zone of the gland, and tumors with a volume > 0.2 mL are palpable at that location. Accordingly, a suspicious palpable nodule is an absolute indication for prostatic biopsy.

TRUS, with a specificity of approximately 36%, is considered an adjunctive test in the diagnosis of prostate cancer. Several studies have shown a detection rate of approximately 20% and a positive predictive value between 30% and 58%. The negative predictive value is 50 to 65%. Several studies have also investigated the sensitivity of TRUS, especially in the important preoperative detection of capsular involvement and seminal vesicle invasion. Extracapsular extension can be detected with a sensitivity of 83% and a specificity of 67%, seminal vesicle invasion with a sensitivity of 43% and a specificity of 86%. Today the undisputed domain of TRUS is the ultrasound-guided transrectal prostate biopsy. The transperineal approach is used mainly in patients who have had a proctectomy.[5]

Prostate cancer usually appears as a hypoechoic area, and this finding should be reproducible in both axial and sagittal planes. In 35% of cases, however, the lesion appears isoechoic or even hyperechoic. Conversely, not every hypoechoic lesion is prostate cancer. Based on studies comparing TRUS findings with histology, it is known that slightly hyperechoic areas in the peripheral zone of the gland may represent normal prostate tissue, acute or chronic prostatitis, atrophy, prostatic infarction, or prostatic intraepithelial neoplasia (PIN).

Accordingly, the following sonographic criteria are considered suggestive of prostate cancer:

- Hypoechoic area with irregular margins located in the peripheral zone
- The abnormal area penetrates through the bright rim of the prostate capsule or extends to the rectal wall.
- Asymmetry of the prostate lobes
- Obliteration of the angle between the prostate and seminal vesicle. Portions of the seminal vesicles not invaded by cancer may show asymmetrical dilatation.

Treatment

The treatment of prostate cancer depends on patient age and health status, PSA, histologic stage (TNM), and tumor grade (Gleason score). Localized prostate cancer is usually treated by primary radical prostatectomy. Other options are modern radiotherapy regimens (high-dose rate [HDR] and low-dose-rate [LDR], brachytherapy with or without percutaneous radiation, or even active surveillance. Metastatic prostate cancer is treated primarily with various forms of antiandrogen therapy. If the tumor becomes resistant to hormone therapy (hormone-refractory prostate cancer, HRPC), various chemotherapeutic agents (taxanes, mitoxantrone) may be administered with palliative intent.[6]

26.2.2 Prostatic Abscess

Diagnosis

Abscess formation in the prostate disrupts its normal zonal architecture. As in other organs, the abscess typically appears hypoechoic with ill-defined margins. The hypoechoic areas sometimes contain internal echoes.

Treatment

Percutaneous needle aspiration can be performed by the transrectal or transperineal route under TRUS guidance. If the aspiration yields putrid fluid, an abscess that is larger than 2 cm should be drained. This is done by dilating the needle tract with Teflon dilators over a guidewire using Seldinger technique. Next, a pigtail catheter is introduced, and 40 mg of gentamicin is instilled into the abscess cavity through the catheter and left there for 1 hour. The contents of the abscess cavity are then drained into a collecting bag. When the drain output reaches zero, the catheter is removed and the site is assessed by endosonography.

An alternative treatment is to open the abscess during a transurethral resection of the prostate (TURP).

26.3 Prostate Biopsy

26.3.1 Introduction

Core needle biopsy of the prostate is usually performed through a transrectal approach. The transperineal approach is less commonly used for prostate biopsy, although it is used routinely for brachytherapy. The biopsy is performed with an 18-gauge needle and a spring-loaded biopsy gun (e.g., Biopty device [Bard]). There is no evidence that biopsy needles cause tumor seeding in patients with prostate cancer. A distinction is made between *targeted* biopsies, which sample selected areas that have been identified by ultrasound or palpation, and *systematic* biopsies, which sample all portions of the prostate according to a standard scheme. The classic sextant biopsy described by Hodges has been abandoned in favor of volume- and age-dependent biopsy strategies such as the Vienna nomogram.

26.3.2 Indications

Prostate biopsy should be performed only if a possible diagnosis of prostate cancer would have therapeutic implications. The correlation between PSA levels and relative risk of prostate cancer was shown to be 6.6 for a PSA level of 0 to 0.5 and 26.9 for a PSA level of 3.1 to 4.[7]

26.3.3 Informed Consent and Preparation

The patient is informed about the risks and benefits of the procedure, and written informed consent is obtained (e.g., Diomed consent form).

We routinely perform a cleansing enema prior to the biopsy. Oral antibiotic prophylaxis with a gyrase inhibitor (1 × 500 mg norfloxacin) is started on the morning of the procedure and is continued once daily for 3 days. After the bowel has been emptied, a local anesthetic is administered (Instillagel [Farco Pharma], 15 mL) for 15 min. The patient is then placed in left lateral decubitus with the knees and hips flexed. First a digital rectal examination is performed to evaluate sphincter tone and palpable findings, followed next by TRUS with volumetry. At our center we generally follow this with a systematic biopsy based on the Vienna nomogram (▶ Fig. 26.1). The retrieved tissue cores are individually fixed in formalin and processed for histologic examination.

26.3.4 Complications and Their Management

Patients with high anal sphincter tone or anal sphincter sclerosis may experience several days' discomfort following use of the endorectal ultrasound probe.

The incidence of complications of transrectal prostate biopsy, regardless of the number of cores harvested, includes the following complications[8]: hematospermia, 37.4%; persistent urethral bleeding > 1 day, 14.5%; rectal bleeding, 2.2%; prostatitis, 1.0%; fever, 0.8%; epididymitis, 0.7%; urosepsis, 0.3%; urinary retention, 0.2%.

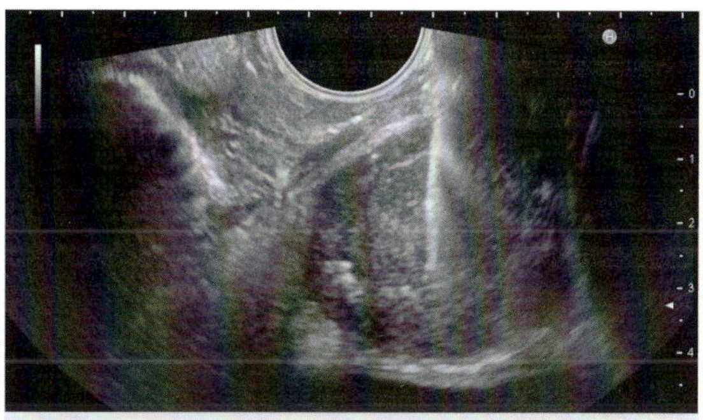

Fig. 26.1 Ultrasound-guided prostate biopsy. The Vienna nomogram is used to determine the optimum number of tissue cores.

The management of complications may include the following measures, depending on the symptoms:

- Chills: hospitalization and treatment with IV antibiotics (e.g., ceftriaxone, 2 g once daily)
- Rectal bleeding: tamponade for 6 to 12 hours (unroll gauze bandage, apply Instillagel before insertion)

26.3.5 Transperineal Biopsy

Following antiseptic preparation and local anesthesia of the perineum in the lithotomy position, the biopsy needle is introduced through the perineal skin. Antibiotic coverage may often be omitted when this approach is used.

26.4 Percutaneous Nephrostomy

26.4.1 Introduction

Percutaneous nephrostomy (PCN) performed under combined fluoroscopic and sonographic guidance has completely superseded the classic surgical technique. The procedure can be done under local anesthesia in most patients. Percutaneous nephrostomy can be successfully performed in 95 to 98% of children and adults who have a dilated renal collecting system. In patients with a nondilated collecting system, the success rate falls dramatically even in the hands of an experienced operator.

26.4.2 Indications

Percutaneous nephrostomy is in competition with ureteral stenting. Its advantages and disadvantages should be weighed against each other for every clinical situation:

- Decompression of hydronephrosis
- Removal of renal pelvic and calyceal stones (percutaneous nephrolitholapaxy, PNL)
- Decompression of the lower urinary tract: unilateral or bilateral percutaneous nephrostomy for management of urinary fistula, palliative PCN for bladder dysfunction due to tumor invasion
- Diagnostic: antegrade pyeloureterography
- Historical: measurement of renal pelvic pressure (Whitaker test)

26.4.3 Relative Contraindications

Coagulation disorders, tumors of the kidney and renal pelvis.

26.4.4 Complications

Transient macrohematuria is usually present. Rare cases may show significant bleeding from the PCN (injury to a large renal vessel in 1–2%, bleeding-associated mortality rate 0.2%). The accidental puncture of a nearby organ (bowel, lung, liver, spleen) is rare. A PCN can be life-saving in patients with septic hydronephrosis but may occasionally exacerbate the septic state due to bacterial release into the circulation.

The nephrostomy tube is subject to possible dislodgment or clogging over time.

26.4.5 Preparations

The preparations for PCN include the following measures:

- The patient is fasted.
- The possible need for intubation is assessed.
- A peripheral IV line is placed.
- Blood count, Quick value, PTT, creatinine, electrolytes are determined.
- Dilatation of the targeted collecting system is checked sonographically.
- Fluoroscopy unit: request in PACS.
- A lead apron is placed over the pelvic region.

26.4.6 Materials and Equipment

Nephrostomy catheters have a central open tip and are slightly shorter than transurethral catheters. One-way polyurethane catheters with a curled end (pigtail catheters) are often used and must be fixed to the skin with a suture. One-way nephrostomy tubes are available in sizes from 6F to 12F. Long-term nephrostomy care should employ a two-way occluding balloon catheter made of silicone with a short, central open tip. Silicone nephrostomy tubes are available in sizes from 10F to 24F. See ▶ Fig. 26.2, ▶ Fig. 26.3.

26.4.7 Technique

The patient is positioned prone or in lateral decubitus. A hollow needle is passed into the posterior inferior calyx

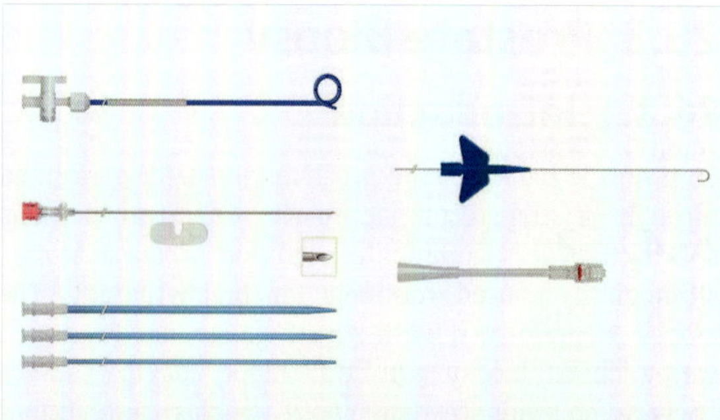

Fig. 26.2 Nephrostomy set (OptiMed) for catheter placement by the classic Seldinger technique for external drainage of urine and viscous fluids. Made from OD material (soft polyurethane). The set consists of: pigtail catheters with two-way stopcock (diameters 7F–16F, length 30 cm), Schüller exchange guidewire (diameter 0.035 inch, length 90 cm, flexible tip, 10 cm, 3-mm J curve, rigid 40-cm shaft, flexible end), dilators (diameters 6F–10F, length 20 cm).

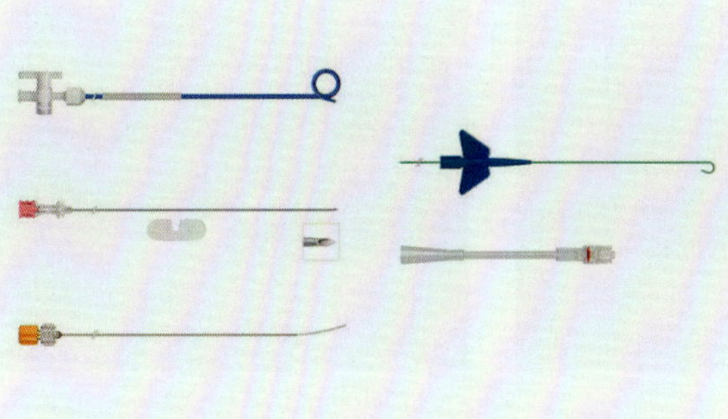

Fig. 26.3 Special nephrostomy set (OptiMed) for catheter placement by the Seldinger technique for external drainage of urine and viscous fluids. The obturator can straighten the drainage catheter without perforating. Made from OD material (soft polyurethane). The set consists of: pigtail catheters with two-way stopcock (diameters 7–9 French, length 30 cm), two-part puncture needle with echogenic tip (diameter 1.3 mm, 17.5-gauge, length 20 cm), two-part obturator with round blunt plastic stiffener (diameters 1.2–1.3 mm), coated PTFE guidewire (diameter 0.035 inch, length 100 cm, flexible tip, 3-mm J curve), rotating male Luer lock adapter.

(▶ Fig. 26.4), and a rigid Seldinger guidewire (Lunderquist wire, Cook Medical Europe) is introduced. Puncture of a posterior calyx provides easy access to the renal pelvis. The needle should be angled laterally 20° to 30° from the perpendicular in the prone patient. Next the tract is dilated to size along the guidewire and the nephrostomy catheter (initial size 8–12F) is advanced into the renal pelvis over the wire. Fluoroscopic guidance is helpful during nephrostomy tube placement.

26.4.8 Anesthesia

First the needle tract is infiltrated with local anesthetic (e.g., mepivacaine 1%, 5–20 mL) down to the renal capsule, then a long yellow (No. 1) anesthesia needle is introduced under sterile conditions after the site has been draped and the needle path defined with the ultrasound probe and needle guide under a sterile cover.

26.4.9 Procedure

Positioning

The patient is positioned prone over an inflatable roll on the urologic procedure table. The ipsilateral side should be flexed forward as much as possible to provide optimum posterior tension. After the needle path has been checked and the collimator adjusted, the skin site is prepped with an antiseptic solution (Braunoderm, Braun Melsungen) and draped. The nephrostomy is illustrated in ▶ Fig. 26.3 (case of the month, www.efsumb.org), and a conventional pigtail catheter placement is shown in ▶ Fig. 26.4.

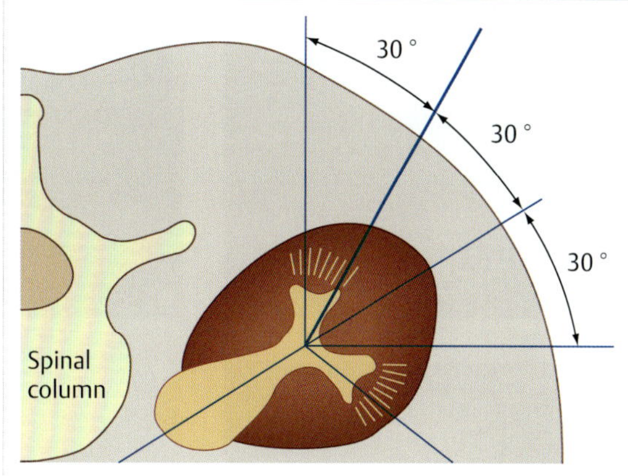

Fig. 26.4 Diagrammatic representation of the angles for directing a needle into the posterior group of calyces for PCN. The needle is angled 20° to 30° laterally to pass through the posterior calyces and into the renal pelvis. Puncturing a lateral group of calyces at this angle will not access the renal pelvis.

Puncture and Nephrostomy Tube Placement

Caution

Do not use fluoroscopy in pregnant patients!

Puncture and tube placement consists of the following steps:

1. Contact gel (Instillagel) is applied to the skin.
2. The sterilized ultrasound probe is positioned for needle guidance into the inferior group of renal calyces.
3. Local anesthesia is applied, and the Schüller needle is advanced into the inferior group of calyces, making sure the needle is directed radially (perpendicular to the renal surface and through a papilla).
4. If necessary, urine is aspirated and sent for bacteriology or cytology.
5. Next a small amount of contrast medium is injected through the needle and its position is checked fluoroscopically.
6. A Seldinger wire is introduced through the puncture needle into the renal pelvis (▶ Fig. 26.5, ▶ Fig. 26.6).
7. Correct placement of the wire is checked by fluoroscopy or ultrasound.
8. The skin is incised with a scalpel down to the fascia, and if necessary the tract is dilated over the guidewire. The PCN tube is then introduced over the wire.
9. Additional contrast medium is injected to define the collecting system.
10. The PCN tube is fixed to the skin with a suture, and if necessary the catheter balloon is inflated for retention in the renal pelvis.
11. Finally the incision is covered with a sterile self-adhesive dressing.

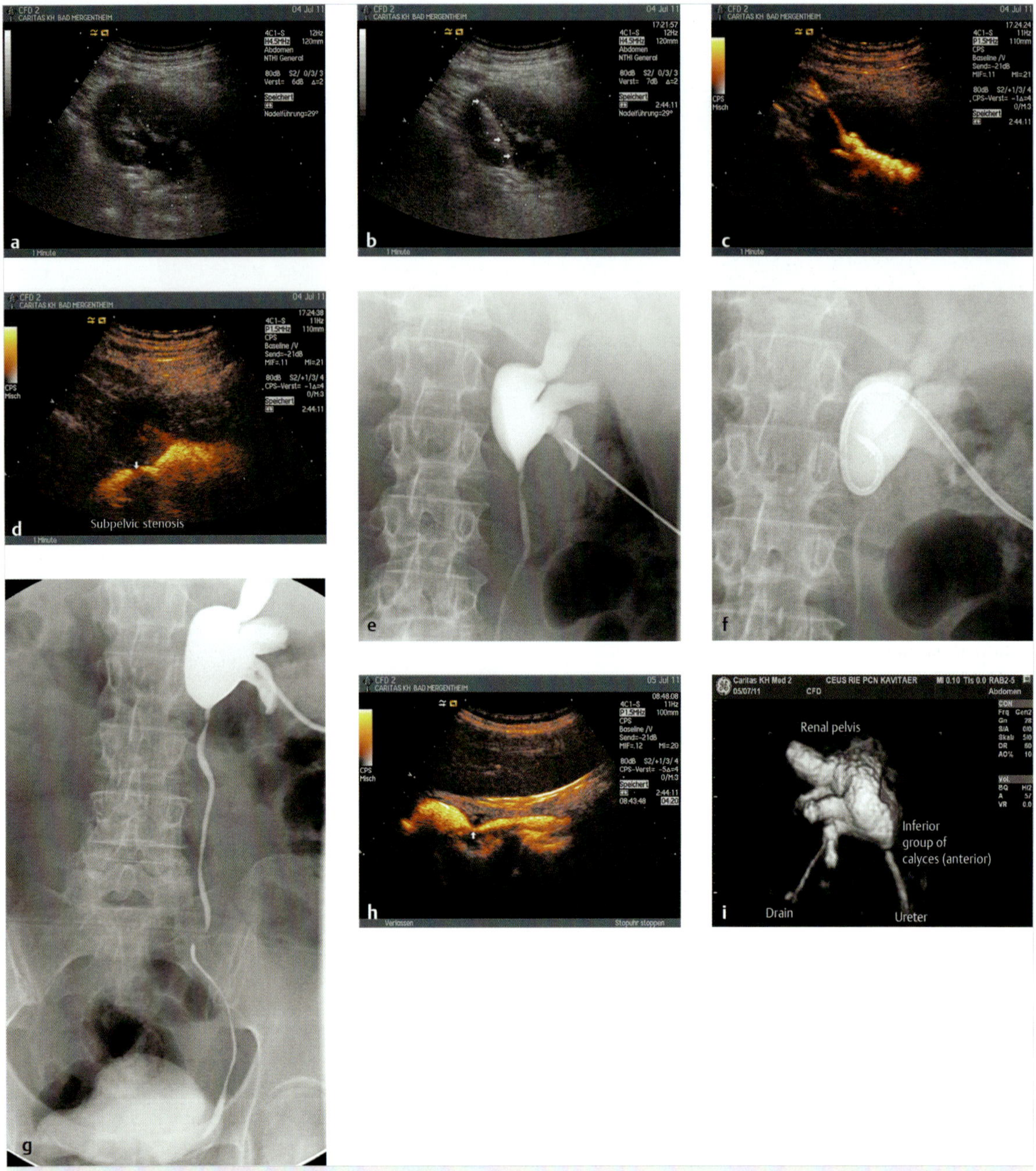

Fig. 26.5 Percutaneous nephrostomy. Ultrasound images of the dilated calyces (**a**) and needle insertion (**b**). SonoVue contrast administration (**c**) demonstrates a presumed subpelvic stenosis (**d**). Note the prone position of the patient and the reverse screen orientation with inferior structures displayed on the left side of the image. Radiographic images are added to confirm correct needle position (**e**), show the placement of the pigtail catheter (**f**), and document the completed, functioning nephrostomy (**g**). Transabdominal contrast-enhanced ultrasound the following day also demonstrates the subpelvic ureteral stenosis (**h**). 3D reconstructed image of the renal pelvis shows the drainage tube, inferior group of calyces, renal pelvis, and ureter (**i**).

Inadequate Dilatation of the Collecting System

If the collecting system is not sufficiently dilated, percutaneous nephrostomy should be withheld and a ureteral catheter should be placed by the transurethral route.

26.4.10 Postoperative Care

- If bleeding occurs, the nephrostomy tube should be clamped off to tamponade the collecting system. This will arrest the bleeding in most cases. If it does not, the nephrostomy tube can be exchanged for a balloon catheter to apply local pressure. If the bleeding still persists,

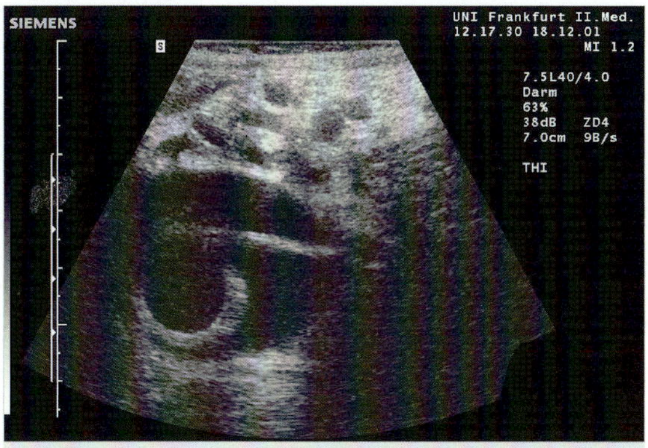

Fig. 26.6 Standard-orientation ultrasound image documents conventional pigtail catheter placement in the renal pelvis.

it can be managed by superselective transcatheter embolization of the injured renal vessels. Nephrectomy is available as a last resort.

- It is important to maintain an accurate balance of input and output. In patients with reactive polyuria (e.g., after decompression of hydronephrosis), input should equal output plus 500 mL (to allow for insensible perspiration). Input in febrile patients should be increased accordingly.
- Patients with pyonephrosis, fever, and chills should receive intravenous antibiotic therapy (e.g., 2 g ceftriaxone).
- Laboratory tests should include hemoglobin level, electrolytes, and retention values.
- Catheter care is also important (*caution:* the tube should be stabilized during dressing changes to avoid dislodgment when the adhesive tape is removed). The nephrostomy tube should be changed every 4 to 6 weeks.

References

[1] Keberle E, Dietrich CF, Wolff JM. Transrektaler Ultraschall der Prostata (TRUSP) und der Samenblasen. In: Dietrich CF, ed. Endoskopischer Ultraschall, eine Einführung. Konstanz: Schnetztor Verlag; 2005: 428–441

[2] McNeal JE. Origin and development of carcinoma in the prostate. Cancer 1969; 23: 24–34

[3] Watanabe H, Igari D, Tanahashi Y, Harada K, Saitoh M. Transrectal ultrasonotomography of the prostate. J Urol 1975; 114: 734–739

[4] Siegel R, Naishadham D, Jemal A. Cancer statistics, 2012. CA Cancer J Clin 2012; 62: 10–29

[5] Hara RY, Jo Y, Fujii T et al. Optimal approach for prostate cancer detection as initial biopsy: prospective randomized study comparing transperineal versus transrectal systematic 12-core biopsy. Urology 2008; 71: 191–195

[6] Heidenreich A, Bellmunt J, Bolla M et al. European Association of Urology. EAU guidelines on prostate cancer. Part 1: screening, diagnosis, and treatment of clinically localised disease. Eur Urol 2011 Jan; 59: 61–71

[7] Thompson IM, Pauler DK, Goodman PJ et al. Prevalence of prostate cancer among men with a prostate-specific antigen level < or =4.0 ng per milliliter. N Engl J Med 2004; 350: 2239–2246

[8] Moran BJ, Braccioforte MH, Conterato DJ. Re-biopsy of the prostate using a stereotactic transperineal technique. J Urol 2006; 176: 1376–1381; discussion 1381

Other Organ Systems

27 Interventional Thyroid Ultrasound . . . 288

28 Musculoskeletal Interventions . . . 304

29 Neurologic Interventions, Ultrasound-Guided Regional Anesthesia . . . 315

30 Ultrasound-Guided Emergency and Vascular Interventions . . . 332

27 Interventional Thyroid Ultrasound

B. Braun, T. Mueller

Ultrasonography is superior to all other imaging modalities (scintigraphy, CT, MRI, PET) for imaging the thyroid gland. Ultrasound is an essential tool in the work-up of thyroid diseases and dysfunction and is the next diagnostic step following the history, physical examination, and key laboratory tests (thyroid-stimulating hormone [TSH], free thyroxine [fT_4], free triiodothyronine [fT_3]).[1]

Ultrasound-guided interventional procedures in the thyroid gland have both diagnostic and therapeutic applications:

- Biopsies:
  - Fine needle aspiration (FNA)
  - Core needle biopsy (CNB)
- Fluid evacuation:
  - Single or repetitive needle aspirations
  - Catheter drainage
- Ablative procedures:
  - Percutaneous ethanol instillation (PEI)
  - Radiofrequency ablation (RFA, performed rarely)
  - Percutaneous laser ablation (PLA, performed rarely)

27.1 Diagnostic Interventions

In the traditional technique of thyroid biopsy, a palpable or visible tumor, nodule, or cyst in the thyroid gland is fixed between the thumb and index finger of one hand while the needle is introduced into the mass with the other hand. Diagnostic accuracy can be increased by making 2 to 6 passes, in each case using a new needle and syringe, and preparing additional smears for evaluation.[2]

Ultrasound guidance has improved this technique. Nonpalpable nodules and lesions can be biopsied, and sonographically suspicious nodules and peripheral vascularized areas in cystic lesions can be accurately targeted while avoiding injury to the trachea, common carotid artery, and jugular vein. Ultrasound visualization of the needle tip allows for continuous and precise monitoring of the needle path. In contrast to palpation-guided biopsies, one needle insertion is generally sufficient. A second pass may be necessary only if the initial aspirate is bloody or when dealing with a large, inhomogeneous mass. Ultrasound guidance has decreased the rate of nondiagnostic biopsies, improved diagnostic accuracy, and reduced costs. Ultrasound-guided FNA biopsy has reduced by 25% the number of suspicious goiters selected for surgery and has increased the rate of carcinomas found in surgical specimens from < 15% to 40 to 50%.[3–6] The guidance of thyroid biopsy by palpation has become obsolete.

27.1.1 Indications

The most frequent indication for thyroid biopsy is the investigation of suspicious thyroid nodules. The sonographic criteria of malignancy are as follows:

- Low echogenicity
- Inhomogeneous echo pattern
- Presence of microcalcifications
- Ill-defined or microlobulated margins
- Irregular intranodal vascularity
- Hard nodule by elastography

A single criterion is not suspicious for malignancy in itself, but two or more criteria warrant a high index of suspicion. The size of the nodule is not a factor.[7,8] Larger malignancies tend to show central cystic transformation, so partially cystic nodules should be biopsied at their periphery. Other factors that influence patient selection for thyroid biopsy are the history (first-degree relative with thyroid cancer, prior radiation exposure), clinical criteria (hoarseness, hard palpable nodule), laboratory findings (calcitonin), and other sonographic criteria (transmural extension, lymphadenopathy).[9]

The **most common indications** for percutaneous thyroid biopsy are:

- Thyroid nodule with clinical, sonographic or scintigraphic criteria suspicious for malignancy (▶ Fig. 27.1a, b)
- Confirmation of diagnosis of subacute granulomatous thyroiditis (▶ Fig. 27.2a, b)
- Confirmation of diagnosis of chronic Hashimoto thyroiditis or investigation of suspected lymphoma (▶ Fig. 27.3)
- Confirmation of diagnosis of acute thyroiditis, identification of infecting organism (▶ Fig. 27.4)
- Symptomatic thyroid cysts before sclerotherapy
- Lymph node enlargement after thyroid cancer surgery

27.1.2 Contraindications

The contraindications to thyroid FNA are as follows:

- Significant coagulopathy (PTT > 50 seconds, INR > 1.6, platelets < 50×10^9/L)
- Lack of therapeutic implications
- Lack of informed consent

27.1.3 Methods

Fine Needle Aspiration (FNA)

Aspiration cytology is the method of choice for differentiating between benign and malignant thyroid nodules.

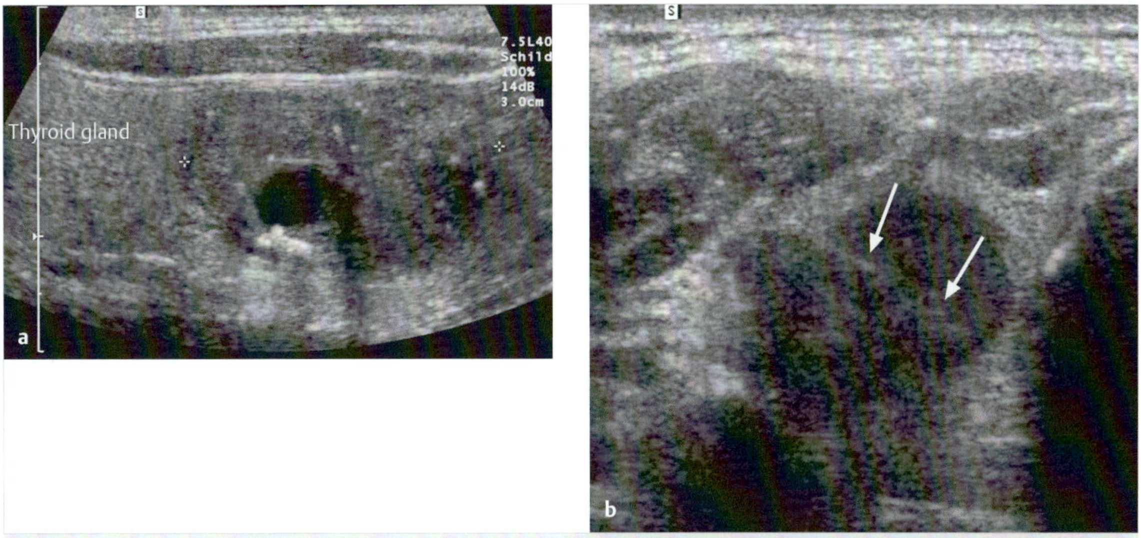

Fig. 27.1
a Medullary thyroid carcinoma displaying multiple sonographic criteria of malignancy: low echogenicity, inhomogeneity, microcalcifications, and ill-defined margins.
b Papillary thyroid carcinoma with marked hypoechogenicity and ill-defined margins. Arrows indicate the 20-gauge needle.

The FNA of suspicious thyroid nodules has a sensitivity of 83% (65–98%) and a specificity of 92% (72–100%). The rate of false-negative findings in the literature ranges from 1.1 to 23.7%.[9–11] The high range of variation is due mainly to differences in the expertise of operators and cytologists. Even small nodules (< 5 mm) can be confidently sampled and classified.[12]

Core Needle Biopsy (CNB)

Generally there will be no difficulty in the cytologic classification of thyroid malignancies when an adequate specimen is obtained and the general cytologic criteria for malignancy are applied (nuclear pleomorphism, nuclear hyperchromasia, irregular nuclear membrane, prominent nucleoles, multinucleated tumor giant cells, marked cellular dissociation).

In the case of anaplastic carcinomas, it can be extremely difficult to make an accurate cytologic or even histologic diagnosis. Accurate classification is important due to differences in prognosis and treatment, as in the differentiation of anaplastic thyroid carcinoma from high-grade lymphoma. A core needle biopsy of the thyroid may be necessary in selected cases to provide a histologic diagnosis based in part on immunohistochemical tests.[9] This is particularly true in patients with thyroid lymphoma[13,14] and in rare cases of sarcoma or hemangioendothelioma.

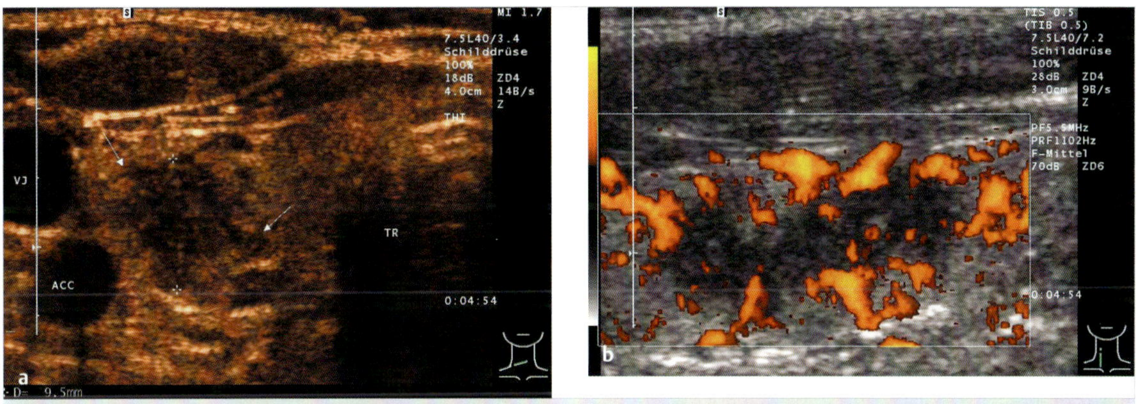

Fig. 27.2
a Transverse scan of the neck in a 45-year-old woman shows an inhomogeneous area in the right thyroid lobe (+ +), which was slightly tender to pressure. Laboratory tests showed elevated C-reactive protein (CRP). The patient had received neck radiation for a cervical hemangioma in childhood. Differential diagnosis: tumor infiltration, subacute thyroiditis. FNA: subacute granulomatous thyroiditis.
b Color Doppler ultrasound (power Doppler) shows hypoechoic inflammatory infiltrates with scant vascularity.

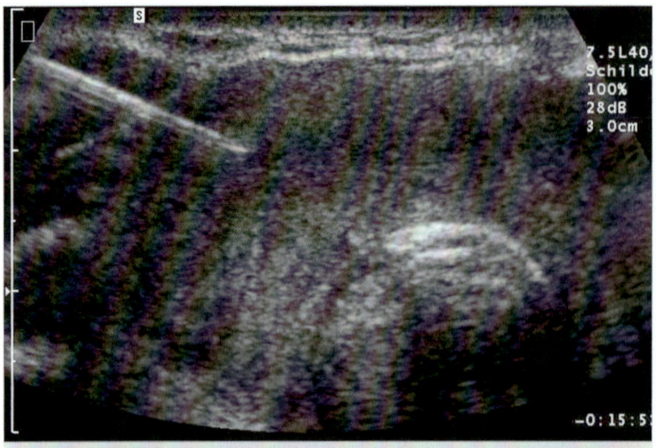

Fig. 27.3 Enlarged, hypoechoic thyroid gland in a patient with rheumatoid arthritis and vitiligo. FNA biopsy was performed using classic technique. Ultrasound displays the oblique needle shaft (left side of image). Cytology and histology detected lymphocytic infiltration: rare form of Hashimoto thyroiditis with thyroid enlargement.

Because of contradictory results on the diagnostic accuracy of CNB versus FNA, the latter is still considered the basic method of choice for the diagnostic evaluation of suspicious thyroid nodules.[15–17]

27.1.4 Complications

Owing to the superficial location of the thyroid gland, compression of the needle tract is sufficient to prevent bleeding even in patients with coagulation disorders. There is no need to discontinue aspirin use before thyroid biopsy.

Hematomas are the most common minor complication of FNA and occur in 0.2% of needle biopsies. Major complications occur only sporadically and have not been documented in large studies.[11,18]

Seeding of tumor cells along the needle tract is a rare occurrence and generally has no significance because even an inoculation metastasis can easily be removed.[19]

Core needle biopsy appears to be associated with a slightly higher rate of minor complications (hematoma, infection) than FNA. No major complications have been reported.[15–17]

27.1.5 Materials and Equipment

Ultrasound Technology

Ultrasound imaging of the thyroid gland requires the use of high-frequency transducers (7.5–12 MHz). A very large goiter with retrosternal extension should additionally be scanned with a curved array at 5 to 7.5 MHz to obtain a more comprehensive view of the mass and its surroundings. The ultrasound probe should have the smallest possible footprint to facilitate needle insertion and guidance in the neck (▸ Fig. 27.5).

Color Doppler imaging (conventional or power Doppler) can clearly display movements of the biopsy needle,

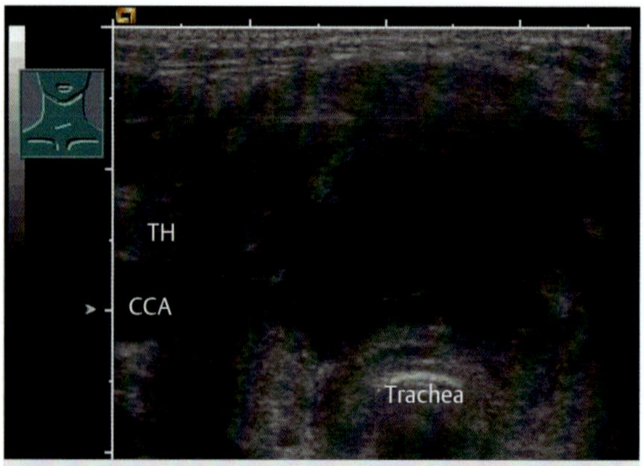

Fig. 27.4 Very tender thyroid gland (TH) in a small child with local warmth and swelling in the neck. FNA cytology and bacteriology indicated acute thyroiditis with abscess formation caused by staphylococcal infection.

fluid aspiration from a cyst, or ethanol injection into a lesion (▸ Fig. 27.6a, b).

For ethanol instillation into autonomous hyperfunctioning thyroid adenomas, we use the vascularity of the nodule on contrast-enhanced ultrasound (CEUS) for guiding a second or third injection. Ethanol is selectively instilled into nodular areas that exhibit vascularity.

Dedicated biopsy transducers have several disadvantages: they are expensive; the angle of needle insertion is difficult to vary; imaging is limited in the area of the transducer orifice; and the biopsy transducer has to be sterilized after each use. In our experience, even side-mounted needle guides are not a helpful aid in performing thyroid biopsies.

Biopsy Materials

Standard biopsy materials and supplies are illustrated in ▸ Fig. 27.7.

We use (economical) 20-gauge hypodermic needles for thyroid FNA, like those commonly used for drawing

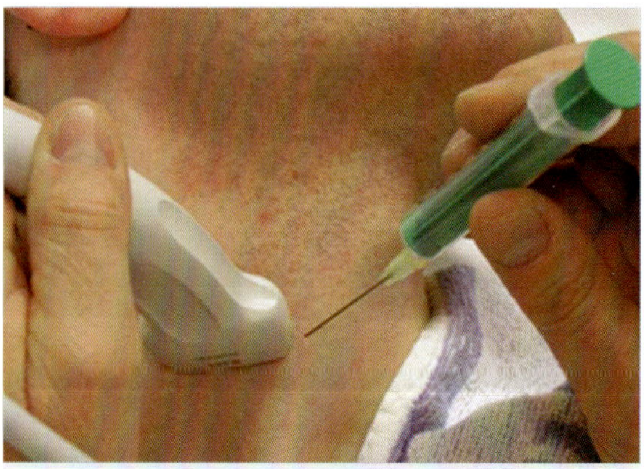

Fig. 27.5 FNA using the long-axis technique. The 20-gauge needle, mounted on a 5-mL syringe, is introduced at a 45° angle to the skin at the narrow end of the ultrasound probe.

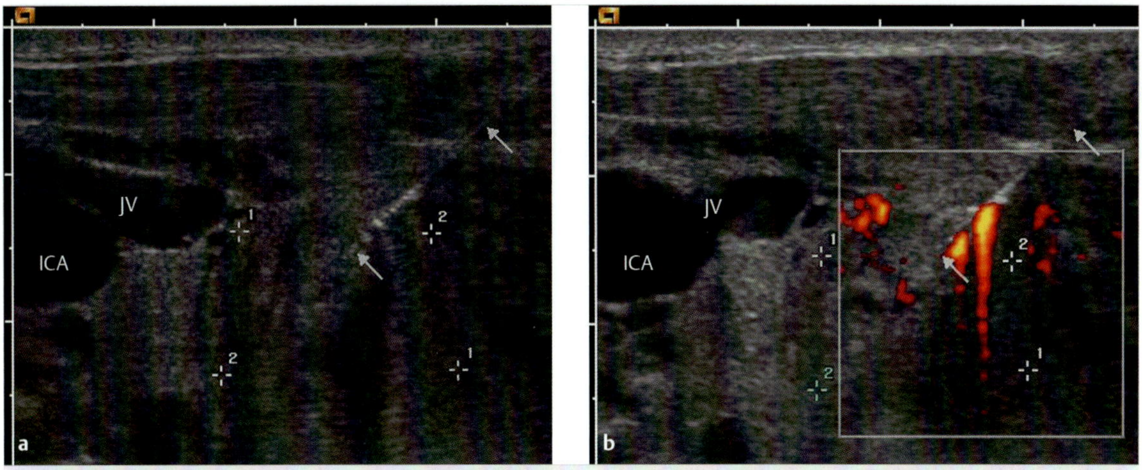

Fig. 27.6
a Transverse scan of the right thyroid lobe. Viewed in the B-mode image, the full length of the needle (arrows) is visible within the inhomogeneous, poorly marginated thyroid nodule (+ +) and in its course through the subcutaneous tissue and neck muscles. The lower arrow indicates the needle tip.
b Brisk movements of the needle produce color artifacts in the color Doppler image, similarly to the aspiration of cyst contents or the injection of alcohol. (ICA, internal carotid artery; JV, right jugular vein.)

blood. They are 0.9 mm in diameter, 4 or 7 cm long, and can be clearly visualized with ultrasound. We use 2- or 5-mL syringes to draw samples for aspiration cytology as well as for therapeutic ethanol instillation. Either 20- or 50-mL syringes are used for the drainage of thyroid cysts, depending on the cyst contents.

Some histologic specimens are obtained with fine needles 0.8 to 0.9 mm in diameter (approximately 21- to 20-gauge). We perform core biopsies with 18-gauge end-cutting needles in an automated biopsy instrument with one-hand operation (Biopince, Argon Medical Devices). The biopsy process is simple and can retrieve long tissue cores whose diameters equal the full luminal diameter of the needle.

27.1.6 Preparation

The purpose of the procedure, possible alternatives, and the steps involved in the procedure are fully explained to the patient with a nurse or other assistant present, and written consent is obtained. The patient is also informed that two or perhaps three passes may have to be made, depending on the quality of the sample, and that thyroid biopsy is comparable to a peripheral venipuncture. Most biopsies are performed on an outpatient basis. Generally the total time required for an ultrasound-guided thyroid biopsy, including preparations, ultrasound examination and postprocedure care, is less than 15 minutes.

Positioning the Patient

The patient is positioned supine with the upper body elevated 45° to 50°. A roll is placed beneath the cervical spine to hyperextend the neck and increase the distance between the lower jaw and the clavicle or sternum. This position also makes it easier to visualize retrosternal portions of the thyroid[20] and allows the sonographer to work in a conventional position.

Recommendations on Selecting the Target Site

While a cyst can be aspirated at any site, selection of the target site is important in the case of solid and suspicious nodules. This has been demonstrated by comparisons of preoperative ultrasound findings with surgical

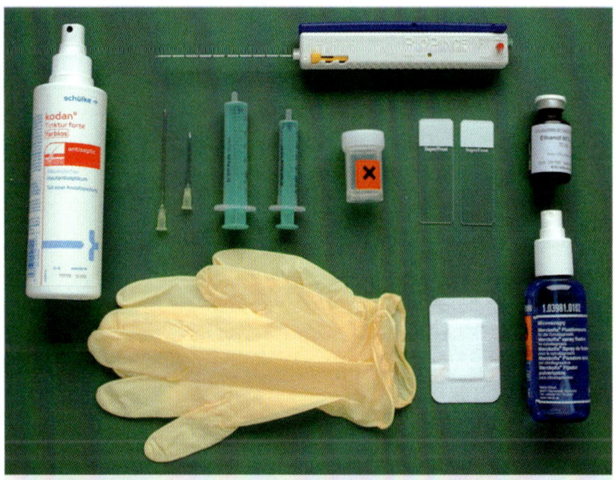

Fig. 27.7 Materials for FNA biopsy, core needle biopsy, and ethanol injection: skin prep solution (Kodan tincture forte [Schülke & Mayr]); 20-gauge needles in two lengths; 5- and 10-mL syringes; 18-gauge automated core biopsy needle (Biopince [Argon Medical Devices]); specimen vessel with 4% formalin; microscope slides; ampule with 10 mL of 96% ethanol; nonsterile gloves; adhesive dressing; and spray fixative (Merckofix [Merck Millipore]).

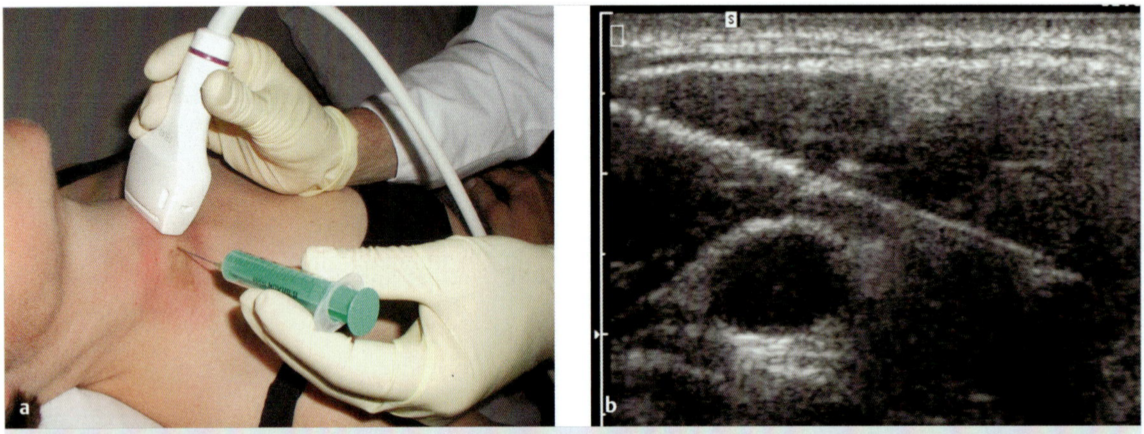

Fig. 27.8 Classic "long-axis" technique for biopsy of a suspicious thyroid nodule.
a The right hand holds the 7.5-MHz transducer while the left hand holds the 10-mL syringe on a 20-gauge needle. The needle is introduced at the narrow end of the transducer and is directed at a low angle to the skin.
b Transverse cervical scan displays the needle as a diagonal echogenic line entering the image from the left side and visible anteriorly to the common carotid artery. The needle tip has entered the hypoechoic thyroid nodule.

specimens. When dealing with a nodule that is suspicious for malignancy, the periphery of the lesion should be biopsied because that is where tumor cells tend to proliferate. Central areas are more likely to be necrotic, resulting in a more difficult cytologic diagnosis.[20,21] Predominantly cystic nodules should be biopsied in a solid area.[22]

Antisepsis

The skin is prepared with an alcohol-based solution after first shaving the site if necessary. The transducer is cleaned and thoroughly disinfected before use (e.g., with alcohol- and aldehyde-free wipes such as Microbac tissues [BODE Chemie]). The needle and syringe are, of course, sterile.

Because the operator does not come into contact with the needle or the patient's skin, it is unnecessary to wear sterile gloves. Disposable gloves should be used, however, to protect against contamination with the patient's blood.

Catheters for draining thyroid cysts and abscesses should be placed under sterile conditions. Sterile drapes, gown, mask, hood, and sterile instrument covers should be used, just as in an operating room.

After the procedure is completed, the transducer is wiped cleaned with a (nonsterile) towel and cleaned with disinfectant wipes.[23–25]

27.1.7 Procedure

Long-Axis Biopsy Technique

Given the relatively small size of the thyroid gland and its proximity to blood vessels and the larynx, it is helpful to visualize the full length of the biopsy needle. The needle is introduced at the narrow end of the transducer, directing it at a low angle to the skin. Ideally the needle should be constantly visible over its full length as a double echogenic line (▶ Fig. 27.6, ▶ Fig. 27.8b).

The needle tip is not always clearly visible in echogenic surroundings, and small back-and-forth movements of the needle can aid visualization. The operator can hold the transducer in either hand, depending on his or her ability to manipulate the syringe and needle with the opposite hand.

Short-Axis Biopsy Technique

In the "short-axis" technique the biopsy needle is introduced at the center of the long edge of the transducer and is directed almost perpendicular to the skin. This technique is sometimes necessary when dealing with small lesions and a difficult access route. It is more difficult because the full length of the needle shaft is not displayed on the screen and the tip can be identified only by rocking the transducer in a "radarlike" sweep (▶ Fig. 27.9a, b; ▶ Fig. 27.10a).

Fine needle Aspiration

FNA does not require local anesthesia.[26] We prefer the bimanual freehand technique with a long-axis probe placement, as it is economical and can be repeated as often as desired. It also permits the needle to be intro duced at any angle.[27]

When the needle has entered the nodule, the plunger of the syringe is drawn back 2 cm^3 to create suction, and the needle is repeatedly advanced and withdrawn 3 or 4 times in a fan-shaped pattern while suction is maintained (▶ Fig. 27.11a, b). It is important to sample the periphery of the nodule, where there should be a higher yield of viable tissue.[20]

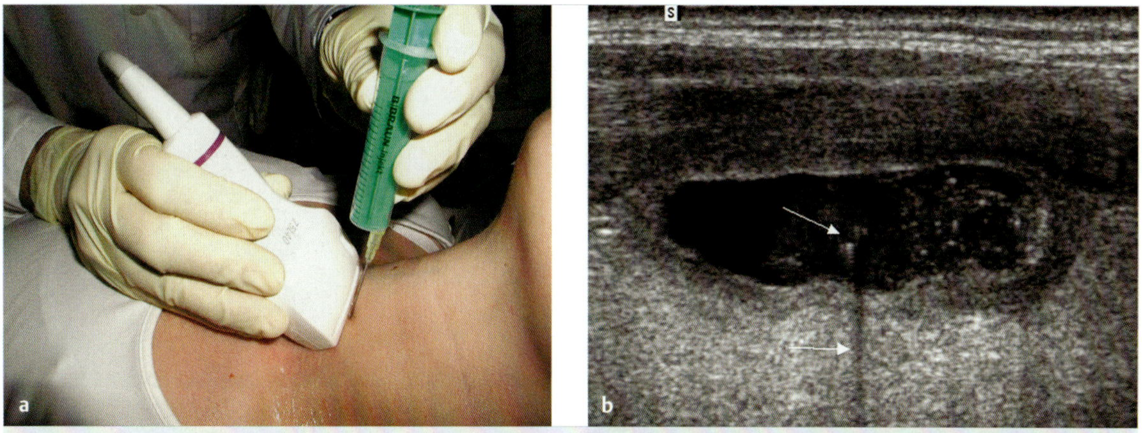

Fig. 27.9 Less common "short-axis" technique for aspirating a thyroid cyst.
a The needle is introduced at the center of the long edge of the transducer.
b The needle tip appears as a high-amplitude echo (upper arrow) with a distal acoustic shadow (lower arrow) within the elliptical cyst, which contains scattered internal echoes. In the moving image, visualization is aided by varying the scan angle and making fast twitching movements of the needle, making the tip easier to identify than in this static image.

The plunger should be released to discontinue suction before the needle is withdrawn, or at least by the time aspirated material appears within the syringe barrel (▶ Fig. 27.12). Releasing the suction in this way will minimize the aspiration of extraneous material into the syringe and prevent tumor seeding of the needle tract.

When the biopsy is completed, the patient places uniform pressure on the puncture site with a sterile pad for several minutes while the physician processes the aspirate.

Preparation of the Aspirate

The operator detaches the syringe from the needle, fills approximately half the syringe with air, and reattaches the needle to the syringe. The needle is then placed bevel-down against the prepared slide, and the harvest is expelled onto the slide in drops. A second slide is used to prepare smears. Further processing of the specimens (air drying or fixed in Merckofix, for example) should be discussed with the cytopathologist. Alcohol fixation of smears should be done *immediately* after the smears are prepared.

An adequate specimen should include at least six groups of well-preserved thyroid epithelial cells consisting of at least 10 cells each.[8]

Aspirated cystic fluid is taken immediately in a fresh state to the cytology laboratory for centrifugation. If this is not possible (e.g., at weekend), the specimen should be stored in a refrigerator.

Drill Technique, Fine Needle Nonaspiration

In this technique the biopsy proceeds initially as described above, and the needle tip is watched on the monitor until it reaches the target site. At that point the transducer is set aside and the syringe is stabilized securely with one hand. With the other hand, the operator grasps the syringe by the plunger (while applying little or no suction) and twists it once or twice on its long axis while advancing it slightly. The syringe–needle unit must be held at a constant angle while this is done. The purpose of "drilling" the needle in this way is to sample a core of thyroid tissue while causing minimal tissue trauma. This technique is somewhat more difficult to learn than fine needle aspiration.

One advantage of the drill technique is that it causes less tissue trauma, resulting in the aspiration of less blood.[20]

Core Needle Biopsy

CNB is preceded by local anesthesia of the skin (0.5–2 mL 2% lidocaine). We use a one-hand biopsy gun with an 18-gauge end-cutting needle. The precise depth of the nodule should be measured before the biopsy so that the throw length can be limited accordingly.

The transducer is placed in a long-axis orientation to provide a full-length view of the biopsy needle, not just the tip (▶ Fig. 27.13a, b).

When the needle has reached the biopsy target, the device is fired to "shoot" the cutting needle to the depth previously set on the handle (13–33 mm). A clip retains the harvested tissue core inside the needle during removal. The tissue core is immersed in 4% formalin.

After the biopsy is completed, the needle track is compressed with a sterile pad for 5 to 10 minutes to prevent a subcutaneous hematoma or bleeding into the thyroid gland. Then an adhesive dressing is applied and the patient is released from the outpatient unit.

27.1.8 Problems

Problems may relate to clear visualization of the needle tip or to the aspiration of (too much) blood-tinged

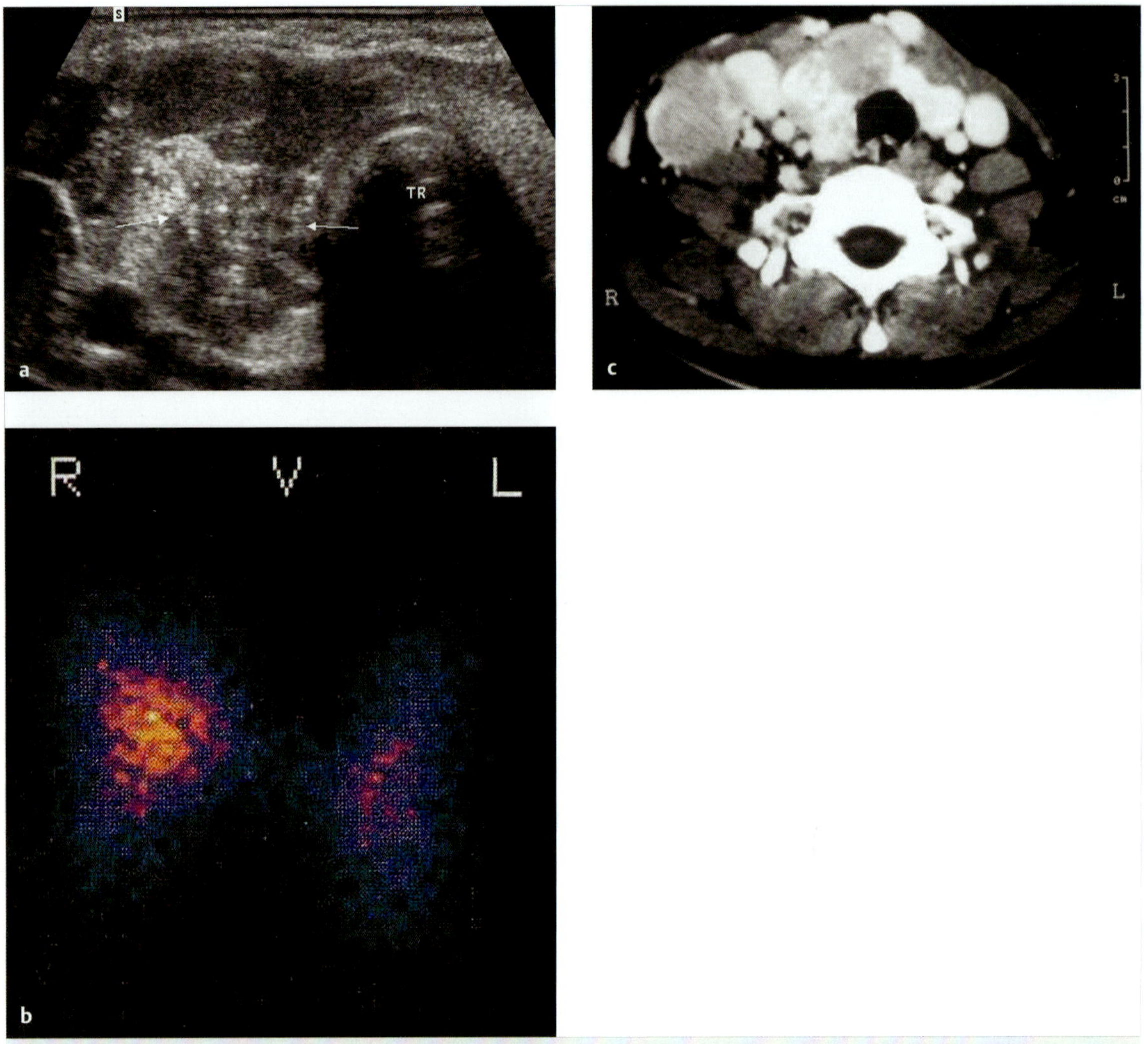

Fig. 27.10 FNA biopsy using the short-axis technique.
a Transverse cervical scan shows the uniformly echogenic normal tissue of the thyroid left lobe on the right side of the image, bordering the trachea (TR). The right lobe has been infiltrated by an inhomogeneous mass (arrows). Small psammomatous body–like echoes of calcium density make it difficult to identify the needle tip, but short twitching movements can define the tip much more clearly in the moving image than in this static image. FNA identified the lesion as mixed follicular papillary thyroid carcinoma.
b Thyroid scintiscan in the same patient appears normal!
c Contrast-enhanced CT was performed elsewhere in the same patient. Note that this type of scan is contraindicated as it interferes with radioiodine therapy after thyroidectomy.

material. Potential problems and their solutions are listed in ▶ Table 27.1.

27.1.9 Pitfalls in Thyroid Biopsy

The results of FNA biopsy depend on the expertise of the sonographer and cytopathologist and also on the patient and his or her underlying disease. As a general rule, larger thyroid nodules are associated with a lower false-negative rate, although the rate climbs back to 50% with nodules > 4 cm.[28]

Cytology may be unable to differentiate between benign follicular neoplasia and follicular carcinoma. Hence when "follicular neoplasia" is detected, the diagnosis should be checked by core needle biopsy or surgical excision.[29] Papillary carcinomas in particular may undergo cystic degeneration and elude cytology.[10,29] Nondiagnostic specimens and/or continued suspicion of malignancy despite a negative biopsy should prompt a repeat FNA, CNB, or excision.[9]

The most frequent causes of **false-positive cytologic findings** ("malignant" cytology from a histologically

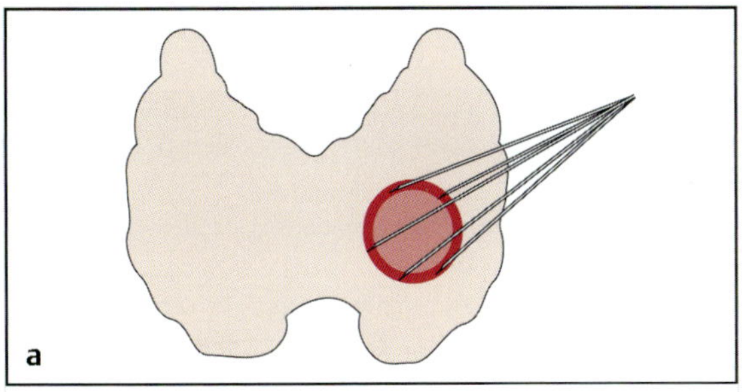
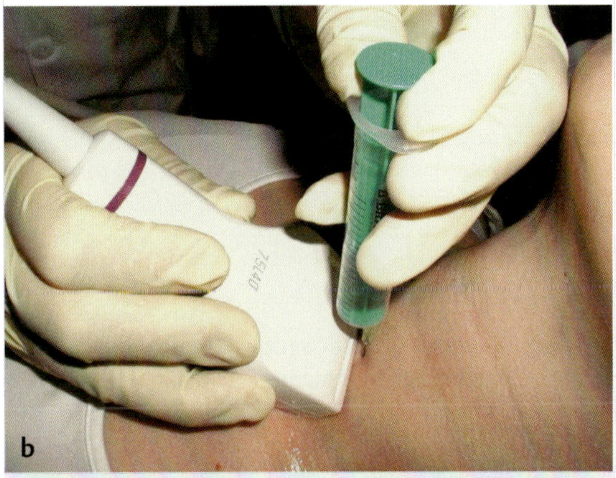

Fig. 27.11
a Diagrammatic representation of fine needle aspiration from the periphery of a thyroid nodule. Suction should be discontinued before the needle is withdrawn from the nodule into normal thyroid tissue.
b Hand position during aspiration: the thumb and index finger of the left hand maintain suction while moving the syringe and needle back and forth under vision.

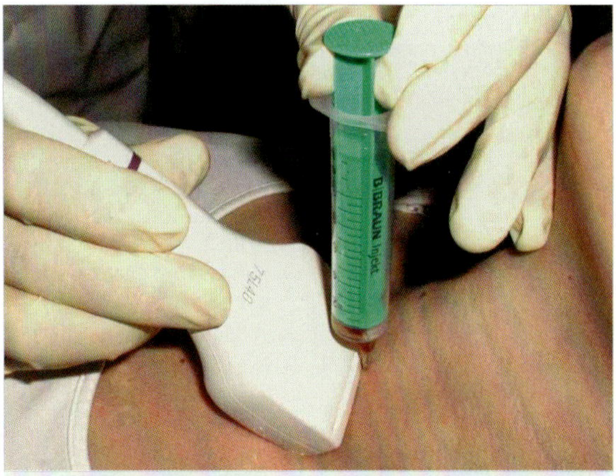

Fig. 27.12 A small amount of blood-tinged aspirate appears inside the barrel of the syringe. The plunger is released, and the syringe is withdrawn without suction.

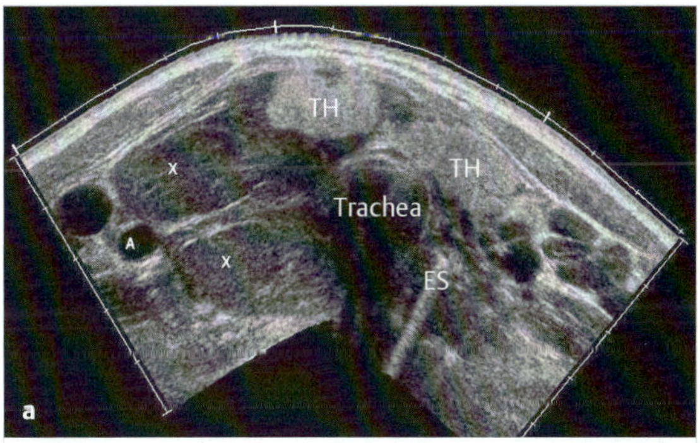

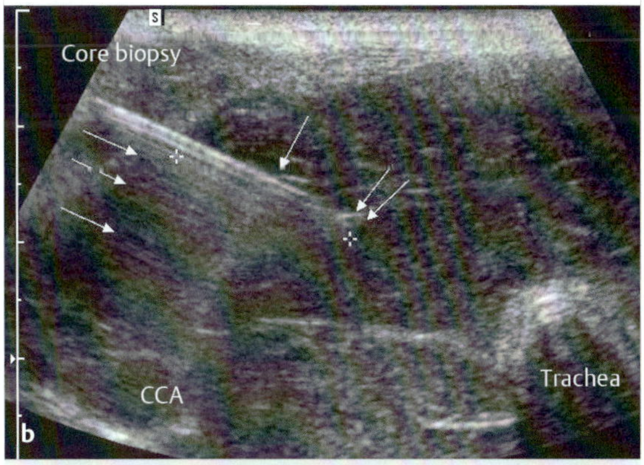

Fig. 27.13
a Core needle biopsy of a thyroid tumor 3 days after an inconclusive fine needle aspiration. Axial panoramic ultrasound scan of the neck. Remnants of normal thyroid tissue (TH) are visible anterior and to the left of the trachea. Hypoechoic tumor invasion (X) is especially prominent in the thyroid right lobe. The reverberations are caused by air in the esophagus. A, cross-section of the right carotid artery; ES, esophagus.
b Long-axis view displays the full length of the needle, introduced obliquely through the skin into the tumor tissue (single arrow, needle shaft; two arrows, needle tip; three arrows, reverberations distal to the needle). Histology and immunohistochemistry revealed thyroid infiltration by malignant lymphoma.

benign lesion) are Hashimoto thyroiditis mistaken for lymphoma (see ▶ Fig. 27.3) and follicular or Hurthle cell adenomas mistaken for papillary carcinoma.

There are numerous ways to help reduce **false-negative findings** in the FNA of focal thyroid lesions:

- Use continuous sonographic guidance using long-axis technique.
- Needle into the lesion fanwise.
- Sample material from the lesion periphery rather than the (necrotic) center.
- Make two or three passes.
- Use proper smear technique.
- Consult with the cytologist on fixation method.
- Involve an experienced cytopathologist.

27.2 Therapeutic Interventions

Therapeutic procedures on the thyroid gland are of two main types: evacuation procedures and destructive (ablative) procedures. The procedures and their indications are reviewed in ▶ Table 27.2.

Table 27.1 Technical problems and their solutions

Problem	Solution
Poor visualization of the needle tip	• Use long-axis technique • Move the transducer in a "radar" sweep • Twitch the needle tip • Use tissue harmonic imaging (THI) • Turn on color Doppler mode and twitch the needle tip • Learning curve, expertise!
No aspirate	• Target a more peripheral portion of the nodule • Core needle biopsy
Bloody aspirate	• Second pass with less or no suction • Use the "drill" technique • Discontinue suction (release the plunger) when aspirate appears in the syringe

Table 27.2 Therapeutic thyroid interventions: indications and procedures

Indications	Evacuation procedures	Ablative procedures
Abscess	Single or repetitive needle aspirations Drainage	
Symptomatic cysts	Single or repetitive needle aspirations Catheter drainage	Percutaneous ethanol injection
Hyperfunctioning nodules		Percutaneous ethanol injection (radiofrequency ablation, percutaneous laser ablation)
"Cold" nodules		(Percutaneous ethanol injection)

27.2.1 Evacuation Procedures

This category includes single or multiple percutaneous fluid aspirations (with a 20-gauge needle) and catheter drainage procedures (using 6F to 8F pigtail catheters).

Indication: Symptomatic Cyst

Most thyroid cysts are benign and result from degenerative changes or intralesional hemorrhage in colloid nodules or adenomas. Because malignancy may also occasionally develop in complex cysts and because malignant tumors may undergo cystic degeneration,[30] malignancy should be excluded before local ablative treatment is performed. Solid components should be biopsied in making this determination.

In the initial examination of a thyroid cyst, therefore, we perform a detailed ultrasound examination that includes color Doppler evaluation of solid peripheral areas. Afterward the cyst is completely evacuated with a 20-gauge needle and the aspirate is examined cytologically (see ▶ Fig. 27.9a, b).

After the needle is removed, the patient compresses the puncture site with a sterile pad for at least 10 minutes. In our experience, approximately 20% of percutaneously aspirated thyroid cysts will not recur owing to irritation of the cyst wall by the penetrating needle, slight intracystic hemorrhage during the procedure (endogenous fibrin glue!), and local compression after the aspiration.

If a symptomatic cyst recurs and tumor cells were excluded in the initial aspirate, the patient is offered the two therapeutic options of surgical treatment or percutaneous ethanol injection.

Indication: Abscess

Thyroid abscesses are a serious acute disease that requires immediate treatment. The diagnosis is established by fine needle aspiration. If pus is obtained, it is sent for microbiologic testing followed by local therapy. Needle aspiration may be adequate for small abscesses (< 3 cm, see ▶ Fig. 27.4), while larger abscesses are drained with 8F pigtail catheters under sonographic guidance according to the general principles of abscess treatment.[31]

27.2.2 Ablative Procedures

Percutaneous Ethanol Injection

Thyroid adenomas are traditionally treated medically, surgically, or by radioiodine therapy. Based on positive experience with ultrasound-guided percutaneous ethanol injection (PEI) for the palliative and curative treatment of small hepatocellular carcinomas, Livraghi et al first reported in 1990 on percutaneous alcohol injections for the treatment of autonomous thyroid adenomas.[32] The procedure, which we modified by injecting smaller amounts of ethanol per session and by using color Doppler ultrasound,[33–35] is now practiced at many centers.

The goal of PEI is to render the autonomous adenoma nonfunctioning. The procedure induces a coagulative necrosis of the parenchyma and local thrombosis of intranodal vessels. Effective PEI will shrink nodules by more than 50% of their initial volume. Solitary adenomas and nodules smaller than 10 cm^3 show better remission rates than nodules larger than 3 to 4 cm in diameter and oligofocal nodules. The degree of vascularity is recognized as a diagnostic criterion for adenoma activity, and the regression of vascularity provides an early prognostic index for the efficacy of PEI. By contrast, it takes several weeks for normalization of TSH levels to occur.[33,34]

Table 27.3 Percutaneous ethanol injection: indications and therapeutic goals

Indication	Goal
Focal autonomy with or without hyperthyroidism	Normalization of thyroid function
Thyroid cyst	Cure
Nonfunctioning ("cold") nodule	Nodule shrinkage
Thyroid cancer (recurrent)	Tumor shrinkage

The primary response rates in our patients are approximately 90%. Partial destruction (approximately 50% mean reduction in nodule volume) is sufficient to reestablish a euthyroid state.[33] Similar response rates have been reported at other centers.[36–39] Long-term results after 12 years' follow-up ($n = 113$) at our center indicate an 80% response rate for toxic adenomas and 73% for pretoxic adenomas. Twelve percent of the patients in each group had a recurrence, and primary treatment results were unsuccessful in 8% and 15%, respectively.

Thus, PEI provides a low-risk, cost-effective alternative to surgery or radioiodine therapy in the curative treatment of unifocal or oligofocal autonomous adenomas with latent or overt hyperthyroidism (see ▶ Table 27.3, ▶ Table 27.4). Since randomized comparative studies have yet to be conducted, PEI is still reserved for selected cases.

The efficacy of this therapy has also been documented in the treatment of thyroid cysts.[40] Symptomatic thyroid cysts are usually ablated by one or two ethanol injections. Pain is less common than in the treatment of autonomous adenomas, and late sequelae such as dysphonia or hypothyroidism have not been observed. The only therapeutic alternative is surgery, which is associated with higher risks (bleeding, recurrent laryngeal nerve damage, hypocalcemia, parenchymal loss with significant hypothyroidism), potentially objectionable scarring, and significantly higher costs.

In a randomized study of cold thyroid nodules, Bennedbaek et al (1998) found that a single ethanol injection into a solitary colloid thyroid nodule was more effective in producing nodule shrinkage and growth control than one year of suppressive thyroxine therapy.[41] We do not use ethanol injection therapy for this indication[42] because cold nodules have a residual risk of malignancy, and the alcohol-induced necrosis and granulomatous scar tissue formation would hamper cytologic and histologic follow-ups. Several reports indicate that PEI can be used palliatively for the shrinkage of recurrent thyroid cancers, but there is a lack of studies with conclusive data.[43] Current international consensus guidelines recommend PEI only for the treatment of cysts based on available long-term results.[9]

▶ Table 27.5 lists situations that would be favorable or unfavorable for the treatment of focal autonomy by PEI.

Table 27.4 Percutaneous ethanol injection: advantages and disadvantages

Advantages	Disadvantages
No surgical complications	Multiple sittings required
No scarring	No comparative studies randomized for standard procedures
No radiation exposure	
Preserves healthy tissue	
No risk of hypothyroidism	
No hypoparathyroidism	
Low cost	

Contraindications

The basic contraindications are the same as those listed under fine needle aspiration of the thyroid.

We do not perform PEI in anticoagulated patients or if the platelet count is less than 80×10^9/L. PEI should not be performed in thyrotoxic crisis without thyrostatic premedication, as it may cause a transient rise in serum thyroid hormone levels.

PEI is contraindicated in the treatment of latent or overt hyperthyroidism in Graves disease and is used only in highly selected cases of multifocal or diffuse autonomy.

Materials and Supplies

Basic materials and supplies are the same as for fine needle aspiration of the thyroid. Supplies should also include 96% alcohol and 0.5 to 2 mL of local anesthetic solution (2% lidocaine).

Table 27.5 Situations favorable or unfavorable for PEI[33,34,38,52]

Favorable situations	Unfavorable situations
One or two adenomas	Large nodular goiter
Adenoma < 4 cm (< 30 mL)	Nodule > 4.5 cm (> 45 mL)
Multimorbidity	Nodule at "exposed" location
Patient refuses surgery and radioiodine therapy	Coagulation disorder
Nodule location: central, good clearance from carotid artery, jugular vein, and recurrent laryngeal nerve	Patient < 20 years of age (?)
Clear visualization by scintigraphy, ultrasound (color Doppler)	
Patient > 40 years of age (?)	

Source: modified from Blank W, Braun B. Ethanol instillation of adenoma of the thyroid gland—a five-year experience. Minimally Invasive Therapy & Allied Technologies 1998;7:581–588, with permission from Informa Healthcare.

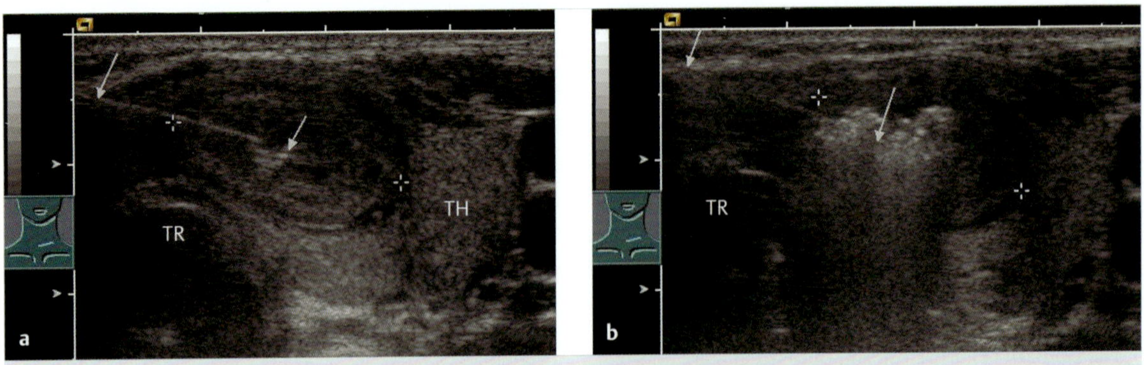

Fig. 27.14
a Ethanol injection into an autonomous adenoma in the thyroid left lobe. The needle has been introduced obliquely from the right side of the neck using classic technique and is visible over its entire length (arrows). The needle tip, marked by reverberations, has been positioned at the center of the nodule (+ +). TR, trachea; TH, normal echogenic thyroid tissue in the left lobe.
b Ethanol injection produces a typical snowstorm pattern, which partially obscures the needle tip (right arrow).

Preparation

Since PEI has an inherently higher complication rate than thyroid FNA, patients require a more comprehensive disclosure of information. Written informed consent should cover the advantages and disadvantages of PEI, alternatives (surgery or radioiodine therapy for autonomous adenoma; surgery for cyst), the principle of the procedure, and the steps involved.

The patient is placed in a semi-sitting position like that for FNA. We prefer to have just one physician perform the procedure, aided by a nurse or physician's assistant.

The patient is told to raise his or her hand or "hum" if pain is felt during the alcohol injection and to lower the hand again when the pain subsides (generally within 20–30 seconds). The patient should avoid swallowing during the injection.

Indication: Adenomas

PEI has the following indications in the treatment of autonomous functioning adenomas (thyroid autonomy):

- Small, solitary nodule (< 15 mL)
- Large nodules prior to radioiodine therapy
- Large nodules or multifocal autonomy (2–3 nodules) in multimorbid patients
- Side effects from thyrostatic drugs
- Iodine-induced hyperthyroidism
- Refusal of surgery or radioiodine therapy
- Hyperthyroidism in pregnancy

Procedure

When the freehand technique is used, one hand holds the transducer while the other hand controls the needle and syringe. This allows the operator to maintain constant control of all cervical structures, vary the scan plane, and control the ethanol injection with better precision.

The steps are as follows:

- The skin is aseptically prepared (e.g., with Kodan tincture forte [Schülke & Mayr], clear), and the transducer is disinfected (e.g., with Microbac tissues [BODE Chemie]).
- The volume of the targeted nodule is determined (height × width × depth × 0.5).
- The skin is numbed with a minimal amount of local anesthetic (0.5–1 mL) to prevent acoustic shadowing while eliminating skin pain during needle movements.
- Only now is the ethanol (96%, 5 mL) drawn into the syringe. The operator should do this personally to avoid any confusion.
- The 20-gauge needle on the alcohol syringe is introduced slowly. The long-axis view (▸ Fig. 27.14a) is ideal for monitoring needle insertion. If a short-axis view is necessary for technical reasons, the position of the needle tip should be checked and documented in two planes.
- When the needle tip is in position, a trial injection of 0.1 mL ethanol is made to produce a "snowstorm" echo pattern and confirm correct placement.
- Only then is the injection continued, instilling no more than 1 mL of ethanol in 30 to 60 seconds. The patient should try not to swallow but may be told to perform an "e" phonation during the injection. The diffusion of the alcohol within the nodule appears in the B-mode image as a spreading "snowstorm" cloud of very high-amplitude echoes (▸ Fig. 27.14b).
- Since the needle tip is obscured by the echo cloud, the initial injection should be made in the deeper portion of the nodule. The needle tip is then retracted slightly to inject the more superficial portions.
- If the patient feels pain during the alcohol injection, they should give the designated hand signal or "hum." The injection is paused until the pain subsides.
- We inject approximately **1 mL of ethanol per centimeter nodule diameter** in one session, according to

subjective tolerance. This dose will not cause too much of a pressure rise inside the nodule—the actual cause of the pain—and it will reduce the risk of alcohol diffusing back through the thyroid capsule toward the recurrent laryngeal nerve or refluxing into the needle tract (and thus into the pain-sensitive subcutaneous tissue).
- When the injection is completed, the syringe and needle are left in place for one additional minute.
- After the needle is removed, the patient lightly compresses the puncture site with a sterile gauze pad for 2 to 3 minutes.
- After that, the patient sits upright and an adhesive dressing is applied. An ice pack is placed over the injection site for 10 to 15 minutes.
- Before the patient leaves the recovery room about 15 minutes later, the treating physician speaks with the patient to assess voice quality and, if necessary, make an appointment for the next session.
- At follow-up several days to one week later, the treatment result is assessed by contrast-enhanced ultrasound. High vascularity indicates portions of the adenoma that were not ablated by PEI (▶ Fig. 27.15).

- PEI therapy is performed 1 or 2 times weekly and is generally concluded after 3 to 5 sessions, depending on nodule size (▶ Fig. 27.16).

Complications

Up to 21% of patients who undergo PEI experience mild neck pain during the first 24 hours after the procedure. Rare complications are transient skin irritation, dysphonia, and pressure sensation. One case of laryngeal necrosis was reported after inadvertent alcohol injection into parathyroid tissue.[36,44]

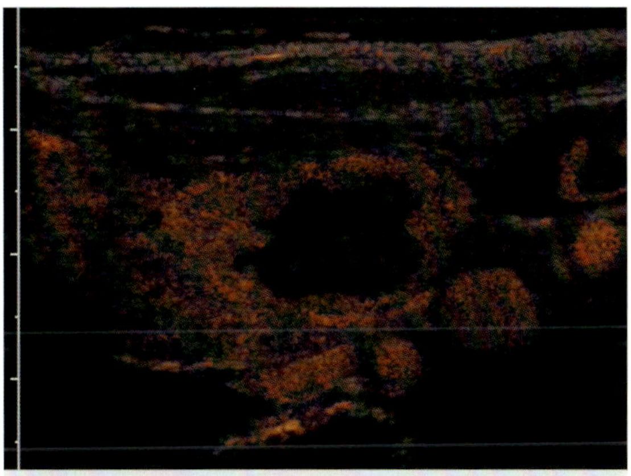

Fig. 27.15 Contrast-enhanced ultrasound 1 week after PEI (low-MI mode, Acuson CPS [Siemens]) shows a large central necrotic zone in the treated adenoma, but the peripheral area is still perfused. Another treatment session was scheduled.

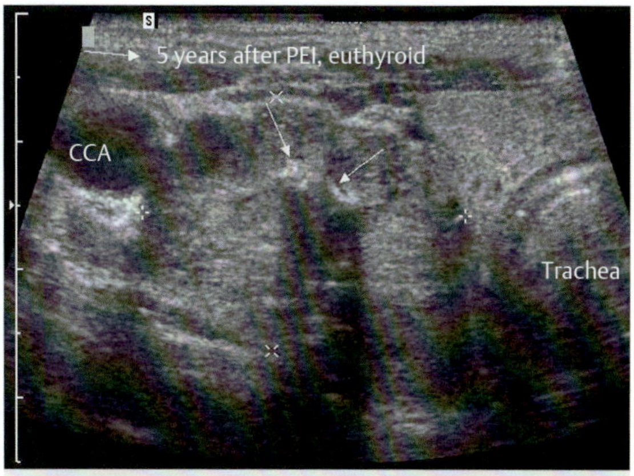

Fig. 27.16 Status 5 years after PEI for nodular goiter and hyperthyroidism. The adenoma (+ +) in the thyroid right lobe has shrunk to 40% of its initial volume and has a central calcified scar (arrows). Homogeneously echogenic thyroid tissue is visible anterior to the trachea. The patient is clinically and chemically euthyroid.

▶ **Neck pain.** Because the needle remains in place for several minutes and is repeatedly moved into different portions of the nodule to improve alcohol distribution and sonographic visualization of the needle tip, the insertion site should be anesthetized with 0.5 to 1 mL of 2% lidocaine.

During the ethanol injection, the patient may experience a local pressure sensation radiating toward the jaw and ipsilateral ear. This is caused by the tension and increased volume of the injected nodule. Whereas Livraghi et al[32] administered more than 10 cm^3 of ethanol in one sitting, we limit the dose to 1 to 5 mL per session. We also reduce pain by instilling the agent extremely slowly and carefully, and when pain occurs we pause the injection (generally for about 30 seconds) until the patient signals that the pain has subsided (see ▶ Table 27.6).

Pain may also be caused by ethanol diffusing back into the needle tract, inciting a chemical irritation of superficial cervical structures (platysma, subcutaneous tissue, skin). The rules for prevention of this are as follows:
- Avoid rapid injection.
- Do not inject too much ethanol in one session (never more than 5 mL).

Table 27.6 Essential points during PEI

Criterion/Observation	Response/Action
Select the proper injection site	Position the needle tip toward the center of the nodule, at least 3–5 mm from its margin.
Confirm the needle position	Check it carefully in two planes.
If the needle tip penetrates the posterior edge of the thyroid gland or the posterior margin of the nodule	Do not inject ethanol (risk of recurrent laryngeal nerve injury!).
Pressure sensation	Pause the ethanol injection.

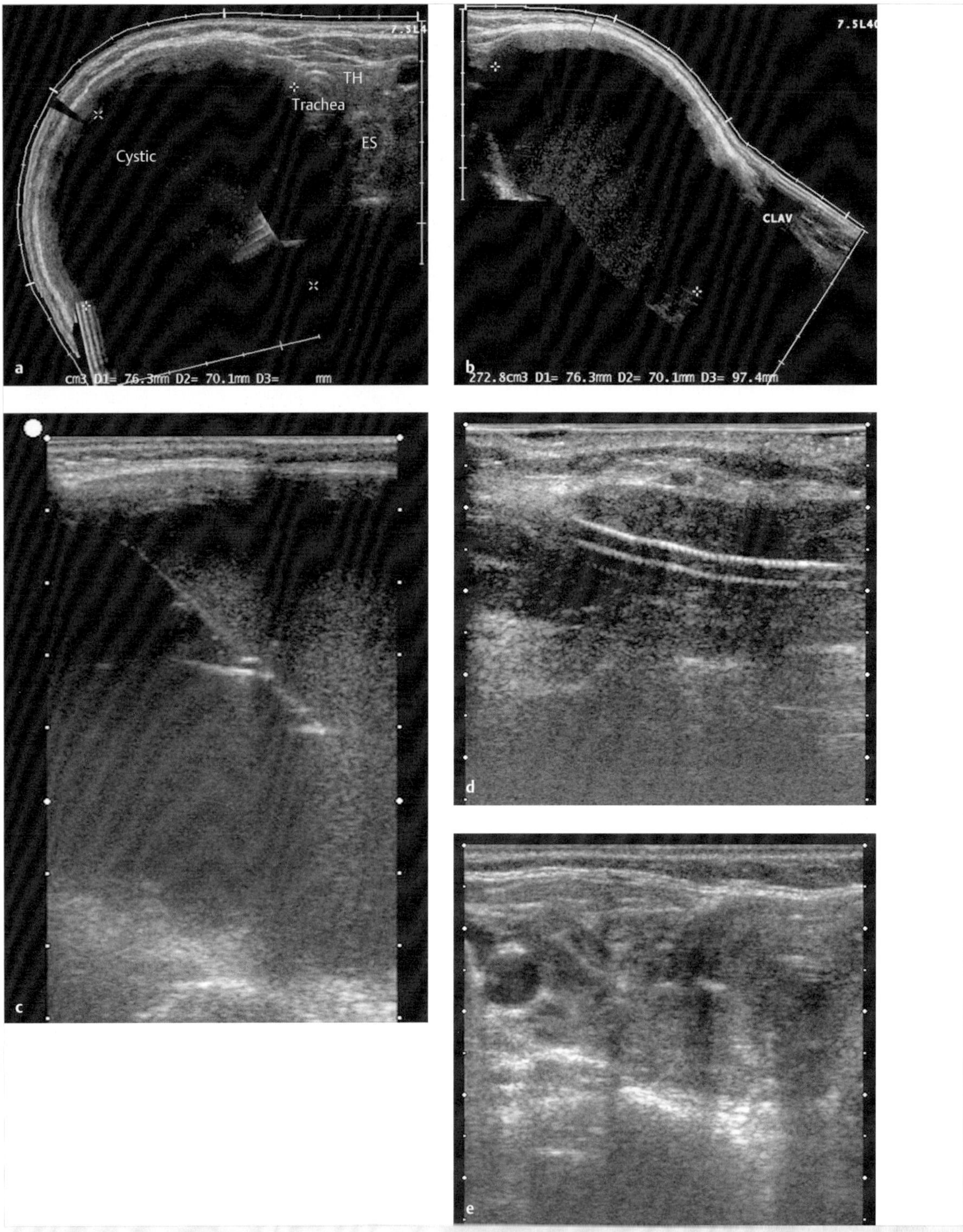

Fig. 27.17
a Axial panoramic scan of a symptomatic cyst in the right thyroid lobe with a volume of 273 mL.
b Longitudinal panoramic scan of the same cyst.
c A primary 14-gauge needle has been introduced into the cyst in the long-axis view. A drainage catheter is subsequently placed over a Seldinger wire.
d The drain appears as parallel echogenic lines.
e The instillation of 70 mL ethanol produces an immediate echogenic transformation of the cyst contents. The drain is no longer delineated.

- Leave the needle in place for 30 to 60 seconds after the injection is completed.
- If desired, slowly inject 0.5 to 1 mL of 2% lidocaine as the needle is withdrawn.
- Place an ice pack on the neck for 10 to 15 minutes after the injection.

▶ **Exacerbation of hyperthyroidism.** An acute rise of serum thyroglobulin levels due to the destruction of thyroid follicles has been documented after PEI, contrasting with only a minimal rise in thyroid hormones.

Elderly patients and cardiac-risk patients in particular should be treated with beta blockers for 5 days before PEI (e.g., 3 × 10 to 20 mg propranolol/day) or with carbimazole for 10 days before PEI (10 to 30 mg/day).

▶ **Ability to drive a motor vehicle.** Studies of percutaneous ethanol injection in the liver did not show a significant rise in blood alcohol levels.[45]

▶ **Adhesions.** Studies after technically correct ethanol instillations showed no scarring or adhesions in the thyroid gland or cervical structures. Later thyroid operations could be performed without difficulty.[46]

Pitfalls in Percutaneous Ethanol Injection

The pitfalls In PEI include the following:

- Undetected malignancy. This is why we do not perform PEI on cold nodules!
- Hot nodules are almost certainly benign.
- We consider that PEI is contraindicated in high-risk patients with prior radiation to the neck or a positive family history of thyroid malignancy. A suspected tumor should first be excluded by diagnostic FNA.
- When dealing with cysts, we first await the cytology result on the aspirate. Only recurrent cysts are treated by PEI.

Indication: Cysts

Percutaneous ethanol instillation is the procedure of choice for symptomatic and recurrent thyroid cysts after the exclusion of malignancy. Cure rates average 82% with a relapse rate of approximately 6%. PEI is more effective than simple needle aspiration or the instillation of saline solution.[40,47]

The steps are as follows:

- We use a one-operator technique in which the sonographer holds the transducer in one hand and inserts the needle with the other.
- When dealing with cysts > 50 mL (▶ Fig. 27.17), we place an 8F pigtail catheter to drain the contents and instill alcohol. The cyst contents should not be drained completely to ensure that the drain side holes will not slip out of the collapsed cyst.
- The needle is displayed in a long-axis view (▶ Fig. 27.17c). The cyst is aspirated with a 20- or 50-mL syringe, depending on the calculated cyst volume, and is almost completely evacuated.
- The needle, whose tip is clearly visible sonographically in the small amount of residual fluid, is stabilized and a syringe with 96% ethanol is connected to it.
- The ethanol is slowly instilled (2–3 minutes), administering a volume equal to 25% to at most 50% of the previously aspirated volume.
- Then the needle is left in place for at least 1 minute. The operator waits for the pressure in the residual cyst to fall in order to avoid ethanol reflux into the needle tract.
- After the needle is removed, the needle tract is lightly compressed for 1 to 2 minutes, an adhesive dressing is applied, and an ice pack is placed on the neck for 10 to 15 minutes.
- If a drain has been placed, the ethanol is aspirated from the cyst after 30 minutes. The drain is left in place until the next day to prevent ethanol seepage into surrounding tissues.

Postprocedure Care and Follow-up

The patient leaves the hospital approximately 30 minutes after the procedure following local inspection of the injection site and the assessment of phonation. We perform an ultrasound follow-up only if there is a recurrent swelling in the neck.

Radiofrequency Ablation; Percutaneous Laser Ablation

Ultrasound-guided radiofrequency ablation (RFA) has been advocated as an alternative to PEI for the treatment of adenomas and malignancies[48,49] and percutaneous laser ablation (PLA) for the treatment of adenomas, cold nodules, and cysts.[50,51] These procedures are considerably more costly and technically complex than PEI. While some randomized studies have indicated good results for both procedures, the majority are based on small case numbers. Consequently, neither RFA nor PLA has become established as a standard procedure in the treatment of thyroid adenomas and malignancies.[9]

References

[1] Braun B, Blank W. Ultrasonography of the thyroid and parathyroid gland [Article in German]. Internist (Berl) 2006; 47: 729–746, quiz 747

[2] Gharib H. Changing concepts in the diagnosis and management of thyroid nodules. Endocrinol Metab Clin North Am 1997; 26: 777–800

[3] Can AS, Peker K. Comparison of palpation-versus ultrasound-guided fine-needle aspiration biopsies in the evaluation of thyroid nodules. BMC Res Notes 2008; 1: 12

[4] Danese D, Sciacchitano S, Farsetti A, Andreoli M, Pontecorvi A. Diagnostic accuracy of conventional versus sonography-guided fine-needle aspiration biopsy of thyroid nodules. Thyroid 1998; 8: 15–21

[5] Gharib H. Changing trends in thyroid practice: understanding nodular thyroid disease. Endocr Pract 2004; 10: 31–39

[6] García-Mayor RV, Pérez Mendez LF, Páramo C et al. Fine-needle aspiration biopsy of thyroid nodules: impact on clinical practice. J Endocrinol Invest 1997; 20: 482–487

[7] Kim EK, Park CS, Chung WY et al. New sonographic criteria for recommending fine-needle aspiration biopsy of nonpalpable solid nodules of the thyroid. AJR Am J Roentgenol 2002; 178: 687–691

[8] Paschke R. Diagnostic work-up of euthyroid nodules: which nodules should undergo fine-needle aspiration biopsy? Relevance of ultrasound [Article in German]. Dtsch Med Wochenschr 2009; 134: 2498–2503

[9] Gharib H, Papini E, Paschke R et al. AACE/AME/ETA Task Force on Thyroid Nodules. American Association of Clinical Endocrinologists, Associazione Medici Endocrinologi, and EuropeanThyroid Association Medical Guidelines for Clinical Practice for the Diagnosis and Management of Thyroid Nodules. Endocr Pract 2010; 16 (Suppl 1): 1–43

[10] Berner A, Pradhan M, Jørgensen L, Heilo A, Grøholt KK. Fine needle cytology of the thyroid gland [Article in Norwegian]. Tidsskr Nor Laegeforen 2004; 124: 2359–2361

[11] Bhatki AM, Brewer B, Robinson-Smith T, Nikiforov Y, Steward DL. Adequacy of surgeon-performed ultrasound-guided thyroid fine-needle aspiration biopsy. Otolaryngol Head Neck Surg 2008; 139: 27–31

[12] Kim DW, Park AW, Lee EJ et al. Ultrasound-guided fine-needle aspiration biopsy of thyroid nodules smaller than 5 mm in the maximum diameter: assessment of efficacy and pathological findings. Korean J Radiol 2009; 10: 435–440

[13] Cha C, Chen H, Westra WH, Udelsman R. Primary thyroid lymphoma: can the diagnosis be made solely by fine-needle aspiration? Ann Surg Oncol 2002; 9: 298–302

[14] Kwak JY, Kim EK, Ko KH et al. Primary thyroid lymphoma: role of ultrasound-guided needle biopsy. J Ultrasound Med 2007; 26: 1761–1765

[15] Harvey JN, Parker D, De P, Shrimali RK, Otter M. Sonographically guided core biopsy in the assessment of thyroid nodules. J Clin Ultrasound 2005; 33: 57–62

[16] Khoo TK, Baker CH, Hallanger-Johnson J et al. Comparison of ultrasound-guided fine-needle aspiration biopsy with core-needle biopsy in the evaluation of thyroid nodules. Endocr Pract 2008; 14: 426–431

[17] Screaton NJ, Berman LH, Grant JW. US-guided core-needle biopsy of the thyroid gland. Radiology 2003; 226: 827–832

[18] Polyzos SA, Anastasilakis AD. Clinical complications following thyroid fine-needle biopsy: a systematic review. Clin Endocrinol (Oxf) 2009; 71: 157–165

[19] Ito Y, Tomoda C, Uruno T et al. Needle tract implantation of papillary thyroid carcinoma after fine-needle aspiration biopsy. World J Surg 2005; 29: 1544–1549

[20] Kim MJ, Kim EK, Park SI et al. US-guided fine-needle aspiration of thyroid nodules: indications, techniques, results. Radiographics 2008; 28: 1869–1886; discussion 1887

[21] Yokozawa T, Fukata S, Kuma K et al. Thyroid cancer detected by ultrasound-guided fine-needle aspiration biopsy. World J Surg 1996; 20: 848–853; discussion 853

[22] Bellantone R, Lombardi CP, Raffaelli M et al. Management of cystic or predominantly cystic thyroid nodules: the role of ultrasound-guided fine-needle aspiration biopsy. Thyroid 2004; 14: 43–47

[23] Merz E. Transducer hygiene—an underrated topic? [Article in English, German]. Ultraschall Med 2005; 26: 7–8

[24] Caturelli E, Villani MR, Schiavone G et al. Safety and low cost of "free-hand" technique with ordinary antisepsis in abdominal US-guided fine-needle punctures: clinical report of a four-year experience. Eur J Ultrasound 1997; 6: 131–134

[25] Robert Koch-Institut. Anforderungen an die Hygiene bei Punktionen und Injektionen. Bundesgesundheitsblatt 2011; 54: 1135–1144

[26] Kim DW, Rho MH, Kim KN. Ultrasound-guided fine-needle aspiration biopsy of thyroid nodules: is it necessary to use local anesthesia for the application of one needle puncture? Korean J Radiol 2009; 10: 441–446

[27] Jakobeit C. Ultrasound-controlled puncture procedures: free-hand puncture versus transducer biopsy puncture. 5 years' experience [Article in German]. Ultraschall Med 1986; 7: 290–292

[28] Pinchot SN, Al-Wagih H, Schaefer S, Sippel R, Chen H. Accuracy of fine-needle aspiration biopsy for predicting neoplasm or carcinoma in thyroid nodules 4 cm or larger. Arch Surg 2009; 144: 649–655

[29] Lee YH, Lee NJ, Kim JH, Suh SI, Kim TK, Song JJ. Sonographically guided fine needle aspiration of thyroid nodule: discrepancies between cytologic and histopathologic findings. J Clin Ultrasound 2008; 36: 6–11

[30] de los Santos ET, Keyhani-Rofagha S, Cunningham JJ, Mazzaferri EL. Cystic thyroid nodules. The dilemma of malignant lesions. Arch Intern Med 1990; 150: 1422–1427

[31] Yeow KM, Liao CT, Hao SP. US-guided needle aspiration and catheter drainage as an alternative to open surgical drainage for uniloculated neck abscesses. J Vasc Interv Radiol 2001; 12: 589–594

[32] Livraghi T, Paracchi A, Ferrari C et al. Treatment of autonomous thyroid nodules with percutaneous ethanol injection: preliminary results. Work in progress. Radiology 1990; 175: 827–829

[33] Blank W, Braun B. Ethanol instillation of adenoma of the thyroid gland – a five-year experience. Minim Invasive Ther Allied Technol 1998; 7: 581–588

[34] Braun B, Blank W. Color Doppler sonography-guided percutaneous alcohol instillation in the therapy of functionally autonomous thyroid nodules [Article in German]. Dtsch Med Wochenschr 1994; 119: 1607–1612

[35] Braun B, Blank W. Ultrasound-guided alcohol instillation in treatment of autonomous thyroid adenoma [Article in German]. Ultraschall Med 1994; 15: 159–162

[36] Janowitz P, Ackmann S. Long-term results of ultrasound-guided ethanol injections in patients with autonomous thyroid nodules and hyperthyroidism [Article in German]. Med Klin (Munich) 2001; 96: 451–456

[37] Lippi F, Ferrari C, Manetti L et al. The Multicenter Study Group. Treatment of solitary autonomous thyroid nodules by percutaneous ethanol injection: results of an Italian multicenter study. J Clin Endocrinol Metab 1996; 81: 3261–3264

[38] Livraghi T, Paracchi A, Ferrari C, Reschini E, Macchi RM, Bonifacino A. Treatment of autonomous thyroid nodules with percutaneous ethanol injection: 4-year experience. Radiology 1994; 190: 529–533

[39] Monzani F, Caraccio N, Goletti O et al. Five-year follow-up of percutaneous ethanol injection for the treatment of hyperfunctioning thyroid nodules: a study of 117 patients. Clin Endocrinol (Oxf) 1997; 46: 9–15

[40] Bennedbaek FN, Hegedüs L. Treatment of recurrent thyroid cysts with ethanol: a randomized double-blind controlled trial. J Clin Endocrinol Metab 2003; 88: 5773–5777

[41] Bennedbaek FN, Nielsen LK, Hegedüs L. Effect of percutaneous ethanol injection therapy versus suppressive doses of L-thyroxine on benign solitary solid cold thyroid nodules: a randomized trial. J Clin Endocrinol Metab 1998; 83: 830–835

[42] Caraccio N, Goletti O, Lippolis PV et al. Is percutaneous ethanol injection a useful alternative for the treatment of the cold benign thyroid nodule? Five years' experience. Thyroid 1997; 7: 699–704

[43] Kim BM, Kim MJ, Kim EK, Park SI, Park CS, Chung WY. Controlling recurrent papillary thyroid carcinoma in the neck by ultrasonography-guided percutaneous ethanol injection. Eur Radiol 2008; 18: 835–842

[44] Mauz PS, Stiegler M, Holderried M, Brosch S. Complications of ultrasound guided percutaneous ethanol injection therapy of the thyroid and parathyroid glands. Ultraschall Med 2005; 26: 142–145

[45] Livraghi T, Lazzaroni S, Pellicanò S, Ravasi S, Torzilli G, Vettori C. Percutaneous ethanol injection of hepatic tumors: single-session therapy with general anesthesia. AJR Am J Roentgenol 1993; 161: 1065–1069

[46] Monzani F, Caraccio N, Basolo F, Iacconi P, LiVolsi V, Miccoli P. Surgical and pathological changes after percutaneous ethanol injection therapy of thyroid nodules. Thyroid 2000; 10: 1087–1092

[47] Del Prete S, Caraglia M, Russo D et al. Percutaneous ethanol injection efficacy in the treatment of large symptomatic thyroid cystic nodules: ten-year follow-up of a large series. Thyroid 2002; 12: 815–821

[48] Jeong WK, Baek JH, Rhim H et al. Radiofrequency ablation of benign thyroid nodules: safety and imaging follow-up in 236 patients. Eur Radiol 2008; 18: 1244–1250

[49] Monchik JM, Donatini G, Iannuccilli J, Dupuy DE. Radiofrequency ablation and percutaneous ethanol injection treatment for recurrent local and distant well-differentiated thyroid carcinoma. Ann Surg 2006; 244: 296–304

[50] Døssing H, Bennedbaek FN, Hegedüs L. Beneficial effect of combined aspiration and interstitial laser therapy in patients with benign cystic thyroid nodules: a pilot study. Br J Radiol 2006; 79: 943–947

[51] Papini E, Bizzarri G, Pacella CM. Percutaneous laser ablation of benign and malignant thyroid nodules. Curr Opin Endocrinol Diabetes Obes 2008; 15: 434–439

[52] Blank W, Braun B. Sonography of the thyroid—part 2: thyroid inflammation, impairmant of thyroid function and interventions [Article in English, German]. Ultraschall Med 2008; 29: 128–149, quiz 150–155

28 Musculoskeletal Interventions

W. Hartung, T. Weigand

Percutaneous interventions on musculoskeletal structures have become well established in both rheumatology and orthopedic surgery and have gained an important role in the diagnosis and treatment of inflammatory and degenerative diseases of the musculoskeletal system. Percutaneous procedures on joints, intra-articular cysts, ganglia, tendon sheaths, and bursae are performed routinely in everyday practice.

Even today, a large percentage of percutaneous procedures are still performed "blind," i.e., the operator is guided by visual and palpable anatomical landmarks in locating the desired route for needle insertion. Several studies have documented the relatively poor precision of "blind" procedures, however. Eustace,[1] for example, found that only 37% of needles had been placed accurately for glenohumeral joint injections. Jones,[2] in a review of 108 joint injections, confirmed correct intra-articular needle placement in just 56 cases (52%), with only a 10% rate of correct needle placements in the subgroup of glenohumeral injections.

Practice

In the light of these findings, "blind" procedures should be limited strictly to joints that are easily accessible and show significant swelling (e.g., a large joint effusion or subdeltoid bursitis).

As the ultrasound imaging of joints has become more widely practiced in rheumatology and orthopedics, ultrasound has emerged as the imaging modality of choice for guiding percutaneous procedures on joints and soft tissues.[3–7] Ultrasound guidance can significantly increase the success rates of both diagnostic and therapeutic interventions.[1] Even the smallest intra-articular effusion (< 1 mL) can be selectively aspirated with high precision.

Moreover, ultrasound-guided joint injections and aspirations can be performed considerably faster than CT- or fluoroscopy-assisted interventions[8] and can be done without radiation exposure to patients or staff.

Two principal techniques are employed in ultrasound-guided musculoskeletal interventions. In one technique the most favorable puncture site is identified sonographically and is marked on the skin with a waterproof marking pen. The needle is then introduced at that site in a separate step. But we prefer the technique described below, in which the needle is introduced under sonographic vision. We believe that this technique is particularly accurate and effective for puncturing small joints and aspirating small fluid volumes.

28.1 Indications and Contraindications

28.1.1 Indications

The indications for ultrasound-guided interventional procedures are basically the same as for all percutaneous procedures on joints and soft tissues.

The general indications are:

- Decompression of joints (reduction of capsular tension) by the aspiration of intra-articular effusions
- Analysis of aspirated material (crystal arthropathies, bacterial effusion, etc.; inflammatory versus non-inflammatory effusion)
- Drug injections (e.g., for local anti-inflammatory treatment of arthritis or activated osteoarthritis, chemical synoviorthesis, etc.)

Special indications are:

- Previous "dry tap" of an ultrasound-detected effusion, with need to retrieve a diagnostic sample
- Needle insertions close to vulnerable anatomical structures (nerves, vessels, etc.), as in the treatment of digital flexor tendon synovitis

28.1.2 Contraindications

- Contraindications to therapeutic joint injections are: Systemic infections
- Skin damage or disease at the injection site
- Tumors about the puncture site
- Fresh fractures near the puncture site
- Suspected bacterial infection of the affected joint
- Prior unsuccessful therapeutic injections in the same region within the previous 6 weeks
- Lack of informed consent
- The following are considered relative contraindications to diagnostic arthrocentesis: Coagulation disorders or anticoagulant therapy (Quick value < 30%, PTT > 50 seconds)
- Note that strong suspicion of septic arthritis does not contraindicate diagnostic arthrocentesis because of the importance of establishing a diagnosis.

28.2 Materials and Equipment

The selection of materials depends partly on the size of the joint and its specific anatomical characteristics (▶ Table 28.1). A small joint such as the MCP (metacarpophalangeal) joint will require a shorter and thinner-gauge needle than a large joint such as the knee. Another consideration is the clinical question, which determines the

Table 28.1 Needles for joint injections and aspirations

Joint region	Manufacturer[a]	Size	Color code	Comment
Small joints (e.g., fingers, toes)	Braun	26G × 1 (0.45 × 25 mm)	Brown	
Medium-sized joints (e.g., wrist, elbow)	Braun	22G × 1¼ (0.7 × 30 mm)	Black	
Large joints (e.g., knee)	Braun	20G × 1½ (0.9 × 40 mm)	Yellow	
Hip	Braun	20G × 2¾ (0.9 × 70 mm)	Yellow	First measure the necessary insertion depth!
		21G × 4¾ (0.8 × 120 mm)	Green	First measure the necessary insertion depth!
Sacroiliac joint	Braun	20G × 2¾ (0.9 × 70 mm)	Yellow	First measure the necessary insertion depth!
		21G × 4¾ (0.8 × 120 mm)	Green	First measure the necessary insertion depth!

[a] Represents products habitually used in our department.

scope of the proposed procedure: will the joint be injected, aspirated, or both? In our experience, an effusion that is echogenic at ultrasound has a high cellularity, indicating the need to use a larger-caliber needle.

No special puncture sets are available for joint interventions. We use ordinary disposable syringes and injection needles (Luer system) that are appropriate for the specific joint region and requirements in ▶ Table 28.1.

For the transducers, we use a probe cover set that includes sterile coupling gel. The size of the cover should fit the length of the linear probe (▶ Table 28.2).

28.3 Procedure

28.3.1 Preparations

Patient position depends on the joint that will be injected or aspirated. Patients are positioned supine for procedures on lower-limb joints and are generally placed in a sitting position for procedures on upper-limb joints (except in patients with circulatory problems, for example). Correct initial positioning of the joint is essential and will help to accomplish the procedure with better speed and accuracy.

Transducer selection depends on joint size. We use a linear probe with a high-frequency bandwidth for small joints (e.g., 8–18 MHz) and a linear probe with a 5- to 10-MHz bandwidth for large and medium-sized joints. In very rare cases we may use a curved array on a hip with a thick soft-tissue envelope, as it will give a larger field of view with better penetration depth due to the low center frequency (3.5 MHz).

The procedure room requires regular cleaning and disinfection of objects and surfaces close to the patient, and additional disinfection is needed after exposure to material contaminated with infectious organisms. The number of staff members in the treatment room during the procedure should be limited to essential personnel. The clothing worn by the physician and assistants should not pose an infection risk, so we don protective clothing that is worn only in the procedure rooms (long-sleeved gown). The hands are cleaned with a hygienic handwash or handrub, and sterile gloves are worn. Conversation should be avoided if possible during the procedure itself, and a mask should always be worn during joint interventions that require a change of syringes.[9]

The injection site and its surroundings should be widely exposed to prevent contamination by clothing items and draped with a sterile towel. They should be antiseptically prepared after any necessary initial cleaning. Any hair that is in the way should be removed with scissors rather than with a razor (which may cause skin injury that promotes infection). The injection site should be generously prepared with antiseptic spray or wipes, thoroughly wetting the skin and leaving the solution in place for at least 1 minute (or perhaps longer; note the manufacturer's recommended contact time).

Sterile, disposable syringes and needles should be used. All sterile-packaged items should be kept sealed until just before the procedure, then opened and laid out ready for

Table 28.2 Ultrasound probe covers

Probe size	Manufacturer	Product ID[a]	Size	Comment
Linear up to 5 cm	Microtek Medical	Ultracover PC1297	8 × 61 cm	
Linear up to 7 cm	Microtek Medical	Ultracover PC1298	10 × 61 cm	
Curved array	Microtek Medical	Ultracover PC1291	13 × 61 cm	Hip joint

[a] Represents products habitually used in our department.

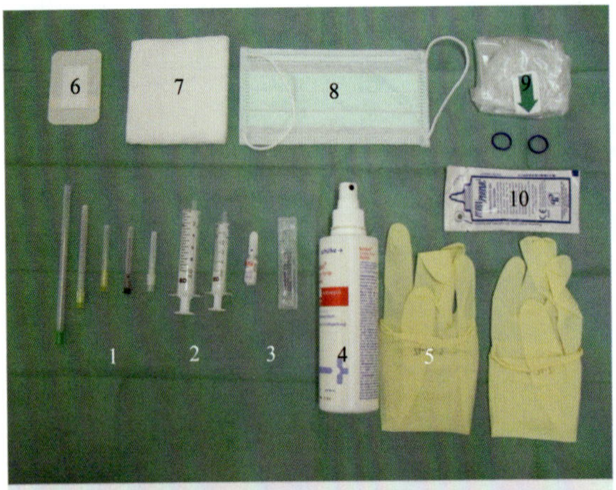

Fig. 28.1 Materials and supplies for ultrasound-guided joint injections and aspirations. **1**: Injection needles (size depends on the joint and indication; small joints require smaller-gauge needles than large joints, and viscous aspirate requires larger needles). **2**: Disposable syringes (for aspiration or injection). **3**: Injectable agent (e.g., triamcinolone or 0.5% lidocaine); an extra needle is required for drawing the agent into the syringe. **4**: Antiseptic spray (for skin preparation and acoustic coupling of the ultrasound probe). **5**: Sterile gloves. **6**: Adhesive dressing to cover the puncture site after the intervention. **7**: Sterile pads. **8**: mask. **9**: Sterile probe cover. **10**: Sterile ultrasound gel.

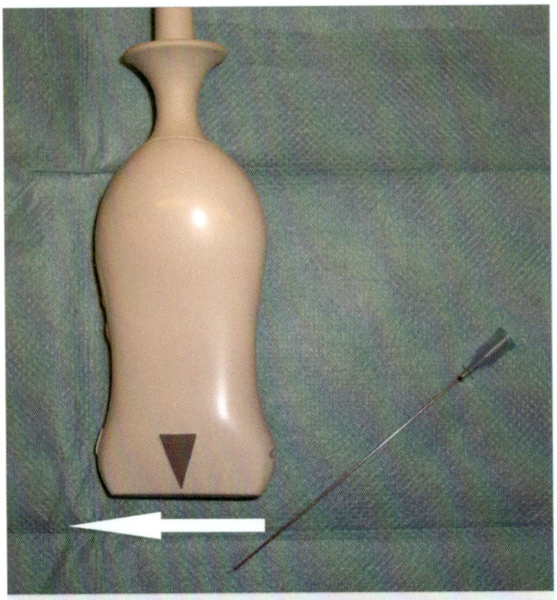

Fig. 28.2 The needle is introduced parallel to the long axis of the ultrasound probe. This provides a long-axis view of the needle shaft (full probe width can be utilized), and the advancing needle tip can be closely monitored. The short-axis technique (probe perpendicular to the needle axis) provides a much more limited view.

use, preferably on a side table covered with a sterile drape (▶ Fig. 28.1). Necessary pharmacologic agents are drawn into the syringes using rigorous sterile technique (the needle used to draw the agent should not be used for the injection!).

Finally a sterile probe cover is placed over the transducer. Some coupling gel is placed into the cover before it is applied.

The needle for an intra-articular injection is *not* introduced through a stab incision.

Caution

If a cold spray is used for cryoanesthesia of the skin, it should never come in contact with the transducer as it could seriously damage the delicate instrument. Consequently, we do not recommend local cryoanesthesia and do not consider it to be necessary.

28.3.2 Overview of Technique

Once an ultrasound-guided musculoskeletal intervention has become routine, it can be practiced by one operator holding both the needle and the ultrasound probe.

When relevant anatomical structures have been identified in two planes, the needle is always directed *parallel to the long axis* of the probe (▶ Fig. 28.2). This technique can display the needle over a long distance (utilizing the full length of the probe) and allows for accurate tracking of the needle tip.

28.3.3 Details of Technique

One operator maintains sonographic guidance while simultaneously performing the intervention itself: the probe is held in one hand ("guide hand") and the needle in the other ("working hand").

This technique requires some precise preliminary work. First the operator images the target region sonographically in the plane of the proposed intervention, taking time to optimize the image quality, penetration depth, focus, and field of view. The necessary needle length is also measured if required. The equipment settings made at this time will be maintained throughout the rest of the procedure. The probe should always be held strictly in one hand.

The probe is acoustically coupled to the skin with antiseptic solution, which is sprayed onto the skin by an assistant as needed. It is unnecessary to place sterile ultrasound gel on the skin, since the generous skin prep will thoroughly wet the skin and ensure good acoustic coupling. Next the targeted structure is displayed sonographically in a long-axis view. The probe should be pressed gently into the soft tissues so that the antiseptic agent will run toward the probe if possible (and away from the needle) and pool around it. This will further reduce the risk of contamination and improve acoustic coupling.

It is unnecessary to make a stab incision in the skin. Local anesthesia is occasionally helpful in anxious patients (e.g., raise a wheal with 1% lidocaine). The empty syringe connected to the puncture needle is held in the "working hand." The needle is introduced using freehand technique. It is inserted into the skin approximately 0.5 to 1 cm from the ultrasound probe. Although the probe is protected with a sterile cover, care should be taken that the probe and needle do not touch each other. The needle is advanced to the intended target site under sonographic guidance.

Next the plunger of the syringe is carefully drawn back to aspirate synovial fluid, for example. If an agent will be injected, the syringe should be changed at this time. It takes skill to disconnect the needle and syringe and reconnect a different syringe with just one hand. If an injection is required, the agent is instilled under sonographic vision and correct needle placement can be checked at that time. Finally the syringe is changed again to flush out any agent still present in the needle bore (e.g., with 1 to 2 mL of 1% lidocaine or 0.9% NaCl), and the needle is removed. Brief compression of the needle tract should be sufficient to prevent bleeding and any leakage of the instilled agent if the soft-tissue envelope is thin. Finally an adhesive dressing is applied to complete the procedure.

Technique at Specific Locations

Joint regions accessible to ultrasound-guided interventions are too numerous to cover individually in this chapter, so we shall illustrate the techniques for several commonly treated joints and tendon sheaths.

All procedures should start with a sonographic assessment of local anatomy, the targeted area, and the location of nearby nerves and blood vessels.

Hip Joint

We perform all injections and aspirations of the hip joint through an anterior approach. The patient is positioned supine with the hip in slight internal rotation (approximately 10°). We use a linear transducer (5–12 MHz).

Following generous skin preparation and the probe preparation described above, the hip is imaged in an anterior longitudinal section by placing the probe in a longitudinal orientation over the femoral neck. This view should display the junction of the femoral head and neck with the target region appearing at the center of the image. The necessary needle length can be accurately estimated from the sonographic image (measure the distance from the skin to the femoral neck). We generally use a needle 12 cm long (0.8 × 120 mm), but a 7-cm needle (0.9 × 70 mm) may be sufficient in thin patients.

By indenting the skin, the probe creates a well that will pool antiseptic solution and improve acoustic coupling. This also lessens the risk of contamination because the solution will flow toward the probe and away from the puncture site.

The needle is introduced parallel to the long axis of the probe, approximately 1 cm caudal to it and angled cephalad approximately 45° to the skin surface (▶ Fig. 28.3a). The needle tip should not be advanced up onto the femoral head, as this could damage the articular cartilage. The optimum needle-tip position is at the junction of the femoral head and neck (▶ Fig. 28.3b). At this point the operator can feel the needle tip come safely into contact with the bone surface. Ultrasound can clearly demonstrate the entry of the needle tip into the distended joint capsule. In that position fluid can be aspirated from the joint and an intra-articular injection can be performed; both steps can be clearly monitored and documented sonographically (▶ Fig. 28.3c).

After an agent (e.g., 1 mL of triamcinolone 40 mg/mL) has been instilled, 1 to 2 mL of 1% lidocaine (or 0.9% NaCl) is additionally injected to flush any residual agent from the needle lumen.

Shoulder

Following preparation of the skin site and ultrasound probe, the optimal puncture site is identified. This site depends partly on the distribution and size of the effusion. The probe is positioned for an anterior transverse scan with the guide hand while the working hand holds the syringe. The needle is introduced approximately 1 cm lateral to the probe (▶ Fig. 28.4a), taking care not to touch the probe with the needle. The needle is advanced in a lateral to medial direction at a 30° to 45° angle under sonographic guidance until the needle tip is precisely within the subdeltoid bursa (▶ Fig. 28.4b). If synovial fluid is being withdrawn on the basis of sonographic findings and for diagnostic purposes, the effusion should be aspirated with an empty syringe. Then the syringe should be disconnected with the working hand before connecting the syringe with the injectable agent and performing the injection. Only in this way can the desired position of the needle be maintained during shifting of the overlying muscles and soft tissues.

Glenohumeral Joint

A needle can be introduced into the glenohumeral joint from the anterior or posterior side. There are three reasons why we always use the posterior approach for ultrasound-guided injections and aspirations of the glenohumeral joint[10]:

- The posterior route poses less risk of injury to nerves, blood vessels, and tendons.
- Ultrasound can more clearly demonstrate key landmarks such as the glenoid, labrum, and humeral head.
- Even very small effusions can be visualized in the posterior recess.

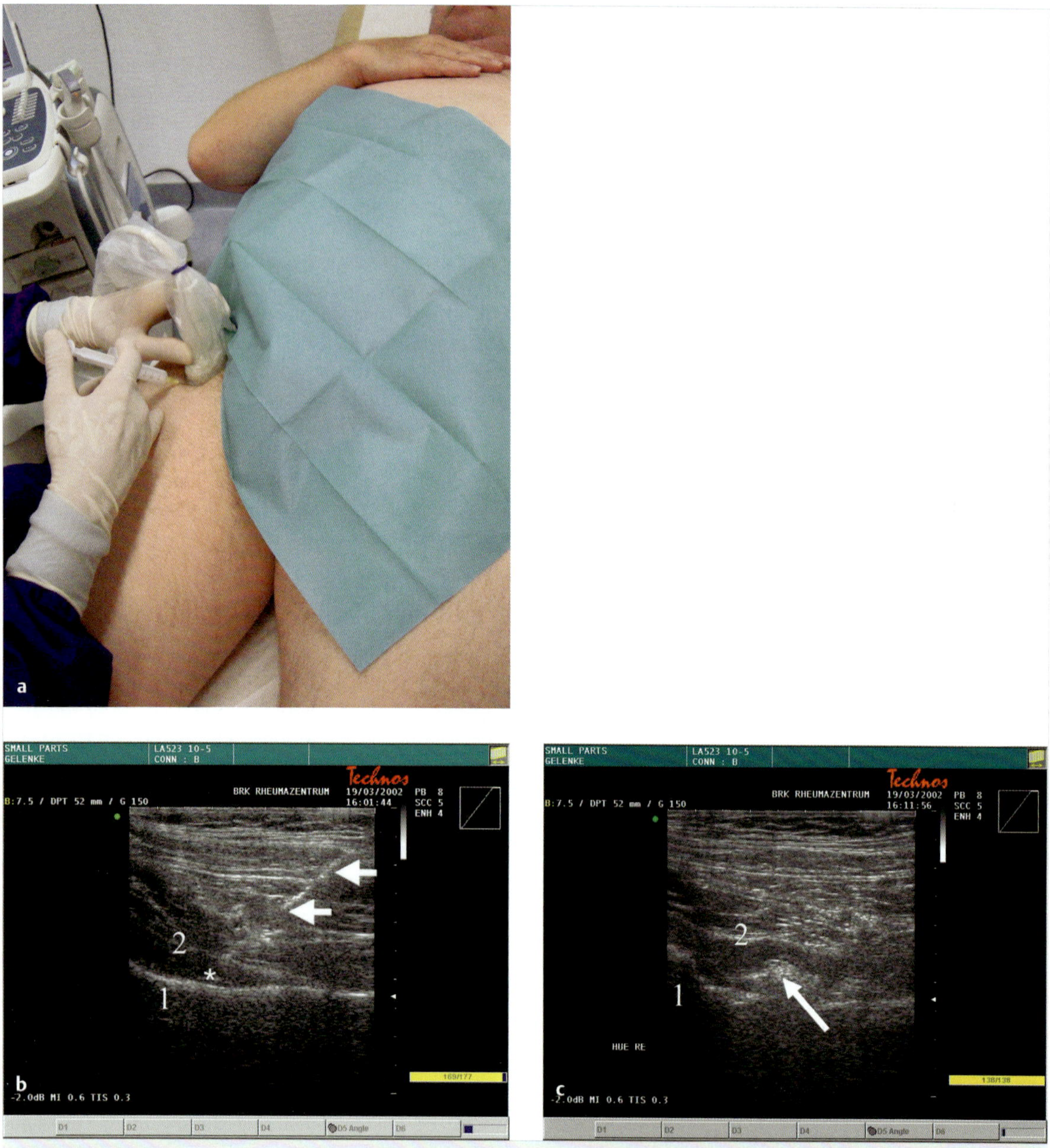

Fig. 28.3 We always perform hip injections and aspirations from the anterior side. Following skin preparation and the placement of a sterile probe cover, the probe is positioned for a long-axis view of the femoral neck. The needle is introduced approximately 1 cm caudal to the probe at an approximately 45° angle to the skin surface.
a The probe should not touch the needle, and the needle tip should not gouge the hyaline cartilage on the femoral head.
b The needle (arrows) has been introduced at an oblique angle and is now advanced into the joint capsule under vision. The needle tip (*) is in the joint capsule. **1**: Femoral neck. **2**: Echo at the joint capsule interface.
c Ultrasound appearance after instillation of triamcinolone. The image confirms precise intra-articular placement of the agent (arrow indicates the high-amplitude echoes produced by the injected solution). **1**: Femur. **2**: Echo at the joint capsule interface.

The operator sits diagonally behind the patient. The patient's upper arm hangs loosely alongside the body in an externally rotated position (which will reveal even small effusions and relax the posterior joint capsule). The needle is introduced in a medial-to-lateral direction at an approximately 60° angle (▶ Fig. 28.5a) while the joint is imaged in a posterior transverse section. Care is taken to display key landmarks: the humeral head, glenoid, labrum, and posterior recess. The needle path runs through the deltoid and infraspinatus muscles into the posterior recess, and the needle tip should be positioned between the glenoid labrum and humeral head

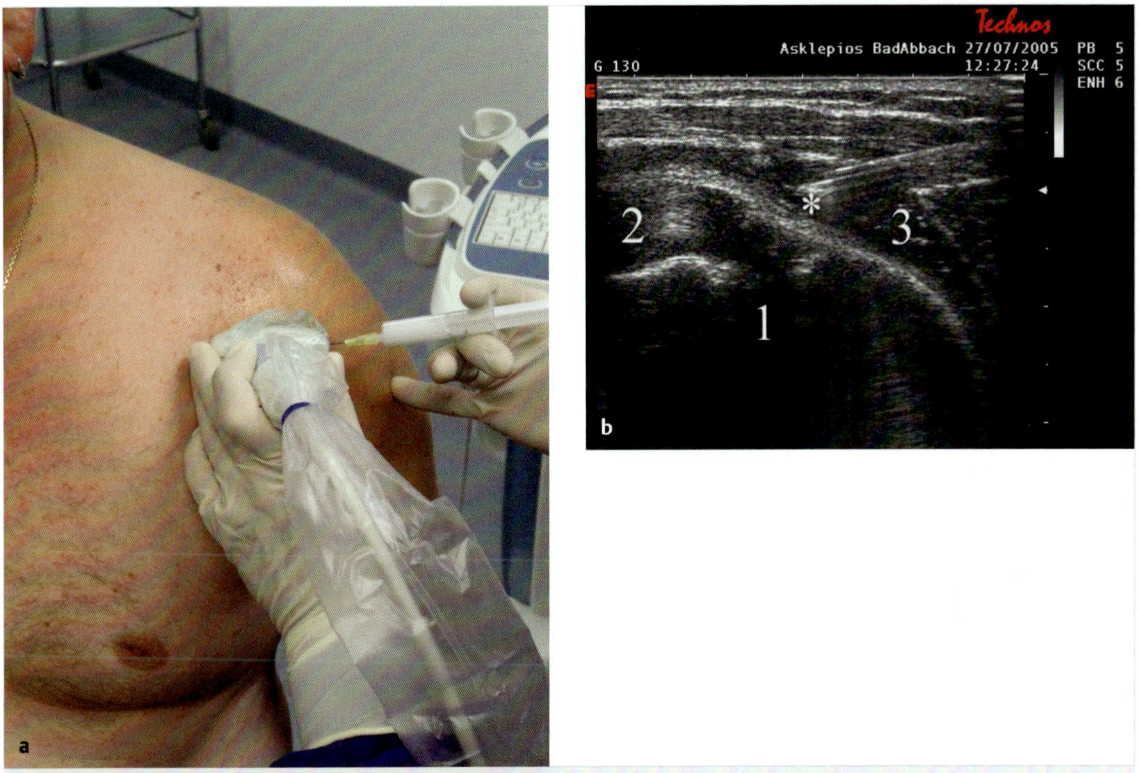

Fig. 28.4 Puncture of the subdeltoid bursa in a patient with rheumatoid arthritis.
a The needle is usually introduced in a lateromedial direction at a 30° to 45° angle under sonographic guidance. This is necessary to ensure an accurate needle position despite significant variations in the overlying muscles and soft tissues.
b The needle is advanced until the tip (✱) is within the subdeltoid bursa (3). Contact with the rotator cuff (2: subscapularis) and humeral head should be avoided. Following accurate needle placement, synovial fluid can be aspirated and/or agents can be instilled.

(▶ Fig. 28.5b). If the angle of insertion of the needle is too steep, the needle tip may not be visualized due to a lack of echo return to the transducer, although it can still be identified indirectly by motion artifacts generated by small-amplitude oscillating movements of the needle. Alternatively, the needle tip can be directly visualized by inserting the needle at a shallower angle (▶ Fig. 28.5b).

28.3.4 Rotator Cuff (Supraspinatus Muscle)

Rotator cuff interventions most commonly involve the supraspinatus muscle, which, for anatomical reasons, is a site of predilection for degenerative changes.[11] After the lesion has been identified, the best access route is determined sonographically. In patients with symptomatic calcifications in the supraspinatus, the rotator cuff is imaged in a lateral longitudinal scan. The needle is angled upward in an inferolateral-to-superomedial direction (▶ Fig. 28.6a) and is advanced under vision into the hyperechoic calcified area (▶ Fig. 28.6b). This may be followed if necessary by targeted "needling" of the calcium deposit, and a local anesthetic-steroid mixture can be instilled.

Hand and Fingers

Flexor Tendon Tenosynovitis in the Carpal Tunnel with Secondary Carpal Tunnel Syndrome

Injection of the carpal tunnel is performed in the sitting patient with the wrist supinated and slightly dorsiflexed (▶ Fig. 28.7a). The physician sits opposite the patient and watches the ultrasound screen. We use a high-frequency linear probe (12–18 MHz). The flexor tendons are imaged in a longitudinal palmar scan that displays the target site in the distal third of the image (try to find a short access route!) (▶ Fig. 28.7b). The median nerve must be positively identified; the plane of needle insertion should be medial to the nerve and directed along the longitudinal axis of the tendon sheaths. It is important to avoid injury to the median nerve as well as any needle contact with the nerve, which would be very painful. The needle is introduced at a very low angle (approximately 10–20°) due to the superficial location of the target structures. The needle is advanced in a distal-to-proximal direction toward the ultrasound probe, entering the skin at a point approximately 5 mm distal to the probe. The needle tip is guided sonographically to the target site, where material

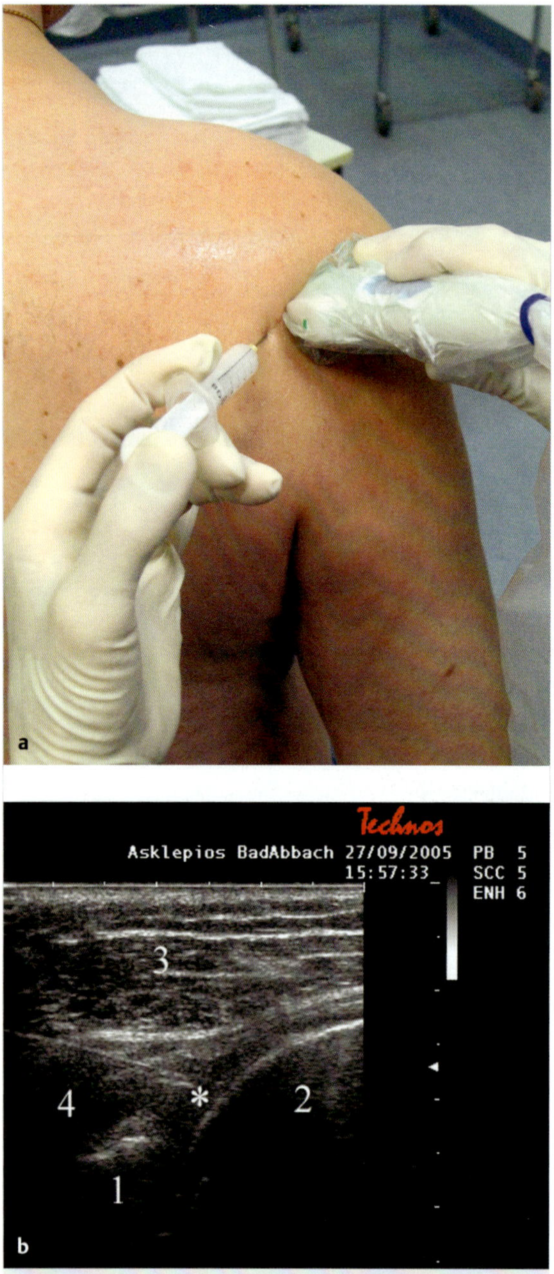

Fig. 28.5 The needle is advanced into the glenohumeral joint from the posterior side. The operator sits diagonally behind the patient. The upper arm hangs loosely at the side in an externally rotated position (to disclose small effusions and relax the posterior joint capsule).

a The needle is introduced in a mediolateral direction at an angle of approximately 60° to 75°.

b Posterior transverse scan displays the joint space between the glenoid (1) and humeral head (2). The needle appears as an echogenic line extending mediolaterally through the deltoid (**3**) and infraspinatus muscles (**4**). The needle tip (✱) is visible in the posterior recess.

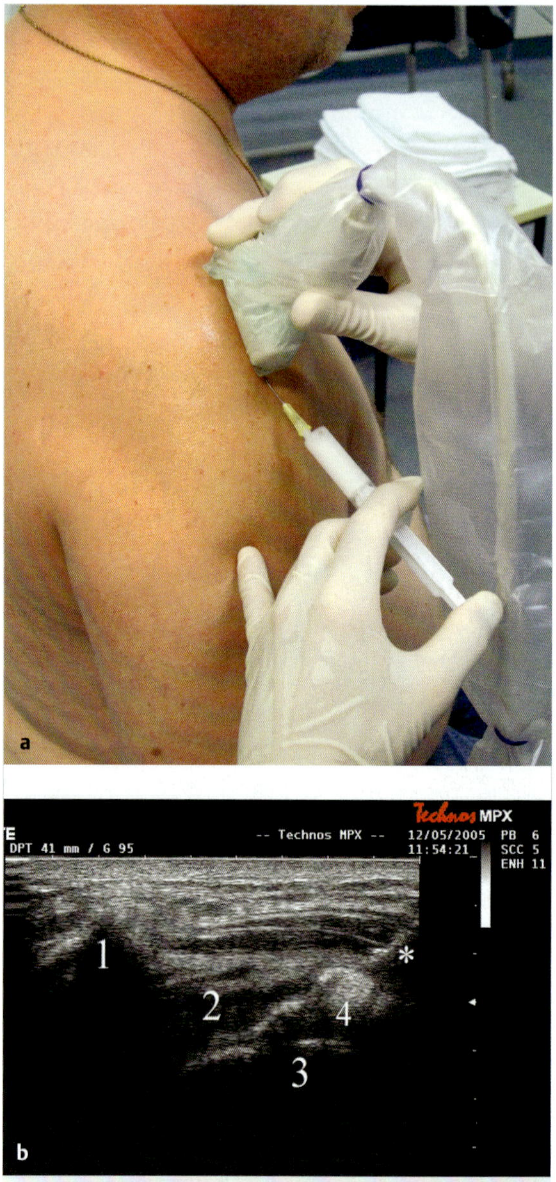

Fig. 28.6 The patient is in a sitting position with the upper arm hanging loosely at the side. The lesion is identified, and the best access route is determined sonographically.

a The needle is introduced medially upward from below.

b Lateral longitudinal scan shows significant calcifications in the supraspinatus muscle of a patient with typical impingement symptoms. The needle (✱) is poorly visualized on the right side of the image due to an unfavorable beam angle, but oscillating needle movements can clearly localize the needle tip to the lesion (4). **1**: Acromion. **2**: Supraspinatus muscle. **3**: Humerus.

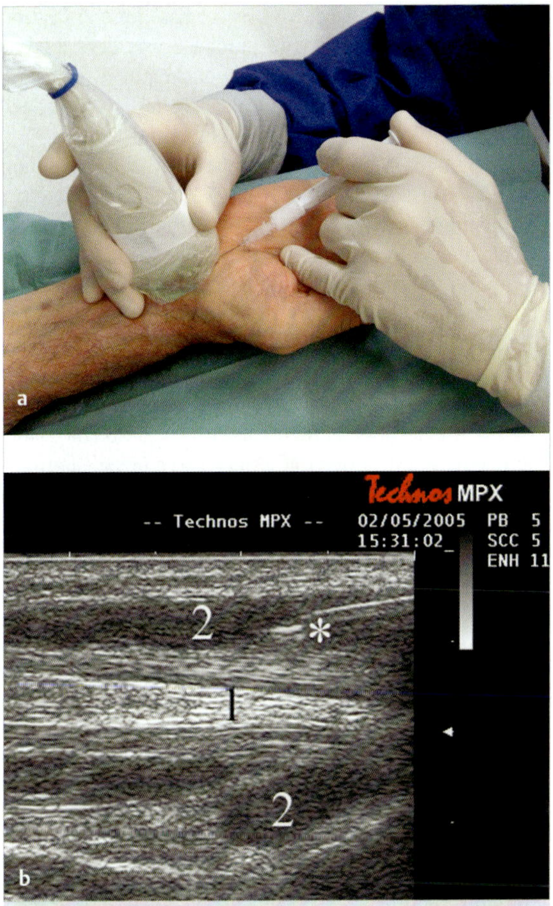

Fig. 28.7 Flexor tendon tenosynovitis in a patient with rheumatoid arthritis and secondary carpal tunnel syndrome.
a The needle is introduced at a very low angle (10–20°) due to the superficial location of the target structures and is angled proximally toward the probe.
b First the median nerve is positively identified, and the scan plane for needle insertion should be medial or lateral to the nerve and directed along the tendon sheath axis to avoid very painful contact of the needle with the nerve. **1**: Flexor tendons. **2**: Distended tendon sheaths. **✱**: Needle tip within the tendon sheath.

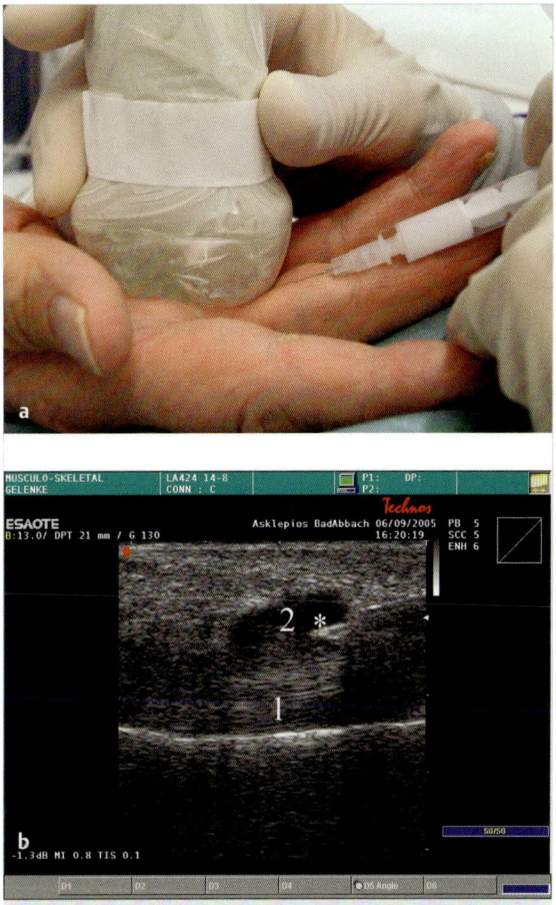

Fig. 28.8 The puncture of flexor tendon sheaths or ganglia is performed in the sitting position. The physician sits opposite the patient while viewing the monitor.
a The needle is introduced at a very low angle (10–20°) due to the superficial location of the target structures and is directed proximally toward the probe.
b The needle tip (**✱**) is precisely within the ganglion (**2**), which measures only 3 mm × 8 mm. The needle does not touch the flexor tendon (**1**).

may be aspirated and a therapeutic agent can be instilled (e.g., 4 mg dexamethasone for an inflammatory rheumatic process).

Injection of a Pulley Ganglion or Digital Flexor Tendons

The injection of hand and finger joints, flexor tendons, or ganglia in the hand is performed in the sitting patient with the hand resting on a small table mounted in front of the patient. The physician sits opposite the patient while viewing the ultrasound screen.

The ganglion or distended flexor tendon sheath is imaged in a longitudinal palmar scan that displays the targeted ganglion or sheath in the distal third of the image (▶ Fig. 28.8b) (try to find a short access route!). The needle is inserted at a very low angle (approximately 10–20°) due to the superficial location of the target. The needle is advanced in a distal-to-proximal direction toward the ultrasound probe, entering the skin approximately 5 mm distal to the probe (▶ Fig. 28.8a). *The needle must not injure the flexor tendon.* The needle is advanced into the ganglion under ultrasound guidance, and a therapeutic agent may be instilled if necessary (e.g., 1 mg dexamethasone for an inflammatory rheumatic process).

Knee

Puncture of a Popliteal Cyst

The patient is positioned prone with the knee slightly flexed (10° with a roll placed beneath the ankle). We use

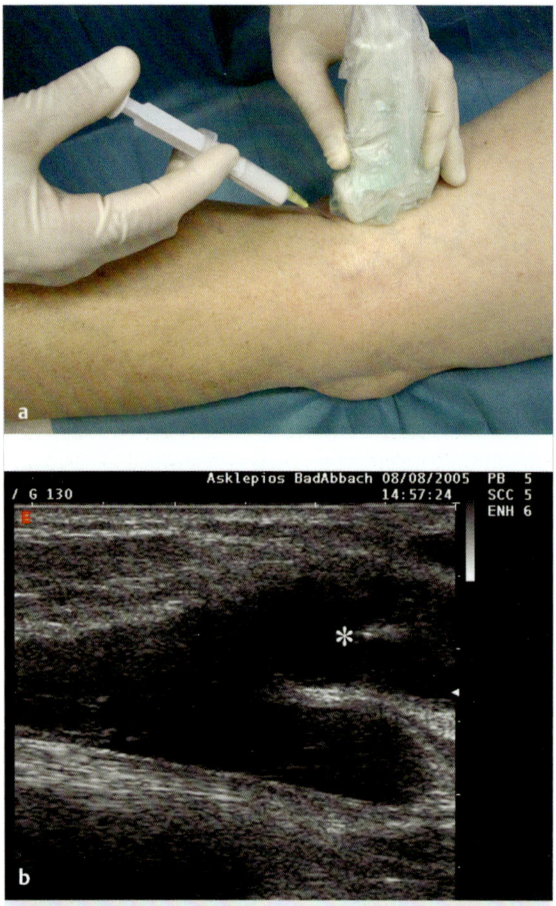

Fig. 28.9 The patient is positioned prone for the aspiration or injection of popliteal cysts.
a The popliteal cyst is imaged in longitudinal section. The needle is introduced in a distal-to-proximal direction.
b The bright echo (✱) with faint reverberations confirms accurate placement of the needle tip in the lumen of the lobulated popliteal cyst.

a linear probe (7–12 MHz). The popliteal cyst is imaged in longitudinal section along its largest dimension. By indenting the skin, the probe creates a low point that will pool antiseptic solution. The needle is angled cephalad and inserted approximately 1 cm distal to the probe in a long-axis orientation (▶ Fig. 28.9a). There should be no difficulty in advancing the needle tip into the cyst lumen under sonographic guidance (▶ Fig. 28.9b), at which point the contents may be aspirated or an agent instilled.

Sacroiliac Joints

Rheumatologists often perform sacroiliac joint injections in patients with active sacroiliitis in a setting of spondyloarthritis. Due to the complex anatomy, these interventions should always be performed with imaging guidance. Ordinarily the joint space is defined fluoroscopically or by CT. The first successful sacroiliac joint injection performed under ultrasound guidance was described in 2003.[12] We favor the technique published by A. Klauser[13] and have been practicing it routinely for more than 4 years.[14] We recommend the following procedure.

The patient is positioned prone on the examination table. We use a linear probe (7–12 MHz) for most patients and a curved array (3.5–5 MHz) for very obese patients.

First the posterior superior iliac spine is identified as a landmark, and the scan plane is oriented to display the spine at the lateral edge of the image. Then the probe is tracked slowly downward to display the additional bony landmarks of the sacrum and sacral crest. The posterior sacroiliac joint space can be defined most clearly at the level of the second sacral foramen (▶ Fig. 28.10a). Now the needle is introduced at a very steep angle (approximately 70–80°) in a medial-to-lateral direction (▶ Fig. 28.10b) and is advanced into the joint space under sonographic vision. Often the needle cannot be directly visualized due to the steep insertion angle, but its position can still be determined very precisely from motion artifacts generated by small oscillating movements of the needle.

28.4 Pitfalls and Complications

Any of the following problems may arise during musculoskeletal interventions.

- Very superficial structures such as the digital flexor tendons require a very low insertion angle so that the needle can be tracked on the screen.
- Connecting and disconnecting the needle with one hand requires training and practice.
- In cases where the needle is not directly visualized due to an unfavorable beam angle, it can be made indirectly visible by oscillating the needle to generate motion artifacts.

To date there have been no published reports of specific complications in musculoskeletal interventions, and none have occurred in any of our patients. We know of no studies that have specifically addressed this issue. One study found no increase in complication rates using a one-hand technique in abdominal ultrasound-guided fine-needle punctures.[15]

Thus, possible complications consist of the adverse events that are known to occur in joint injections and aspirations: Bleeding may occur depending on the joint, puncture site, and needle path. There is also a risk of injury to tendons or the hyaline cartilage surface, and there is always a potential risk of iatrogenic joint infection. Published reports on the incidence of iatrogenic infections vary widely and range from 1:1,000[16] and 1:20,000[17] to 1:35,000.[18] When the above technical principles are followed, however, the risks to the patient should be extremely low.

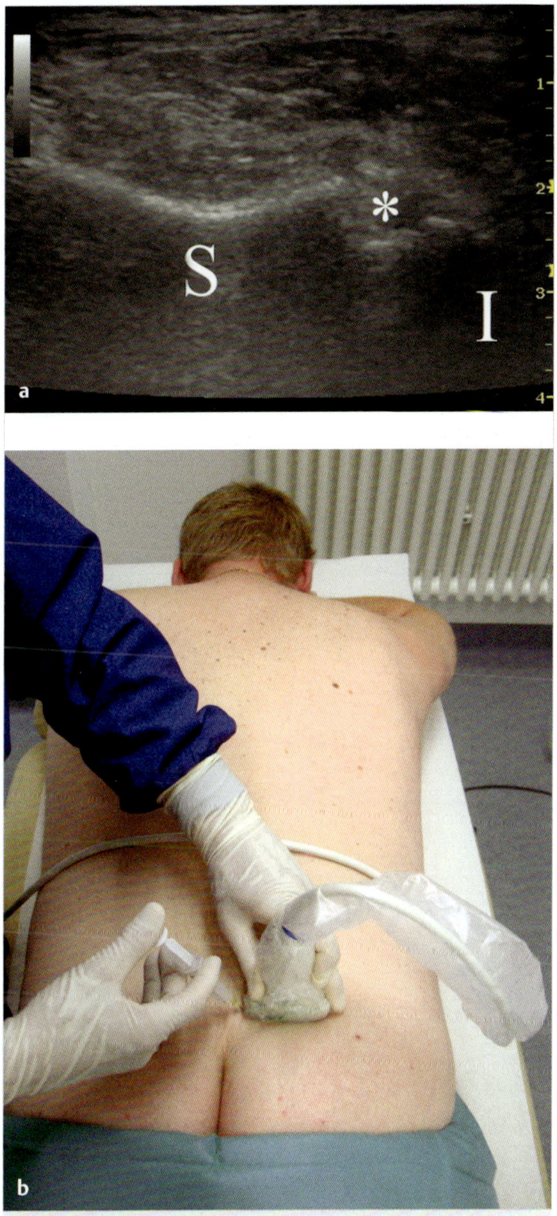

Fig. 28.10 Sacroiliac joint injection.
a The sacrum (S) and ileum (I) provide excellent sonographic landmarks. The sacroiliac joint space (✱) can be identified between them.
b The needle is inserted at a very steep angle in the medial-to-lateral direction. The needle tip should always be positioned precisely over the joint space. Because the space is very narrow and because of possible ossification, the needle cannot always be advanced into the joint space.

28.5 Postprocedure Care

The injection site is covered with a simple adhesive dressing to prevent contamination of the wound and clothing. The patient should be informed about the possible occurrence of complaints, complications, and side effects and told what to do if they arise (which is to return at once). Especially after chemical or radiosynoviorthesis, it is likely that a reactive effusion will develop and may require needle aspiration. Some flushing may occur after therapeutic corticosteroid injections. Weight-bearing joints should not be overused (patients are often tempted to overuse joints made painless by local anesthetic injection!). The hip joint in particular should bear no weight for 24 hours after the procedure because of its particular anatomy. Complete joint rest is also advised for 24 hours after chemical or radiosynoviorthesis. Any kind of balneotherapy to the joint (medicinal baths, mud baths, etc.) should be avoided on the day of the procedure to minimize the risk of infection. All needles and syringes should be properly disposed of to reduce the risk of injury or infection.

References

[1] Eustace JA, Brophy DP, Gibney RP, Bresnihan B, FitzGerald O. Comparison of the accuracy of steroid placement with clinical outcome in patients with shoulder symptoms. Ann Rheum Dis 1997; 56: 59–63

[2] Jones A, Regan M, Ledingham J, Pattrick M, Manhire A, Doherty M. Importance of placement of intra-articular steroid injections. BMJ 1993; 307: 1329–1330

[3] Adler RS, Sofka CM. Percutaneous ultrasound-guided injections in the musculoskeletal system. Ultrasound Q 2003; 19: 3–12

[4] Cunnington J, Marshall N, Hide G et al. A randomized, double-blind, controlled study of ultrasound-guided corticosteroid injection into the joint of patients with inflammatory arthritis. Arthritis Rheum 2010; 62: 1862–1869

[5] Grassi W, Farina A, Filippucci E, Cervini C. Sonographically guided procedures in rheumatology. Semin Arthritis Rheum 2001; 30: 347–353

[6] Koski JM. Ultrasound guided injections in rheumatology. J Rheumatol 2000; 27: 2131–2138

[7] Micu MC, Bogdan GD, Fodor D. Steroid injection for hip osteoarthritis: efficacy under ultrasound guidance. Rheumatology (Oxford) 2010; 49: 1490–1494

[8] Rutten MJ, Collins JM, Maresch BJ et al. Glenohumeral joint injection: a comparative study of ultrasound and fluoroscopically guided techniques before MR arthrography. Eur Radiol 2009; 19: 722–730

[9] Gemeinsame Leitlinie der Deutschen Gesellschaft für Orthopädie und orthopädische Chirurgie (DGOOC), des Berufsverbands der Ärzte für Orthopädie (BVO), und des Arbeitskreises "Krankenhaushygiene" der AWMF. WMF Guideline Registry 029/006: Intraartikuläre Punktion und Injektionen [Intra-Articular Punctures and Injections]. AWMF Online; 2008 http://www.awmf.org/leitlinien/detail/ll/029-006.html accessed February 20, 2014)

[10] Schmidt WA, Schicke B, Krause A. Which ultrasound scan is the best to detect glenohumeral joint effusions? [Article in German]. Ultraschall Med 2008; 29 (Suppl 5): 250–255

[11] Aina R, Cardinal E, Bureau NJ, Aubin B, Brassard P. Calcific shoulder tendinitis: treatment with modified US-guided fine-needle technique. Radiology 2001; 221: 455–461

[12] Pekkafahli MZ, Kiralp MZ, Başekim CC et al. Sacroiliac joint injections performed with sonographic guidance. J Ultrasound Med 2003; 22: 553–559

[13] Klauser A, De Zordo T, Feuchtner G et al. Feasibility of ultrasound-guided sacroiliac joint injection considering sonoanatomic landmarks at two different levels in cadavers and patients. Arthritis Rheum 2008; 59: 1618–1624

[14] Hartung W, Ross CJ, Straub R et al. Ultrasound guided sacroiliac joint injection in patients with established sacroiliitis: precise injection verified by MRI scanning does not predict clinical outcome. Rheumatology 2010; 49: 1479–1482

[15] Caturelli E, Giacobbe A, Facciorusso D et al. Free-hand technique with ordinary antisepsis in abdominal US-guided fine-needle punctures: three-year experience. Radiology 1996; 199: 721–723

[16] Kendall PH. Local corticosteroid injection therapy. III. Ann Phys Med 1963; 7: 31–38

[17] Pal B, Morris J. Perceived risks of joint infection following intra-articular corticosteroid injections: a survey of rheumatologists. Clin Rheumatol 1999; 18: 264–265

[18] Bernau H, Heeg P. Haftpflichtprozess. Gelenkinfektion. Chir Praxis 1989; 40: 3–8

29 Neurologic Interventions, Ultrasound-Guided Regional Anesthesia

H. H. Wilckens, A. Ignee, M. Kaeppler, H. Boehrer, C. F. Dietrich

Ultrasonography is increasingly employed as an imaging and guidance modality for regional anesthesia and is becoming an important tool in the everyday practice of anesthesiology.

When ultrasound-guided nerve blocks were introduced in the mid-1990s, the advantages of this new technique were obvious.[1,2] Ultrasound guidance enables the operator to visualize targeted structures and selectively block them. A large number of ultrasound-guided nerve block techniques were described in subsequent years.

The clinical application of ultrasound-guided nerve blocks requires state-of-the-art imaging equipment and an adequate level of training. The operator should be well versed in the anatomy of the targeted structures and have the technical expertise necessary to image the structures of interest with the ultrasound machine.

29.1 History and Development

After Carl Koller performed the first ocular local anesthesia in 1884, the practice of regional anesthesia relied for more than a century on surface landmarks, reference lines, and intersecting lines for orientation purposes. But human anatomy is highly variable and cannot always be accurately predicted, with the result that many peripheral nerve blocks were unsuccessful. Sonography was introduced as a means of solving this problem. A Doppler ultrasound blood-flow detector was first used in 1978 to facilitate the supraclavicular brachial plexus block.[3] Sonography was first used for the direct imaging guidance of a brachial plexus block in 1994, again using the supraclavicular approach.[1]

During the past 10 years, ultrasound technology has continued to evolve in its application to regional anesthesia techniques. New scanners and software have also been developed with the goal of facilitating peripheral nerve blocks.

▸ **Published data.** Since the first ultrasound-guided peripheral regional anesthesia was performed in 1994,[1] this field has continued to develop from year to year. Ultrasound guidance has resulted in higher success rates, lower complication rates, and improved patient safety and comfort.[4–7] Several randomized studies and case series have been published in the past decade dealing with the improvement of ultrasound-guided peripheral nerve blocks.

29.2 Indications

Regional anesthesia can be used in surgical patients either as an adjunct to general anesthesia or as a standalone anesthesia procedure when possible contraindications are taken into account.

Procedures in the distribution of the brachial plexus (e.g., a radial fracture or shoulder arthroscopy) can be performed by targeting the anesthesia to specific nerves that are visualized with ultrasound.[8] Of course, this same principle can be applied to procedures in the distribution of the lumbosacral plexus, such as the ultrasound-guided placement of a femoral nerve catheter during major knee surgery.[9]

Ultrasound can also direct the placement of a catheter for postoperative analgesia[10] and to facilitate postoperative mobilization of the treated limb. Single-shot techniques should employ long-acting local anesthetics and should be supplemented by the use of nonopioid analgesics (e.g., ibuprofen, diclofenac, metamizole).

29.3 Contraindications

29.3.1 Patient Refusal

Refusal of informed consent is recognized as a general absolute contraindication to the use of regional anesthesia.

29.3.2 Clinically Overt Coagulopathy and Anticoagulant Medication

Clinically overt coagulation disorders are generally a contraindication to proximal peripheral nerve blocks, although a nerve block may still be performed in selected cases where the benefit outweighs the risk.

Regarding the use of anticoagulant medications, there are no randomized studies or guidelines like those for spinal anesthesia techniques, except for the psoas compartment block. Only recommendations have been published. There are some illustrative case reports, however, showing that peripheral nerve block catheters were used safely in patients on anticoagulant medication.[11] On the other hand, there is an increased theoretical risk that injury to the epineurium will cause hematoma or microhematoma formation in patients on anticoagulant medication.

The German Society of Anesthesiology and Intensive Care Medicine has published recommendations on the use of peripheral nerve blocks for regional anesthesia in patients receiving thromboembolic prophylaxis. Available data form the basis of the following guidelines for peripheral nerve blocks in settings of thromboembolic prophylaxis and antithrombotic medication[12]:

1. Whenever possible, the same precautionary measures followed for spinal anesthesia should also apply to peripheral nerve blocks.
2. If these measures cannot be implemented, a careful risk–benefit analysis should be conducted for each individual case. Considerations in performing a peripheral nerve block in a patient on anticoagulant medication should be discussed with the patient and documented in writing.
3. All techniques that involve a deliberate vascular puncture (e.g., transarterial techniques) should be avoided.
4. Patients taking aspirin, NSAIDs, or low-molecular-weight heparin (in the absence of other coagulation-inhibiting agents and no clinical signs of coagulopathy) are considered better candidates for regional anesthesia than patients treated with fondaparinux, clopidogrel, or ticlopidine.
5. Superficial nerve blocks that are easily accessible to compression, and the very rare blocks that require vascular puncture, can be performed more safely in patients on anticoagulant medication than can deep nerve blocks in joints not accessible to compression. The following blocks can usually be performed safely in patients on thromboembolic prophylaxis or antiplatelet drugs:
   - Axillary plexus block (excluding the transarterial technique)
   - Interscalene plexus block (use only techniques that do not risk vertebral artery puncture, such as the Meier technique)
   - 3-in-1 block (femoral nerve block)
   - Distal sciatic nerve block (posterior or lateral approach)
   - All nerve blocks about the elbow and knee and distal to those joints

29.3.3 Infections at the Puncture Site

An infection at the puncture site is an absolute contraindication, although ultrasound can be used to locate a different puncture site that is outside the infected area but still gives access to the site of the desired nerve block. Catheter placement is contraindicated in patients with a systemic infection (and possible bacteremia).[13,14]

29.3.4 Neurologic Deficit

An existing neurologic deficit in the area of the proposed peripheral nerve block is only a relative contraindication. Precise, detailed documentation and evaluation of the patient's neurologic status is essential. An immediate postoperative evaluation of neurologic function is necessary to exclude a reversible cause.[15]

29.4 Needle Insertion Techniques

29.4.1 Out-of-Plane versus In-Plane Technique

In the out-of-plane technique, the needle is inserted and advanced in a short-axis plane perpendicular to the ultrasound image plane (▶ Fig. 29.1). The needle is imaged in cross-section as an echogenic structure with a distal acoustic shadow. In most cases only the needle tip can be visualized. The angle of needle insertion is adjusted according to the depth of the target structures: the needle is inserted at a low angle for superficial blocks and at a steeper angle for deeper blocks. A steeper insertion angle allows better visualization of the needle tip than a flatter angle.

In the in-plane technique, the needle is inserted in a long-axis view that is in-plane with the ultrasound beam (▶ Fig. 29.2). The entire needle can be visualized, but only if the plane of needle insertion precisely coincides with the ultrasound image plane. In this technique the needle tip can be localized at any time, significantly reducing the risk of neurovascular injury.[16] A low insertion angle will provide better needle visualization than a steeper angle. The distance from the insertion site to the target structure is 2 to 3 times longer in the in-plane technique than in the out-of-plane technique.

29.5 Ultrasound Imaging of Nerves and Muscles

29.5.1 Nerves

Given the multitude of neural structures that exist in the human body, nerves have a variety of ultrasound

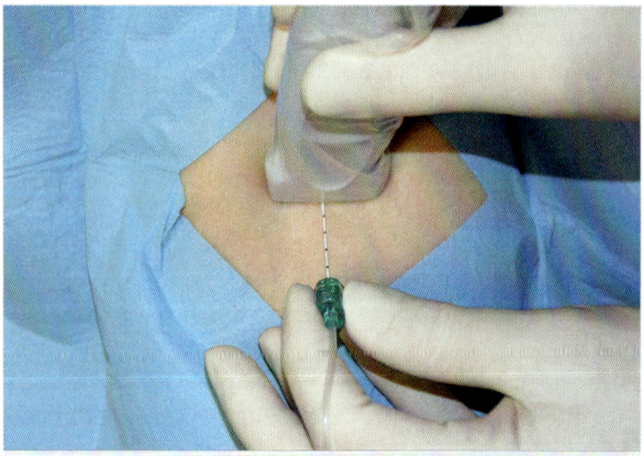

Fig. 29.1 Out-of-plane technique of needle insertion.

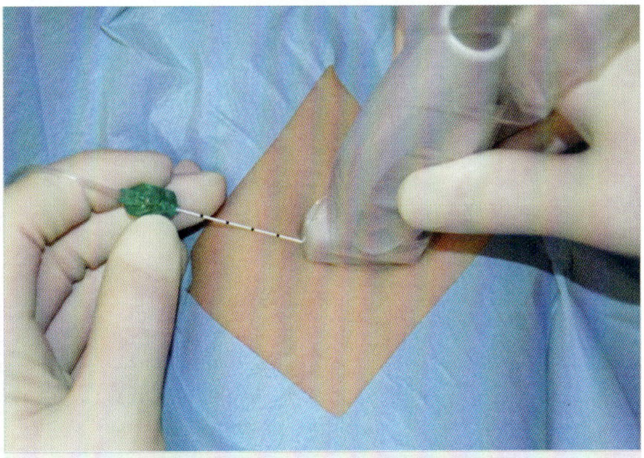

Fig. 29.2 In-plane technique of needle insertion.

appearances depending on their location. Proximal nerves appear as hypoechoic structures with a hyperechoic rim (e.g., interscalene brachial plexus C5 to T1). Nerves at more distal sites appear hyperechoic (e.g., ulnar nerve) due to a larger proportion of connective tissue between the neurons. But echogenicity also varies with the ultrasound beam angle, a phenomenon known as *anisotropy*. Nerves also present typical geometric shapes at ultrasound, which may be described as round, oval, or triangular. Thus, the exact description of a nerve imaged with ultrasound depends on its geometry and echogenicity.

29.5.2 Muscles

Muscles appear sonographically as heterogeneous structures with interspersed hyperechoic lines (intramuscular septa) or as homogeneous structures. Generally speaking, muscles have a fibrolamellar appearance when imaged with ultrasound.

29.6 Materials and Equipment

29.6.1 Ultrasound Machines

A number of manufacturers offer ultrasound systems specially designed for use in anesthesiology (e.g., ▶ Fig. 29.3). Nerve blocks can be guided with small portable ultrasound machines or with larger stationary systems, which often provide better contrast resolution.

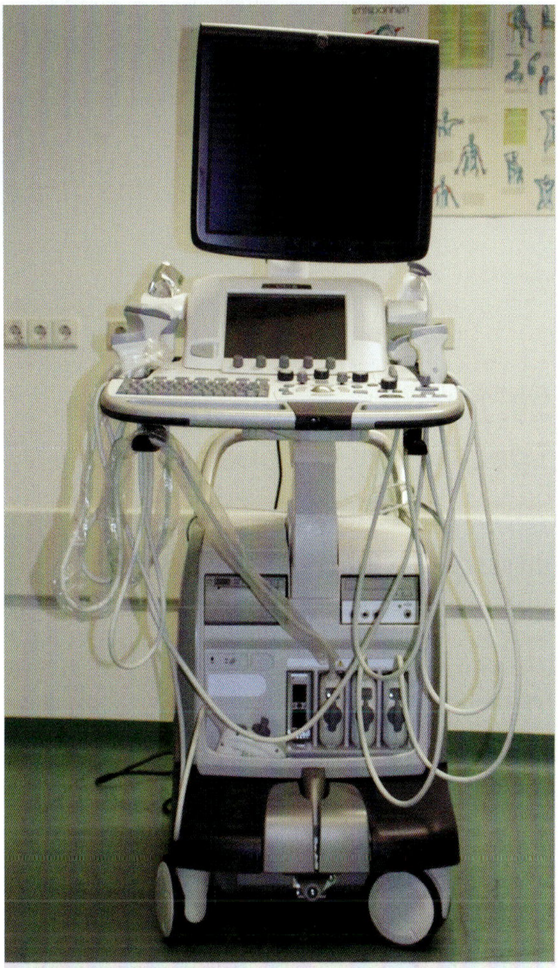

Fig. 29.3 Logiq E9 ultrasound system.

29.6.2 Anesthesia Needles and Catheters

Manufacturers such as Pajunk and Braun supply a variety of different injection needles and catheters for use in regional anesthesia (▶ Fig. 29.4, ▶ Table 29.1). These devices may consist of single-injection needles, with or without nerve stimulation, or catheter sets for administering continuous regional anesthesia.

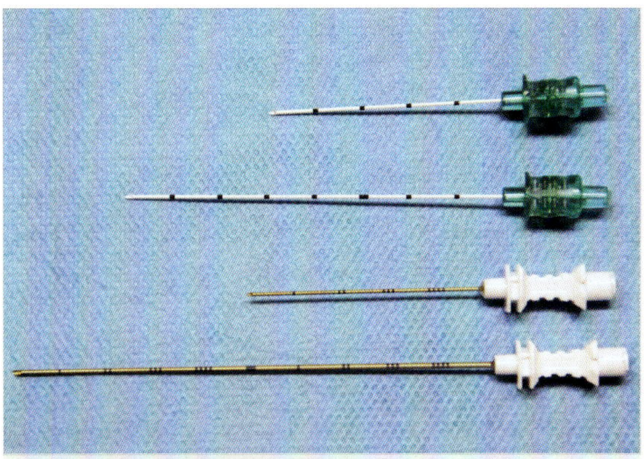

Fig. 29.4 Regional anesthesia needles.

Table 29.1 Injection needles for use with ultrasound guidance

Company	Needle gauge	Needle length (mm)	Needle tip	Special features
Pajunk	22	50	Faceted bevel, Sprotte	"Cornerstone" reflectors reflect ultrasound beam without energy loss
Braun	22	50/80	15° bevel geometry, 30° bevel geometry	
Pajunk	19	50	Faceted bevel, Sprotte, Tuohy	Suitable for catheter technique
Pajunk	19	100	Faceted bevel, Sprotte, Tuohy	Suitable for catheter technique

29.7 Regional Anesthesia at Specific Sites: Upper Limb

29.7.1 Brachial Plexus

Interscalene Brachial Plexus Block

The interscalene brachial plexus block was first described by Winnie in 1970.[17] It is used for the reduction of shoulder dislocations, for shoulder arthroscopy, for shoulder replacement arthroplasty as an adjunct to general anesthesia, and for intra- and postoperative shoulder mobilization. The technique can also be used for procedures on the lateral clavicle and upper arm. Whether the block is used alone or combined with general anesthesia depends on the operation, since the inside of the upper arm is partially supplied by portions of the intercostobrachial nerve (T12), requiring an additional block. An incomplete block during shoulder surgery[18] is attributable to incomplete anesthesia of the suprascapular nerve (C5). But all the roots of the brachial plexus (C5–T1) can be visualized with ultrasound and can be selectively blocked under sonographic guidance.

Indications

The indications for an interscalene brachial plexus block are as follows:

- Reduction of a shoulder dislocation
- Anesthesia and analgesia for shoulder surgery and for operations involving the lateral clavicle and upper arm

Contraindications

The interscalene brachial plexus block has the following contraindications:

- Contralateral phrenic nerve palsy
- Contralateral recurrent laryngeal nerve palsy

Complications

Possible complications include the following:

- Horner syndrome (blockade of the stellate ganglion: myosis, ptosis, and enophthalmos)
- Phrenic nerve palsy: the phrenic nerve (C4) runs down the anterior border of the anterior scalene muscle.
- Recurrent laryngeal nerve palsy
- Bezold–Jarish reflex: in some patients, the beach-chair position used for shoulder surgery evokes bradycardia and hypotension that may lead to circulatory collapse and cardiac arrest.[19]

Patient Position

The patient is positioned supine with the head resting on a soft gel cushion and turned slightly toward the contralateral side. The skin site is aseptically prepared as described in Chapter 8.

Sonography

To define the neural structures of the brachial plexus, the transducer is placed parallel to the clavicle in the supraclavicular fossa. The subclavian artery is identified as a pulsating vascular structure. The pleura appears as a hyperechoic structure below the subclavian artery. The brachial plexus appears lateral to the subclavian artery as a cluster of small hypoechoic structures with a hyperechoic outer rim (▶ Fig. 29.5). Sliding the transducer cephalad will trace the brachial plexus into the interscalene groove and display 3 to 5 hypoechoic round or oval structures arranged in a string-of-beads pattern: the C5–T1 nerve roots. The needle is advanced in a lateral-to-medial direction using either the out-of-plane or in-plane technique. Injecting 20 mL of local anesthetic is usually sufficient to block the nerve roots. Following spread of the local anesthetic, a catheter can additionally be placed to facilitate postoperative mobilization of the shoulder and arm.

Literature on the Interscalene Brachial Plexus Block

Goebel et al[20] conducted a randomized, placebo-controlled study in 70 patients to investigate postoperative analgesia following the placement of an interscalene plexus catheter. The patients who received 0.2% ropivacaine by continuous infusion for postoperative analgesia

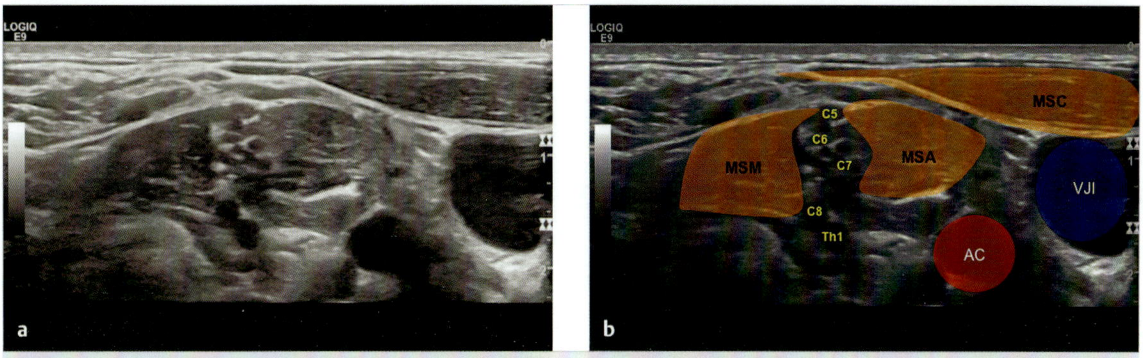

Fig. 29.5 a, b Ultrasound appearance of the interscalene portion of the brachial plexus (C5–T1).MSC, sternocleidomastoid muscle; MSM, middle scalene (MSM); MSA, anterior scalene; AC, carotid artery; VJI, internal jugular vein.

had less need for opioid rescue medication during the first 24 hours after shoulder surgery than the group of patients who received a 0.9% saline solution via the catheter. The interscalene plexus block and catheter placement were performed under ultrasound guidance.

Mariano et al[21] studied 32 patients who also received an interscalene plexus catheter for postoperative analgesia, but the posterior approach described by Pippa[22] was used. The nerve block was performed with ultrasound assistance. The study indicates that either approach can provide an effective blockade of the interscalene brachial plexus.

Supraclavicular Brachial Plexus Block

The supraclavicular technique of the brachial plexus block was first described by Kulenkampff in 1911. Because this approach entails a risk of pneumothorax due to its proximity to the pleura, several attempts have been made to refine the technique.[23,24] Ultrasound guidance can be used to direct the needle to the target site under vision and minimize the risk of this complication.

Indications

The supraclavicular brachial plexus block is used to produce anesthesia and analgesia of the upper arm, forearm, and hand (e.g., humeral shaft fracture, elbow fracture or dislocation).

Contraindications

The supraclavicular nerve block has the following contraindications:

- Contralateral phrenic nerve palsy
- Contralateral recurrent laryngeal nerve palsy

Complications

Possible complications are as follows:

- Pneumothorax
- Horner syndrome
- Phrenic nerve palsy
- Recurrent laryngeal nerve palsy

Patient Position

The patient is positioned supine with the head placed on a soft gel cushion and turned slightly toward the contralateral side. The skin site is prepared as described in Chapter 8.

Sonography

The anesthesiologist stands at the head of the table and places the transducer in the supraclavicular fossa parallel to the clavicle. The subclavian artery is identified as a pulsating echo-free structure (▶ Fig. 29.6). Just below the subclavian artery, the first rib appears as a hyperechoic line with an acoustic shadow. Lateral to the subclavian artery are small, hypoechoic oval structures representing the nerve bundle of the supraclavicular plexus. Angling the transducer reveals a second hyperechoic white line, offset from the first, which represents the pleura. It is critically important to identify both lines in order to distinguish the pleura from the first rib and reduce the risk of pneumothorax. Angling the transducer alters the ultrasound image as the hyperechoic line with the posterior shadow moves laterally and the second hyperechoic line appears below the subclavian artery. The needle is inserted in a lateral-to-medial direction using the in-plane technique, which is preferred as it gives better visualization of the needle tip. Just 20 mL of local anesthetic is sufficient to produce adequate anesthesia and analgesia, making certain that both the posterior and anterior portions of the supraclavicular plexus are anesthetized. The needle is initially directed toward the first rib to avoid piercing the pleura. Then the needle is retracted and the anterior branches of the supraclavicular plexus are anesthetized.

Literature on the Supraclavicular Brachial Plexus Block

Perlas et al[25] studied 510 patients who received a supraclavicular brachial plexus block for upper limb surgery. A

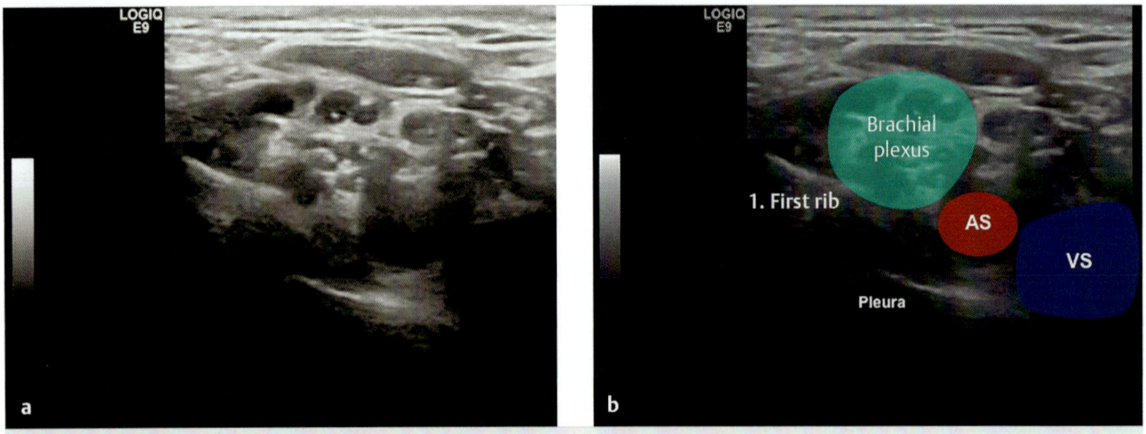

Fig. 29.6 a, b Subclavian vein (VS), subclavian artery (AS), lateral brachial plexus.

successful block was achieved in 94.6% of the cases reviewed. A medial-to-lateral approach was used in 361 patients and a lateral-to-medial approach in 149. The medial-to-lateral approach was associated with 2 cases of iatrogenic vascular injury and 2 cases of postoperative numbness that persisted for days after the surgery. No puncture-related complications occurred with the lateral-to-medial approach. There were no instances of pneumothorax in either group. We accordingly also prefer the lateral-to-medial approach. The needle was introduced by the in-plane approach for better visualization of the needle tip.

29.7.2 Infraclavicular Brachial Plexus Block

The infraclavicular brachial plexus block is a simple method of producing anesthesia and analgesia of the upper limbs. It is useful in cases where a high arm block is desired for surgery. The needle is inserted using the in-plane technique. One disadvantage of the infraclavicular nerve block is the risk of iatrogenic pleural injury and the development of pneumothorax. One advantage from an anatomical standpoint is the more proximal level of the approach. In contrast to the axillary approach, this eliminates the need for separate anesthesia of the musculocutaneous nerve, which emerges from the lateral fascicle.

Indications

Indications for the infraclavicular brachial plexus block are anesthesia and analgesia from the distal upper arm to the hand.

Contraindications

The infraclavicular brachial plexus block has the following contraindications:

- Contralateral pneumothorax
- Contralateral phrenic nerve palsy
- Contralateral recurrent laryngeal nerve palsy
- Previous contralateral pneumonectomy

Complications

Possible complications include:

- Pneumothorax
- Horner syndrome
- Phrenic nerve palsy
- Recurrent laryngeal nerve palsy

Patient Position

The patient is positioned supine with the arm either abducted 90° or left in its neutral position. The skin site is prepared as described in Chapter 8.

Sonography

The transducer is placed in the infraclavicular fossa, and the axillary artery is identified. Lateral to the axillary artery is the brachial plexus with its mixed hyperechoic and hypoechoic structure. Medial to the axillary artery is the axillary vein (▶ Fig. 29.7). Above the artery are two pennate structures identified as the pectoralis major and minor muscles. Angling the transducer laterally displays the pleural apex, a parabolic line running along the axillary vein. The in-plane technique is used for better needle tip visualization, and the target site is located just below the axillary artery. Injection of the local anesthetic should be followed by appearance of the "double bubble" sign,[26] the local anesthetic appearing as an echo-free oval collection below the axillary artery.

Literature on the Infraclavicular Brachial Plexus Block

Tran et al[27] conducted a prospective randomized study in 88 patients undergoing upper limb surgery to investigate the differences between a single ultrasound-guided

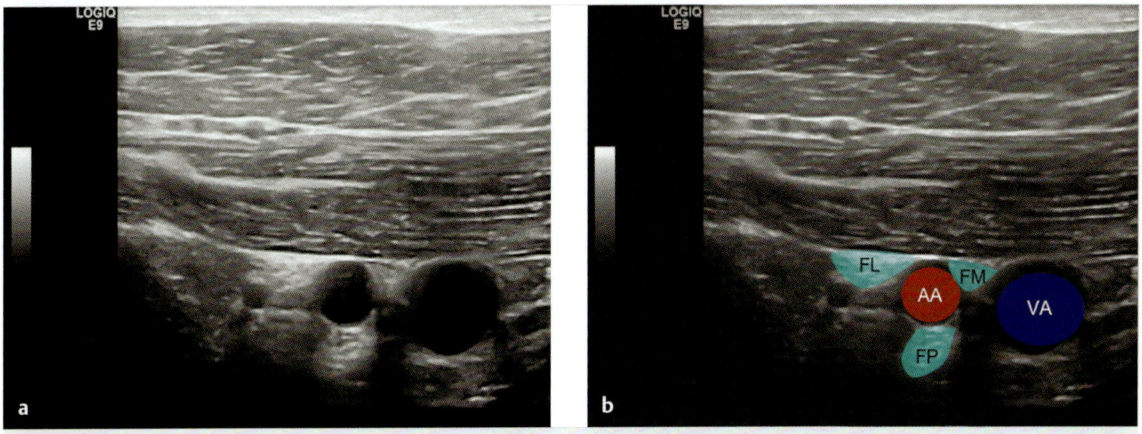

Fig. 29.7 a, b Axillary artery (AA) and, medial to it, the axillary vein (VA). FP, posterior fascicle; FM; medial fascicle; FL, lateral fascicle.

injection of local anesthetic below the axillary artery compared with one injection above and one below the axillary artery. No significant differences were found in performance or onset time, and both methods had the same success rates. The in-plane technique was used for better visualization of the needle tip.

29.7.3 Axillary Brachial Plexus Block

The axillary brachial plexus block is the most commonly used nerve block for upper limb surgery. Hirschel first noted in 1911 that a percutaneous injection in the axilla could anesthetize the brachial plexus. The method published by De Jong in 1961 is still used today[28] for operations on the upper limb. In 1989, an ultrasound machine was used for the first time to direct an axillary plexus block in 10 patients.[29] The use of ultrasound guidance increased the success rate of axillary plexus blocks from 81.9% using nerve stimulation or a transarterial technique to 91.6% in the ultrasound-guided group ($P = 0.003$). Usage of local anesthetic decreased from 46.7 ± 17.1 mL to 39.8 ± 6.4 mL ($P < 0.0001$). Also, the total time spent in the preparation room was significantly reduced from 40.1 ± 27.3 minutes to 30.6 ± 14.2 minutes ($P < 0.0001$).[30,31] Ultrasound can also display the patient's specific anatomy so that anesthesia can be accurately targeted to the ulnar, median, radial, and musculocutaneous nerves.[32]

Indications

Indications for the axillary brachial plexus block are anesthesia and analgesia for the distal upper arm, elbow, forearm, and hand (e.g., radial fracture, carpal tunnel syndrome).

Contraindications

There are no specific contraindications relating to the method.

Complications

Possible complications are vascular punctures and nerve injuries.

Patient Position

The patient is positioned supine with the arm abducted 90° at the shoulder and flexed 90° at the elbow. The skin site is prepared as described in Chapter 8. The needle can be introduced using either the out-of-plane or in-plane technique.

Sonography

The axillary artery is imaged in cross-section. The axillary plexus is highly variable in its anatomy,[32] and individual nerves can be identified by angling and sliding the transducer. The venous vessels are usually in a compressed state during imaging, so care should be taken that local anesthetic is not inadvertently injected into one of the compressed vessels.

Identification of the short head of the biceps brachii muscle closer to the transducer and the coracobrachialis muscle farther from the transducer aids in identifying the musculocutaneous nerve. This typically appears as a flat hyperechoic structure between the two muscles, although variants may be encountered[33] (▶ Fig. 29.8). The other three nerves can usually be imaged as hyperechoic or hypoechoic elliptical structures grouped around the axillary artery. The median nerve is at approximately the 11 o'clock position, the ulnar nerve at the 2 o'clock position, and the radial nerve at the 5 o'clock position.[32]

Literature on the Axillary Brachial Plexus Block

The axillary plexus block is perhaps the most common peripheral nerve block used for anesthesia in upper limb operations. Given the anatomical variations that exist in

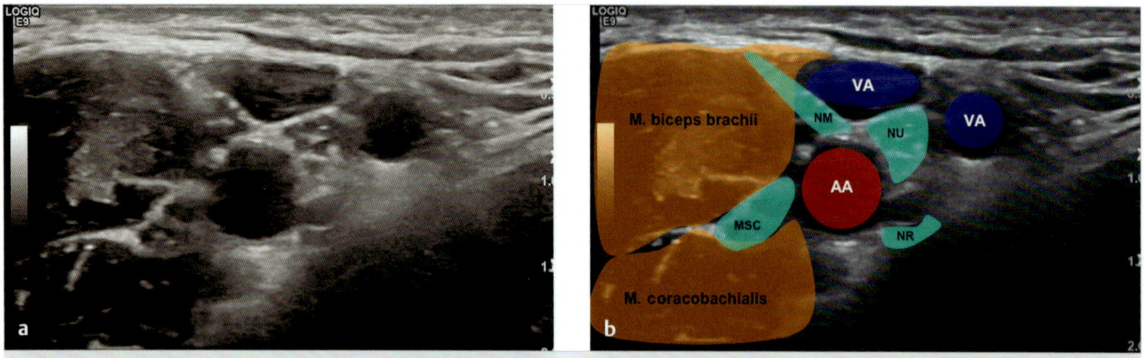

Fig. 29.8 a, b Axillary brachial plexus. The musculocutaneous nerve (NMC) is visible between the biceps brachii and coracobrachialis muscles. The structures grouped around the axillary artery (AA) are the median nerve (NM), ulnar nerve (NU), radial nerve (NR), and axillary vein (VA).

the axilla,[32] the success rates associated with the use of nerve stimulators or the transarterial technique[28] were significantly lower than in ultrasound-guided axillary plexus blocks.[30] In a randomized study of 188 patients, Chan et al[5] found that the success rate of the axillary plexus block was significantly improved by ultrasound guidance.

29.8 Regional Anesthesia at Specific Sites: Lower Limb

29.8.1 Lumbosacral Plexus

Psoas Compartment Block

The psoas compartment block, first described in 1976,[34] is a technique that blocks the femoral nerve, obturator nerve, and lateral femoral cutaneous nerve with a single targeted injection. The psoas compartment block has numerous risks that must be considered. One is the possibility of an intrathecal injection. Since regional anesthesia employs a greater volume of local anesthetic than does spinal anesthesia, this error could cause total spinal anesthesia with risk of respiratory failure and cardiac arrest. The proximity of the kidney to the injection site also poses a risk of renal injury, and a retroperitoneal hematoma could result from injury to nearby vessels.[35] Ultrasound, with its ability to visualize structures of interest, can minimize the risks. One problem has been the inability of ultrasound to accurately define the lumbar plexus,[36] but the latest generation of scanners can visualize the lumbosacral plexus in thin patients. A curved-array transducer (abdominal transducer) may be helpful for this application.

Indications

The psoas compartment block has the following indications:

- Anesthesia and analgesia of the femoral nerve, obturator nerve, and lateral femoral cutaneous nerve
- Combined with a sciatic nerve block, the psoas compartment block can also provide anesthesia for lower limb surgery below the hip. This combination is necessary because the psoas compartment injection can block only the nerve fibers from L2 to L4/L5 while the sciatic nerve carries fibers from L4 to S2/S3. The combination ensures a complete block.

Contraindications

Contraindications to the psoas compartment block are anticoagulant medication (see Chapter 29.3; same guidelines apply as in spinal or epidural anesthesia) and coagulation disorders.

Complications

Possible complications are as follows:

- Accidental spinal anesthesia (high or total), epidural anesthesia
- Renal injury
- Retroperitoneal hematoma
- Psoas abscess

Patient Position

The patient is placed in the lateral position with the operative side to be blocked uppermost and the arm raised above the head. The skin site is prepared as described in Chapter 8.

Sonography

The iliac crest is palpated on the side to be blocked, and a perpendicular line is dropped from there to the spinal column to locate the L4 vertebral body. The transducer is now placed at the level of L4 approximately 5 cm lateral to the spinous processes, first placing it in a horizontal orientation in line with the transverse processes. The psoas major and its bordering structures (kidney, erector spinae, quadratus lumborum) must be identified by

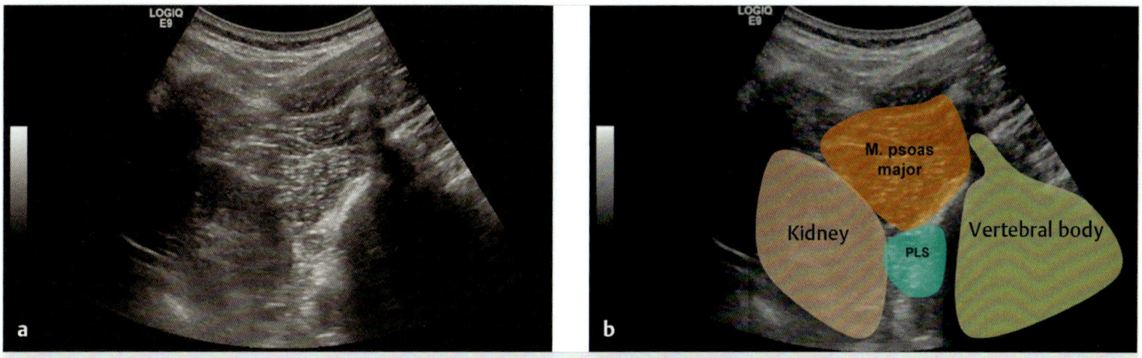

Fig. 29.9 a, b Psoas compartment block. PLS, lumbosacral plexus.

sliding the transducer to the L3 and L2 levels and also to L5 (▶ Fig. 29.9). Landmarks are the transverse processes of the vertebral bodies, which appear as acoustic shadows in the ultrasound image. Given the deep location of the target site, needle insertion should be aided by the use of a needle guide attachment or biopsy transducer. A needle length up to 120 mm may be required.

29.8.2 Femoral Nerve Block

The femoral nerve block is a simple, low-risk procedure. Winnie was the first author to mention the femoral "3-in-1" block in 1973.[37] The rationale is that the three nerves (femoral nerve, obturator nerve, and lateral femoral cutaneous nerve) run in a common fascial sheath before separating below the inguinal ligament. Winnie stated that an injection just below the inguinal ligament could block all three nerves.

Lang showed, however, that this technique will block the obturator nerve in only about 4% of cases.[38] Marhofer showed in 1997 that ultrasound guidance could improve the onset time and quality of the block.[2]

Indications

The femoral nerve block has the following indications:

- When used alone, this block is adequate only for minor surgical procedures in the distribution of the femoral nerve (e.g., mesh graft removal).
- Postoperative pain control after procedures on the knee or femur (e.g., knee replacement, cruciate ligament reconstruction)
- Combined with a sciatic nerve block for procedures on the distal thigh and lower leg above the foot

Contraindications

There are no strict contraindications, although strict criteria should be applied in selecting patients undergoing femoral bypass surgery.

Complications

No complications are known.

Patient Position

The patient is positioned supine with the leg to be blocked in slight external rotation and abduction and the knee slightly flexed. The skin site is prepared as described in Chapter 8.

Sonography

First the femoral artery is identified sonographically as a round, pulsating hypoechoic structure (▶ Fig. 29.10). For this step the transducer is placed at the level of the inguinal ligament and oriented at right angles to the course of the femoral artery. Medial to that vessel is the femoral vein, which, unlike the artery, is compressible. Lateral to the femoral artery is a conspicuous structure of mixed echogenicity; this is the femoral nerve. The pennate structure of the iliopsoas muscle can also be identified lateral to the femoral artery. The femoral nerve usually occupies a lateral-to-medial depression visible in the course of the anterior muscle fascia.

The needle can be inserted using either the out-of-plane or in-plane technique, but the out-of-plane technique is preferred owing to the relatively short path from the skin surface to the nerve, which will facilitate catheter placement.

Literature on the Femoral Nerve Block

In a study of 40 patients, Mariano et al[39] investigated the time to femoral nerve catheter placement by ultrasound guidance compared with the use of a nerve stimulator. The catheter could be placed more quickly in the ultrasound group than in the nerve stimulator group. No vascular punctures occurred in the ultrasound group, whereas four punctures occurred in the nerve stimulator group. The in-plane technique was used for needle insertion.

29.8.3 Obturator Nerve Block

The obturator nerve block can be used for urologic endoscopic procedures or for pain control in knee operations.

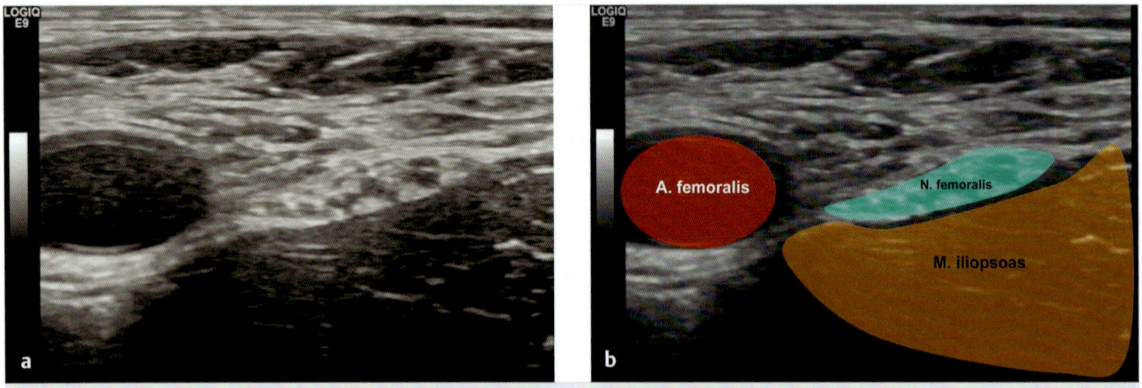

Fig. 29.10 a, b The femoral nerve is displayed lateral to the femoral artery with the iliopsoas muscle below.

Indications

- Adjunct for pain control in knee operations
- Transurethral resection of the bladder or prostate

Contraindications

There are no contraindications to the obturator nerve block.

Complications

No complications are known.

Patient Position

The patient is positioned supine with the leg to be blocked in slight external rotation and abduction. The skin site is prepared as described in Chapter 8.

Sonography

First the femoral artery is identified in the inguinal region. Medial to it is the compressible femoral vein. The transducer is first slid distally and then medially toward the adductor muscle group. The pectineus muscle appears laterally. Next to it is the adductor longus, and below that the adductor brevis and adductor magnus, each separated from the others by a hyperechoic line. Between the adductor longus and brevis is the anterior branch of the obturator nerve, appearing as a hyperechoic oval structure in the hyperechoic tissue. If the nerve is difficult to define, visualization may be improved by angling the transducer. Between the adductor brevis and the adductor magnus is the posterior branch of the obturator nerve, also appearing as a hyperechoic oval structure (▶ Fig. 29.11). Often the two branches cannot be imaged simultaneously and the transducer must be angled to define both branches separately in the ultrasound image.

The needle is inserted in a lateral-to-medial direction using the in-plane technique. In our experience it is better to visualize and block the posterior branch first, then retract the needle to anesthetize the anterior branch. If the anterior branch were blocked first, the local anesthetic would tend to obscure the posterior branch. The obturator nerve can be blocked by ultrasound guidance alone without the need for nerve stimulation.[40]

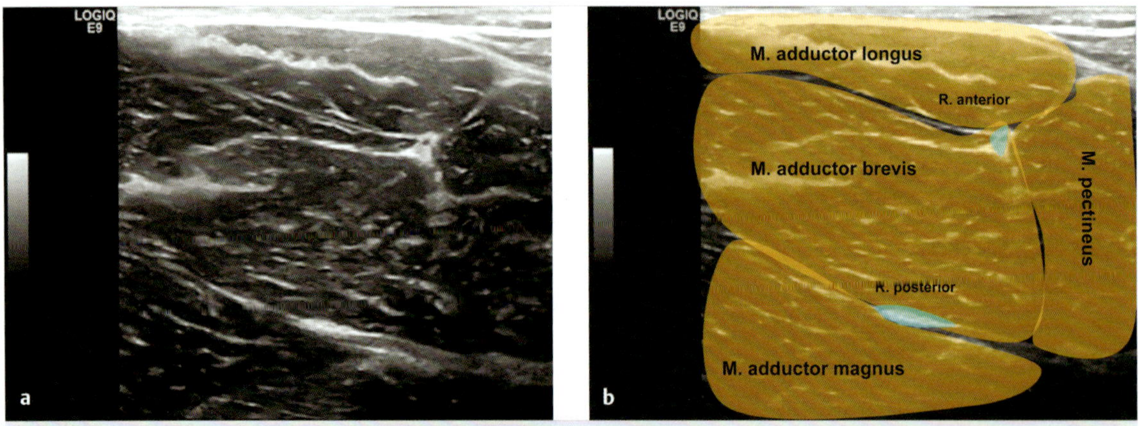

Fig. 29.11 a, b The anterior and posterior branches of the obturator nerve and their relation to adductor longus, brevis and magnus.

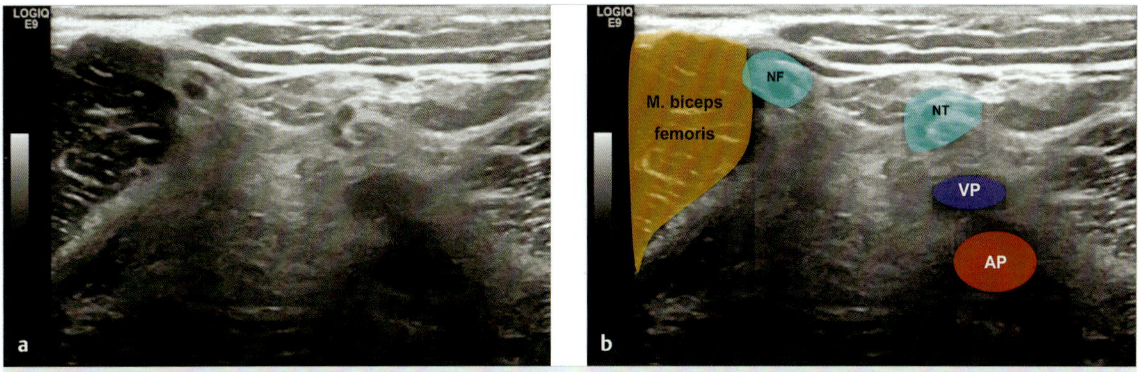

Fig. 29.12 a, b The tibial part (NT) and fibular part (NF) of the sciatic nerve are visible above the popliteal artery (AP) and popliteal vein (VP). The biceps femoris appears laterally.

Literature on the Obturator Nerve Block

In a study of 30 patients undergoing knee surgery, Sinha et al[40] showed that blocking the obturator nerve under ultrasound guidance without the additional use of nerve stimulation had the same success rates as obturator nerve blocks aided by nerve stimulation.[41]

29.8.4 Sciatic Nerve Block

Many approaches are available for anesthetizing the sciatic nerve, which can be blocked anywhere in its course. A quality ultrasound scanner can trace the nerve from the gluteal region into the popliteal fossa.[42,43] The course of the nerve deepens at various sites, making it inaccessible to imaging with a high-frequency probe. A curved array (abdominal transducer) may have to be used in very muscular patients. We prefer to block the sciatic nerve in the popliteal fossa, because the tibial nerve and fibular nerve can also be selectively and separately anesthetized at that level. This requires turning the patient to a lateral position, however. In cases where patient mobility is restricted, the sciatic nerve can be blocked through an anterior approach.[44]

Indications

Indications for the sciatic nerve block are as follows:

- Surgical procedures on the distal lower leg down to the foot (usually combined with a saphenous nerve block)
- Surgical procedures anywhere in the leg when combined with a psoas compartment block or femoral nerve block

Contraindications

There are no contraindications to the sciatic nerve block.

Complications

No complications are known.

Patient Position

The patient is placed in a lateral position with the leg to be blocked uppermost and with the lowermost leg flexed at the knee. A pad is placed between both legs. The leg to be blocked is extended at the knee, and the foot is supported on a padded rest. The skin site is prepared as described in Chapter 8. The operator sits behind the patient.

Sonography

The transducer is placed in the popliteal fossa and oriented to image the popliteal vein in cross-section. The popliteal vein appears as a round, echo-free structure that is easily compressed (▶ Fig. 29.12). The popliteal artery appears below it as another round, echo-free, pulsating structure. When the popliteal vein has been compressed and only the popliteal artery can be seen, the tibial nerve can be identified as a round hyperechoic structure lateral to the artery. The transducer is now slid laterally toward the head of the fibula. The biceps femoris is identified, and the fibular nerve appears as a hypoechoic round or oval structure below the biceps femoris insertion. The transducer is moved proximally to the level where both nerves unite, and the anesthesia needle is introduced at that level. The needle may be advanced using the out-of-plane or in-plane technique. The in-plane technique can be used from the medial or lateral side. We prefer the out-of-plane approach because it shortens the distance from the skin surface to the nerve.

Literature on the Sciatic Nerve Block

Danelli et al[45] conducted a prospective, randomized study in 44 patients undergoing lower limb surgery. Sciatic nerve block was directed by nerve stimulation in 22 of the patients and by ultrasound guidance in the remaining 22. The onset time of sensory and motor block, success rate, and need for intraoperative fentanyl supplementation were evaluated. Patient satisfaction and procedure-related

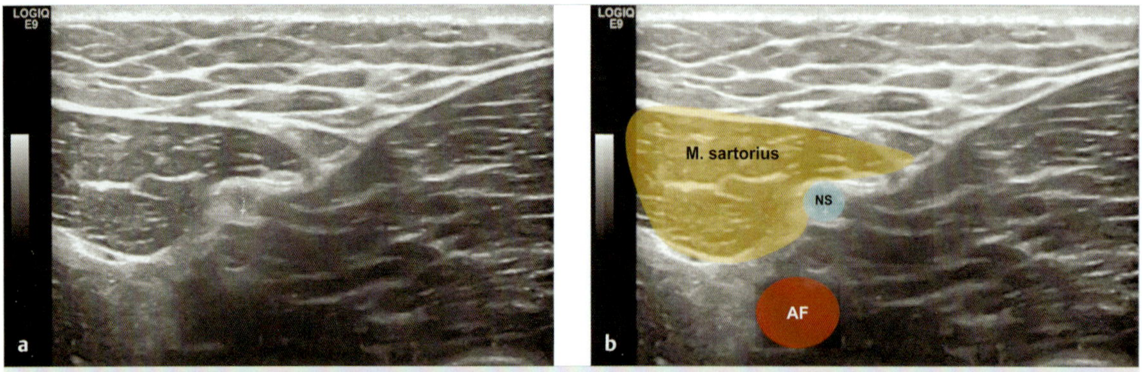

Fig. 29.13 a, b The saphenous nerve (NS) and sartorius muscle (tub-shaped) are imaged in the middle third of the thigh. The femoral artery (AF) appears below the saphenous nerve.

pain were also documented. The needle was advanced using in-plane technique. The onset times for sensory and motor blocks were comparable in both groups. The success rate was higher for ultrasound guidance than for nerve stimulation. Ultrasound guidance reduced the time needed to perform the block and was associated with less procedural pain.

29.8.5 Saphenous Nerve Block

The saphenous nerve is a terminal sensory branch of the femoral nerve. It courses in the adductor canal with the femoral vessels and runs between the sartorius and vastus medialis muscles to the medial side of the knee. It is distributed to the medial border of the foot, accompanied by the long saphenous vein. The infrapatellar branch of the saphenous nerve follows a curved path below the patella.

Indications

The saphenous nerve block has the following indications:

- Surgical procedures on the lower leg and foot when combined with a sciatic nerve block (e.g., forefoot amputation in multimorbid patients)
- Blocking the infrapatellar branch to relieve pain after knee arthroscopy

Contraindications

There are no contraindications to the saphenous nerve block.

Complications

No complications are known.

Patient Position

The patient is positioned supine with the leg in slight external rotation and abduction. The skin site is prepared as described in Chapter 8.

Sonography

The first step is to locate the femoral artery, which appears as a round echo-free structure in the inguinal region. It is used as a landmark and is traced distally until a tub-shaped pennate structure appears in the middle third of the leg. This is the sartorius muscle, which marks the level at which the saphenous nerve can be blocked (▶ Fig. 29.13). The saphenous nerve appears as a hypoechoic oval structure at the inferior border of the sartorius. The needle is introduced using in-plane technique,[46] which provides a clear view of the needle tip and reduces the risk of puncturing the femoral artery.

Literature on the Saphenous Nerve Block

Tsai et al[46] studied the efficacy of an ultrasound-guided subsartorial approach to the saphenous nerve block in a retrospective series of 39 patients. The block was performed using in-plane technique and had a success rate of 77%.

29.8.6 Lateral Femoral Cutaneous Nerve Block

The lateral femoral cutaneous nerve is a pure sensory nerve branch. It crosses the iliacus muscle in the iliac fossa, then passes through the lacuna musculorum approximately 1 cm medial to the anterior superior iliac spine and is distributed to the skin on the lateral thigh. With modern ultrasound scanners, it is now possible to identify and block even very small nerves. Complete anesthesia of the leg can be produced by blocking the lateral femoral cutaneous nerve at the level of the anterior superior iliac spine in addition to blocking the femoral nerve, sciatic nerve, and obturator nerve. This nerve block can also be used for the successful treatment of meralgia paresthetica.[47]

Indications

Indications for the lateral femoral cutaneous nerve block are as follows:

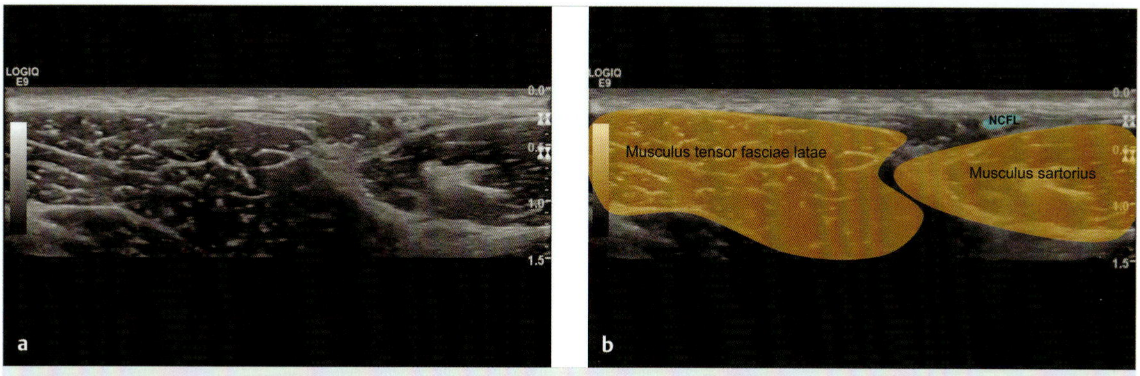

Fig. 29.14 a, b Lateral femoral cutaneous nerve (NFCL) imaged above the sartorius muscle.

- Adjunct for producing complete anesthesia of the leg; can also be used with a tourniquet for surgery under regional anesthesia alone
- Treatment of meralgia paresthetica (lateral femoral cutaneous nerve compression syndrome characterized by burning and needle-prick pains and numbness on the anterolateral aspect of the thigh)

Contraindications

There are no contraindications to the lateral femoral cutaneous nerve block.

Complications

No complications are known.

Patient Position

The patient is positioned supine with the leg in a neutral position. The skin site is prepared as described in Chapter 8.

Sonography

The anterior superior iliac spine is first palpated and then imaged by placing the transducer at right angles to the iliac spine. The bony anterior superior iliac spine appears sonographically as a bright echo with a posterior acoustic shadow. The transducer is now rotated downward on its medial side to display the sartorius muscle and tensor fasciae latae, both of which originate from the anterior superior iliac spine. With the transducer rotated downward, it is slid distally in that position until the lateral femoral cutaneous nerve appears above the sartorius muscle as an oval hypoechoic structure containing several small hypoechoic fascicles (▶ Fig. 29.14). This structure is also called a honeycomb pattern.[48] The needle is advanced in a lateral-to-medial direction using in-plane technique.

29.9 Summary

▶ Table 29.2 lists the various nerve blocks together with their technique, local anesthetic agent, and indications.

Table 29.2 Commonly used nerve and plexus blocks

Block	Needle insertion technique	Direction of needle insertion	Local anesthetic	Conditions and procedures
Interscalene brachial plexus block	Out-of-plane technique	Craniocaudal between the scalene muscles	0.2% ropivacaine, 20 mL, plus general anesthesia 1.5% prilocaine, 30 mL	Shoulder dislocation Shoulder surgery, operations on the lateral clavicle and upper arm
Supraclavicular brachial plexus block	In-plane technique	Transducer perpendicular to clavicle, lateral-to-medial needle insertion	1.5% prilocaine, 20–30 mL, with or without general anesthesia	Humeral shaft fracture Elbow fracture or dislocation
Infraclavicular brachial plexus block	In-plane technique	Transducer in infraclavicular fossa, perpendicular to and just below the clavicle; needle is inserted inferiorly in lateral-to-medial direction	1.5% prilocaine, 20–30 mL	Ulnar groove syndrome Forearm fracture Carpal tunnel syndrome

(Continued on next page.)

Table 29.2 (continued) Commonly used nerve and plexus blocks

Block	Needle insertion technique	Direction of needle insertion	Local anesthetic	Conditions and procedures
Axillary brachial plexus block	Out-of-plane technique	Transducer perpendicular to axillary artery; four nerves are individually identified	1.5% prilocaine, 30–40 mL	Forearm fracture Carpal tunnel syndrome Arthroscopic wrist surgery
Psoas compartment block	In-plane technique	Transducer horizontal to transverse processes of spine; surrounding structures are visualized (kidney, psoas major, lumbosacral plexus)	1.5% prilocaine, 30–40 mL	Femoral neck fracture, hip replacement when combined with sciatic nerve block
Femoral nerve block	Out-of-plane technique	Transducer parallel to inguinal ligament; femoral nerve is identified	0.25% bupivacaine, 20 mL, plus general anesthesia 0.2% ropivacaine for postoperative analgesia 1.5% prilocaine, 10 mL	Knee replacement Cruciate ligament reconstruction Arthrolysis
Obturator nerve block	In-plane technique	Femoral artery imaged in cross-section, transducer slid medially; adductors are identified; anesthesia is targeted to nerve branches	1.5% prilocaine, 10 mL	Useful as a supplemental block for knee operations
Sciatic nerve block	Out-of-plane technique	Popliteal vessels imaged in cross-section at level of popliteal fossa; anesthesia is targeted to the tibial nerve and fibular nerve	0.25% bupivacaine, 20 mL, plus general anesthesia 1.5% prilocaine, 20 mL 0.375% bupivacaine, 10 mL	Forefoot amputation when combined with saphenous nerve block
Saphenous nerve block	In-plane technique	Sartorius muscle and femoral artery imaged in cross-section in lower third of thigh	1.0% prilocaine, 10 mL	See sciatic nerve block
Lateral femoral cutaneous nerve block	In-plane technique		1.5% prilocaine, 6–7 mL	Treatment of meralgia paresthetica Analgesia for toleration of an intraoperative tourniquet

References

[1] Kapral S, Krafft P, Eibenberger K, Fitzgerald R, Gosch M, Weinstabl C. Ultrasound-guided supraclavicular approach for regional anesthesia of the brachial plexus. Anesth Analg 1994; 78: 507–513

[2] Marhofer P, Schrögendorfer K, Koinig H, Kapral S, Weinstabl C, Mayer N. Ultrasonographic guidance improves sensory block and onset time of three-in-one blocks. Anesth Analg 1997; 85: 854–857

[3] la Grange P, Foster PA, Pretorius LK. Application of the Doppler ultrasound bloodflow detector in supraclavicular brachial plexus block. Br J Anaesth 1978; 50: 965–967

[4] Bloc S, Mercadal L, Garnier T et al. Comfort of the patient during axillary blocks placement: a randomized comparison of the neurostimulation and the ultrasound guidance techniques. Eur J Anaesthesiol 2010; 27: 628–633

[5] Chan VW, Perlas A, McCartney CJ, Brull R, Xu D, Abbas S. Ultrasound guidance improves success rate of axillary brachial plexus block. Can J Anaesth 2007; 54: 176–182

[6] Gianesello L, Pavoni V, Coppini R et al. Comfort and satisfaction during axillary brachial plexus block in trauma patients: comparison of techniques. J Clin Anesth 2010; 22: 7–12

[7] O'Donnell BD, Ryan H, O'Sullivan O, Iohom G. Ultrasound-guided axillary brachial plexus block with 20 milliliters local anesthetic mixture versus general anesthesia for upper limb trauma surgery: an observer-blinded, prospective, randomized, controlled trial. Anesth Analg 2009; 109: 279–283

[8] Chan VW, Peng PW, Kaszas Z et al. A comparative study of general anesthesia, intravenous regional anesthesia, and axillary block for outpatient hand surgery: clinical outcome and cost analysis. Anesth Analg 2001; 93: 1181–1184

[9] Fredrickson MJ, Danesh-Clough TK. Ambulatory continuous femoral analgesia for major knee surgery: a randomised study of ultrasound-guided femoral catheter placement. Anaesth Intensive Care 2009; 37: 758–766

[10] Wang AZ, Gu L, Zhou QH, Ni WZ, Jiang W. Ultrasound-guided continuous femoral nerve block for analgesia after total knee arthroplasty: catheter perpendicular to the nerve versus catheter parallel to the nerve. Reg Anesth Pain Med 2010; 35: 127–131

[11] Plunkett AR, Buckenmaier CC, III. Safety of multiple, simultaneous continuous peripheral nerve block catheters in a patient receiving therapeutic low-molecular-weight heparin. Pain Med 2008; 9: 624–627

[12] Gogarten W, Van Aken H, Büttner J, Riess H, Wulf H, Buerkle H. Rückenmarksnahe Regionalanästhesien und Thromboembolieprophylaxe/ antithrombotische Medikation. A&I Anästhesiologie und Intensivmedizin 2007; 48: S109–S124
[13] Capdevila X, Pirat P, Bringuier S et al. French Study Group on Continuous Peripheral Nerve Blocks. Continuous peripheral nerve blocks in hospital wards after orthopedic surgery: a multicenter prospective analysis of the quality of postoperative analgesia and complications in 1,416 patients. Anesthesiology 2005; 103: 1: 035-1-0-45
[14] Neuburger M, Breitbarth J, Reisig F, Lang D, Büttner J. Complications and adverse events in continuous peripheral regional anesthesia Results of investigations on 3,491 catheters [Article in German]. Anaesthesist 2006; 55: 33–40
[15] Horlocker TT, O'Driscoll SW, Dinapoli RP. Recurring brachial plexus neuropathy in a diabetic patient after shoulder surgery and continuous interscalene block. Anesth Analg 2000; 91: 688–690
[16] Bigeleisen P, Wilson M. A comparison of two techniques for ultrasound guided infraclavicular block. Br J Anaesth 2006; 96: 502–507
[17] Winnie AP. Interscalene brachial plexus block. Anesth Analg 1970; 49: 455–466
[18] Yang WT, Chui PT, Metreweli C. Anatomy of the normal brachial plexus revealed by sonography and the role of sonographic guidance in anesthesia of the brachial plexus. AJR Am J Roentgenol 1998; 171: 1631–1636
[19] Campagna JA, Carter C. Clinical relevance of the Bezold-Jarisch reflex. Anesthesiology 2003; 98: 1250–1260
[20] Goebel S, Stehle J, Schwemmer U, Reppenhagen S, Rath B, Gohlke F. Interscalene brachial plexus block for open-shoulder surgery: a randomized, double-blind, placebo-controlled trial between single-shot anesthesia and patient-controlled catheter system. Arch Orthop Trauma Surg 2010; 130: 533–540
[21] Mariano ER, Afra R, Loland VJ et al. Continuous interscalene brachial plexus block via an ultrasound-guided posterior approach: a randomized, triple-masked, placebo-controlled study. Anesth Analg 2009; 108: 1688–1694
[22] Pippa P, Cominelli E, Marinelle C, Aito S. Brachial plexus block using the posterior approach. Eur J Anaesthesiol 1990; 7: 411–420
[23] Brown DL, Cahill DR, Bridenbaugh LD. Supraclavicular nerve block: anatomic analysis of a method to prevent pneumothorax. Anesth Analg 1993; 76: 530–534
[24] Korbon GA, Carron H, Lander CJ. First rib palpation: a safer, easier technique for supraclavicular brachial plexus block. Anesth Analg 1989; 68: 682–685
[25] Perlas AM, Lobo GM, Lo NM, Brull RM, Chan VWS, Karkhanis RM. Ultrasound-guided supraclavicular block: outcome of 510 consecutive cases. Reg Anesth Pain Med 2009; 34: 171–176
[26] Tran QH, Charghi R, Finlayson RJ. The "double bubble" sign for successful infraclavicular brachial plexus blockade. Anesth Analg 2006; 103: 1048–1049
[27] De Tran QH, Bertini PM, Zaouter CM, Muñoz LM, Finlayson RJM. A prospective, randomized comparison between single- and double-injection ultrasound-guided infraclavicular brachial plexus block. Reg Anesth Pain Med 2010; 35: 16–21
[28] De Jong RH. Axillary block of the brachial plexus. Anesthesiology 1961; 22: 215–225
[29] Ting PL, Sivagnanaratnam V. Ultrasonographic study of the spread of local anaesthetic during axillary brachial plexus block. Br J Anaesth 1989; 63: 326–329
[30] Lo N, Brull R, Perlas A et al. Evolution of ultrasound guided axillary brachial plexus blockade: retrospective analysis of 662 blocks. Can J Anaesth 2008; 55: 408–413
[31] O'Donnell BD, Iohom G. An estimation of the minimum effective anesthetic volume of 2% lidocaine in ultrasound-guided axillary brachial plexus block. Anesthesiology 2009; 111: 25–29
[32] Christophe JL, Berthier F, Boillot A et al. Assessment of topographic brachial plexus nerves variations at the axilla using ultrasonography. Br J Anaesth 2009; 103: 606–612
[33] Remerand F, Laulan J, Couvret C et al. Is the musculocutaneous nerve really in the coracobrachialis muscle when performing an axillary block? An ultrasound study. Anesth Analg 2010; 110: 1729–1734
[34] Chayen D, Nathan H, Chayen M. The psoas compartment block. Anesthesiology 1976; 45: 95–99
[35] Touray ST, de Leeuw MA, Zuurmond WWA, Perez RSGM. Psoas compartment block for lower extremity surgery: a meta-analysis. Br J Anaesth 2008; 101: 750–760
[36] Kirchmair L, Entner T, Wissel J, Moriggl B, Kapral S, Mitterschiffthaler G. A study of the paravertebral anatomy for ultrasound-guided posterior lumbar plexus block. Anesth Analg 2001; 93: 477–481
[37] Winnie AP, Ramamurthy S, Durrani Z. The inguinal paravascular technic of lumbar plexus anesthesia: the "3-in-1 block". Anesth Analg 1973; 52: 989–996
[38] Lang SA, Yip RW, Chang PC, Gerard MA. The femoral 3-in-1 block revisited. J Clin Anesth 1993; 5: 292–296
[39] Mariano ER, Loland VJ, Sandhu NS et al. Ultrasound guidance versus electrical stimulation for femoral perineural catheter insertion. J Ultrasound Med 2009; 28: 1453–1460
[40] Sinha SKM, Abrams JHM, Houle TTP, Weller RS. Ultrasound-guided obturator nerve block: an interfascial injection approach without nerve stimulation. Reg Anesth Pain Med 2009; 34: 261–264
[41] Kardash K, Hickey D, Tessler MJ, Payne S, Zukor D, Velly AM. Obturator versus femoral nerve block for analgesia after total knee arthroplasty. Anesth Analg 2007; 105: 853–858
[42] Bruhn J, Van Geffen GJ, Gielen MJ, Scheffer GJ. Visualization of the course of the sciatic nerve in adult volunteers by ultrasonography. Acta Anaesthesiol Scand 2008; 52: 1298–1302
[43] Perlas A, Brull R, Chan VWS, McCartney CJL, Nuica A, Abbas S. Ultrasound guidance improves the success of sciatic nerve block at the popliteal fossa. Reg Anesth Pain Med 2008; 33: 259–265
[44] Tsui BCH, Ozelsel TJ. Ultrasound-guided anterior sciatic nerve block using a longitudinal approach: "expanding the view". Reg Anesth Pain Med 2008; 33: 275–276
[45] Danelli G, Fanelli A, Ghisi D et al. Ultrasound vs nerve stimulation multiple injection technique for posterior popliteal sciatic nerve block. Anaesthesia 2009; 64: 638–642
[46] Tsai PB, Karnwal A, Kakazu C, Tokhner V, Julka IS. Efficacy of an ultrasound-guided subsartorial approach to saphenous nerve block: a case series. Can J Anaesth 2010; 57: 683–688
[47] Tumber PS, Bhatia A, Chan VW. Ultrasound-guided lateral femoral cutaneous nerve block for meralgia paresthetica. Anesth Analg 2008; 106: 1021–1022
[48] Hurdle MF, Weingarten TN, Crisostomo RA, Psimos C, Smith J. Ultrasound-guided blockade of the lateral femoral cutaneous nerve: technical description and review of 10 cases. Arch Phys Med Rehabil 2007; 88: 1362–1364

30 Ultrasound-Guided Emergency and Vascular Interventions

T. Mueller, C. Jenssen

30.1 Emergency Interventions

Ultrasonography has assumed an increasingly important role in emergency and critical care medicine in recent years. After the history and physical examination, ultrasound is the method of choice for the investigation of a medical acute abdomen.[1] In surgical emergencies it is used in the FAST protocol (focused assessment with sonography for trauma) within the framework of ATLS (advanced trauma life support) and is practiced under a number of other acronyms (FASTER, p-FAST, EFAST, etc.). Ultrasound is used in emergency settings for the rapid detection of free fluid in the abdomen, pleural space, or pericardium. Abdominal ultrasound provides a specificity > 90% with a variable sensitivity ranging from 31 to 83%.[2–6] FAST has not yet demonstrated a survival benefit in trauma patients,[7] although its primary use in an algorithm with secondary CT is advocated in equivocal cases.[8]

Ultrasound provides a technology that "comes to the patient" in critical care situations. Diagnostic uses are paramount, with one study finding that ultrasound-guided interventions accounted for just 0.25% of all indications.[9] Ultrasound had immediate diagnostic or therapeutic implications in 5.5% of cases and short-term implications in another 20%.

Ultrasound is fast, mobile, economical, and highly sensitive for the detection of free fluids. Consequently, percutaneous interventions should be integrated into the examination:

- Diagnostic interventions, followed if necessary by immediate therapeutic interventions, in patients with suspected hemorrhage (hemothorax, hemoperitoneum), empyemas, or abscesses
- Drainage procedures in life-threatening situations (pericardial tamponade, tension pneumothorax)
- Establishing access to central and peripheral veins and arteries

Several international ultrasound societies have proposed or instituted multilevel training programs for emergency sonography. All of these programs include ultrasound-guided interventions in the initial training phase.[10–13]

30.1.1 Indications

A number of urgent indications for interventional procedures are recognized in emergency and critical care medicine. They are summarized in ▶ Table 30.1.

Almost all ultrasound-guided interventions in emergency medicine are also practiced in "routine" situations.

Table 30.1 Indications for ultrasound-guided emergency and vascular interventions

Indication	Goals	Method
Fluid in the pleural space	Determine etiology	Aspirate with 20-gauge needle under ultrasound guidance
Hemothorax	Establish drainage, improve dyspnea, prevent organized hematoma formation	Place 12–14F drain under ultrasound guidance
Thoracic empyema	Establish drainage, improve dyspnea, prevent sepsis	Place 12–14F drain under ultrasound guidance
Pneumothorax Tension pneumothorax	Expand the lung, improve dyspnea	Place 8F drain under ultrasound guidance
Intra-abdominal free fluid	Determine etiology	Aspirate with 20-gauge needle under ultrasound guidance
Spontaneous bacterial peritonitis	Establish drainage, improve dyspnea, prevent sepsis	Place 10–12F drain under ultrasound guidance
Fluid in the pericardium	Differential diagnosis	Aspirate with 20-gauge needle under ultrasound guidance
Pericardial tamponade	Establish drainage, prevent pump failure	Place 14-gauge catheter under ultrasound guidance
Abscess, empyema	Confirm suspected diagnosis	Aspirate with 20-gauge needle under ultrasound guidance
	Therapeutic drainage	Place 8–12F drain under ultrasound guidance
Venous access	Rapid, uncomplicated placement of a secure central venous line	Ultrasound guidance in long- or short-axis view
Arterial cannula	Arterial pressure measurement, BGA	Ultrasound guidance in long- or short-axis view
Pseudoaneurysm	Obliterate the pseudoaneurysm	Ultrasound-guided thrombin injection

In this chapter, accordingly, we shall focus our attention on specific issues relating to emergency settings and will otherwise refer the reader to chapters dealing with specific body regions.

Ultrasound can also be used for control purposes before or after critical care interventions: Studies indicate that imaging the neck before a percutaneous dilatational tracheostomy warrants a change of puncture site in 24 to 36% of cases. The rate of major complications can be reduced from 4% to 0%, while the rate of minor complications remains approximately the same (0.7% versus 1%) and the rate of cuff perforations falls from 10% to 0.9%. Ultrasound guidance can also prevent placing the tracheostomy tube too high.[14–16]

The correct placement of a conventionally placed endotracheal tube can be reliably confirmed by the "sliding lung sign," or relative sliding of the visceral and parietal pleura seen at ultrasound. This sign is absent over a nonventilated lung.[17,18]

Ultrasound can reliably detect the presence of a feeding tube for enteral nutrition in the small intestine. This method appears to be particularly useful in children as a means of avoiding radiation exposure.[19,20]

30.1.2 Contraindications

Possible alternatives (CT-guided intervention, surgical intervention) should also be considered in emergencies. No comparative studies have yet been done on the different options that are available in emergency settings. Fewer contraindications exist in emergencies, and it is important to make an individual risk assessment in a patient with impaired coagulation, for example. Physicians still have the obligation to disclose necessary information, except in the case of an acutely life-threatening, unstable situation or an unconscious patient. The timing and scope of the disclosure depend on the severity and urgency of the intervention.

Two basic contraindications remain:

- Refusal of informed consent
- Lack of practical implications

30.1.3 Materials and Equipment

Ultrasound Technology

"Bedside ultrasound" and "point-of-care ultrasound" are terms that describe the capability to examine patients almost anywhere using portable devices. The advantage of portable scanners is that they can be delivered quickly to the patient and can even be taken to accident sites by rescue personnel.[21] Many authors stress the time gained by use of mobile devices in the hospital—which usually means that ultrasound machines are absent at strategically important sites like the emergency room and intensive care unit.

In principle, ultrasound equipment should be available that can image and document relevant structures with optimum quality in every situation. Portable machines are inferior to high-end systems in terms of image quality.[22,23]

No comparative prospective studies have yet been done on interventions with portable ultrasound scanners. One small series ($n = 12$) reported good results with hand-carried ultrasound-guided pericardiocentesis and thoracentesis.[24] In our experience, the success of an ultrasound-guided intervention depends to a substantial degree on the familiarity of the operator with the machine, regardless of its portability.

Superficial interventions in arteries and veins are guided with a 7.5- to 10-MHz linear transducer, while a standard curved-array "abdominal" transducer is used for paracentesis. We also use a high-frequency linear transducer for the aspiration of small pleural effusions.

Interventional Materials

A limited array of interventional materials and supplies are used in emergency settings (▶ Table 30.2). Procedures are simplified by using as few different materials as possible to solve a maximum number of problems.

Practice

- Ultrasound machines and interventional equipment belong at the emergency treatment site.
- Physicians on duty must be familiar with the materials and equipment.

Table 30.2 Necessary interventional materials in the emergency room and intensive care unit

Goal	Materials
Diagnostic aspiration (effusion, abscess, empyema, hemorrhage)	20-gauge needles in 4- and 7-cm lengths 10-mL and 20-mL syringes
Drain insertion (chest, abdomen)	8–14F pigtail catheters Scalpels Initial puncture needles Seldinger wires Dilators Three-way stopcocks Luer lock bag Reservoirs with water seal (Or: ready-to-use sets)
Drain insertion (pericardium)	14-gauge single-lumen CVC sets Three-way stopcocks 50-mL perfusor syringes Luer lock bag (Or: ready-to-use sets)
CVC placement	Standard CVC sets
Arterial cannula	Standard arterial indwelling cannulas
Aneurysm obliteration	20-gauge needles in 4- and 7-cm lengths 1-mL syringes with fine scale (insulin syringes) Thrombin

Abbreviation: CVC, central venous catheter.

30.1.4 Antisepsis

The principles of antisepsis are reviewed in Chapter 8.

The patient's skin is shaved if necessary and prepared with an alcohol solution. The transducer must be thoroughly cleaned and disinfected before use (e.g., with alcohol- and aldehyde-free wipes). Since the operator will not touch the needle or the patient's skin in a diagnostic intervention, it is unnecessary to wear sterile gloves. Disposable gloves are worn, however, to prevent contamination with the patient's blood.[25]

Following use, the transducer is cleaned with a (nonsterile) towel and again disinfected with antiseptic wipes.

Vascular interventions and the drainage of abscesses and effusions must be performed under sterile conditions. Sterile drapes, gloves, gown, mask, cap, and sterile device covers (for transducer and keyboard) are essential, just as in an operating room.

30.1.5 Problems and Complications

Emergency ultrasonography takes several minutes of calm, steady concentration and should always employ sterile technique. Problems arise when the operator is unfamiliar with the ultrasound machine, space is confined, vision is poor, or multiple concurrent actions are being carried out on the patient (see ▶ Table 30.3).

The complications that may arise in emergency interventions are of the same nature as those in elective settings. To date there have been no systematic studies comparing the complication rates of interventions in emergency settings versus normal conditions. Time pressure, unstable patients, a hectic environment, confined space, and hygienic issues suggest that complication rates are likely to be higher. The complication rates of thoracentesis in ICU patients range from 1.3% to 18% and are comparable to the rates reported in routine settings.[26,27]

Table 30.3 Problems and proposed solutions

Problem	Possible solutions
Difficulty operating a device	Train all ER and ICU staff members in the operation of the device. Bring along a familiar, portable device.
Difficult ambient conditions	Darken the room. Pause other actions. Call for assistance.
Difficult patient conditions	Improve position if possible. Move patient to a (semi)sitting position for thoracentesis. Move patient to a supine position for abdominal puncture. Use sedation if required.
Uncertain needle path	Look for a different approach. Reposition the patient. Summon experts. Consider alternative procedures.
Difficult asepsis	Diagnostic intervention: employ aseptic skin preparation, ensure transducer disinfection. Use sterile "operating room" technique for drains and vascular access.

30.1.6 Intra-abdominal Free Fluid

A differential diagnosis must be made quickly, and its scope depends on the patient's history. If the pattern of injury is unclear in a patient with blunt abdominal trauma, or if no organic injuries can be found but emergency ultrasound detects the presence of free fluid, a diagnosis of *hemoperitoneum* should be confirmed. The sensitivity of ultrasound for detecting intra-abdominal free fluid in the FAST evaluation of trauma patients varies greatly in published studies—as does the proficiency of the examiners. If fluid can be detected, an immediate *ultrasound-guided fine needle aspiration* should be performed to investigate the cause (hemoperitoneum, ascites, urine). This intervention takes only a few minutes and may be crucial in directing further actions.

In patients with an acute abdomen and/or sepsis and intra-abdominal free fluid, the diagnostic aspiration of ascites can provide a rapid diagnosis and may facilitate the decision for emergency laparotomy by detecting bowel contents, pancreatogenic ascites, purulent fluid, or blood.

Bacterial peritonitis (spontaneous or secondary) should be urgently excluded in patients with hepatic cirrhosis, ascites, and sudden clinical deterioration. Again, immediate needle aspiration may be rewarding as a granulocyte count > 240/µL establishes a diagnosis of spontaneous bacterial peritonitis.[28]

There is no emergency indication for the immediate catheter drainage of intra-abdominal free fluid. Even for spontaneous bacterial peritonitis, there have been no studies comparing patients treated by catheter drainage versus antibiotics only.

Procedure

The steps in the procedure are as follows:

1. Locate the ideal puncture site (easily accessible, no interposed vessels, significant fluid volume).
2. Introduce the 20-gauge needle under long- or short-axis ultrasound guidance without prior local anesthesia.
3. The detection of blood or bloody ascites may warrant (exploratory) laparotomy.
4. Ascites should be investigated by chemical and microbiological analysis.

Caution

Free fluid in the abdomen of emergency room patients requires immediate diagnostic aspiration.

Abscess, Empyema

Abscesses and empyemas (e.g., acute cholecystitis, infected pancreatic pseudocyst) are an urgent but rarely emergent indication for percutaneous drainage. They should always be treated on the same day. This allows enough time to perform these procedures "semielectively" in a calm atmosphere. The puncture and drainage techniques are described in Chapter 15.

30.1.7 Intrathoracic Free Fluid

A **hemothorax** may require immediate surgical intervention (e.g., for an aortic dissection), depending on the pattern of injury. Primary chest tube placement is a reasonable option in cases where acute bleeding may have stopped but the patient still has significant respiratory compromise. With a long-standing hemothorax, significant adhesions may develop between the pleural layers.

Large (more than 1/2 hemithorax), loculated effusions and empyemas with a pH < 7.2 or positive microbial stain or culture also require immediate chest tube drainage (▶ Fig. 30.1).[29,30]

Traditionally, hemothorax and empyema are treated with a large-bore thoracostomy tube that requires prior blunt surgical dissection of the drainage tract. Pigtail catheters (8–14F) can be placed faster and more easily. They have success rates of 42 to 80% for the drainage of empyema and up to 100% for traumatic hemothorax.[26,31] We therefore primarily use 10F to 12F drains. An early diagnosis and early initiation of treatment are important because the later formation of septa and adhesions will prevent percutaneous therapy.

If treatment is unsuccessful (no significant improvement in 3 days, clogged drain, poor output), the tube should be promptly exchanged for a large-bore catheter or replaced by thoracoscopic therapy.[30]

Empyemas can also be treated by instilling fibrinolytic agents (streptokinase, urokinase) into the pleural cavity. This treatment achieves higher cure rates than saline irrigation. The role of drainage compared with primary thoracoscopic therapy cannot be definitively assessed at present.[29,32]

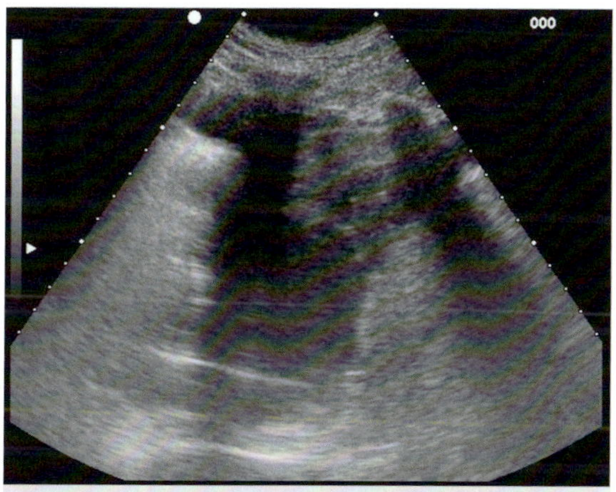

Fig. 30.1 Right posterior infrascapular ultrasound scan of a hemothorax following multiple rib fractures (motorcycle accident). An inhomogeneous, hypoechoic fluid collection is visible in the pleural space.

Procedure

The steps in the procedure are as follows:

1. Place the patient in a sitting position if possible.
2. Locate the ideal puncture site (easily accessible, superior rib border, significant fluid volume).
3. Introduce the 20-gauge needle (diagnostic) under long- or short-axis ultrasound guidance without prior local anesthesia.
4. Then administer local anesthesia if required.
5. Make a stab incision.
6. Introduce a pigtail catheter along the superior rib border using trocar technique. With large effusions, the skin site can be marked under sonographic guidance and the needle inserted without continuous imaging (▶ Fig. 30.1, ▶ Fig. 30.2).
7. Connect a three-way stopcock and reservoir with water seal; suction may be applied if needed (15 cm H_2O).
8. Analyze the aspirate according to etiology: infectious → microbiology, Ziehl-Neelsen stain, pH, WBC, clinical chemistry; traumatic → Hb; malignant: → cytology.

30.1.8 Pneumothorax

Ultrasound is more sensitive than standard chest radiographs in the diagnosis of pneumothorax[33,34] and therefore is an effective guidance modality for treatment. While ultrasound cannot display the position of the drain in the pneumothorax, it can determine whether pneumothorax is actually present at the proposed puncture site.

Adequate drainage can usually be obtained with 7F to 9F pigtail catheters, which have an 84 to 97% success rate for drainage periods of 2 to 4 days. Single or repeated needle aspiration is an alternative for idiopathic pneumothorax.[35,36] If a drainage tube is placed, an oblique intra- and subcutaneous tunnel should be developed to prevent recurrence after drain removal (see also Chapter 24).

Procedure

1. Elevate the upper body 30 to 45°.
2. Localize free air by ultrasound and administer local anesthesia at the typical Monaldi site (second or third intercostal space in the midclavicular line) or at an atypical site if the pneumothorax is incomplete or accompanied by adhesions.

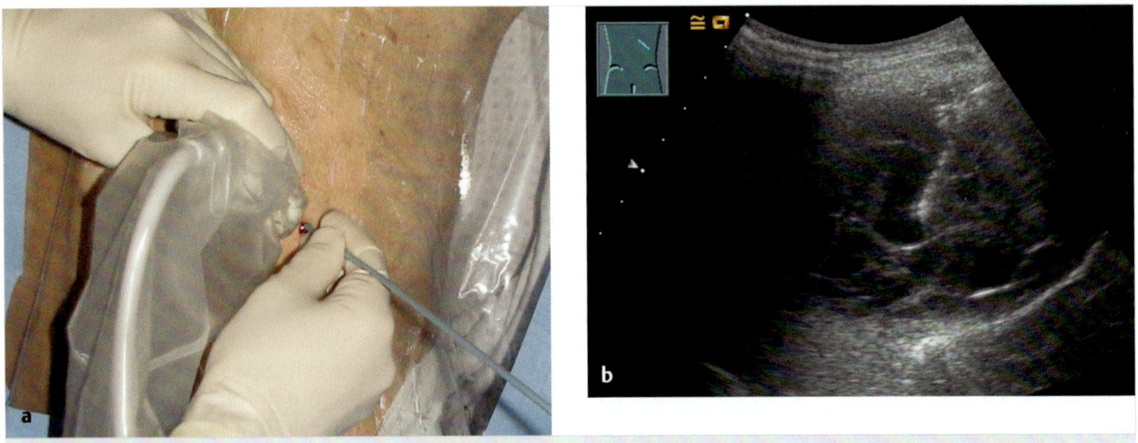

Fig. 30.2 Drainage of an empyema in a severely dyspneic patient under sonographic guidance using the trocar technique.
a Transducer placement and drain insertion using sterile technique.
b Corresponding ultrasound image. The drain appears as a linear echo entering the image from the right side. Multiple septa have already formed within the empyema, appearing as echogenic lines.

3. Make a stab incision.
4. Introduce an 8F to10F pigtail catheter along the superior rib border using trocar technique.
5. Connect a three-way stopcock and water-seal suction at 15 cm H_2O.

30.1.9 Pericardial Fluid

Pericardial tamponade is a life-threatening condition that may have a malignant, infectious, postoperative, or occasionally a traumatic etiology. Echocardiography typically shows "swinging heart" motion within the pericardium (▶ Fig. 30.3). The right atrium and possibly the left atrium show diastolic collapse, and the right ventricle may collapse at end diastole. Even small effusions may be life threatening: the clinical parameters of hypotension, tachycardia with a paradoxical pulse (i.e., pulse diminished on inspiration), and distended neck veins are considered indications for pericardiocentesis. An aortic dissection should first be excluded as the cause, as it would necessitate primary surgical treatment.[37] Ultrasound has a sensitivity of 100% and specificity of 96.9% in the detection of traumatic pericardial effusion.[38]

Caution

With fluid in the pericardium: rule out aortic dissection!

Ultrasound guided drainage has been described as safe and effective in several clinical series, with success rates of 97 to 99.1%. Major complications (1.3%) are ventricular injury, hemopneumothorax, and sustained ventricular tachycardia (3%) while minor complications have a reported incidence of 3.5% in the largest published series.[39,40]

The ideal puncture site is not necessarily subxiphoid, which was once considered standard. With ultrasound guidance, the needle can be introduced at the site where the effusion volume is greatest and the distance from the skin surface is short with no critical intervening structures. The injection of NaCl or HES (hydroxyethyl starch), for example, will produce a "white cloud" that accurately marks the position of the puncture needle and drain (▶ Fig. 30.4, ▶ Fig. 30.5).[41]

We use a single-lumen 14-gauge central venous catheter for pericardial drainage, since all physicians are familiar with its use. Pericardiocentesis sets usually include approximately 8F drains and dilators (e.g., from Cook Medical). It is not necessary to have an ECG lead attached

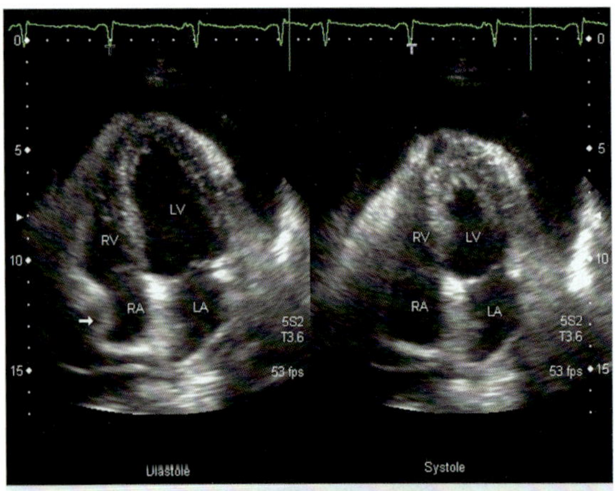

Fig. 30.3 Hemodynamically significant pericardial effusion with a "swinging heart" pattern in a breast cancer patient. The swinging heart in the pericardial sac shows diastolic collapse of the right atrium (arrow at left) and end-diastolic collapse of the right ventricle. (Source: image courtesy of Dr. M. H. Hust, Reutlingen, Germany.)

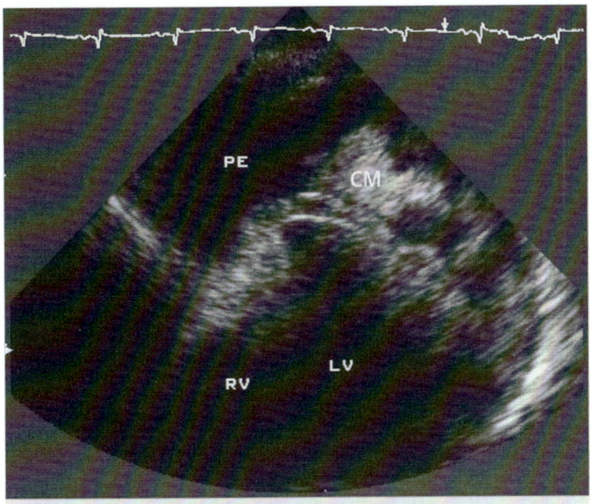

Fig. 30.4 HES is injected to check the position of the puncture needle. The solution acts like contrast medium (CM) to produce a visible "white cloud." LV, left ventricle; PE, pericardial effusion; RV, right ventricle. (Source: image courtesy of Dr. M. H. Hust, Reutlingen, Germany.)

to the needle hub when ultrasound guidance and skin surface leads are used.

Procedure

1. Elevate the upper body 30 to 45°.
2. Start ECG monitoring.
3. Administer local anesthesia under sonographic guidance.
4. Make a stab incision.
5. The needle is usually introduced under sonographic guidance. On entering the pericardial sac, inject agitated NaCl or HES to check the needle position.

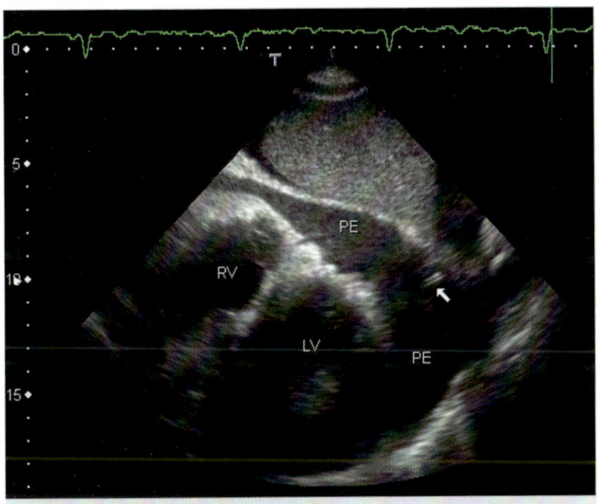

Fig. 30.5 Pericardiocentesis in situ. The drainage catheter appears as a tram-track echo at the tip of the arrow. LV, left ventricle; PE, pleural effusion; RV, right ventricle. (Source: image courtesy of Dr. M. H. Hust, Reutlingen, Germany.)

6. Change to Seldinger wire and insert a drain primarily or after dilating the tract.
7. Recheck placement by injecting NaCl or HES.
8. The aspiration of bright red blood may indicate puncture of a coronary artery, the right ventricle, or the left ventricle if an apical approach was used.
9. Analyze the aspirate according to etiology: infectious → microbiology, Ziehl-Neelsen stain; traumatic (or bloody aspirate) → Hb; malignant → cytology.

30.2 Percutaneous Vascular Interventions

30.2.1 Vascular Access

Central venous catheterization was traditionally done "blindly" on the basis of designated anatomical landmarks. Ultrasound improved this technique by allowing the operator to image the target vessel in two planes and then mark its course on the skin, followed again by a "blind" needle insertion (▶ Fig. 30.6a, b). In any case, the target vessel must be imaged sonographically before the intervention in order to detect any positional anomalies and avoid puncturing a thrombosed vein (▶ Fig. 30.7).

On the basis of the results of two meta-analyses, central venous catheter placement *under continuous ultrasound guidance* results in fewer placement attempts and fewer malplacements in the internal jugular vein, subclavian vein, and femoral vein of adults and the internal jugular vein of children, reducing overall complication rates from 10.2% to 4.6%. The differences in time to catheter placement and costs (including device acquisition) were not clinically relevant compared with the landmark technique.[42–44]

Another study showed that real time ultrasound guidance also reduced complications relative to the landmark technique under emergency conditions using a portable scanner.[45] Central venous catheterization under ultrasound guidance has been incorporated into the British guidelines of the National Institute for Health and Care Excellence.[46]

The needle can be visualized in a long-axis view with the vessel imaged in longitudinal section, or a short-axis orientation can be used. In the short-axis view the needle cross-section appears as a punctate echo. The needle tip can be identified only by gently oscillating the transducer. The long-axis view displays the full length of the needle, making it easier to avoid penetration of the posterior vessel wall (▶ Fig. 30.8, ▶ Fig. 30.9).

The **internal jugular vein** is the vessel most often catheterized and is excellent for learning the ultrasound guidance technique. Even physicians unfamiliar with general diagnostic ultrasound can quickly master the long-axis imaging technique with a little practice. It takes some practice to work synchronously with both hands, i.e., holding the transducer in one hand while inserting the needle with the other.

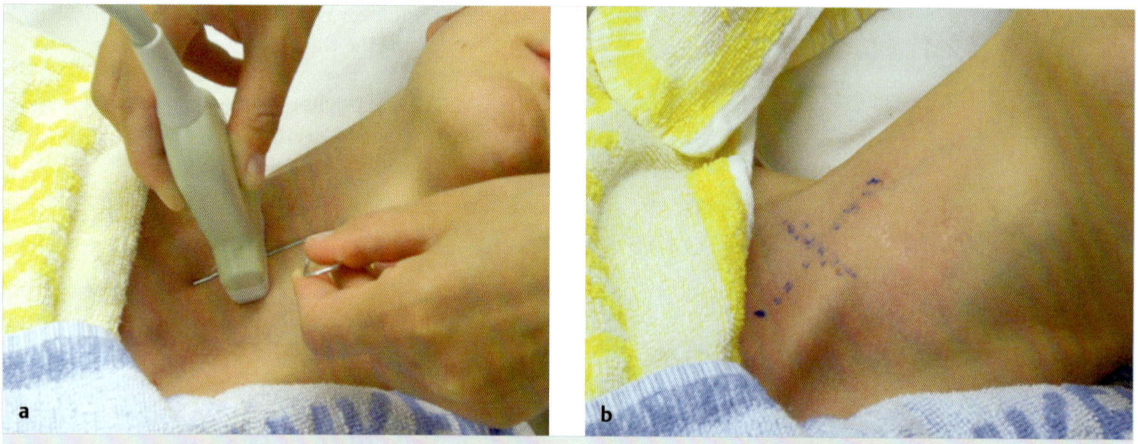

Fig. 30.6 a, b Ultrasound-assisted landmark technique. The right internal jugular vein is imaged in two planes, and its course and the puncture site are marked on the skin with a waterproof marker. The paperclip beneath the transducer is oriented along the course of the vein.

There are very few occasions where a central venous catheter must be placed within a few minutes without benefit of an ultrasound machine. Given the smaller number of placement attempts and needle redirections, placement of a central venous catheter (CVC) under continuous ultrasound imaging guidance should be standard practice. It can significantly reduce the incidence of complications.

Practice

Continuous ultrasound guidance reduces errors in CVC placement and should be standard practice.

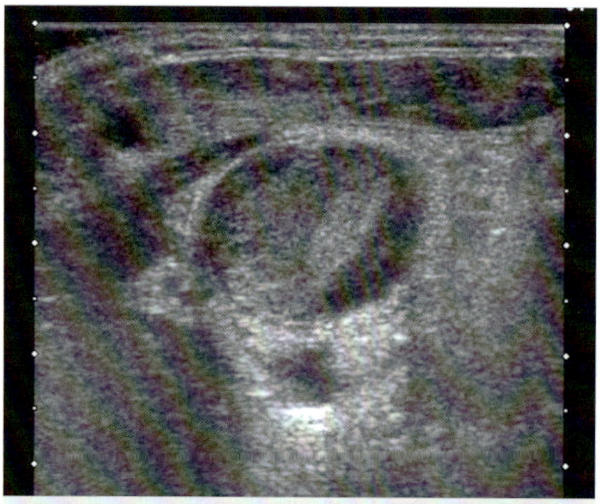

Fig. 30.7 Short-axis view (cross-section) of the left internal jugular vein. The vessel is noncompressible and filled with echogenic material: thrombosis in a breast cancer patient. The catheter was inserted on the opposite side.

Procedure

1. Help from an assistant in sterile attire is ideal.
2. Place the transducer in a sterile probe cover.
3. The operator should wear sterile operating room attire.
4. The patient is positioned supine. A head-down tilt may be added to improve venous filling.
5. For puncture of the internal jugular vein, the operator stands behind the patient's head with the ultrasound machine next to the patient. For puncture of the subclavian vein, the operator stands on the ipsilateral side next to the patient (▶ Fig. 30.8a).
6. First image the vessel in a long-axis (longitudinal) view and short-axis (cross-sectional) view.
7. Inspect the vessel and its surroundings (atypical location? thrombi? venous valves?).
8. Image the vessel in a long-axis view proximal to the puncture site.
9. Administer local anesthesia under sonographic guidance.
10. Introduce the needle using Seldinger technique in a long-axis view that shows the full needle path. Insertion of the puncture needle and wire is monitored on the screen. After that, any tract dilation and exchange for the CVC can be done with or without real-time ultrasound guidance (▶ Fig. 30.8b–d, ▶ Fig. 30.9).

Even deep or nonpalpable *peripheral veins* can be reliably catheterized in (obese) adults and children with difficult intravenous access when ultrasound guidance is used.[47,48] With a tourniquet on the upper arm, the vein is imaged in a long-axis view proximal to the puncture site. The operator holds the transducer in one hand while introducing the needle with the other (▶ Fig. 30.10). Skin antisepsis and transducer disinfection are sufficient for the

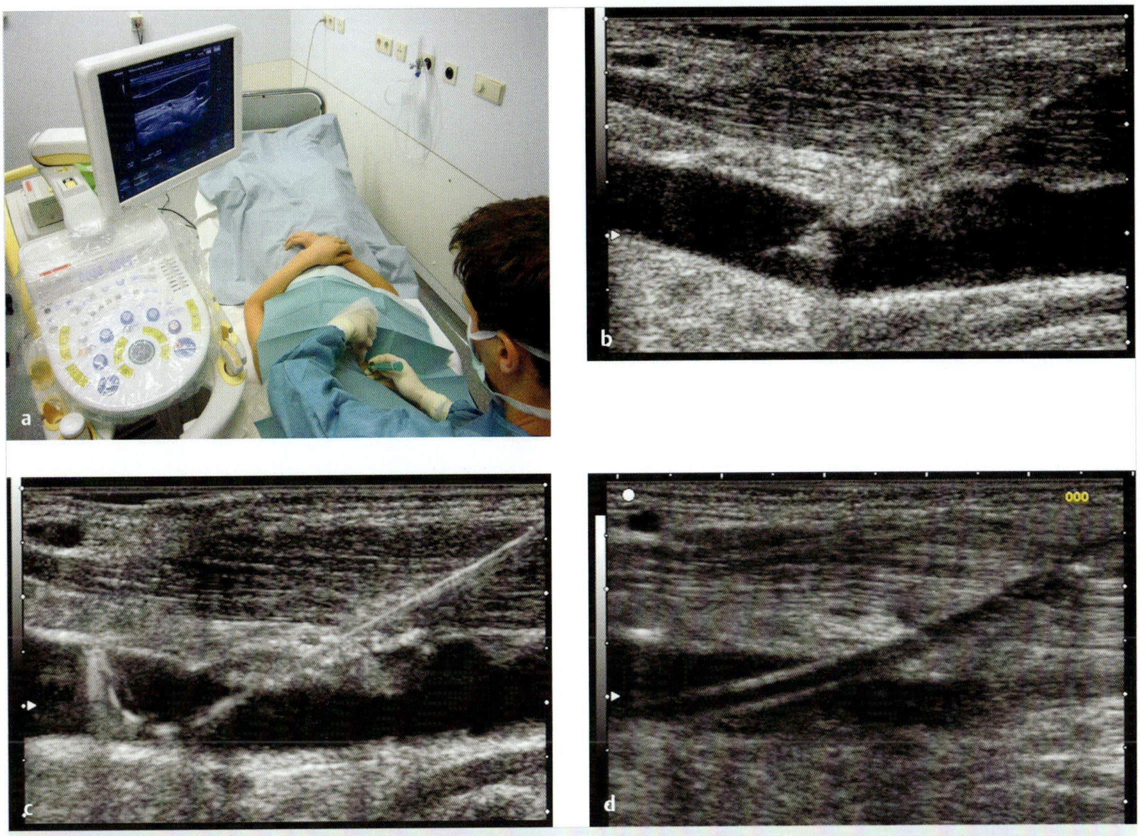

Fig. 30.8 Central venous catheter placement.
a Sterile conditions for catheterization of the right internal jugular vein. The operator in sterile attire sits behind the patient's head and has a clear view of both the monitor and puncture site. Sterile covers have been placed on the keyboard and transducer.
b Puncture of the right internal jugular vein: the needle is clearly visualized in the long-axis view, which avoids perforating the posterior vessel wall.
c The advancing guidewire is clearly visualized.
d The double-wall echoes from the CVC (here a single-lumen dialysis catheter) are clearly visible in the vessel lumen.

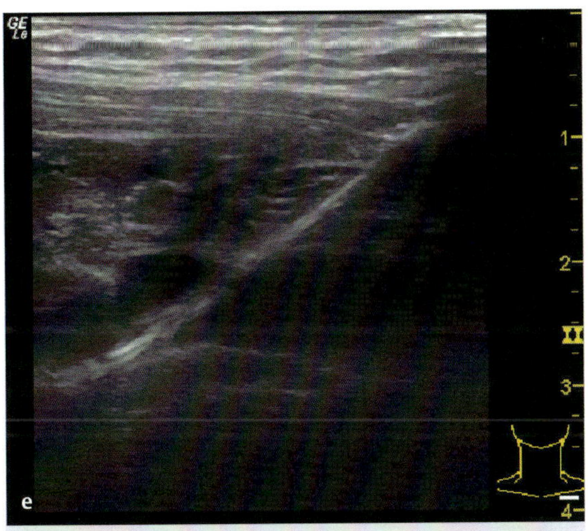

Fig. 30.9 Long-axis view of the catheter advancing in the subclavian vein. (Source: image courtesy of Dr. C. Rex, Reutlingen, Germany.)

placement of a simple indwelling venous cannula, taking care not to touch the transducer with the cannula.

Ultrasound can also be used successfully for **arterial cannulation** (blood gas analysis, invasive blood pressure measurement). For this application we usually introduce the needle in a short-axis view (▶ Fig. 30.11). Before the puncture, the patency of both forearm arteries (radial and ulnar arteries) is assessed by color Doppler ultrasound to avoid inducing critical ischemia in the hand.

Practice

If multiple attempts or needle redirections are necessary in peripheral venous catheterizations: use ultrasound.

Endovascular Therapies

Poorly palpable femoral pulses, adhesions in the groin region, and morbid obesity may be responsible for the

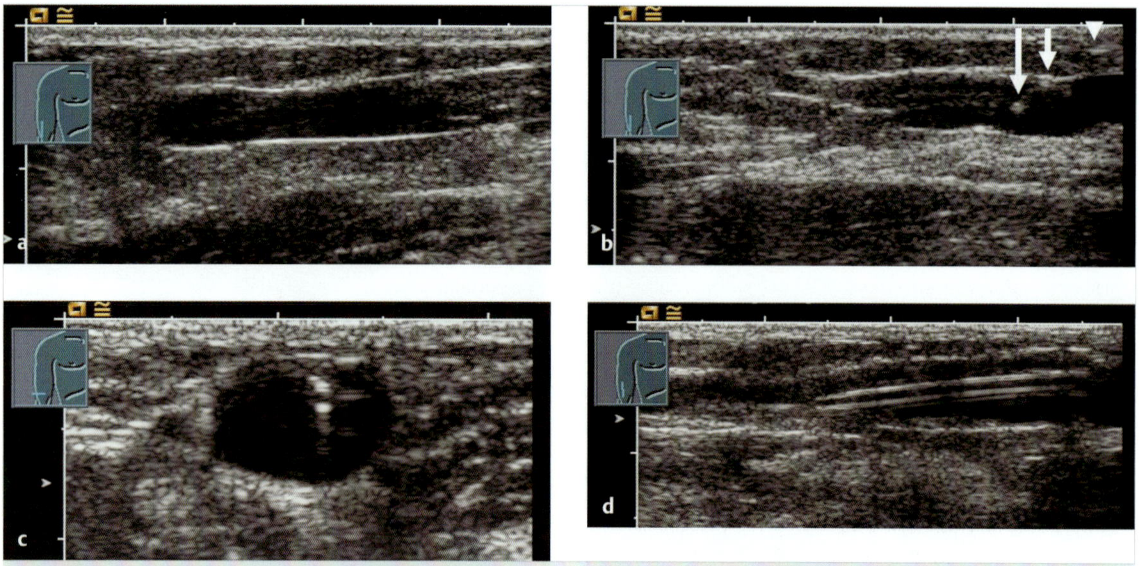

Fig. 30.10 Puncture of a peripheral vein at the elbow. No veins are palpable in an obese arm.
a Ultrasound clearly shows a (nonpalpable) cephalic vein at the elbow. The vein is surprisingly superficial.
b The indwelling venous cannula appears fragmentary in the long-axis view, but the tip (left arrow) can be positively identified.
c Short-axis view.
d Long-axis view after stabilizing the metal cannula and advancing the plastic cannula. The walls of the plastic cannula are clearly visualized, and its intraluminal advance can be monitored.

failure of **femoral artery puncture** during angiography. The CW Doppler ultrasound guidance of femoral artery puncture in patients with weak or absent femoral pulses was first described in 1980.[49] A recent randomized prospective study showed that ultrasound-guided retrograde femoral arterial access was significantly superior to fluoroscopic guidance with regard to speed and safety.[50] In cases that required large-bore sheath systems (20F or larger) for the endovascular placement of aortic stent grafts, ultrasound guidance was found to reduce vascular complications, significantly shorten the procedure time, and improve the success of percutaneous access closure.[51] In cases where antegrade puncture of the common femoral artery was not possible due to obesity or scarring ("hostile groin"), puncture of the superficial femoral artery guided by color duplex ultrasound (CDU) was found to be technically easier and faster and was associated with less radiation exposure and fewer complications than CDU-guided common femoral artery puncture.[52]

It was first reported in the early 1990s that a complete vascular intervention in the lower limb could be per-

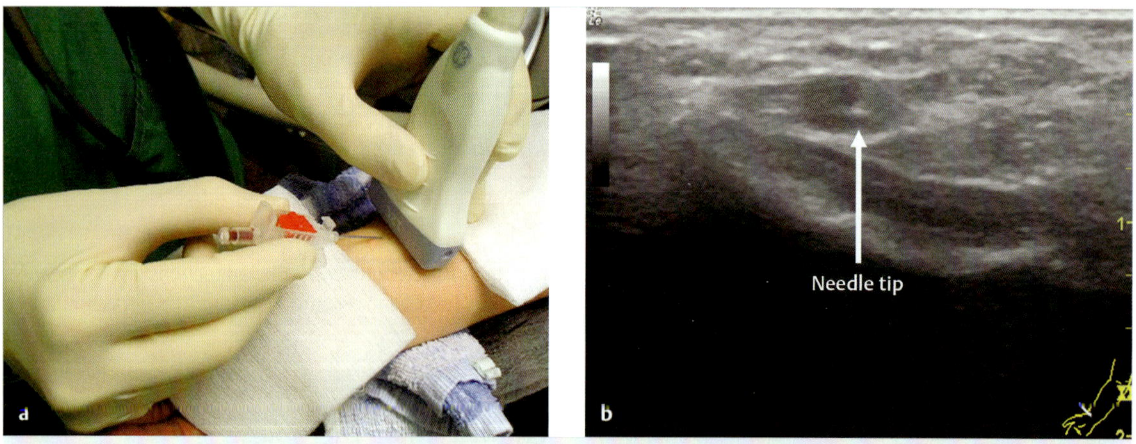

Fig. 30.11 Cannulation of the radial artery. In the short-axis orientation (**a**) the needle tip (**b**) appears only as a punctate echo. (Source: image courtesy of Dr. C. Rex, Reutlingen, Germany.)

formed under CDU guidance alone.[53–57] Since then several groups of authors have shown, some in large case numbers, that the CDU-guided endovascular therapy (percutaneous transluminal angioplasty [PTA] and stenting) of femoropopliteal and crural vascular occlusions and stenoses was technically feasible, safe, and effective. Both the arterial puncture and the crossing of vascular lesions with a wire can be performed under ultrasound guidance. The selection of balloon length and diameter is directed by sonographic measurements, and the positioning and expansion of balloons and stents are done under sonographic guidance. The efficacy of the angioplasty can be assessed during the procedure itself without contrast injection. The results are comparable to those reported with fluoroscopic guidance.[58–61]

Stent angioplasty of atherosclerotic *renal artery stenosis* is controversial. In a comparative study of 30 patients with renal artery stenosis and severe renal insufficiency, a group of Italian authors showed that the PTA stenting of renal artery stenosis under CDU guidance was as effective as the standard DSA technique and was even superior in terms of renal functional outcomes.[62]

Case reports have also been published on the successful CDU-guided interventional treatment of aortoiliac artery occlusions,[63,64] long segmental femoral artery occlusions,[65] infrainguinal bypass stenosis,[66] popliteal artery aneurysms,[67] carotid stenosis,[68] as well as dialysis fistula stenosis and brachial stenosis in the forearm during or after the creation of a dialysis fistula.[60,69–72] CDU guidance can also direct the intra-abdominal thrombolysis of acute and subacute thrombotic femoropopliteal occlusions.[73,74]

Materials

Ultrasound-guided endovascular therapies employ the same materials and equipment ordinarily used for angiographic interventions. Balloon insufflation can be performed with distilled water instead of radiographic contrast medium. Sterile covers should be placed over the transducer and the control panel of the ultrasound machine. Sterile ultrasound gel or an antiseptic spray should be used for acoustic coupling.

Basic Steps in CDU-Guided Interventions

1. The operator should be aided by an assistant in sterile attire.
2. The transducer should be placed in a sterile probe cover.
3. The operator should wear sterile attire.
4. Generally the procedure is done in the catheterization laboratory or operating room with a fluoroscopic unit available if needed.
5. The position of the operator and equipment depends on the intervention (antegrade or retrograde vascular access).
6. The targeted vascular segment is precisely mapped by CDU.
7. The vessel is imaged in longitudinal section.
8. Local anesthesia is administered under sonographic guidance.
9. The vessel is punctured using Seldinger technique in a long-axis view that displays the full needle path. Insertion of the puncture needle, initial wire, sheath, and interventional wire are all done under ultrasound guidance.
10. Image the vessels proximal to the vascular lesion, then move the transducer to the lesion itself and cross it with the wire under ultrasound guidance (▸ Fig. 30.12a–c).
11. Base the PTA balloon and/or stent selection on sonographic measurements of the lesion and of the vessel lumen proximal and distal to the lesion.
12. Exchange the guide catheter and wire using Seldinger technique, aided by fluoroscopic guidance if needed.
13. Advance the balloon over the indwelling guidewire, cross the lesion under ultrasound control, and expand the balloon under ultrasound guidance (with distilled water, ▸ Fig. 30.12d, e). A stent can be deployed if necessary.
14. Immediately evaluate the lesion: lumen width, peak flow velocity, qualitative assessment of Doppler spectrum; dissection?, recoiling? (▸ Fig. 30.12f).
15. Repeat the dilation or assess the need for stent placement (failed repeat PTA, dissection, recoiling).

Specific Complications, Advantages and Disadvantages

No specific complications of CDU-guided vascular interventions are known. A prospective study found no significant differences in complication rates between CDU guided and fluoroscopically guided vascular interventions (12.5% versus 18.3%, $P = 0.4$). As expected, renal function impairment occurred only in the fluoroscopically guided interventions (6.7% of patients). The technical success rate of CDU-guided femoropopliteal angioplasties in this study was slightly less than that of fluoroscopically guided angioplasties (84.6% versus 98.1%, $P = 0.001$) while the 12-month patency rates were similar. Technical failures related to problems with ultrasound visualization of the interventional material, especially in the presence of significant calcifications.[58]

Other disadvantages of CDU guidance are incomplete visualization of the overall anatomy of the crural arteries, limited visualization of the pelvic axis and retroperitoneal vessels, and relatively poor guidance in crossover interventions. As a result, up to 10% of cases require the additional use of fluoroscopy or the use of very low contrast medium doses.[58]

Decisive advantages of CDU-guided vascular interventions are decreased radiation exposure to patients and staff,

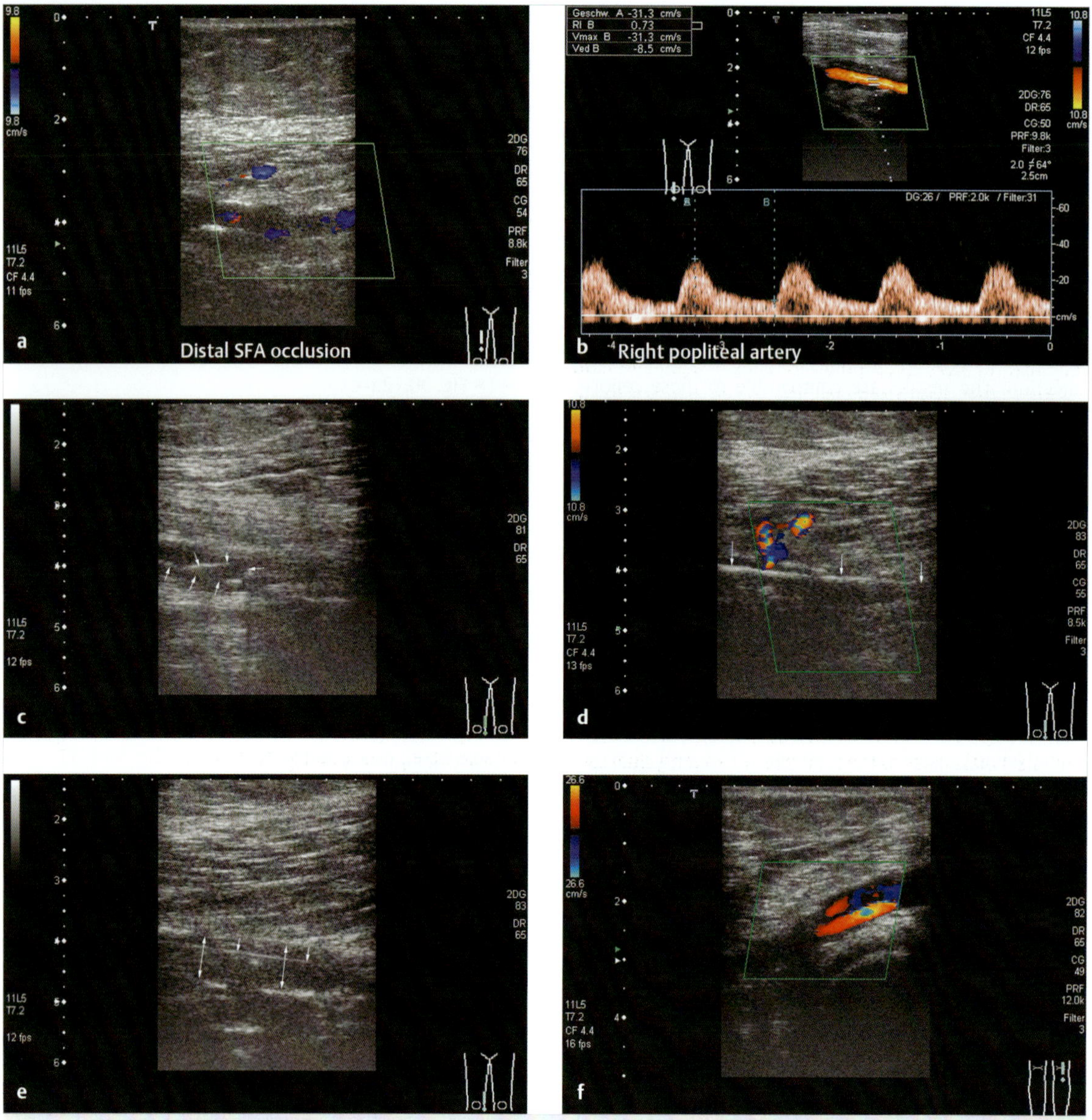

Fig. 30.12 CDU-guided arterial vascular intervention in an 82-year-old obese woman with diabetic nephropathy and Fontaine stage III peripheral arterial occlusive disease (PAOD): hypoechoic subtotal occlusion of the distal right superficial femoral artery (**a**) with a postocclusive signal in the popliteal artery (**b**; peak systolic velocity = 0.3 m/s). Ultrasound clearly demonstrates the 35-inch Terumo wire before crossing the occlusion (**c**; arrow indicates the curled-back catheter tip) and the 80 mm × 5 mm balloon catheter, matched to the sonographic morphology of the occlusion, before PTA (**d**, arrows; CDU shows large collaterals proximal to the occlusion) and during balloon PTA (**e**; double arrows highlight the diameter of the water-filled balloon; arrows indicate the guidewire). Image after PTA shows a dissection in the first popliteal segment (**f**).

no risk of contrast-induced nephropathy (approximately 15% in angiographic procedures),[75,76] and no risk of contrast allergies. Other advantages have also been described: faster and safer arterial access, less risk of subintimal dissection and vascular perforation, improved capability for antegrade interventions through an ipsilateral approach, less risk of access-related complications, improved access to proximal occlusions of the superficial femoral artery, and the real-time detection of complications or failed recanalization (dissection, recoiling, embolism).[50,58,59,64]

Note

CDU-guided vascular interventions require detailed preliminary sonographic vascular mapping!

30.2.2 Ultrasound-Guided Treatment of Pseudoaneurysms

An arterial pseudoaneurysm (false aneurysm) is a confined rupture of all three layers of the artery wall. It may result from an iatrogenic puncture (especially in percutaneous vascular interventions) or may be anastomotic, posttraumatic, or (post)inflammatory.

The incidence of pseudoaneurysms is 0.05 to 2% after diagnostic angiography and 2 to 8% after endovascular interventions.[77,78] Risk factors are the use of large introducer systems (≥ 7F), long and complex interventions, very high or very deep puncture sites, inadequate compression after sheath removal, the use of arterial closure systems, combined treatment with antiplatelet drugs and anticoagulants, and patient-specific factors.[77–79] Potential complications are enlargement, rupture, and infection. Complex pseudoaneurysms with an arteriovenous fistula (AVF) may be encountered.

Diagnosis

Pseudoaneurysms present clinically with a painful swelling at the puncture site accompanied by an abnormal bruit. The diagnosis is based upon:

- The sonographic detection of a hypoechoic (uni- or multilobular) mass close to the puncture site (aneurysmal sac)
- The color duplex detection of flow signals in all or portions of the mass (usually a pulsatile, swirling flow pattern)
- The Doppler detection of typical bidirectional flow with rapid systolic inflow and decelerated diastolic outflow (high resistance, turbulence) in the connecting tract between the parent artery and pseudoaneurysm (▶ Fig. 30.13)[77,80]

Unlike a pseudoaneurysm, an arteriovenous fistula shows a low-resistance type of flow pattern with absence of bidirectional flow. Marked arterial flow modulation is found in the affected vein.[77]

At diagnosis the examiner should describe the extent of the aneurysm (longitudinal axis, depth, width), the size of the perfused or thrombosed portions, morphology (unilobular, multilobular), the length and width of the connecting tract, the Doppler waveform (differentiation from AVF), flow characteristics in the affected artery and accompanying vein, and the peripheral Doppler index.

Posttreatment ultrasound should document absence of flow in the pseudoaneurysm, flow characteristics in the affected artery and vein, and the peripheral Doppler index.

Indications for Treatment, Therapeutic Procedure

Small pseudoaneurysms (≤ 20 mm) in patients who have mild symptoms and are not on anticoagulant or antiplatelet drugs will undergo spontaneous thrombosis in approximately 50% of cases. Ultrasound follow-up is required.[81,82] If treatment is necessary, options include (ultrasound-guided) compression, ultrasound-guided para-aneurysmal saline injection, ultrasound-guided thrombin injection, other ultrasound-guided injection techniques, bridging the rupture site with a covered stent, and vascular surgery (▶ Fig. 30.14).

Vascular surgery has a relatively high morbidity and mortality. In 2009 a retrospective analysis of 79 femoral pseudoaneurysms treated by vascular surgery, complications arose in 71% of the patients and the mortality rate was 3.8%.[83] A Cochrane Review in 2009 showed that **compression therapy** is effective, regardless of whether ultrasound guidance is used.[84] The success rate of ultrasound-guided compression therapy was 72.1% in a large case series (281 patients). Negative predictors of successful compression therapy were anticoagulation (success rate only 30%) and pseudoaneurysm size.[85]

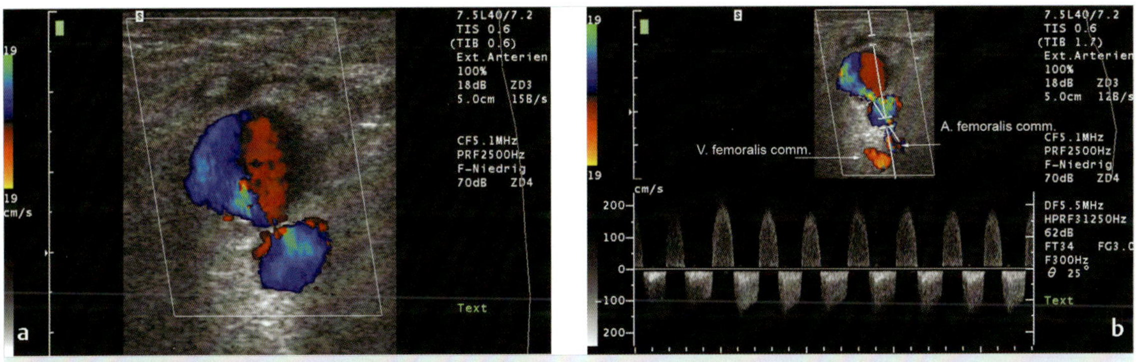

Fig. 30.13 Femoral pseudoaneurysm 10 days after PTA of a contralateral superficial femoral artery stenosis and 2 days after resumption of oral anticoagulants in addition to aspirin.
a Color Doppler shows an hourglass-shaped (loculated) pseudoaneurysm with a reversal of blood flow direction at the apex of the pseudoaneurysm.
b Doppler spectrum shows a typical waveform sampled from the connecting tract to the common femoral artery.

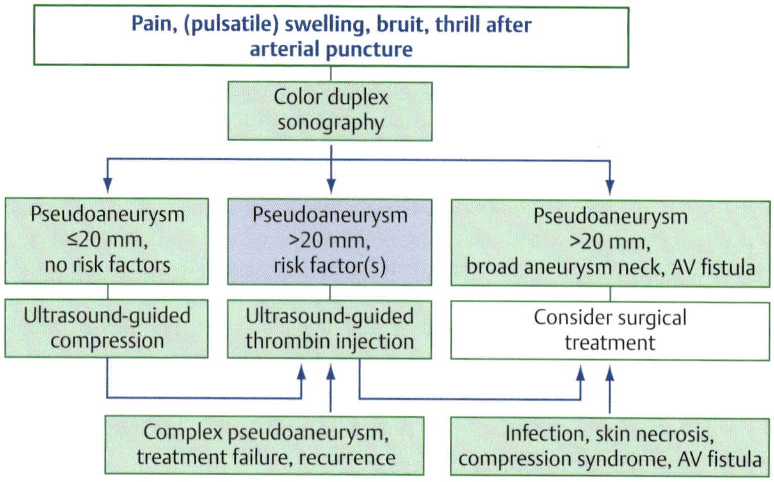

Fig. 30.14 Diagnostic and therapeutic algorithm for an arterial pseudoaneurysm.

Percutaneous thrombin injection is superior to a single session of ultrasound probe compression.[84] Ultrasound-guided thrombin injection has reported success rates of 91 to 100% (average in published series, 97.5%).[78] Risk factors for recurrence are obesity, combined antiplatelet drug therapy, and anticoagulation.

Materials

The **ultrasound probe compression** of pseudoaneurysms can be most effectively accomplished with a curved-array transducer with color duplex capability.

Thrombin injection can be guided with a high-frequency linear transducer, a low-frequency curved-array transducer, or a special biopsy transducer depending on local anatomy. A 20- to 22-gauge needle can be used. Thrombin is usually injected with a 1-mL Luer lock syringe. Our agent of choice is human thrombin. Bovine thrombin is cheaper but has a stronger allergenic potential and an indeterminate risk of prion transmission. In any case, this type of therapy involves an off-label use. Sporadic cases have also been treated by fibrinogen injection and by the ultrasound-guided placement of removable coils.[86]

Technique of Ultrasound-Guided Compression

Successful ultrasound-guided probe compression was first reported in 1991.[87] After a detailed sonomorphologic evaluation of the pseudoaneurysm, the transducer (selected according to size and local anatomy) is positioned directly over the connecting tract or aneurysm neck, and pressure is applied and gradually increased until it stops the flow.

The transducer position and compression angle should be sufficient to stop blood flow in the pseudoaneurysm with a minimum amount of pressure while preserving blood flow through the artery. A constant pressure is maintained for approximately 10 minutes and then slowly reduced under color duplex control. If flow recurs, the pressure is immediately increased again until the

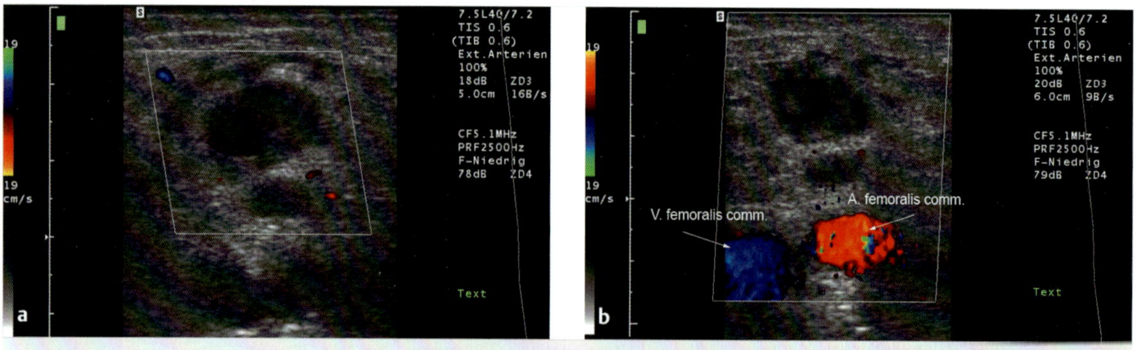

Fig. 30.15 Complete thrombosis of the femoral pseudoaneurysm shown in ▶ Fig. 30.13 after termination of oral anticoagulation and ultrasound-guided compression for 100 minutes (!).
a Both chambers in the pseudoaneurysm are obliterated.
b Flow is detected only in the femoral vessels.

flow signal ceases. In our experience it takes 20 to 45 minutes of probe compression for the blood within the pseudoaneurysm to clot, depending on the size and shape of the pseudoaneurysm and the effects of anticoagulant therapy. A retrospective study found that the average compression time to occlusion was 33 (10–120) minutes (▶ Fig. 30.15).[88]

Technique of Ultrasound-Guided Perilesional injection Therapy

A seldom-practiced but simple and low-cost option for pseudoaneurysm treatment is the ultrasound-guided perilesional injection of saline solution. It is preceded by antiseptic preparation of the skin site and transducer (sterile probe cover). A 22-gauge injection needle is positioned close to the aneurysm neck under ultrasound guidance, and isotonic saline solution (20–80 mL) is injected until enough fluid has pooled to significantly reduce blood flow in the aneurysm.[89,90] This is followed by external ultrasound probe compression, which is continued until blood flow ceases within the pseudoaneurysm.

Technique of Ultrasound-Guided Intralesional Injection Therapy

Percutaneous thrombin injection for the obliteration of pseudoaneurysms was first described in 1986[91] and was later performed with ultrasound guidance. The injection is preceded by antiseptic preparation of the skin site and transducer (sterile probe cover). A 20- or 22-gauge needle is advanced into the pseudoaneurysm under ultrasound guidance. It is recommended that the needle be positioned in the "inflow tract" but at an adequate distance from the aneurysm neck. When correct placement of the needle tip has been confirmed, human thrombin solution is injected (▶ Fig. 30.16).

An insulin or tuberculin syringe should be used for the injection. Only a small amount of thrombin is needed to obliterate the pseudoaneurysm: doses as small as 20 to 800 IU are often sufficient.[77,92] The necessary dose can be accurately estimated from the maximum diameter of the pseudoaneurysm. Less than 500 IU is generally enough for pseudoaneurysms up to 15 mm in diameter.[93] The agent can also be delivered in small, successive divided doses.

The cessation of blood flow in the pseudoaneurysm occurs within seconds after the injection and can be verified in real time by color duplex imaging. With a loculated pseudoaneurysm, thrombin injection into the chamber closest to the connecting tract is most effective. In lesions with a broad neck, it is probably best to obliterate the most superficial chamber first. Afterward the other chambers will usually thrombose as well, although a second or third injection may occasionally be necessary for the deeper chambers.

Most experience has been reported for ultrasound-guided thrombin injections in iatrogenic femoral and brachial pseudoaneurysms. However, numerous case reports have shown that this procedure can be just as successful for posttraumatic and postinflammatory pseudoaneurysms, regardless of location as long as the lesion is accessible to fine needle puncture under ultrasound guidance (▶ Fig. 30.17).

Specific Complications, Contraindications, Advantages and Disadvantages

Complications of ultrasound-guided compression therapy are very rare. Isolated cases of pain-induced vasovagal response, aneurysm rupture, skin necrosis, or deep venous thrombosis have been described.[85] The hematoma that results from lesion obliteration may become infected following intra- and perilesional injection therapy. Complications of ultrasound-guided thrombin injection occurred in 1.3% of the cases (17 of 1,329) reported in 14 published series.[78]

The leakage of small amounts of thrombin into the arterial circulation distal to the origin of the pseudoaneurysm is probably common but usually causes no adverse effects. One study found that echo contrast medium injected into the pseudoaneurysm before the thrombin injection entered the arterial circulation in 58% of cases.[94]

Clinically significant arterial emboli are very rare, however (0.5% in a total of 1,329 patients reviewed in 14 case series).[78] The presence of an AVF is considered a contraindication to ultrasound-guided thrombin injection due to the high risk of deep lower-extremity venous thrombosis caused by thrombin migration. But injection therapy is an acceptable option even for selected complex pseudoaneurysms with an AVF if external compression can keep thrombin from entering the deep venous system (▶ Fig. 30.18)

Thrombin injection is not recommended for the treatment of pseudoaneurysms at surgical anastomoses or of mycotic pseudoaneurysms. All methods of ultrasound-guided percutaneous therapy are contraindicated in the presence of infection, skin necrosis, or a local compression syndrome (ischemia, peripheral nerve irritation).[78] Allergic reactions may occur on reexposure to bovine thrombin.

Ultrasound-guided compression has several advantages over manual or mechanical (pressure dressing, FemoStop; St. Jude Medical) compression without ultrasound guidance. With large and complex pseudoaneurysms, only ultrasound guidance can target the compression to the aneurysm neck or connecting tract and also assess the necessary degree of compression. Only ultrasound-guided compression therapy (▶ Fig. 30.15) can be accurately controlled for duration and intensity and limited to the minimum necessary occlusion time. Compression therapy is painful, and the patients will generally require strong analgesic medication.

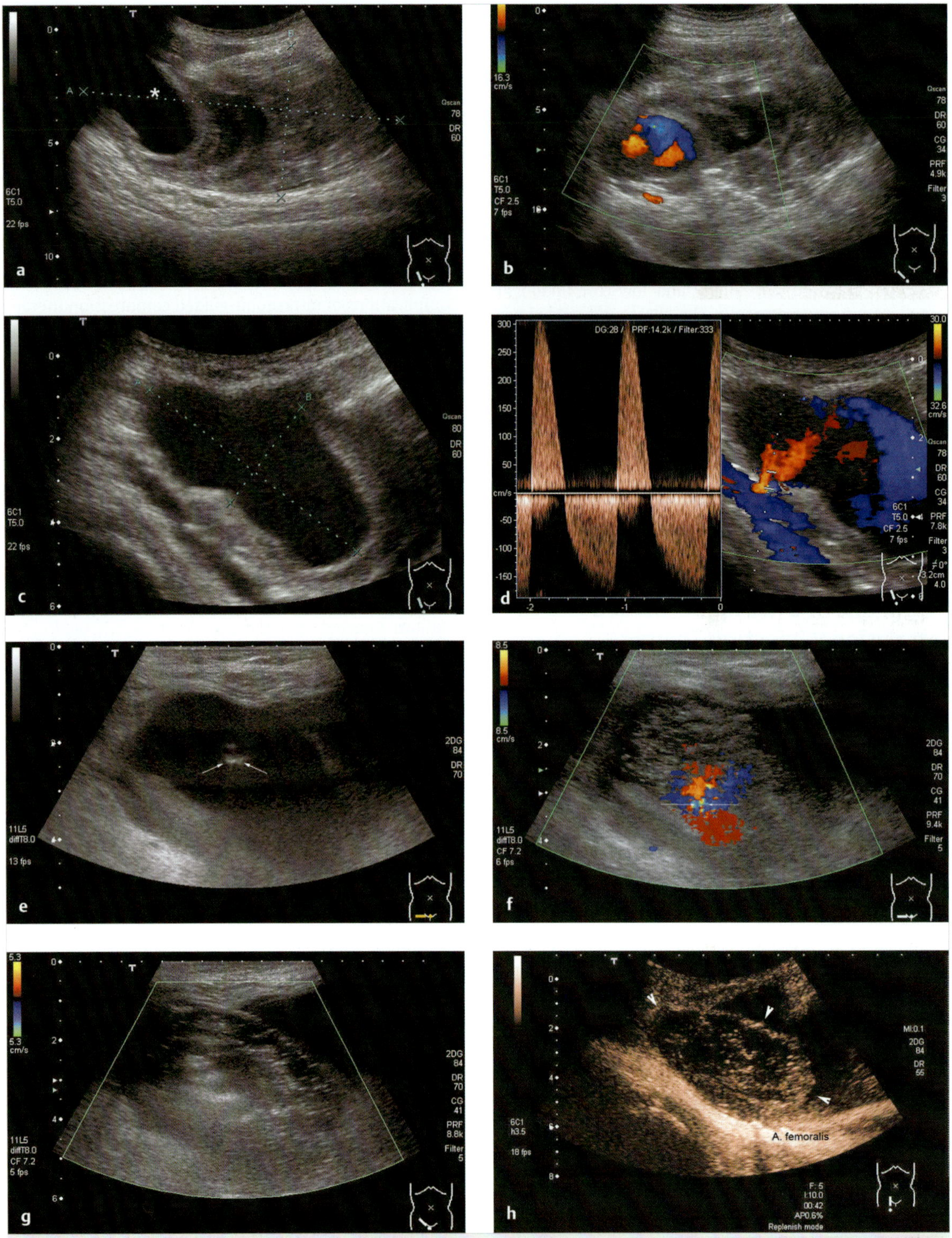

Fig. 30.16 Very large femoral pseudoaneurysm 4 weeks (!) after a coronary intervention in an 83-year-old man on dual antiplatelet therapy (**a**). Only the portions near the artery are perfused (asterisk in **a**; color flow in **b**; calipers in **c**). Typical Doppler spectral findings (**d**). A fine needle is introduced into the pseudoaneurysm (**e**, arrows indicate needle tip). Thrombin injection causes a cessation of blood flow (**f**, **g**; arrows in **f** indicate needle tip). SonoVue injection clearly delineates the formerly perfused portion of the aneurysm (**h**; arrowheads) with no further signs of vascularization. The femoral vessels are patent.

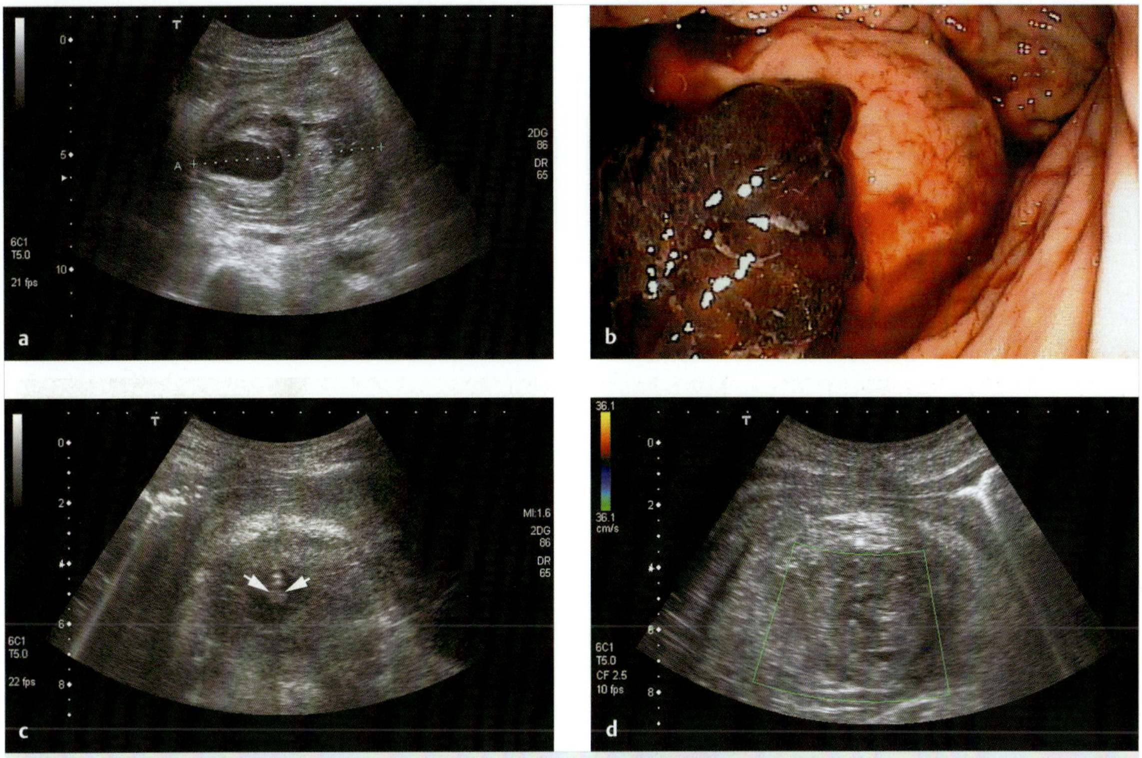

Fig. 30.17 Ultrasound-guided percutaneous treatment of a large visceral pseudoaneurysm by thrombin injection.
a Large splenic artery aneurysm following acute pancreatitis.
b The lesion presents clinically as upper gastrointestinal bleeding from an impression in the posterior stomach wall.
c Ultrasound-guided percutaneous transgastric fine needle insertion (arrows indicate the needle tip) and thrombin injection.
d Cessation of flow in the pseudoaneurysm.

The advantages and disadvantages of ultrasound-guided percutaneous treatment methods are listed in ▶ Table 30.4. A diagnostic and therapeutic algorithm is shown in ▶ Fig. 30.14.

Caution

Thrombin injection has a success rate of 94—100% in the treatment of pseudoaneurysms! It is an off-label use, however.

We recommend approximately 2 hours' bed rest and 24 hours' limited physical activity after successful compression or obliteration therapy. Whenever possible, anticoagulant therapy should not be resumed until the day after the procedure. If anticoagulant therapy must be continued or the risk of recurrence is high for other reasons, it is good practice to apply a pressure dressing for approximately 6 hours after the intervention. Ultrasound follow-up is necessary immediately after the procedure is completed, on the following day or within the first two days, and in cases where symptoms recur.

30.3 Endosonographically Guided Vascular Interventions

30.3.1 Indications and Treatment Goals

To date, the following EUS-guided vascular interventions have been described in the form of case reports or clinical series:

- Obliteration of visceral pseudoaneurysms by EUS-guided injection of thrombin, Gelfoam, and microcoils.[95,96]
- Treatment of recurrent variceal bleeding by EUS-guided intravascular injection (cyanoacrylate, thrombin, fibrin glue, microcoils) of perforator veins or bleeding varices (▶ Fig. 30.19).[95,97,98]
- EUS-assisted sclerotherapy, obliteration, or ligation of esophageal and gastric varices (review of the literature in reference [99]).
- Treatment of recurrent, nonvariceal gastrointestinal bleeding that cannot be managed endoscopically (Dieulafoy lesions, pseudoxanthoma elasticum, peptic ulcer, gastrointestinal stromal tumor) by the intravascular

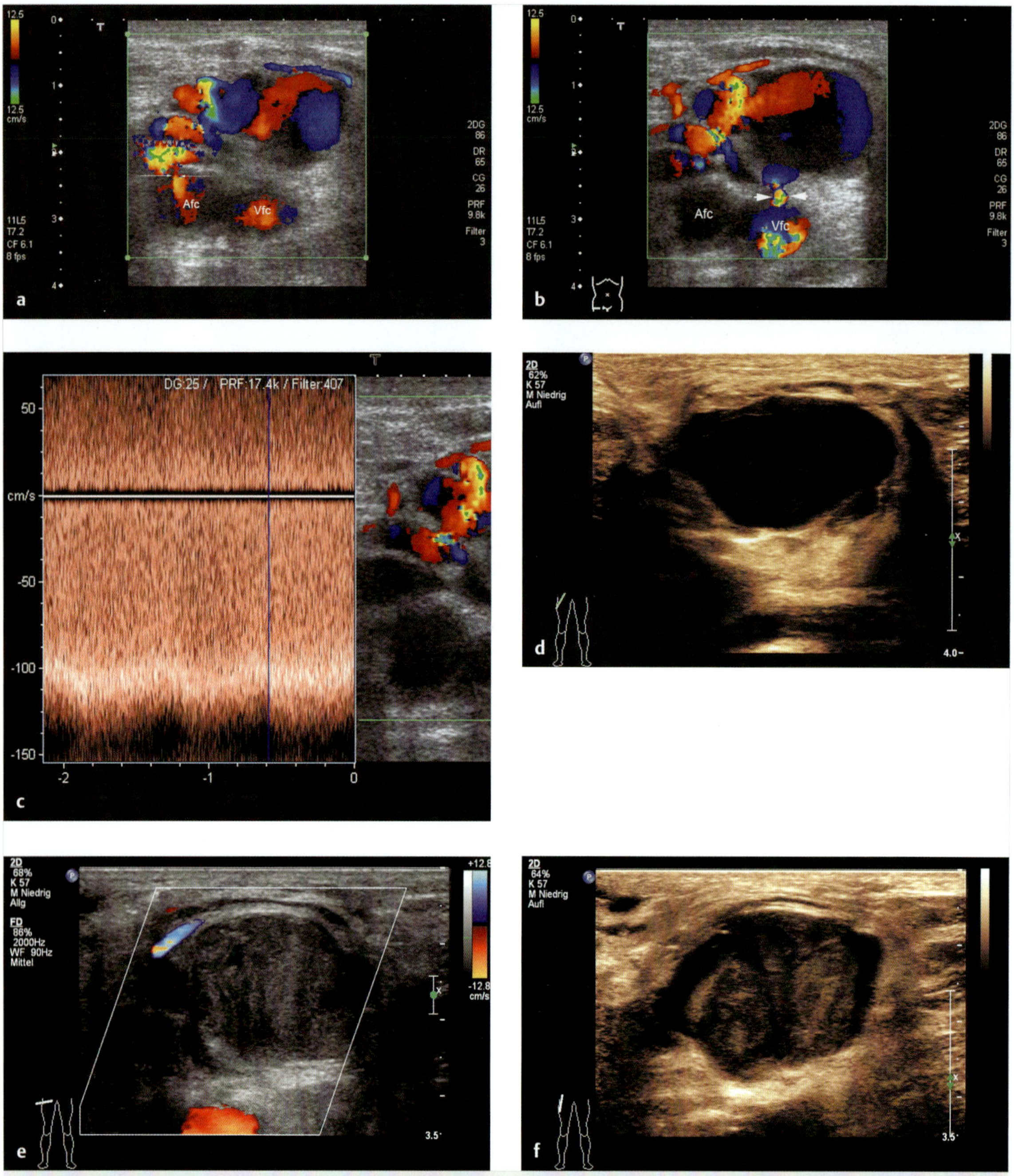

Fig. 30.18 Complex femoral pseudoaneurysm after percutaneous coronary intervention in a patient on dual antiplatelet therapy.
a Communication of the multilocular pseudoaneurysm with the common femoral artery (Afc) (arrows indicate the neck of the pseudoaneurysm). Vfc, common femoral vein.
b Additional communication with the femoral vein, forming an AVF (arrows).
c Doppler spectral analysis.
d After vascular surgical consultation and disclosure of the thrombosis risk to the patient, thrombin injection therapy was performed. The pseudoaneurysm is echo-free in the B-mode image before the injection.
e A very small amount of thrombin (0.3 mL) was injected into the first chamber near the arterial neck of the aneurysm. The color duplex image several minutes later documents complete thrombosis of the pseudoaneurysm.
f B-mode image of the result shows echogenic material in the pseudoaneurysm. Femoral vein thrombosis was prevented by manual compression of the AVF during and 2 minutes after the injection.

Table 30.4 Advantages, disadvantages, and specific risks of various methods for the treatment of femoral pseudoaneurysms in percutaneous vascular interventions

Method	Advantages	Disadvantages	Specific risk
Compression	Modest material requirements	Low efficacy, high patient discomfort	Low (rupture, skin necrosis, venous thrombosis?)
Ultrasound-guided compression	Low material costs, high efficacy	Long procedure time, operator fatigue, high mechanical stress to transducer	Low (pain, rupture, skin necrosis)
Perilesional injection therapy	Low material costs, high efficacy	None	Very low (infection?)
Intralesional injection therapy	Short procedure time, very high efficacy	High material costs	Low (distal arterial occlusion [embolism], venous thrombosis, infection, rupture)
Surgery	Very high efficacy	Very high material and personnel costs, long procedure time	Significant (bleeding, infection, wound dehiscence, thrombosis, anesthesiology risk)

injection of fibrin glue, cyanoacrylate, or 99% alcohol (▶ Fig. 30.20).[95,100]

- EUS-guided transesophageal diagnostic interventions in the heart (pericardial effusion, pericardial tumor, tumor of left atrium).[101–103]
- EUS-guided angiography (portal vessels, hepatic veins, aorta and branch vessels), the EUS-guided creation of an intrahepatic portosystemic shunt, EUS-guided portal vein obliteration before partial hepatectomy, and transesophageal interventions on the coronary vessels and cardiac valves have so far been evaluated only in experimental animals, and their clinical relevance cannot yet be predicted.[103–109]

Materials

EUS-guided hemostasis is usually performed with 22-gauge FNA needles, which can be used to deliver epinephrine solution, sclerosing agents, thrombin solution, fibrin glue, cyanoacrylate, or even coils. A newly developed prototype of a forward viewing interventional echoendoscope may facilitate endosonographic vascular interventions in the future.[110] Animal studies showed that 25-gauge needles were suitable for CO_2 angiography, while only 22- or 19-gauge needles were practical for injecting radiographic contrast media.[106,107] Other animal studies found that EUS-guided vascular interventions using Seldinger technique required the use of 19-gauge needles.[104,105] While 25-gauge needles did not cause any visible vascular injury or bleeding at necropsy, 22-gauge needles left a visible puncture mark with no evidence of active bleeding. The 19-gauge needle, on the other hand, caused a localized hematoma of the vessel's wall with associated intra-abdominal bleeding in 1 of 5 animals.[107]

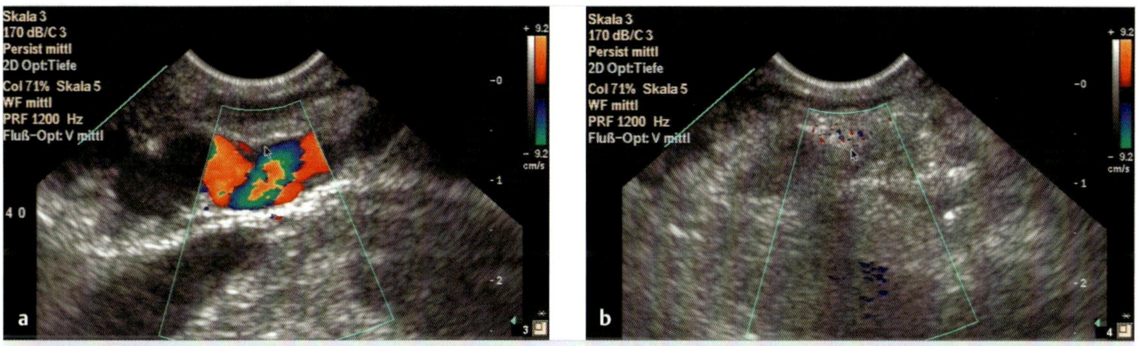

Fig. 30.19 EUS-guided intravascular injection treatment in a case of recurrent variceal bleeding.
a A man 41 years of age had alcoholic cirrhosis of the liver and recent twice-daily bleeding episodes from large cardia varices despite repeated attempts at endoscopic obliteration by histoacryl injection. A TIPS (transjugular intrahepatic portosystemic shunt) was contraindicated due to poor liver function.
b EUS-guided intravascular injection of fibrin glue was the first treatment that stopped the bleeding (arrow: echogenic and color artifacts caused by intravascular fibrin glue). Color duplex image confirms cessation of flow. (Source: images courtesy of Dr. C. Jürgensen, Berlin.)

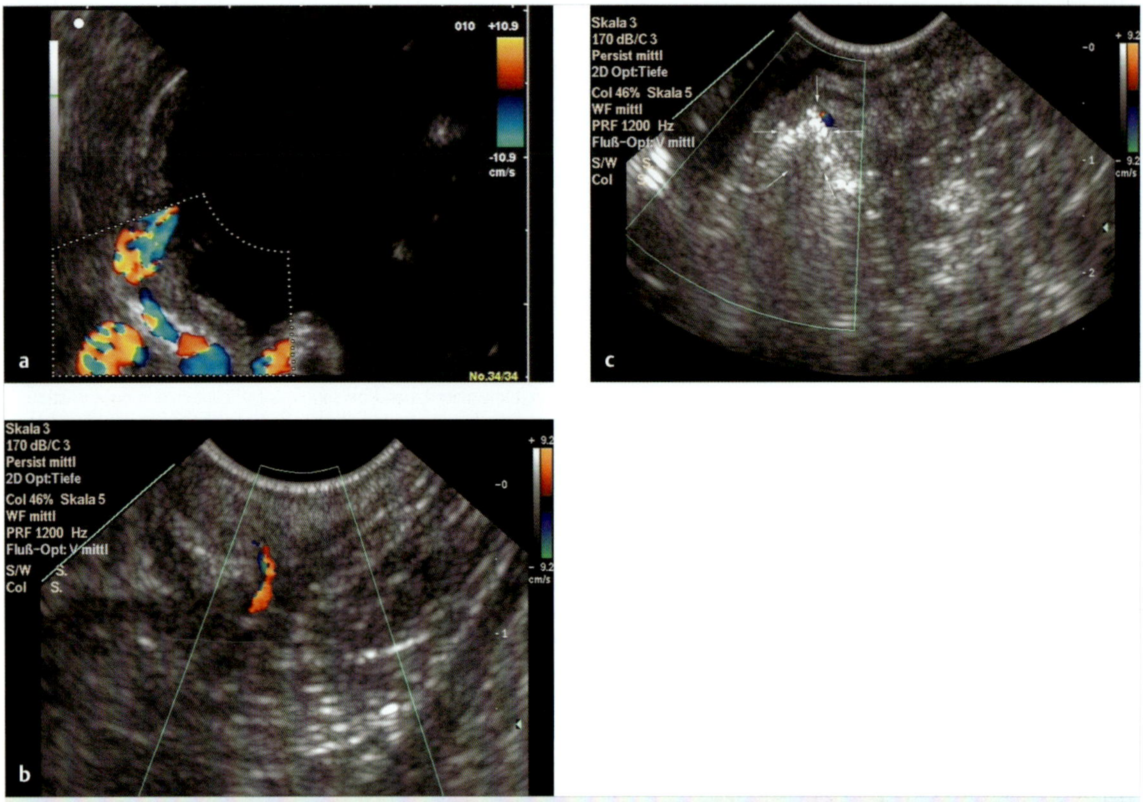

Fig. 30.20 EUS-guided intravascular treatment in a case of recurrent, nonvariceal gastrointestinal bleeding.
a A man 51 years of age had recurrent upper gastrointestinal bleeding of unknown cause. Radial endosonography reveals the source of the bleeding: large-caliber submucous arterial vessels in pseudoxanthoma elasticum.
b, c After the vessels were also imaged with a linear transducer, fibrin glue was injected into the vessels under EUS guidance (arrows: high-amplitude echoes from submucous fibrin glue). The patient was free of any further bleeding episodes for 12 months after treatment. (Source: images courtesy of Dr. C. Jürgensen, Berlin.)

Specific Complications, Contraindications, Advantages, and Disadvantages

On the basis of the small case numbers to date, no serious complications of EUS-guided vascular interventions have yet been published. In theory, however, these procedures could lead to severe ischemic complications, bleeding, or infection. One advantage of EUS guidance is the ability to treat vascular lesions that are poorly accessible or inaccessible by the percutaneous route. Another advantage over endoscopic techniques is the ability to achieve intravascular hemostasis under sonographic guidance. One disadvantage is the long needle lengths and small needle diameters, which create a high resistance to injection.

Caution

EUS-guided vascular interventions are experimental! They should be performed only by experts in highly selected cases after meticulous informed consent.

Evaluating the Result; Postprocedure Care

The treatment result can be assessed endosonographically during the intervention itself. Additional follow-ups are scheduled at frequent intervals and rely on transabdominal ultrasound, another sectional imaging modality, or endoscopy. Postprocedure care is similar to that following the endoscopic treatment of gastrointestinal bleeding or percutaneous vascular interventions.

References

[1] Meuwly JY, Felley C, Vuilleumier H, Schnyder P, Hewig U. Ultrasound examination of non-traumatic acute abdomen [Article in German]. Ultraschall Med 2002; 23: 13–21

[2] Bahner D, Blaivas M, Cohen HL et al. American Institute of Ultrasound in Medicine. AIUM practice guideline for the performance of the focused assessment with sonography for trauma (FAST) examination. J Ultrasound Med 2008; 27: 313–318

[3] Blackbourne LH, Soffer D, McKenney M et al. Secondary ultrasound examination increases the sensitivity of the FAST exam in blunt trauma. J Trauma 2004; 57: 934–938

[4] McKenney M, Lentz K, Nunez D et al. Can ultrasound replace diagnostic peritoneal lavage in the assessment of blunt trauma? J Trauma 1994; 37: 439–441

[5] Hokema F, Donaubauer B, Busch T, Bouillon B, Kaisers U. Initial management of polytraumatized patients in the emergency department [Article in German]. Anasthesiol Intensivmed Notfallmed Schmerzther 2007; 42: 716–723

[6] Rippey JC, Royse AG. Ultrasound in trauma. Best Pract Res Clin Anaesthesiol 2009; 23: 343–362

[7] Stengel D, Bauwens K, Sehouli J et al. Emergency ultrasound-based algorithms for diagnosing blunt abdominal trauma. Cochrane Database Syst Rev 2005: CD004446

[8] Grundmann RT, Petersen M, Lippert H, Meyer F. The acute (surgical) abdomen – epidemiology, diagnosis and general principles of management [Article in German]. Z Gastroenterol 2010; 48: 696–706

[9] Schacherer D, Klebl F, Goetz D et al. Abdominal ultrasound in the intensive care unit: a 3-year survey on 400 patients. Intensive Care Med 2007; 33: 841–844

[10] Policy Statement ACEP American College of Emergency Physicians. Emergency ultrasound guidelines. Ann Emerg Med 2009; 53: 550–570

[11] Grau T, Mäcken T, Strunk H. Appendix 13: Intensive care ultrasound – minimum training requirements for the practice of medical ultrasound in Europe. Ultraschall Med 2009; 30: 414–417

[12] Neri L, Storti E, Lichtenstein D. Toward an ultrasound curriculum for critical care medicine. Crit Care Med 2007; 35 (Suppl): S290–S304

[13] Osterwalder J, Simanowski J, Breitkreuz R et al. Vorschlag für ein 3-Länder-übergreifendes Ausbildungskonzept und Curriculum Notfallsonographie. Unpublished manuscript; 2010

[14] Kollig E, Heydenreich U, Roetman B, Hopf F, Muhr G. Ultrasound and bronchoscopic controlled percutaneous tracheostomy on trauma ICU. Injury 2000; 31: 663–668

[15] Sustić A, Kovac D, Zgaljardić Z, Zupan Z, Krstulović B. Ultrasound-guided percutaneous dilatational tracheostomy: a safe method to avoid cranial misplacement of the tracheostomy tube. Intensive Care Med 2000; 26: 1379–1381

[16] Yavuz A, Ceken K, Yilmaz M et al. Advantage of ultrasound in percutaneous dilatational tracheostomy. Ultraschall Med 2005; 26: P: 147

[17] Chun R, Kirkpatrick AW, Sirois M et al. Where's the tube? Evaluation of hand-held ultrasound in confirming endotracheal tube placement. Prehosp Disaster Med 2004; 19: 366–369

[18] Weaver B, Lyon M, Blaivas M. Confirmation of endotracheal tube placement after intubation using the ultrasound sliding lung sign. Acad Emerg Med 2006; 13: 239–244

[19] Greenberg M, Bejar R, Asser S. Confirmation of transpyloric feeding tube placement by ultrasonography. J Pediatr 1993; 122: 413–415

[20] Hernández-Socorro CR, Marin J, Ruiz-Santana S, Santana L, Manzano JL. Bedside sonographic-guided versus blind nasoenteric feeding tube placement in critically ill patients. Crit Care Med 1996; 24: 1690–1694

[21] Ruesseler M, Kirschning T, Breitkreutz R, Marzi I, Walcher F. Prehospital and emergency department ultrasound in blunt abdominal trauma. Eur J Trauma Emerg Surg 2009; 35: 341–346

[22] Blaivas M, Brannam L, Theodoro D. Ultrasound image quality comparison between an inexpensive handheld emergency department (ED) ultrasound machine and a large mobile ED ultrasound system. Acad Emerg Med 2004; 11: 778–781

[23] Ziegler CM, Seitz K, Leicht-Biener U, Mauch M. Detection of therapeutically relevant diagnoses made by sonography of the upper abdomen: portable versus high-end sonographic units—a prospective study. Ultraschall Med 2004; 25: 428–432

[24] Osranek M, Bursi F, O'Leary PW et al. Hand-carried ultrasound-guided pericardiocentesis and thoracentesis. J Am Soc Echocardiogr 2003; 16: 480–484

[25] Caturelli E, Villani MR, Schiavone G et al. Safety and low cost of 'free hand' technique with ordinary antisepsis in abdominal US-guided fine-needle punctures: clinical report of a four-year experience. Eur J Ultrasound 1997; 6: 131–134

[26] Liang SJ, Tu CY, Chen HJ et al. Application of ultrasound-guided pigtail catheter for drainage of pleural effusions in the ICU. Intensive Care Med 2009; 35: 350–354

[27] Mayo PH, Goltz HR, Tafreshi M, Doelken P. Safety of ultrasound-guided thoracentesis in patients receiving mechanical ventilation. Chest 2004; 125: 1059–1062

[28] Lee HH, Carlson RW, Bull DM. Early diagnosis of spontaneous bacterial peritonitis: values of ascitic fluid variables. Infection 1987; 15: 232–236

[29] Koegelenberg CF, Diacon AH, Bolliger CT. Parapneumonic pleural effusion and empyema. Respiration 2008; 75: 241–250

[30] Kolditz M, Höffken G. Management des parapneumonischen Ergusses und des Pleuraempyems. Der Pneumologe 2008; 5: 219–228

[31] Silverman SG, Mueller PR, Saini S et al. Thoracic empyema: management with image-guided catheter drainage. Radiology 1988; 169: 5–9

[32] Cameron R, Davies HR. Intra-pleural fibrinolytic therapy versus conservative management in the treatment of parapneumonic effusions and empyema. Cochrane Database Syst Rev 2004; 2: CD002312

[33] Blank W, Braun B. Ultraschalldiagnostik bei Pneumothorax. Ultraschall Klin Prax 1989; 1 (Suppl): 66

[34] Wilkerson RG, Stone MB. Sensitivity of bedside ultrasound and supine anteroposterior chest radiographs for the identification of pneumothorax after blunt trauma. Acad Emerg Med 2010; 17: 11–17

[35] Henry M, Arnold T, Harvey J Pleural Diseases Group, Standards of Care Committee, British Thoracic Society. BTS guidelines for the management of spontaneous pneumothorax. Thorax 2003; 58 (Suppl 2): ii39–ii52

[36] Herth FJF. Pneumothorax: Klinik, Diagnostik und Behandlung. Der Pneumologe 2008; 5: 239–246

[37] Isselbacher EM, Cigarroa JE, Eagle KA. Cardiac tamponade complicating proximal aortic dissection. Is pericardiocentesis harmful? Circulation 1994; 90: 2375–2378

[38] Rozycki GS, Feliciano DV, Ochsner MG et al. The role of ultrasound in patients with possible penetrating cardiac wounds: a prospective multicenter study. J Trauma 1999; 46: 543–551; discussion 551–552

[39] Kil UH, Jung HO, Koh YS et al. Prognosis of large, symptomatic pericardial effusion treated by echo-guided percutaneous pericardiocentesis. Clin Cardiol 2008; 31: 531–537

[40] Tsang TS, Enriquez-Sarano M, Freeman WK et al. Consecutive 1127 therapeutic echocardiographically guided pericardiocenteses: clinical profile, practice patterns, and outcomes spanning 21 years. Mayo Clin Proc 2002; 77: 429–436

[41] Silvestry FE, Kerber RE, Brook MM et al. Echocardiography-guided interventions. J Am Soc Echocardiogr 2009; 22: 213–231, quiz 316–317

[42] Hind D, Calvert N, McWilliams R et al. Ultrasonic locating devices for central venous cannulation: meta-analysis. BMJ 2003; 327: 361–367

[43] Froehlich CD, Rigby MR, Rosenberg ES et al. Ultrasound-guided central venous catheter placement decreases complications and decreases placement attempts compared with the landmark technique in patients in a pediatric intensive care unit. Crit Care Med 2009; 37: 1090–1096

[44] Wigmore TJ, Smythe JF, Hacking MB, Raobaikady R, MacCallum NS. Effect of the implementation of NICE guidelines for ultrasound guidance on the complication rates associated with central venous catheter placement in patients presenting for routine surgery in a tertiary referral centre. Br J Anaesth 2007; 99: 662–665

[45] Leung J, Duffy M, Finckh A. Real-time ultrasonographically-guided internal jugular vein catheterization in the emergency department increases success rates and reduces complications: a randomized, prospective study. Ann Emerg Med 2006; 48: 540–547

[46] NICE-Leitlinie 2002. Guidance on the use of ultrasound locating devices for placing central venous catheters. 2002 (http://www.nice.org.uk/nicemedia/pdf/Ultrasound_49_GUIDANCE.pdf)

[47] Doniger SJ, Ishimine P, Fox JC, Kanegaye JT. Randomized controlled trial of ultrasound-guided peripheral intravenous catheter placement versus traditional techniques in difficult-access pediatric patients. Pediatr Emerg Care 2009; 25: 154–159

[48] Mills CN, Liebmann O, Stone MB, Frazee BW. Ultrasonographically guided insertion of a 15-cm catheter into the deep brachial or basilic vein in patients with difficult intravenous access. Ann Emerg Med 2007; 50: 68–72

[49] Kaufman SL. Femoral puncture using Doppler ultrasound guidance: aid to transluminal angioplasty and other applications. AJR Am J Roentgenol 1980; 134: 402

[50] Seto AH, Abu-Fadel MS, Sparling JM et al. Real-time ultrasound guidance facilitates femoral arterial access and reduces vascular complications: FAUST (Femoral Arterial Access With Ultrasound Trial). JACC Cardiovasc Interv 2010; 3: 751–758

[51] Arthurs ZM, Starnes BW, Sohn VY, Singh N, Andersen CA. Ultrasound-guided access improves rate of access-related complications for totally percutaneous aortic aneurysm repair. Ann Vasc Surg 2008; 22: 736–741

[52] Marcus AJ, Lotzof K, Howard A. Access to the superficial femoral artery in the presence of a “hostile groin”: a prospective study. Cardiovasc Intervent Radiol 2007; 30: 351–354

[53] Cluley SR, Brener BJ, Hollier LH et al. Ultrasound-guided balloon angioplasty is a new technique for vascular surgeons. Am J Surg 1991; 162: 117–121

[54] Cluley SR, Brener BJ, Hollier L et al. Transcutaneous ultrasonography can be used to guide and monitor balloon angioplasty. J Vasc Surg 1993; 17: 23–30; discussion 30–31

[55] Ramaswami G, al-Kutoubi A, Nicolaides AN, Dhanjil S, Griffin M, Ryan MF. Peripheral transluminal angioplasty under ultrasound guidance: initial clinical experience and prevalence of lower limb lesions amenable to ultrasound-guided angioplasty. J Endovasc Surg 1995; 2: 27–35

[56] Ramaswami G, al-Kutoubi A, Nicolaides AN et al. Duplex controlled angioplasty. Eur J Vasc Surg 1994; 8: 457–463

[57] Ramaswami G, Nicolaides AN, Vilkomerson D. Principles of angioplasty guidance using ultrasound. J Cardiovasc Surg (Torino) 1996; 37 (Suppl 1): 27–31

[58] Ahmadi R, Ugurluoglu A, Schillinger M, Katzenschlager R, Sabeti S, Minar E. Duplex ultrasound-guided femoropopliteal angioplasty: initial and 12-month results from a case controlled study. J Endovasc Ther 2002; 9: 873–881

[59] Ascher E, Hingorani AP, Marks N. Duplex-guided balloon angioplasty of lower extremity arteries. Perspect Vasc Surg Endovasc Ther 2007; 19: 23–31

[60] Bacchini G, La Milia V, Andrulli S, Locatelli F. Color Doppler ultrasonography percutaneous transluminal angioplasty of vascular access grafts. J Vasc Access 2007; 8: 81–85

[61] Katzenschlager R, Ahmadi A, Minar E et al. Femoropopliteal artery: initial and 6-month results of color duplex US-guided percutaneous transluminal angioplasty. Radiology 1996; 199: 331–334

[62] Cianci R, Lavini R, Letizia C et al. Low-contrast medium doses for ultrasound imaging during renal revascularization by PTA-stenting. J Nephrol 2004; 17: 520–524

[63] Cook C, Rees M. Ultrasound and fluoroscopic-guided angioplasty over the aortic bifurcation in a patient with previous severe reaction to contrast medium. J Endovasc Ther 2001; 8: 648–651

[64] Kawarada O, Yokoi Y, Takemoto K. Practical use of duplex echo-guided recanalization of chronic total occlusion in the iliac artery. J Vasc Surg 2010; 52: 475–478

[65] Banerjee S, Das TS, Brilakis ES. Transcutaneous ultrasound-guided endovascular crossing of infrainguinal chronic total occlusions. Cardiovasc Revasc Med 2010; 11: 116–119

[66] Marks N, Ascher E, Hingorani AP. Treatment of failing lower extremity arterial bypasses under ultrasound guidance. Perspect Vasc Surg Endovasc Ther 2007; 19: 34–39

[67] Ascher E, Gopal K, Marks N, Boniscavage P, Shiferson A, Hingorani A. Duplex-guided endovascular repair of popliteal artery aneurysms (PAAs): a new approach to avert the use of contrast material and radiation exposure. Eur J Vasc Endovasc Surg 2010; 39: 769–773

[68] Ascher E, Marks NA, Schutzer RW, Hingorani AP. Duplex-assisted internal carotid artery balloon angioplasty and stent placement: a novel approach to minimize or eliminate the use of contrast material. J Vasc Surg 2005; 41: 409–415

[69] Ascher E, Hingorani A, Marks N. Duplex-guided balloon angioplasty of failing or nonmaturing arterio-venous fistulae for hemodialysis: a new office-based procedure. J Vasc Surg 2009; 50: 594–599

[70] Liang HL, Pan HB, Chung HM et al. Restoration of thrombosed Brescia-Cimino dialysis fistulas by using percutaneous transluminal angioplasty. Radiology 2002; 223: 339–344

[71] Marks N, Ascher E, Hingorani AP. Duplex-guided repair of failing or nonmaturing arterio-venous access for hemodialysis. Perspect Vasc Surg Endovasc Ther 2007; 19: 50–55

[72] Napoli M, Montinaro A, Russo F et al. Early experiences of intraoperative ultrasound guided angioplasty of the arterial stenosis during upper limb arteriovenous fistula creation. J Vasc Access 2007; 8: 97–102

[73] Higgins JN. Technical report: the use of ultrasound in positioning a catheter for thrombolysis of an occluded prosthetic femoropopliteal graft. Clin Radiol 1994; 49: 351–353

[74] Katzenschlager R, Ahmadi A, Atteneder M et al. Colour duplex sonography-guided local lysis of occlusions in the femoro-popliteal region. Int Angiol 2000; 19: 250–254

[75] Schillinger M, Haumer M, Mlekusch W, Schlerka G, Ahmadi R, Minar E. Predicting renal failure after balloon angioplasty in high-risk patients. J Endovasc Ther 2001; 8: 609–614

[76] Solomon R. The role of osmolality in the incidence of contrast-induced nephropathy: a systematic review of angiographic contrast media in high risk patients. Kidney Int 2005; 68: 2256–2263

[77] Hanson JM, Atri M, Power N. Ultrasound-guided thrombin injection of iatrogenic groin pseudoaneurysm: Doppler features and technical tips. Br J Radiol 2008; 81: 154–163

[78] Webber GW, Jang J, Gustavson S, Olin JW. Contemporary management of postcatheterization pseudoaneurysms. Circulation 2007; 115: 2666–2674

[79] Ates M, Sahin S, Konuralp C et al. Evaluation of risk factors associated with femoral pseudoaneurysms after cardiac catheterization. J Vasc Surg 2006; 43: 520–524

[80] Middleton WD, Dasyam A, Teefey SA. Diagnosis and treatment of iatrogenic femoral artery pseudoaneurysms. Ultrasound Q 2005; 21: 3–17

[81] Kent KC, McArdle CR, Kennedy B, Baim DS, Anninos E, Skillman JJ. A prospective study of the clinical outcome of femoral pseudoaneurysms and arteriovenous fistulas induced by arterial puncture. J Vasc Surg 1993; 17: 125–131; discussion 131–133

[82] Toursarkissian B, Allen BT, Petrinec D et al. Spontaneous closure of selected iatrogenic pseudoaneurysms and arteriovenous fistulae. J Vasc Surg 1997; 25: 803–808; discussion 808–809

[83] San Norberto García EM, González-Fajardo JA, Gutiérrez V, Carrera S, Vaquero C. Femoral pseudoaneurysms post-cardiac catheterization surgically treated: evolution and prognosis. Interact Cardiovasc Thorac Surg 2009; 8: 353–357

[84] Tisi PV, Callam MJ. Treatment for femoral pseudoaneurysms. Cochrane Database Syst Rev 2009; 2: CD004981

[85] Eisenberg L, Paulson EK, Kliewer MA, Hudson MP, DeLong DM, Carroll BA. Sonographically guided compression repair of pseudoaneurysms: further experience from a single institution. AJR Am J Roentgenol 1999; 173: 1567–1573

[86] Bellmunt S, Dilmé J, Barros A, Escudero JR. Compression assisted by removable coils as a new treatment for iatrogenic femoral pseudoaneurysms. J Vasc Surg 2011; 53: 236–238

[87] Fellmeth BD, Roberts AC, Bookstein JJ et al. Postangiographic femoral artery injuries: nonsurgical repair with US-guided compression. Radiology 1991; 178: 671–675

[88] Cox GS, Young JR, Gray BR, Grubb MW, Hertzer NR. Ultrasound-guided compression repair of postcatheterization pseudoaneurysms: results of treatment in one hundred cases. J Vasc Surg 1994; 19: 683–686

[89] Finkelstein A, Bazan S, Halkin A et al. Treatment of post-catheterization femoral artery pseudo-aneurysm with para-aneurysmal saline injection. Am J Cardiol 2008; 101: 1418–1422

[90] Gehling G, Ludwig J, Schmidt A, Daniel WG, Werner D. Percutaneous occlusion of femoral artery pseudoaneurysm by para-aneurysmal saline injection. Catheter Cardiovasc Interv 2003; 58: 500–504

[91] Cope C, Zeit R. Coagulation of aneurysms by direct percutaneous thrombin injection. AJR Am J Roentgenol 1986; 147: 383–387

[92] Olsen DM, Rodriguez JA, Vranic M, Ramaiah V, Ravi R, Diethrich EB. A prospective study of ultrasound scan-guided thrombin injection of femoral pseudoaneurysm: a trend toward minimal medication. J Vasc Surg 2002; 36: 779–782

[93] Thees-Laurenz R, Kappes-Schädler C, Mertiny E, Wüstner M. Perkutane ultraschallgesteuerte Thrombininjektion vei iatrogenem A. spurium. Ist eine Bestimmung der zum Verschluss benötigten Thrombinmenge möglich? Ultraschall Med 2010; 31: S22

[94] Grewe PH, Mügge A, Germing A et al. Occlusion of pseudoaneurysms using human or bovine thrombin using contrast-enhanced ultrasound guidance. Am J Cardiol 2004; 93: 1540–1542

[95] Levy MJ, Chak A EUS 2008 Working Group. EUS 2008 Working Group document: evaluation of EUS-guided vascular therapy. Gastrointest Endosc 2009; 69 (Suppl): S37–S42

[96] Lameris R, du Plessis J, Nieuwoudt M, Scheepers A, van der Merwe SW. A visceral pseudoaneurysm: management by EUS-guided thrombin injection. Gastrointest Endosc 2011; 73: 392–395

[97] Romero-Castro R, Pellicer-Bautista F, Giovannini M et al. Endoscopic ultrasound (EUS)-guided coil embolization therapy in gastric varices. Endoscopy 2010; 42 (Suppl 2): E35–E36

[98] Romero-Castro R, Pellicer-Bautista FJ, Jimenez-Saenz M et al. EUS-guided injection of cyanoacrylate in perforating feeding veins in gastric varices: results in 5 cases. Gastrointest Endosc 2007; 66: 402–407

[99] El-Saadany M, Jalil S, Irisawa A, Shibukawa G, Ohira H, Bhutani MS. EUS for portal hypertension: a comprehensive and critical appraisal of clinical and experimental indications. Endoscopy 2008; 40: 690–696

[100] Levy MJ, Wong Kee Song LM, Farnell MB, Misra S, Sarr MG, Gostout CJ. Endoscopic ultrasound (EUS)-guided angiotherapy of refractory gastrointestinal bleeding. Am J Gastroenterol 2008; 103: 352–359

[101] Larghi A, Stobinski M, Galasso D, Amato A, Familiari P, Costamagna G. EUS-guided drainage of a pericardial cyst: closer to the heart (with video). Gastrointest Endosc 2009; 70: 1273–1274

[102] Romero-Castro R, Rios-Martin JJ, Gallego-Garcia de Vinuesa P et al. Pericardial tumor diagnosed by EUS-guided FNA (with video). Gastrointest Endosc 2009; 69: 562–563

[103] Fritscher-Ravens A, Ganbari A, Mosse CA, Swain P, Koehler P, Patel K. Transesophageal endoscopic ultrasound-guided access to the heart. Endoscopy 2007; 39: 385–389

[104] Buscaglia JM, Dray X, Shin EJ et al. A new alternative for a transjugular intrahepatic portosystemic shunt: EUS-guided creation of an intrahepatic portosystemic shunt (with video). Gastrointest Endosc 2009; 69: 941–947

[105] Giday SA, Clarke JO, Buscaglia JM et al. EUS-guided portal vein catheterization: a promising novel approach for portal angiography and portal vein pressure measurements. Gastrointest Endosc 2008; 67: 338–342

[106] Giday SA, Ko CW, Clarke JO et al. EUS-guided portal vein carbon dioxide angiography: a pilot study in a porcine model. Gastrointest Endosc 2007; 66: 814–819

[107] Magno P, Ko CW, Buscaglia JM et al. EUS-guided angiography: a novel approach to diagnostic and therapeutic interventions in the vascular system. Gastrointest Endosc 2007; 66: 587–591

[108] Matthes K, Sahani D, Holalkere NS, Mino-Kenudson M, Brugge WR. Feasibility of endoscopic ultrasound-guided embolization of the splenic vein. Endoscopy 2007; 39 (Suppl 1): E3–E4

[109] Matthes K, Sahani D, Holalkere NS, Mino-Kenudson M, Brugge WR. Feasibility of endoscopic ultrasound-guided portal vein embolization with Enteryx. Acta Gastroenterol Belg 2005; 68: 412–415

[110] Elmunzer BJ, Pollack MJ, Trunzo JA et al. Initial evaluation of a novel, prototype, forward-viewing echoendoscope in a porcine arterial bleeding model (with video). Gastrointest Endosc 2010; 72: 611–614

Other Applications of Interventional Ultrasound

31 Extravascular Use of Ultrasound Contrast Agents . . . 354

32 Volume Navigation . . . 359

33 Palliative Interventions and the Role of Ultrasonography in Palliative Care . . . 364

31 Extravascular Use of Ultrasound Contrast Agents

A. Ignee, G. Schuessler, C. F Dietrich

Ultrasound contrast agents (UCAs) are widely used in everyday clinical practice. The majority of indications are for their intravenous use. As early as 1986, however, the first study was published on the extravascular or intracavitary use of UCAs in the renal collecting system.[1] The first in vivo reports were published in 2000.[2]

Since then, studies have been published on the following applications, which fall under the general heading of extravascular contrast-enhanced ultrasound (EVCEUS):

- Voiding sonography (excretory sonography)
- Hysterosalpingo-contrast sonography (HyCoSy)
- Biliary tract:
  - via endoscopic retrograde cholangiography (ERC)[3]
  - via percutaneous transhepatic cholangiography and drainage (PTCD)[4]
- Fistulography[5]

Analogously to the use of conventional radiographic contrast media, UCAs can also be used to improve the visualization of physiologic cavities (e.g., the pleura and peritoneal cavity) and nonphysiologic cavities (e.g., abscesses and cystic lesions), especially during interventional procedures. Imaging of the upper and lower gastrointestinal tract can also be enhanced with UCAs administered by swallowing, injection, or enema.

31.1 Approved Indications

UCAs are approved for intravascular use. They have not been approved for any other indications except voiding sonography with SHU508A (Levovist, Bayer Schering Pharma). Thus, the benefit to the patient must be weighed against possible risks before these agents are used for extravascular imaging, and detailed informed consent must be obtained.

31.2 Contraindications and Complications

To date only a few complications have resulted from the intravenous use of UCAs. In a retrospective multicenter Italian study that included more than 23,000 examinations, the absolute number of adverse events was 29 (0.0086%), 2 of which were severe (1 bronchospasm, 1 allergic shock). No fatal events occurred.[6] Thus, given the very low complication rate of intravenous use and the very low dose used in extravascular applications, it is reasonable to conclude that complications are extremely rare during the extravascular use of UCAs.

31.3 Technique

Intravenous UCAs are administered in an extremely low dose. For example, 1 mL of SonoVue (Bracco Imaging) contains 1 to 5×10^8 microbubbles, and 1.2 mL is adequate for intravenous imaging on modern ultrasound machines. UCAs are generally diluted for extravascular use. Since this is not an approved application, no official dose recommendations are available.

When a contrast agent is injected at a local concentration that is too high, it produces a shadowing artifact that may obscure image details distal to the ultrasound transducer.[7] The administered dose must be reduced, therefore. If too much contrast agent has already been injected, higher-energy ultrasound pulses can be transmitted to reduce the concentration of the microbubbles to a reasonable level.

In the few studies on voiding sonography (vesicoureteral reflux) that have been published to date, concentrations of 1 mL SonoVue in 120 to 210 mL of saline solution (calculated for 2- to 5-year-old children) were injected into the bladder of the pediatric patients.[8,9] This represents a dilution factor of 100 to 200.

For the oral administration of UCAs, 2 to 4 drops of SonoVue are mixed with 200 mL of tap water. For esophageal enhancement the patient can take one mouthful while sitting up, then lie back and swallow the solution while supine. For gastric enhancement all of the solution is swallowed (personal empirical recommendations).

For lower distribution volumes (e.g., in the biliary tract), a reasonable dilution is 0.1 mL of SonoVue per 20 mL of saline solution.[4] Very large distribution volumes (ascites, large pleural effusions) require a higher contrast dose, and one whole ampule of SonoVue should be injected.

If the main goal of the investigation is to determine whether or not contrast medium can enter a cavity (fistulography, vesicoureteral reflux), higher concentrations may be used. The main concern in this case is not image aesthetics but the appearance (or nonappearance) of the contrast medium.

In this chapter we will present the most important extravascular applications of UCAs while referring the reader to the appropriate chapters.

31.4 Use of Ultrasound Contrast Agents in Physiologic Body Cavities

31.4.1 Voiding Sonography for the Detection of Vesicoureteral Reflux

Vesicoureteral reflux is a relatively common disorder in children and may lead to the deterioration of renal function, so that early diagnosis is essential.

Voiding sonography determines whether intravesical contrast medium enters the pyelocalyceal system during micturition, which would confirm vesicoureteral reflux. This requires catheterization of the urethra, generally followed by the injection of a contrast agent. Levovist has been approved for this indication. SonoVue offers many technical advantages over Levovist but has not been approved.

Voiding sonography had advantages over radiography in its ability to define renal anatomy without exposure to ionizing radiation. It should also be noted that vesicoureteral reflux is not a constant phenomenon and may elude detection by a radiographic "snapshot."

The male urethra can be imaged by perineal ultrasound to detect urethral stenosis.[10]

31.4.2 Contrast-Enhanced Ultrasound for Evaluating Tubal Patency

Female infertility tests may include the assessment of tubal patency. Laparoscopy with dye insufflation is considered the gold standard but is invasive. Another method is radiographic hysterosalpingography. Hysterosalpingo-contrast sonography (HyCoSy) was introduced at a relatively early stage to avoid radiation exposure. It did not employ commercial contrast medium but involved the intrauterine injection of saline solution that was shaken to create air bubbles. But several more recent studies have shown that the use of UCAs can improve the test and increase its sensitivity.[11–13]

Antibiotic prophylaxis is given before the examination (e.g., 200 mg doxycycline 30 minutes before the test or 500 mg azithromycin daily 2 days before the test continued until the day of the test). An 8F balloon catheter is introduced into the cervix. Then SonoVue is diluted with saline solution (1.2 mL SonoVue in 5–10 mL saline) and injected into the uterine cavity.[14]

31.4.3 Imaging the Peritoneal Cavity with UCAs (for Detection of Ascites)

Paracentesis is necessary in patients who have diuretic resistance or experience adverse effects from diuretics (e.g., exacerbation of preexisting renal failure). When an ultrasound contrast agent is injected into the peritoneal cavity, the agent is distributed throughout all communicating spaces. This effect is supported by patient movements (e.g., walking around). If septa are present, they will confine the agent to localized areas. A whole ampule should be injected due to the high distribution volume, and the agent does not have to be diluted.

Foschi et al reported on seven patients with cirrhotic ascites and pleural effusion. In five patients they were able to document the passage of UCA from the peritoneal to the pleural cavity. This allowed them to confirm the presumptive diagnosis of hydrothorax, which was reconfirmed by nuclear medicine scans. These findings made it easier or possible to proceed with operative treatment. The authors administered two ampules of SonoVue.[15] Three-dimensional imaging methods can be used (▶ Fig. 31.1).

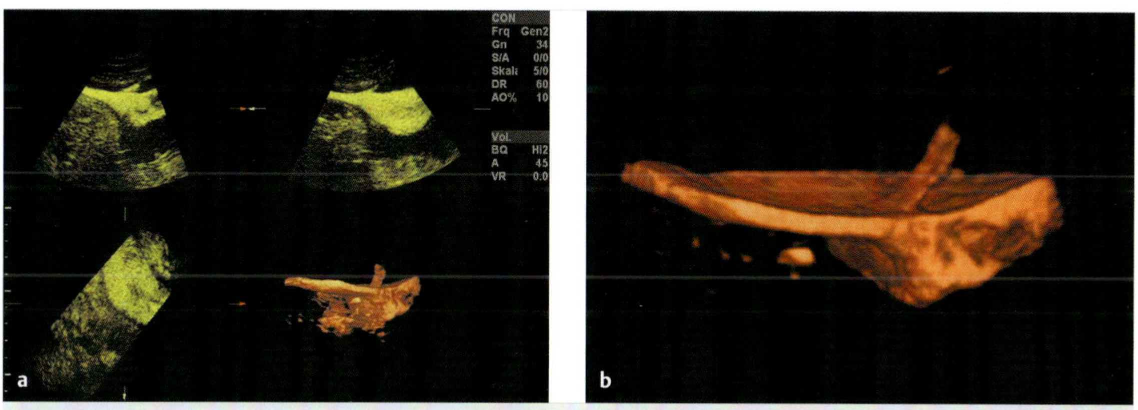

Fig. 31.1 a, b Three-dimensional position check of an ascites drain with a paracentesis needle following postoperative peritonitis with chronic ascites.

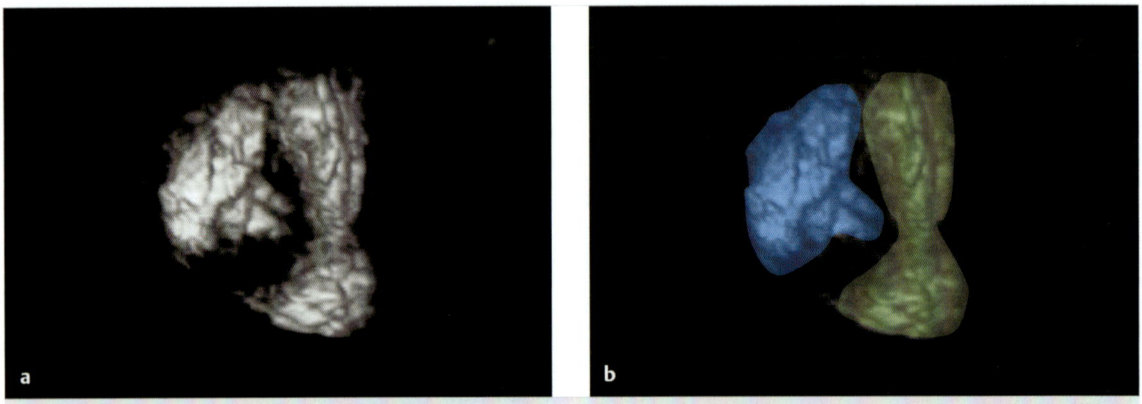

Fig. 31.2 a, b Images from a 74-year-old man with progressive dysphagia. The original image is shown in **a**; in **b** the esophagus is dyed green and the diverticulum is dyed blue. Supraclavicular ultrasound showed a prominent gas-filled structure behind the carotid artery and thyroid gland. The image after oral ultrasound contrast revealed a communication with the esophagus with contrast retention in the cavity. The patient is in good health following surgical resection.

31.4.4 Biliary Tract

UCAs in Percutaneous Transhepatic Cholangiography and Drainage (PTCD)

PTCD is addressed in Chapter 20.

UCAs in Endoscopic Retrograde Cholangiography (ERCP)

Zuber-Jerger et al reported on a patient with a body mass index > 50 kg/m^2. She was suffering from symptomatic choledocholithiasis and could not undergo conventional ERC. The authors therefore performed bedside endoscopy with a duodenoscope and injected SonoVue into the bile duct through a conventional papillotome. This method successfully defined the intrahepatic bile ducts and revealed the stenosis, followed by a sphincterotomy and stone extraction. The authors postulate that the method could also be used in pregnant patients.[3]

31.4.5 UCAs in Enterography

Orally Administered UCAs

Goals

Indications for the oral administration of UCAs are limited to structures accessible to ultrasonography, comparable to the indications for conventional fluoroscopy. The advantages of contrast-enhanced ultrasound are the capability for real-time imaging, the absence of radiation exposure, and rapid accessibility during a conventional ultrasound examination.

Technique

Two to four drops of SonoVue in 200 mL of water provide adequate visualization as far as the duodenum. Larger contrast volumes (e.g., 1 ampule in 500 mL water) must be administered to define lower portions of the intestinal tract. The patient is instructed to walk around 10 minutes after drinking the solution (▶ Fig. 31.2).

31.4.6 CEUS Gastrography—Percutaneous Injection of UCA into the Stomach to Assess Gastrostomy Placement

The use of contrast-enhanced ultrasound (CEUS) in percutaneous gastrostomy is covered in Chapter 21.

31.5 Use of Ultrasound Contrast Agents in Nonphysiologic Body Cavities

31.5.1 Ultrasound Fistulography

The contrast agent is injected into a fistulous opening to define the sinus tract and perhaps identify the body cavity that communicates with the fistula. Blunt-tipped probes can be used for this purpose. A pragmatic solution is to use green or pink indwelling venous cannulas without a metal stylet.

A variety of ultrasound methods may be used. Perianal fistulas can be imaged by perineal ultrasound using conventional linear or curved-array transducers.[16,17] These probes still have the best contrast sensitivity and are easy to use (Case of the Month at www.EFSUMB.org). Another option is endorectal or endovaginal ultrasound. When UCAs are used in contrast-specific imaging mode, the endorectal probes must be able to support this mode. Heinrich et al reported on the evaluation of rectovaginal fistulas after the injection of Echovist (a right-heart contrast agent from Schering) using transvaginal ultrasound and nonspecific imaging. The dose was not stated.[18] Chew and others investigated anal fistulas with transrectal ultrasound by instilling Levovist into the fistulas. Again, the dose was not reported.[5] Volkmer and his group used endorectal ultrasound after intravesical injection of Levovist to demonstrate presumed vesicoenteric fistulas. The authors used 4 g of Levovist in 200 mL of saline solution.[19]

As far as dose is concerned, it may be argued that there is no need to dilute the solution due to the "yes/no" nature of the investigation. But for economical and aesthetic reasons, our group still uses the customary dilution for extravascular imaging (0.1 mL SonoVue in 20 mL saline solution). If the result is negative, we inject another, undiluted, milliliter into the orifice.

31.5.2 Percutaneous Injection of UCAs for Abscess Imaging

This subject is covered in Chapter 15.

31.5.3 UCAs for Demonstrating Pancreatitis-Associated Cystic Lesions after EUS-Guided Biopsy

Goals

Contrast-enhanced endoscopic ultrasound with a low mechanical index and contrast-specific imaging (contrast-enhanced low MI endoscopic ultrasound, CELMIEUS) was first described in 2005[20] and has been commercially available since 2009.[21] The indications and limitations have not previously been defined.

Software and hardware developments now allow us to consider possible extravascular applications of this technique. The following indications may be promising:

- Injection of UCAs during the fine needle aspiration cytology of indeterminate cystic pancreatic lesions to detect a communication with the pancreatic duct
- Injection of UCAs after the puncture of pancreatitis-associated cystic lesions to detect a communication with other cavities (e.g., the omental bursa). This could also be combined with a percutaneous sonographic technique (▶ Fig. 31.3).
- Injection of UCAs to confirm intraductal needle placement during EUS-guided biliary drainage

Technique

EUS-guided punctures are usually performed with a 22-gauge needle. Therapeutic procedures are done with 19-gauge needles since they can accommodate a 0.035-inch wire. Both gauges can be used to inject agents. UCAs are rarely injected through a 25-gauge needle, as the lumen may be small enough to cause microbubble disruption. This hypothesis has yet to be confirmed, however.

31.6 Summary

Extravascular contrast-enhanced ultrasound (EVCEUS) is technically feasible and has been employed under study conditions. It has not yet been approved for any applications other than voiding urosonography with Levovist. Adverse effects of UCAs are extremely rare with conventional use and are presumably even less common with extravascular use.

Several studies have been published on the following subjects:

- Voiding urosonography for the diagnosis of vesicoureteral reflux[22]
- Hysterosalpingo-contrast sonography (HyCoSy)[11,13]

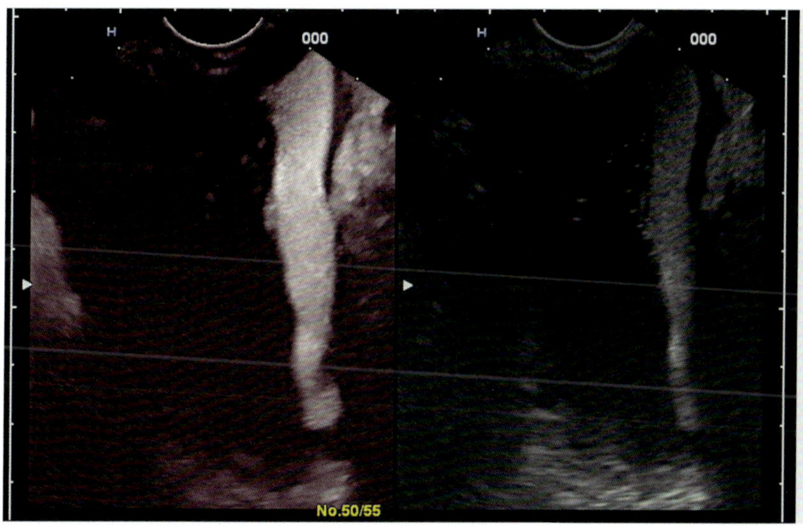

Fig. 31.3 Injection of an ultrasound contrast solution into a large pseudocyst for localization and to detect communications. The difficulty in this case is to achieve an adequate distribution of contrast agent in the lesion. This requires the injection of an adequate contrast volume.

Several published case reports or case series have dealt with:

- UCA injection into the biliary tract during PTCD[4]
- UCA injection into the biliary tract during ERCP[3]
- UCA injection into enteric fistulas[5]

Feasibility has been demonstrated for the following additional applications:

- Oral administration of UCAs
- Intraperitoneal injection of UCAs
- Percutaneous injection of UCAs into the stomach

Prospective studies are needed to document the utility of these applications. Approval would be desirable.

References

[1] Meyer-Schwickerath M, Fritzsch T. Sonographic imaging of the kidney cavity system using a ultrasonic contrast medium [Article in German]. Ultraschall Med 1986; 7: 34–36

[2] Farina R, Arena C, Pennisi F, Di Benedetto V, Politi G, Di Benedetto A. Vesico-ureteral reflux: diagnosis and staging with voiding color Doppler US: preliminary experience. Eur J Radiol 2000; 35: 49–53

[3] Zuber-Jerger I, Endlicher E, Schölmerich J, Klebl F. Endoscopic retrograde cholangiography with contrast ultrasonography. Endoscopy 2008; 40 (Suppl 2): E202

[4] Ignee A, Baum U, Schuessler G, Dietrich CF. Contrast-enhanced ultrasound-guided percutaneous cholangiography and cholangiodrainage (CEUS-PTCD). Endoscopy 2009; 41: 725–726

[5] Chew SS, Yang JL, Newstead GL, Douglas PR. Anal fistula: Levovist-enhanced endoanal ultrasound: a pilot study. Dis Colon Rectum 2003; 46: 377–384

[6] Piscaglia F, Bolondi L. Italian Society for Ultrasound in Medicine and Biology (SIUMB) Study Group on Ultrasound Contrast Agents. The safety of Sonovue in abdominal applications: retrospective analysis of 23188 investigations. Ultrasound Med Biol 2006; 32: 1369–1375

[7] Dietrich CF, Ignee A, Hocke M, Schreiber-Dietrich D, Greis C. Pitfalls and artifacts using contrast enhanced ultrasound. Z Gastroenterol 2011; 49: 350–356

[8] Kis E, Nyitrai A, Várkonyi I et al. Voiding urosonography with second-generation contrast agent versus voiding cystourethrography. Pediatr Nephrol 2010; 25: 2289–2293

[9] Papadopoulou F, Anthopoulou A, Siomou E, Efremidis S, Tsamboulas C, Darge K. Harmonic voiding urosonography with a second-generation contrast agent for the diagnosis of vesicoureteral reflux. Pediatr Radiol 2009; 39: 239–244

[10] Berrocal T, Gayá F, Arjonilla A. Vesicoureteral reflux: can the urethra be adequately assessed by using contrast-enhanced voiding US of the bladder? Radiology 2005; 234: 235–241

[11] Boudghène FP, Bazot M, Robert Y et al. Assessment of Fallopian tube patency by HyCoSy: comparison of a positive contrast agent with saline solution. Ultrasound Obstet Gynecol 2001; 18: 525–530

[12] Tamási F, Weidner A, Domokos N, Bedros RJ, Bagdány S. ECHOVIST-200 enhanced hystero-sonography: a new technique in the assessment of infertility. Eur J Obstet Gynecol Reprod Biol 2005; 121: 186–190

[13] Lanzani C, Savasi V, Leone FP, Ratti M, Ferrazzi E. Two-dimensional HyCoSy with contrast tuned imaging technology and a second-generation contrast media for the assessment of tubal patency in an infertility program. Fertil Steril 2009; 92: 1158–1161

[14] Exacoustos C, Di Giovanni A, Szabolcs B, Binder-Reisinger H, Gabardi C, Arduini D. Automated sonographic tubal patency evaluation with three-dimensional coded contrast imaging (CCI) during hysterosalpingo-contrast sonography (HyCoSy). Ultrasound Obstet Gynecol 2009; 34: 609–612

[15] Foschi FG, Piscaglia F, Pompili M et al. Real-time contrast-enhanced ultrasound—a new simple tool for detection of peritoneal-pleural communications in hepatic hydrothorax. Ultraschall Med 2008; 29: 538–542

[16] Barreiros AP, Hirche TO, Ignee A, Nürnberg D, Dietrich CF. Indications and limitations of perineal ultrasound examination. Scand J Gastroenterol 2010; 45: 764–765

[17] Braden B, Ignee A, Hocke M, Palmer RM, Dietrich C. Diagnostic value and clinical utility of contrast enhanced ultrasound in intestinal diseases. Dig Liver Dis 2010; 42: 667–674

[18] Henrich W, Meckies J, Friedmann W. Demonstration of a recto-vaginal fistula with the ultrasound contrast medium Echovist. Ultrasound Obstet Gynecol 2000; 15: 148–149

[19] Volkmer BG, Nesslauer T, Küfer R, Löffler M, Maier S, Gottfried HW. [Diagnosis of vesico-intestinal fistulas by contrast medium enhanced 3-D ultrasound]. Ultraschall Med 2001; 22: 81–86

[20] Dietrich CF, Ignee A, Frey H. Contrast-enhanced endoscopic ultrasound with low mechanical index: a new technique. Z Gastroenterol 2005; 43: 1219–1223

[21] Dietrich CF. Contrast-enhanced low mechanical index endoscopic ultrasound (CELMI-EUS). Endoscopy 2009; 41 (Suppl 2): E43–E44

[22] Darge K. Voiding urosonography with ultrasound contrast agents for the diagnosis of vesicoureteric reflux in children. I. Procedure. Pediatr Radiol 2008; 38: 40–53

32 Volume Navigation

C. F Dietrich, A. Ignee, M. Hoepfner

The term "volume navigation" in ultrasonography refers to the technical capability to reproducibly determine the exact position in space of a specific sectional plane or anatomical site and use that information for image fusion, position marking, or the 3D guidance of interventions.

Volume navigation requires a tracking system that continuously monitors the transducer position and beam direction in real time with adequate precision. The purpose of this system is to align the images produced by ultrasound and some other sectional imaging modality in order to make use of additional important anatomical information obtained with that imaging modality prior to the interventional procedure and at the same time to exploit the advantages of ultrasound (higher spatial resolution, real-time imaging, easier biopsy guidance).[1,2]

Publications to date have described fusion applications for imaging the coronary arteries, liver, and anorectal region and for guiding neurosurgical procedures.[2–11]

32.1 How Tracking Works

Magnetic fields are produced by a small, cube-shaped transmitter placed close to the patient. Inside the transmitter are three concentric, coreless coils arranged mutually perpendicular to one another. The three coils are excited in turn with a direct current pulse. Each coil is pulsed 80 times/second to alternately generate three orthogonal magnetic fields (▶ Fig. 32.1).

A sensor within range of the transmitter detects the magnetic fields and delivers an output signal whose intensity is proportional to the orientation angle of the sensor relative to the field lines and its distance from the transmitter. Because the angle of incidence of the magnetic field lines rotates 90° at fixed intervals (every 4.2 milliseconds), the output signal from the sensor will tend to vary accordingly. The relationship of the three output levels to one another can then be used to calculate the orientation of the sensor relative to the transmitter. This relationship is easily understood by considering the case of a constant output signal. This can occur only if all three magnetic fields impinge upon the sensor at an identical angle, i.e., at a 45° angle in the x, y, and z axes. This defines its orientation relative to the transmitter.

The angle of the incident field lines can be determined with even greater precision by mounting several (usually three) magnetic field detectors at angles to one another inside one sensor housing.

To determine not just the orientation of the sensor but also its distance from the transmitter (i.e., its position in space), the cumulative intensity of the three signals is measured and compared with a reference value. Since the amplitude of the field declines exponentially with distance from the transmitter, this function can be used to determine the position of the sensor in space.

A tracking system of this kind can monitor the exact three-dimensional position and location of the transducer in real time and make the spatial coordinates available for other linkages.

32.2 Position Marking

The continuous monitoring of transducer position and beam direction allows the examiner to mark points of special interest within the sectional image (e.g., suspicious structures) so that they can be located again from a different perspective, at a different time, or following treatment. This can be done simply by placing a cursor at the center of the targeted structure during the examination. Because the tracking system captures the position and beam direction of the transducer while the cursor position supplies additional information on the lateral and axial relationship of the structure to the transducer, the absolute position of the tagged feature is defined uniquely in three-dimensional space.

When the sectional plane is altered or the region of interest is revisited at a later time, the position marker will reappear on the screen when the active field of view approaches the previously tagged position. The size and shape of the marker symbol indicate the distance to the target, allowing the examiner to very quickly direct the scan plane precisely through the structure of interest.

32.3 Fusion with CT, MRI, or PET Volume Data Sets

One of the most important applications of volume navigation is the precise fusion of live ultrasound images with anatomically corresponding sections from a previously acquired CT, MRI, or PET volume data set. Before the start of the ultrasound examination, the data sets are imported via a network or portable storage device (USB stick, CD, DVD) and loaded into the image memory of the ultrasound system. The data transfer is done in standard DICOM format and generally takes less than 1 minute.

To ensure precise image fusion, the spatial coordinates of the tracking system must be matched to those of the imported volume for each new patient. This image registration can be done quickly and easily by selecting a salient image from the CT, MRI, or PET volume and then imaging the same plane sonographically in the patient. The identity of the sections is confirmed by clicking a button, which matches the coordinate systems of both modalities.

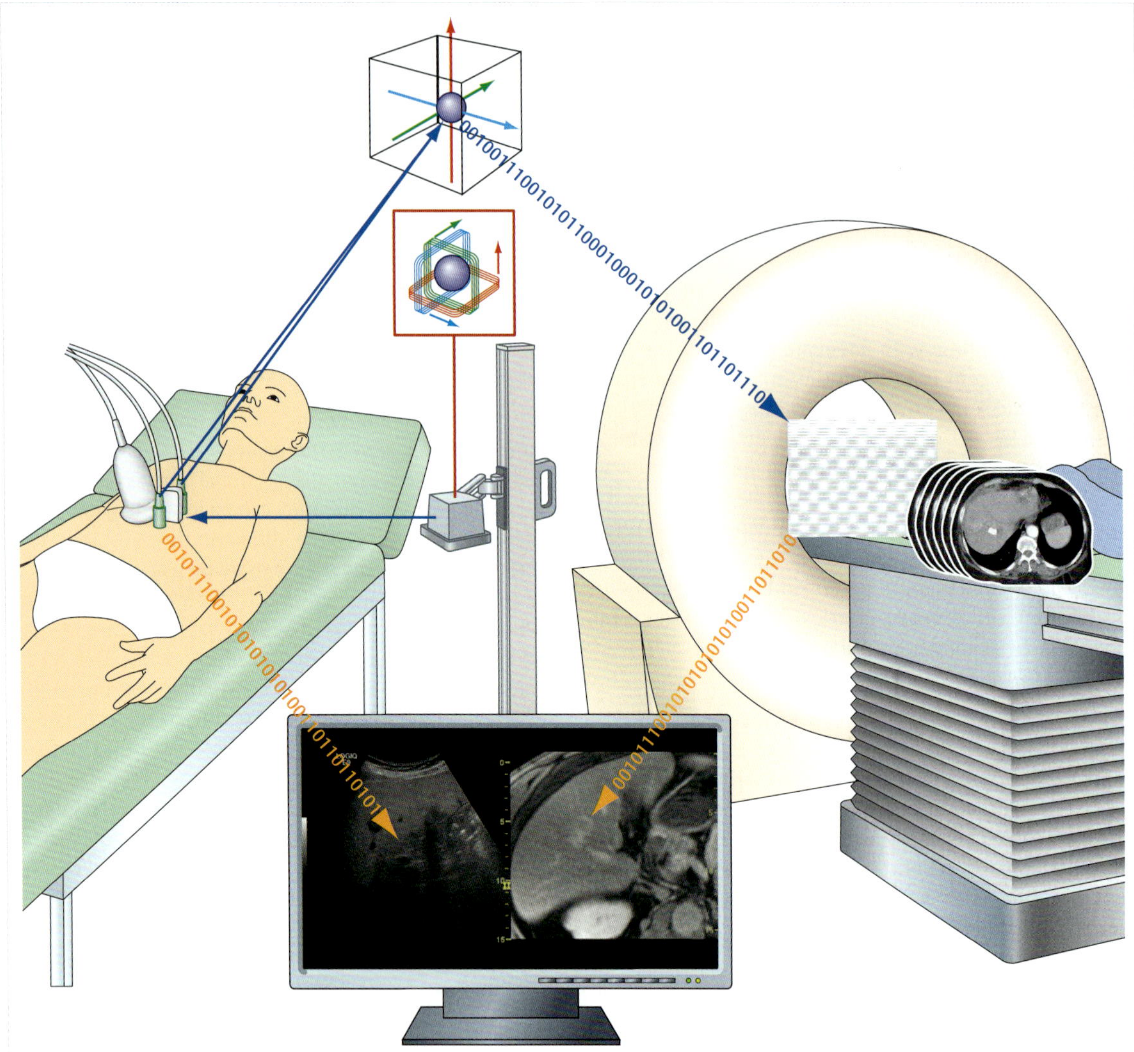

Fig. 32.1 Fusion imaging. A tracking system composed of a stationary magnetic field generator and two sensors mounted on the ultrasound transducer monitors the position, location, and beam direction of the transducer during the ultrasound examination. These spatial coordinates are used to extract a corresponding anatomical section from a previously acquired CT or MRI volume data set and display it side-by-side with or overlaid onto the ultrasound image.

Image registration using markers is more technically complex but also more precise.[12] In this method salient reference points visible in images from both modalities are marked as corresponding. When this process is repeated in several planes, the two coordinate systems will be precisely mapped onto each other in all spatial axes. This preliminary registration process takes approximately 10 minutes[2] but may take less time as the learning curve progresses. The process of matching corresponding anatomical planes will be simplified in the near future by the placement of external markers before performing a CT scan (this is not possible with MRI because of magnetic components). With this small external equipment, the fusion process is accomplished automatically by the machine and the patient has freedom of body movement during the investigation.

Once image registration is completed, the fused ultrasound examination can begin. The data on transducer location and position captured by the tracking system are transferred to the CT, MRI, or PET image memory and are used to extract a section that precisely matches the ultrasound image on the screen. The sections can be displayed side-by-side or can be overlaid. Any change in transducer position and beam direction is instantly registered and changes the image plane and its display with virtually zero time lag. Thus, the two images are matched precisely and continuously in their anatomical location and position, so that suspicious structures can be evaluated from numerous, identical perspectives using a variety of scan techniques.

Fusion imaging not only works in solid organs but is particularly useful in regions where ultrasound imaging conditions are poor (e.g., meteorism in pancreatitis, colon lesions, etc.).

The use of contrast-enhanced ultrasound in fusion imaging appears to be especially promising. In the case of

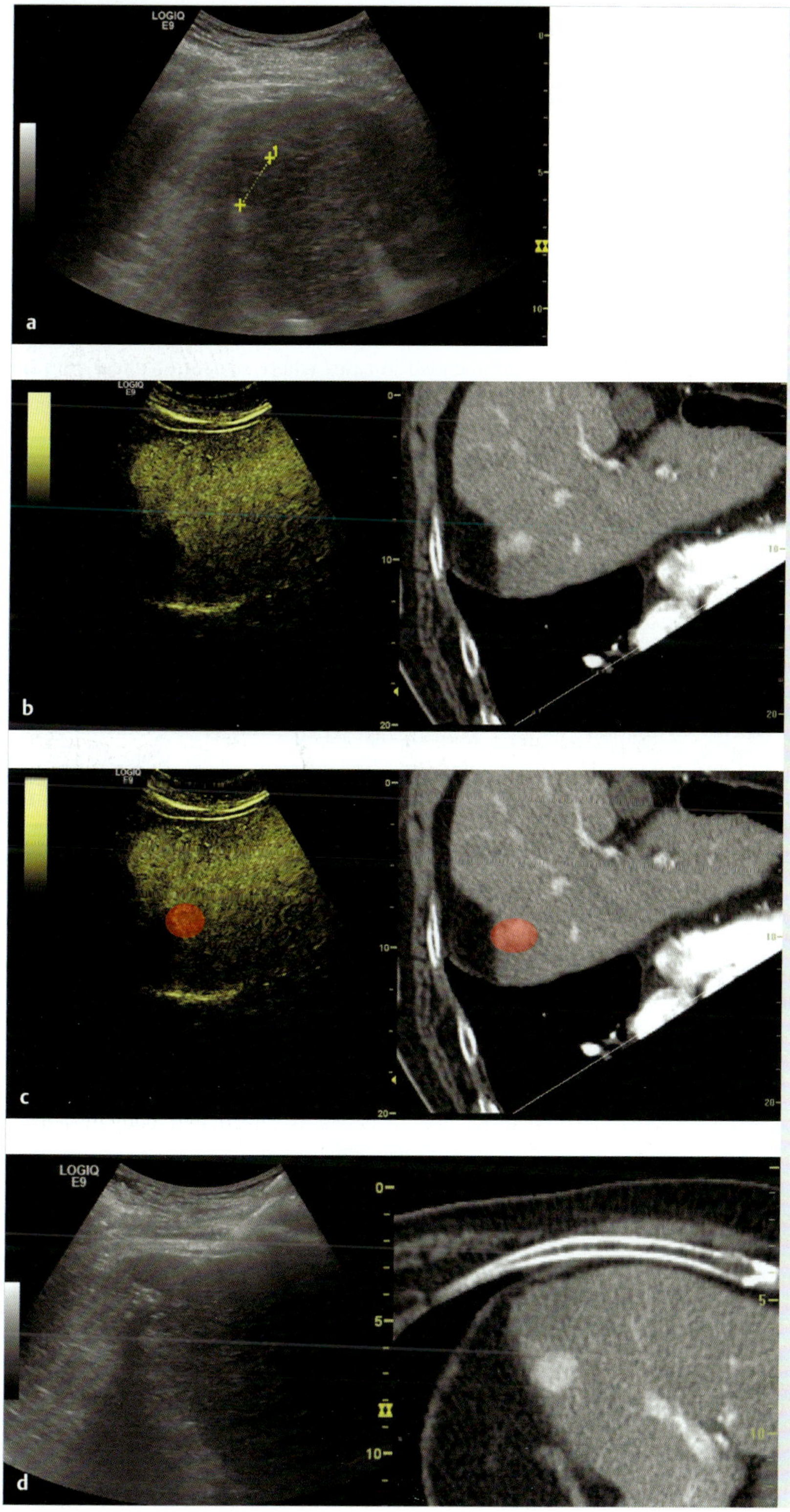

Fig. 32.2 Follow-up after ablation of a hepatocellular carcinoma.
a Nodular mass in close proximity to the ablation zone.
b, c Fusion imaging with CT and contrast-enhanced ultrasound.
d Fusion imaging-guided biopsy for histologic confirmation and repeat radiofrequency ablation.

focal lesions visible only by CT, MRI, or PET, the fusion of contrast-enhanced ultrasound with another modality will allow the perfusion characteristics of the lesion to be assessed while it is viewed from an identical perspective.

32.4 Fusion with Archived Ultrasound Volume Data

As well as CT and MRI data sets, pretherapeutic or preinterventional ultrasound volume data sets can be fused with current sonograms to assess the efficacy of a treatment or procedure.

Of course, this type of fusion is possible only if the initial data were acquired in a 3D ultrasound examination. This is necessary to ensure that a valid reference image corresponding to an arbitrary transducer position can be reconstructed during postinterventional follow-up.

32.5 Magnetic Field–Assisted Needle Tracking and Guidance

New microsensors 0.9 mm in diameter are opening up new possibilities in needle guidance based on the use of magnetic field–assisted tracking. When inserted temporarily into the lumen of a trocar system, the miniaturized sensor can detect the pulsating magnetic field from the transmitter, similarly to the sensors mounted on the ultrasound transducer. But the intraluminal sensor delivers signals different from those of the transducer-mounted sensors, depending on the distance and relative orientations of the trocar and transducer. From this difference the system can calculate the position of the trocar tip and the prospective needle path. Both are then superimposed onto the live ultrasound image and are visible even before the trocar is introduced into the body. This allows the operator to aim the trocar along the virtual target line while it is still extracorporeal and to introduce the trocar at any site desired. Thanks to the tracking system, the real-time position of the trocar tip can be seen throughout the procedure and there is less need to rely on echo return from the needle.

If a 3D scan is performed immediately before the intervention, aided by the tracking system, and the volume data are stored in memory, another interesting possibility arises: introducing the needle *next to* the active scan plane, rather than within it. Even though the needle track is outside the scan field of view, the needle position, prospective needle path and surrounding structures are still displayed on the screen. This is because a virtual sectional image can be extracted from the stored volume data based on the spatial information from the magnetic field sensors in the trocar and displayed side-by-side with the active sectional image. The active and virtual sectional images intersect at the target site, where the needle tip will also generate a primary echo in the live image, providing additional control of the tip position.

This technique, known as off-plane needle tracking, is recommended in cases where structures underlying the transducer face would hamper or prevent direct access.

32.6 Illustrative Images and Case Reports

32.6.1 Case Report 1

An 82-year-old man had undergone radiofrequency ablation of a hepatocellular carcinoma, and follow-up CT detected a recurrence. Subsequent abdominal ultrasound, performed first without contrast, revealed a nodular mass close to the ablation zone (▶ Fig. 32.2a). Fusion imaging with CT and contrast-enhanced ultrasound was then performed, and the two modalities correlated the finding (▶ Fig. 32.2b, c). Subsequent biopsy was guided by fusion imaging and provided histologic confirmation of the recurrence. Repeat radiofrequency ablation was performed successfully.

32.6.2 Case Report 2

A 76-year-old woman was undergoing treatment for an exacerbation of chronic obstructive lung disease. Routine ultrasound scans disclosed a renal mass 15 mm in diame-

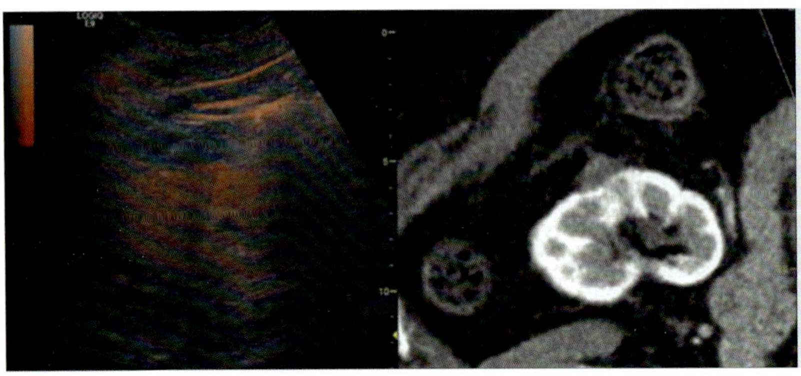

Fig. 32.3 Follow-up examination in a 76-year-old woman 3 days after radiofrequency ablation of a clear-cell renal cell carcinoma of the left kidney 15 mm in diameter. Because the patient had severe chronic obstructive lung disease, interventional treatment was performed.

ter. The indeterminate lesion was identified by core needle histology and was treated by radiofrequency ablation due to significant comorbidity (▶ Fig. 32.3). Contrast-enhanced ultrasound correlated with postoperative CT confirmed complete ablation of the tumor.

References

[1] Ewertsen C, Henriksen BM, Torp-Pedersen S, Bachmann Nielsen M. Characterization by biopsy or CEUS of liver lesions guided by image fusion between ultrasonography and CT, PET/CT or MRI. Ultraschall Med 2011; 32: 191–197

[2] Ewertsen C. Image fusion between ultrasonography and CT, MRI or PET/CT for image guidance and intervention – a theoretical and clinical study. Dan Med Bull 2010; 57: B4172

[3] Kaplan I, Oldenburg NE, Meskell P, Blake M, Church P, Holupka EJ. Real time MRI-ultrasound image guided stereotactic prostate biopsy. Magn Reson Imaging 2002; 20: 295–299

[4] Christensen AF, Nielsen BM, Engelholm SA. Three-dimensional endoluminal ultrasound-guided interstitial brachytherapy in patients with anal cancer. Acta Radiol 2008; 49: 132–137

[5] Cothren RM, Shekhar R, Tuzcu EM, Nissen SE, Cornhill JF, Vince DG. Three-dimensional reconstruction of the coronary artery wall by image fusion of intravascular ultrasound and bi-plane angiography. Int J Card Imaging 2000; 16: 69–85

[6] Fuller DB, Jin H, Koziol JA, Feng AC. CT-ultrasound fusion prostate brachytherapy: a dynamic dosimetry feedback and improvement method. A report of 54 consecutive cases. Brachytherapy 2005; 4: 207–216

[7] Porter BC, Rubens DJ, Strang JG, Smith J, Totterman S, Parker KJ. Three-dimensional registration and fusion of ultrasound and MRI using major vessels as fiducial markers. IEEE Trans Med Imaging 2001; 20: 324–329

[8] Penney GP, Blackall JM, Hamady MS, Sabharwal T, Adam A, Hawkes DJ. Registration of freehand 3D ultrasound and magnetic resonance liver images. Med Image Anal 2004; 8: 81–91

[9] Lindner D, Trantakis C, Renner C et al. Application of intraoperative 3D ultrasound during navigated tumor resection. Minim Invasive Neurosurg 2006; 49: 197–202

[10] Miller D, Heinze S, Tirakotai W et al. Is the image guidance of ultrasonography beneficial for neurosurgical routine? Surg Neurol 2007; 67: 579–587, discussion 587–588

[11] Wein W, Röper B, Navab N. Automatic registration and fusion of ultrasound with CT for radiotherapy. Med Image Comput Comput Assist Interv 2005; 8: 303–311

[12] Ewertsen C, Ellegaard K, Boesen M, Torp-Pedersen S, Bachmann Nielsen M. Comparison of two co-registration methods for real-time ultrasonography fused with MRI: a phantom study. Ultraschall Med 2010; 31: 296–301

33 Palliative Interventions and the Role of Ultrasonography in Palliative Care

D. Nuernberg

33.1 Content and Goals of Palliative Care

Palliative care is playing an increasingly important role in contemporary medicine. Given the fact that many cancers and other diseases are incurable or only partially curable, great importance is attached to the amelioration of suffering. The goal of palliative care is not to cure a disease or combat its causes but to relieve its symptoms. In the truest sense of the word, then, palliative care should wrap a "protective cloak" (Latin *pallium* = cloak or cover) around patients to provide comfort, to shield them from inappropriate procedures, and especially to relieve pain. In this sense, palliation includes all actions (medical, nursing, social, psychological) involved in the management of incurable diseases that shorten life expectancy. It is particularly important to relieve distressing physical symptoms such as pain, dyspnea, and eating difficulties. In some cases the requirements for symptom abatement must remain modest.[1–3] The main goals of palliative care are to:

- Prolong life
- Manage symptoms
- Address spiritual and psychosocial needs
- Provide palliative nursing care

On the basis of the WHO definition of 2002,[4] this concept has been expanded to include:

- Greater emphasis on the patient's **quality of life**
- The **earlier initiation of the palliative care**, which is started concurrently with therapies aimed at prolonging life

What is the specific role of ultrasonography in the palliative care setting ("palliative ultrasound")?[5]

1. Ultrasound is a valuable diagnostic tool in the detection of palliative conditions (palliative staging).
2. Ultrasound is a relatively low-cost means of monitoring palliative care patients and identifying situations that require palliative intervention.
3. A number of palliative interventions can be performed under ultrasound guidance.
4. These interventions can be performed not only as inpatient procedures but also in outpatient settings and at home.
5. Finally, ultrasound examinations can provide care and comfort for palliative patients until the end of life.

33.2 Ultrasound in Palliative Staging, Follow-Up, and Palliative Treatment Monitoring

The natural history of cancer is marked by a progression of typical stages. Ultrasound plays a major role in diagnosis, staging, and treatment monitoring and is the only follow-up imaging study that conforms to consensus guidelines for all tumor entities.[6]

A large percentage of oncologic diseases are incurable, however. The patient eventually enters a stage in which the disease (e.g., pancreatic cancer) is no longer curable and palliative treatment options become a priority concern.[7]

Except in cases of colorectal cancer, the detection of hepatic metastases means that the disease has reached a palliative stage. Ultrasound has high sensitivity (> 90%) in the detection of these lesions. It is considerably less sensitive in the detection of peritoneal carcinomatosis (approximately 50–60%). Ultrasound in a palliative treatment setting is useful for evaluating clinical progression and can accurately assess therapeutic response based on criteria such as the size of hepatic metastases or peritoneal fluid volume. Thus, ultrasound can contribute significantly to making the prognostic assessment that is so important for patients and their families. In cases where the primary intent of care is palliative, ultrasound should be used in subsequent follow-up examinations whenever possible, one goal being to economize on resources. One important goal of **palliative staging** is to spare the patient an unnecessary intervention, operation, or chemotherapy by demonstrating that the procedure will not benefit the patient and will only cause adverse side effects and raise false hopes.

In cases where primary cancer treatment has been successful, the patient is placed on **oncologic follow-up**. The goal of this follow-up is to achieve long-term remission through:

- The early detection and curative treatment of metastasis
- The detection and curative treatment of recurrent disease

Imaging follow-ups have these additional goals:

- The detection of a possible second tumor
- The evaluation of treatment response

Today, of course, general follow-up care is considered to have a more comprehensive scope in line with the

Table 33.1 Proven benefit of surgical treatment (or early detection with a different treatment option) in patients with hepatic metastases

Benefit has been documented for the detection or resection of hepatic metastases	Benefit has not been documented for the detection or resection of hepatic metastases
Colorectal cancer +	Stomach –
Lung – (+)	Breast –
NET (neuroendocrine tumor) (+)	Pancreas –
Lymphoma +	Bile ducts –
	Kidney –

principles of "caring medicine." But ultrasound follow-ups in the narrow sense are concerned mainly with the detection of hepatic metastases. What benefit does this hold for the affected patient? Strictly speaking, a benefit exists only if surgical resection of the metastases is still technically possible and would also provide a survival benefit for the patient (▶ Table 33.1).

When a disease is diagnosed as incurable during primary staging or later in its course, ultrasound also has a special role in **palliative treatment monitoring**. For many interventions ultrasound is a noninvasive, universally available, and cost-effective procedure that is ideal for monitoring and documenting response to palliative therapy.

Classic examples of palliative treatment monitoring are stent evaluation in patients with a malignant biliary obstruction, the assessment of ascites in peritoneal carcinomatosis, and evaluating pancreatic tumor response to chemotherapy. The guideline for palliative chemotherapy states that upper abdominal ultrasound is the modality of choice for evaluating tumor response during the course of palliative chemotherapy (▶ Fig. 33.1, ▶ Fig. 33.2 and ▶ Table 33.2).[7]

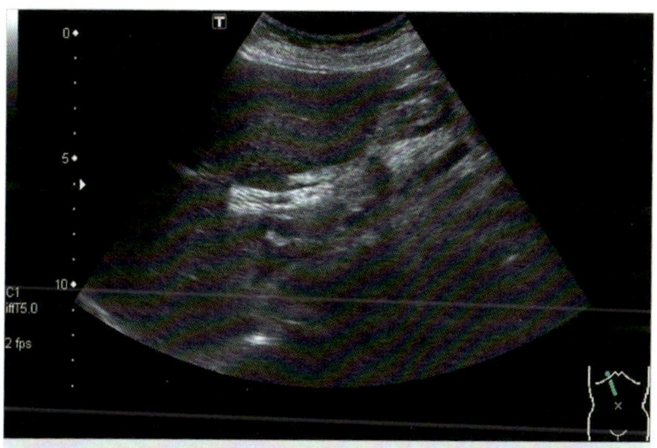

Fig. 33.1 Biliary stent monitoring. Ultrasound after metal stent placement in a patient with bile duct cancer excludes further obstruction of the proximal biliary tract. (Source: image courtesy of Dr. Albrecht Holle, University of Rostock, Germany.)

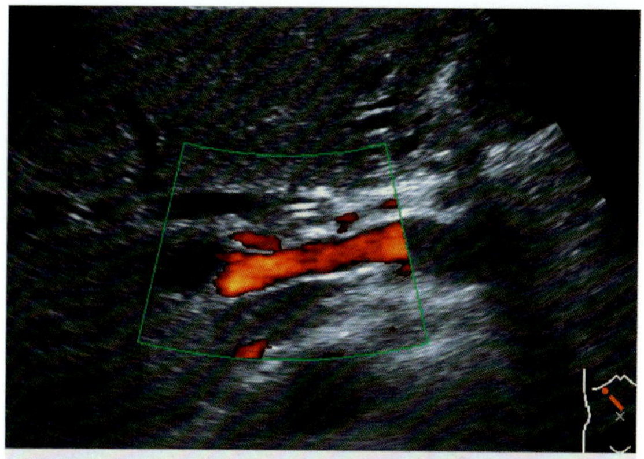

Fig. 33.2 Follow-up image after stenting and during palliative chemotherapy in a patient with pancreatic cancer.

33.3 Ultrasound-Guided Palliative Interventions

33.3.1 Palliative Diagnostic Interventions

Even when a palliative situation is suspected on the basis of clinical and imaging findings, diagnostic confirmation is often required. This is done to provide prognostic confirmation for the patient and physician and may also be important for instituting specific palliative oncologic treatment (chemotherapy or radiation).

Diagnostic Fine Needle Aspiration of Hepatic Metastases

If it is already evident before the intervention that curative treatment is no longer possible or is unlikely to be successful, it is essential to inform the patient about the goals of the diagnostic procedure. A primary goal is to furnish a histologic diagnosis that will show whether hepatic lesions actually originated from the known primary tumor or have a different etiology. It may also show a potential for successful chemotherapy in patients with multiple lesions.

Diagnostic Fine Needle Aspiration of Pancreatic Cancer

The guideline for the diagnosis and treatment of exocrine pancreatic cancer[7] states that biopsy confirmation is mandatory before any specific palliative treatment is performed. This is true regardless of whether the cancer is locally advanced, inoperable, or has already metastasized. The confirmation may be cytologic or histologic, the goal being to ensure that the proper treatment is matched to the disease. Tissue sampling by endosonographic biopsy

Table 33.2 Palliative ultrasound-guided interventions

Diagnostic/ therapeutic	Procedure	Indications, goals, comments	Chapter
Diagnostic	FNA pancreatic cancer[a]	Confirm diagnosis before palliative chemotherapy	12
	FNA HCC	HCC (> 5 cm) before TACE or chemotherapy; HCC (< 5 cm) before HiTT or PEIT	12, 18, 19
	FNA hepatic metastasis	Before ablative treatment (HiTT), before palliative chemotherapy	12, 18, 19
	FNA ascites	Before palliative chemotherapy or local treatment	13, 22
	FNA pleural effusion	Before palliative chemotherapy or pleurodesis	12, 24
	FNA lung cancer[a]	Before chemoradiation	12, 24
Therapeutic	PTCD[a]	Palliative biliary tract decompression in patients with bile duct carcinoma, liver cancer, or pancreatic cancer	20
	PEG	Impassable esophageal stricture due to esophageal cancer, for example	21
	Nephrostomy	Decompression in patients with a bladder tumor or pelvic tumor where retrograde catheterization cannot be performed	26
	Ascites therapy, paracentesis	Temporary decompression and local chemotherapy	13, 22
	Thoracentesis	Temporary decompression, possible induction of pleurodesis	12, 24
	Celiac plexus block[a]	Relieve the pain of pancreatic cancer	22
	Ablation of HCC	For HCC < 5 cm, 1–3 lesions	18, 19
	Ablation of hepatic metastasis	For metastasis < 5 cm, 1–3 lesions	18, 19
	Ablation of renal tumor	For tumors < 5 cm and general palliative settings (e.g., geriatric patients)	18, 19

Abbreviations: FNA, fine needle aspiration; HCC, hepatocellular carcinoma; HiTT, high-frequency induced thermotherapy; TACE, transarterial chemoembolization; PEIT, percutaneous ethanol injection therapy; PTCD, percutaneous transhepatic cholangiodrainage.
[a] EUS guidance is preferred in some cases.

is preferred as it eliminates the risk of needle tract seeding (see Chapter 9). But if the lesion is easily accessible percutaneously, a traditional percutaneous biopsy will provide roughly the same yield with less effort and at considerably lower cost.

Diagnostic Fine Needle Aspiration of Malignant Effusions

Ascites in a cancer patient should not always be interpreted as peritoneal carcinomatosis. It may result from coexisting heart failure or portal vein thrombosis, especially in patients with hepatic, pancreatic, or biliary tumors. It was noted in Chapter 13 that multiple needle aspirations are often necessary to make a diagnosis. It may be appropriate to proceed with laparoscopy if the procedure will have therapeutic implications. Similar considerations apply to pleural effusions (see Chapter 24).[8]

33.3.2 Specific Palliative Therapeutic Interventions

Classic examples of palliative therapeutic interventions include external drainage procedures in existing cavity systems such as percutaneous transhepatic cholangiodrainage (PTCD), palliative nephrostomy or gastrostomy, and paracentesis. This category also includes palliative tumor ablation therapy (radiofrequency ablation [RFA], high-frequency induced thermotherapy [HiTT], percutaneous ethanol injection therapy [PEIT]).

Palliative PTCD

(See Chapter 20.) If the obstructed biliary tract cannot be drained adequately through an internal approach via endoscopic retrograde cholangiography, it should be decompressed by external drainage or external–internal drainage. The main goal of this drainage is to prevent and control jaundice-related itching and to protect and sustain liver function by preventing cirrhosis due to biliary obstruction. The main indications for palliative PTCD are pancreatic cancer and bile duct cancer, as well as intra- and extrahepatic metastatic obstructions. Recurrent tumors of the stomach after a prior gastrectomy may also cause obstruction not accessible to internal drainage. The goal of an external procedure is always conversion to external–internal drainage or to internal drainage alone. This will succeed if the tumor stricture can be crossed with a wire and catheter under fluoroscopic control. With well-organized PTCD access, there should be no difficulty in flushing and changing the drain at regular intervals. The external insertion of a metal stent across the tumor stricture is occasionally recommended. Because this procedure has a high complication rate, it is important to assess its potential benefit for the individual patient (see Chapter 9). External drainage alone is highly unsatisfactory from a medical standpoint and is poorly tolerated by most patients.

Palliative Ultrasound-Guided Percutaneous Endoscopic Gastrostomy

The technique of insertion in ultrasound-guided percutaneous endoscopic gastrostomy is described in Chapter 21. This procedure is indicated whenever a tumor blocks endoscopic access to the stomach and it would be too risky to establish temporary access across the lesion. This situation is most commonly encountered in patients with very advanced esophageal cancer or infiltrating lung cancer. Ultrasound-guided PEG is less invasive than open surgical gastrostomy and thus provides a true alternative in palliative settings.

Ultrasound tracking is an effective alternative when transillumination is not available. Thus it helps to achieve a successful PEG placement in cases where endoscopic access is established but the site cannot be transilluminated. Ultrasound also has a role in diagnosing PEG-related complications. It can detect possible displacement of the retention plate as well as abscesses and inflammatory infiltration in the abdominal wall. Contrast-enhanced ultrasound is almost equivalent to fluoroscopy in its ability to detect leakage.

Palliative Paracentesis

(See Chapter 13.) One palliative treatment option is to decompress a malignant effusion by percutaneous needle aspiration or drainage. This procedure is straightforward and complications are rare even in outpatient settings. Usually it is of only temporary benefit, however. Relief of painful distension and dyspnea for 7 to 10 days is considered a good response that justifies repeating the procedure. Concomitant palliative chemotherapy or even local chemotherapy can significantly prolong the benefit of paracentesis.[8–11]

Palliative Tumor Ablation

The techniques and indications for the local ablative treatment of liver tumors were described fully in Chapter 19. The Berchtold HiTT electrode and other ablative treatments are mainly a palliative option. RFA and other ablation techniques are also used to treat metastases (especially from colorectal cancer) up to 5 cm in diameter. Their effectiveness can be accurately assessed by contrast-enhanced ultrasound (CEUS).

33.4 Portable Ultrasound in Specialized Ambulatory Palliative Care[12]

In 2009, a program was instituted in Germany to improve the outpatient care of palliative patients within the framework of “specialized ambulatory palliative care” (SAPV). The goals of this improved palliative care program for patients with incurable diseases are as follows:

- Provide **ambulatory medical care at home** for incurably ill patients during the last stage of life.
- **Preserve the quality of life.**
- **Avoid medically unnecessary interventions** and unnecessary hospital admissions.

Palliative care teams (PCTs) with qualified palliative care physicians, including hospital-based physicians, have been created that can bring portable ultrasound technology into the home. The use of small, portable ultrasound machines allows the palliative care physician not only to examine the patient at home but also to perform an intervention if necessary (▶ Fig. 33.3). This particularly applies to the palliative drainage of effusions (ascites, pleural effusion). This level of care can avoid hospital referrals along with unnecessary and stressful patient transfers.

33.5 Palliative Ultrasound in Caring Medicine

As a modern method of examination, ultrasound has a special role to play in an age of very brief doctor–patient contacts and anonymous medicine. Greiner[13,14] and others have noted that, by its very nature, diagnostic ultrasound creates an intimacy between examiner and patient that is rarely experienced today. It not only fosters a trusting atmosphere but it is also one of the last instances of direct, personal skin contact combined with conversation, information, and undivided care and concern.

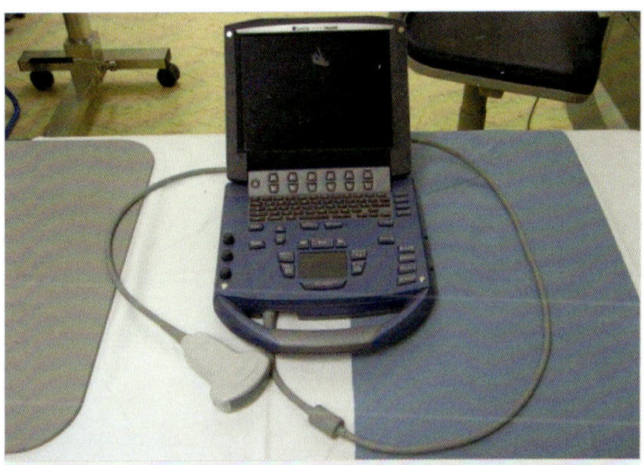

Fig. 33.3 A portable ultrasound machine is excellent for guiding palliative paracentesis in the home.

Patients in palliative care should undergo as few uncomfortable high-tech procedures as possible. There is here a natural conflict between medical technology and palliative care. Often doctors are confronted either with a determined refusal of high-tech medicine or the opposite extreme of patients placing high expectations on the seemingly boundless capabilities of 21st-century medical technology. A major challenge to palliative care physicians is to strike a balance between developing a caring attitude and a trusting atmosphere for physical examination ("touch medicine") and the often unrealistic hopes that are tied to each additional imaging procedure.

There is also "the dilemma of high-tech medicine," which often raises hopes that cannot be fulfilled and may result in alienation and a loss of trust (a growing discrepancy between hope and reality).[1,2] Clinical ultrasound is a very personal solution that offers a good compromise between necessary technology and caring human contact. Mathis[15] pointed out that the acceptance of diagnostic ultrasound remains high even in incurably sick patients who may reject other measures. This surely relates to the fact that ultrasound is a clinical tool in which the proximity of the human examiner and technological know-how together forge a close relationship between patient and examiner.

Given the palliative care applications described above, ultrasound represents an ideal clinical examination tool that combines high diagnostic efficiency with a potential for caring human contact. Palliative care focuses on the relief of suffering, and ultrasound is an ideal palliative instrument for aiding diagnosis and follow-up (monitoring), directing interventions, and providing human contact until the end of life. In this respect ultrasonography must be recognized as a true form of psychosocial support.

33.6 Conclusions

- Ultrasound imaging has numerous applications in palliative care.
- Palliative interventional procedures can relieve symptoms while causing minimal patient discomfort.
- Ultrasound can provide for caring human contact in palliative care.

References

[1] Aulbert E, Nauck F, Radbruch L. Lehrbuch der Palliativmedizin. 2nd ed. Stuttgart: Schattauer; 2007

[2] Huseboe S, Klaschik E. Palliativmedizin. 5th ed. Heidelberg: Springer; 2009

[3] Kloke M, Reckinger K, Kloke O. Grundwissen Palliativmedizin. Cologne: Deutscher Ärzteverlag; 2009

[4] World Health Organization. WHO Definition of Palliative Care. http://www.who.int/cancer/palliative/definition/en/2011

[5] Nürnberg D. Sonographie in der Palliativen Care. 2009 Ultrasound Tri-National Meeting, Salzburg. Ultraschall in Med 2009

[6] Schmiegel W, Pox C, Reinacher-Schick A et al. Federal Committee of Physicians and Health Insurers. S3 guidelines for colorectal carcinoma: results of an evidence-based consensus conference on February 6/7, 2004 and June 8/9, 2007 (for the topics IV, VI and VII). Z Gastroenterol 2010; 48: 65–136

[7] Adler G, Seufferlein T, Bischoff SC et al. S3-Guidelines "Exocrine pancreatic cancer" 2007 [Article in German]. Z Gastroenterol 2007; 45: 487–523

[8] Nürnberg D. Peritonealraum. In: Schmidt G, Greiner L, Nürnberg D, eds. Sonografische Differenzialdiagnose. Stuttgart: Thieme; 2010

[9] Armstrong DK, Bundy B, Wenzel L et al. Gynecologic Oncology Group. Intraperitoneal cisplatin and paclitaxel in ovarian cancer. N Engl J Med 2006; 354: 34–43

[10] Glockzin G, Ghali N, Lang SA, Agha A, Schlitt HJ, Piso P. Peritoneal carcinomatosis. Surgical treatment, including hyperthermal intraperitoneal chemotherapy [Article in German]. Chirurg 2007; 78: 1100,1102–1106,1108–1110

[11] Ross GJ, Kessler HB, Clair MR, Gatenby RA, Hartz WH, Ross LV. Sonographically guided paracentesis for palliation of symptomatic malignant ascites. AJR Am J Roentgenol 1989; 153: 1309–1311

[12] Voltz R. Palliativmedizin – Eine Disziplin für den "ganzen Menschen." Deutsches Ärzteblatt 2008; 105: A80–A82

[13] Greiner L. Sono-psychology. Ultraschall Med 2009; 30: 94–95

[14] Greiner L. Sono-Psychology. EFSUMB European Course Book. EFSUMB; 2010: http://www.efsumb.org/ecb/ecb-ch021-sonopsychology.pdf

[15] Mathis G, Hackspiel S, Gehmacher O. Was empfinden Palliativpatienten bei der bettseitigen Sonografie? Ultraschall Med 2007; 28: DOI:10.1055/s-2007-989104

Index

Note: Page numbers set bold or italic indicate headings or figures, respectively.

1

1-deamino-8-D-arginine vasopressin (DDAVP), *see* desmopressin
16S rDNA assay 71

A

abdominal compartment syndrome 21, **153**
abdominal diagnostic interventions **120**
abdominal fluid collections
- emergency interventions **332**
- localized **133**
- paracentesis **128**
- predilection sites *128*, **128**
- rare **131**

ablative procedures, local, *see* local ablative procedures
abscess drainage 20, 23, **102**, **119**, **144**
- *See also* individual abscesses
- abscess localization **148**
- assistants **148**
- biliary tract communication 149, *150*
- catheter drainage *151*, 152, **152**
- catheter insertion 149
- catheter placement **149**, *150*
- combined procedures **153**
- compartment syndrome **153**
- complications **102**, **158**
- contraindications **147**
- devices **146**
- drain displacement 159
- drain removal **154**
- historical considerations **144**
- imaging modality selection **144**
- indications **147**
- irrigation **154**, **159**
- local anesthesia **148**
- multiple abscesses **153**
- needle aspiration 149, **151**
- needle insertion, initial *149*, **149**
- patient preparation **147**
- postprocedure care **154**
- preparation **148**
- recurrence rate 144
- skin preparation **148**
- specific diseases **154**
- specimen processing **154**
- suture fixation *153*, **153**
- table setup *148*
- technique **148**
- treatment options **148**

abscess(es) **80**, 145, *145*
- *See also* individual abscesses
- diagnosis **80**
- drainage, *see* abscess drainage
- etiology **144**
- pathogenesis 144
- treatment **80**

access needles, endosonography 226, 228, *229*
access routes, as relative risk **94**
accessories **29**, 111, *111*
- decontamination **85**
- endoscopic ultrasound 225

accessory spleen 257
acquired hemostatic disorders **91**
activated partial thromboplastin time (aPTT) 22
active electrode, RFA 189, *189*, 192
acute thyroiditis 288, *290*
acute viral hepatitis 120
adhesions 239, 244
ADP-receptor antagonists 90
adrenal biopsy **100**, *125*, **125**
adrenal metastasis 125, *125*
Aggrastat (tirofiban) 36
air-drying artifacts 52, *52*
Aixstent appliances 232
albendazole *170*, 174, 176
alcohol-induced hepatitis 121
alpha fetoprotein (AFP) 182
alpha1-antitrypsin deficiency 120–121
alveolar echinococcosis 168–169, *170*
ambulatory procedures **38**
amebiasis **156**
amebic liver abscess **78**, **156**, *160*
- causes 77
- clinical features **156**
- diagnosis **78**, **156**
- drainage 78
- sonographic features 145
- treatment **78**, **156**

American Society of Anesthesiologists (ASA) classification 35, 114
amniocentesis 2, *2*, *8*, 138
ampicillin 77, 80
Amsterdam stents 230–231
amyloidosis 256
analgesia 35, **35**
- monitoring 36

anaphylactic reaction, PAIR-induced **177**
anaplastic thyroid carcinoma 289
anchor systems *25*, **25**, *26*
angiography, EUS-guided 248
anisotropy 317
antibiotic prophylaxis
- EUS-guided cholangiodrainage 244
- interventional endosonography 234
- liver tumor radiofrequency ablation **187**
- percutaneous sonographic gastrostomy **220**
- peripancreatic fluid collection drainage 240
- prostate biopsy 281
- transrectal prostatic biopsy 93

antibiotics, *see* individual drugs
- for irrigation, abscess drainage 154
- pyogenic liver abscess 155

anticoagulant therapy
- interruption/discontinuation **36**, 89–90, **90**
- pseudoaneurysms and 345
- regional anesthesia contraindication **315**
- resumption 91
- reversal **90**

antiplatelet therapy
- as contraindication 94, **94**
- discontinuation/interruption 89, **90**, 250, 263, 274

antisepsis
- emergency interventions **332**
- hands, *see* hand antisepsis
- microbiological testing 68
- skin preparation 68, 84
- thyroid biopsy **292**

antithrombotic medication 316
appendicitis, abscess drainage **155**
arterial cannulation 337, *338*
arteriovenous fistula *97*, 99, 278, 341
ascites **79**
- benign vs. malignant 131, 133, *133*
- cancer patients 366
- cirrhosis **130**
- diagnosis 79
- differential diagnosis 129, **129**
- emergency interventions 332
- exudative **129**
- hemoperitoneum 130, *131*
- local ablative procedures contraindication 180
- localized fluid collection vs. **133**
- noninfectious causes 79
- pancreatitis **131**
- paracentesis indications **129**
- pathogenesis **129**
- PTCD contraindication 199
- ruptured cysts **132**
- septic (pyogenic) abscess **157**
- ultrasound contrast agents use **355**
- ultrasound morphology 129, *129*, 130, *130*

aspiration biopsy, history 2
aspiration needles, EUS 227, *228*
aspirin 36, 90, 250, 316
assistance/assisting personnel **109**
- diagnostic ultrasound **110**
- duties **109**
- patient care responsibilities 110
- principles **109**

atypical mycobacteria 75, 77
auramine stain **70**, *71*
autoimmune hepatitis 120–121
Autovac biopsy system **142**, 263, *263*
axillary brachial plexus 321, *322*
axillary brachial plexus block **321**, *322*, 327

B

B-cell lymphomas 46
B-mode scanning, history 3
bacterial liver abscess **77**
balloon dilators **229**, *230*, **241**, 244
basket-tipped catheters 28, *29*
bedside ultrasound 331
benzimidazoles 174
benzodiazepine antagonists 35–36
benzodiazepines 35
beta blockers 301
Bezold–Jarish reflex 318
bile leakage **132**, **135**, *136*, 158
biliary disease **155**
biliary drains 199
biliary-cutaneous fistula creation 206
biliomas 122
Biomol biopsy system **143**
BioPince biopsy system 18, **142**, 263, *263*, 269
biopsy, *see* individual procedures/techniques
- chest, indications 261
- clinical applications 7
- compound scanners 4, *5*
- for pathology/cytology **40**
- materials/equipment **37**, 110–111, *111*
- multiple tissue sampling 16
- needles, *see* needle(s)
- principles **13**
- procedure types **40**
- technical evolution **4**
- techniques **13**, *14*
-- historical aspects 2, 13

biopsy guns 6, 143, 263, *263*, 276
biopsy transducers *4*, *14*, **14**, *140*
- advantages/disadvantages 14
- evolution 4
- frequency range 15
- long needle path length 138
- musculoskeletal interventions 305
- needle guide 4, *6*
- paracentesis 133
- percutaneous renal biopsy *275*, 276
- sector scanner adapter 4, *7*
- thoracic interventions 261
- thyroid biopsy 290

- transrectal ultrasonography of the prostate 280
- ultrasound-guided amniocentesis 2, *2*

bipolar radiofrequency ablation 189
bladder tamponade 99
bleeding complications 9, 22, **87**
- abscess drainage 158
- clinical significance **87**
- detection 95, *96*
- diathermy devices 233
- EUS-guided biopsies 237, 250
- incidence **87**
- local ablative procedures 182
- management 95
- musculoskeletal interventions 312
- needle tract, flow along 95, *96*
- percutaneous nephrostomy 282, 284
- percutaneous transhepatic cholangiodrainage 208
- peripancreatic fluid collection drainage 239, 242
- postinterventional care 95
- prevention **92**
- radiofrequency ablation **192**, 193
- renal biopsy 277
- risk predictors **87**

blind biopsy 13
blood artifacts 52, *53*
blood culture systems 69
bnx needle exchange system 226
Bosniak type III indeterminate cystic mass 165–166
brachial plexus blocks **318**
breast cancer **89**
Budd–Chiari syndrome 120–121
Burkitt lymphoma 46

C

capillary hemangiomas 255
caps (hair coverings) 83
carbon-fiber-reinforced plastic needles 15
cardiac pacemakers 187
cardiology 7
carpal tunnel syndrome *311*
catheters, *see* drainage catheters
cavernous hemangiomas 255
cefazolin 78, 80
cefotaxime 80
ceftriaxone 79–81, 155
cefuroxime 78–81
celiac ganglia 247, *247*
celiac plexus blockade (CPB) **246**
- complications 247, **247**, 249
- indications/treatment goals **246**
- materials **247**
- postinterventional care **247**
- results assessment **247**, 249
- technique **247**, *248*

celiac plexus neurolysis (CPN) **246**
- complications 249
- indications **246**
- materials **247**
- postinterventional care **247**
- results assessment **247**, 249
- technique **247**, *248*

cell blocks **54**, 227
cell counts, ascites 79
CelonPOWER system 191, *191*, **191**
- applicator positioning **191**, 192
- protective medium injection 191, *191*
- resistance-controlled automatic power 191
- RFA technique **192**
- track ablation **192**

central venous catheterization
- blind needle insertion 335
- landmark technique 335, *336*
- needle visualization *337*
- procedure **336**, *337*

centrocyte-like cells 46
cephalosporins 155
chest wall 260, *260*
- fluid collections 264

chest wall lesions **264**
- biopsy 264, *265*

Chiba needle 16, *142*
- abscess drainage 151, *152*
- biopsy technique *18*, *141*, **142**
- holder 142, *142*
- liver cyst aspiration 164

chloroquine phosphate 78, 157
cholangiocellular carcinoma (CCC) 121
cholecystitis **102**
cholecystotomy **103**
cholesterol stones litholysis 159
cholinesterase 182
Christmas tree (Tannenbaum) stents 230
chyloperitoneum **132**
ciprofloxacin 77
cirrhosis 121–122, **130**, **134**
clarithromycin 78
clavulanic acid 77, 80
clopidogrel 36, 89–90
coagulation testing **21**, **36**, 89, 95, 263
coagulopathies **93**, 94, **157**, **315**
coarse needles 15
cold thyroid nodules 297
College of American Pathologists cytopathology reporting guidelines 63
color Doppler ultrasound (CDU)
- femoral artery puncture 338
- pseudoaneurysms 341, *341*
- thoracic tumors 262, *262*
- thyroid biopsy 290, *291*
- vascular interventions 339, **339**, *340*

colorectal cancer 42
colorectal liver metastases **185**
combined histologic-cytologic analysis 138–139
complications **86**
- *See also* individual complications, individual procedures
- biopsy number and **86**
- detection **95**, *96*
- examiner experience and **86**
- frequent **86**
- management **95**
- organ-specific 86
- prevention **89**
-- patient selection **89**
-- risk assessment **89**
-- risk factor modification **90**
- rates **86**
- risk factors **86**
- risk reduction techniques **92**
- specific **89**
- specific biopsy sites **95**
- specific interventions **101**
- treatment **95**

compound scanners 4, *5*
compression therapy, pseudoaneurysms 341, 347
computed tomography (CT)
- abscess drainage **146**
- cystic echinococcosis **173**
- liver tumors, local ablative procedures **186**
- ultrasound fusion **359**

ComVi stent **212**
congenital hemostatic disorders **92**
consent forms **32**, 33
consumption coagulopathy (disseminated intravascular coagulation) 157
contraindications **93**, 94
- *See also* individual procedures
- absolute 94
- relative 94–95
- specific biopsy sites **95**
- specific interventions **101**

contrast agents, *see* ultrasound contrast agents (UCAs)
contrast allergy 200
contrast-enhanced low MI endoscopic ultrasound (CELMIEUS) 357
contrast-enhanced ultrasound (CEUS)
- echinococcosis **172**
- fusion imaging 361
- liver biopsy guidance 122
- percutaneous ethanol injection, thyroid 290, 299, *299*
- postinterventional bleeding detection 95, *98*
- RFA efficacy assessment 193, *194*
- thoracic tumors 262, *262*
- tubal patency assessment **355**

core needle biopsy **138**
- abdomen **138**
- bleeding complications 87
- chest wall lesions 264
- historical background **138**
- local anesthesia 141
- lymph node metastasis 45
- needle path length **138**
- needle path obstructions **139**
- needle type used **138**, **141**
- sedation 141
- subpleural lung lesions 266, *268*
- techniques **138**
- thyroid **289**, 290–291, **293**, *295*

core needles **138**
coronary heart disease 180, 182
covered metal stents 231, *231*
covering, protective **82**
CRE balloon dilators *230*
CRE wire-guided balloon dilation catheter 230
crush artifacts 52, *52*
culture techniques **71**
CUP syndrome 121
curved-array transducers 275, *275*
cutting biopsy 6, **142**
cutting biopsy needles **18**, 262, 291, 293
cyst(s)
- drainage **102**
- echinococcosis 169
- kidney, *see* renal cysts
- liver, *see* liver cysts
- thyroid, *see* thyroid cysts

cystic echinococcosis
- calcification 172, *175*
- clinical manifestations 169
- complications 169
- cyst rupture 169
- diagnosis 168
- epidemiology 168, *168*
- treatment **173**, 175
- WHO classification, *see* WHO classification

cystic renal masses 165
Cysto-Gastro Set 232
Cystofix system 29, *29*
cystotomes 228, **232**, *233*, **241**
cytocentrifugation (Cytospin) *50*, **50**
- solid lesion aspirates **54**

cytochemistry 56, 59
cytology **40**
- accessories *111*
- histology vs. 5, **40**
- stains 59

Cytospin, *see* cytocentrifugation

D

decompensated right heart failure **130**
dehydroemetine 78, 157
dentures 111, *112*
desmopressin
- acquired hemostatic disorders 91
- postinterventional bleeding 95
- pre-renal biopsy 274

diagnostic interventions, *see* individual interventions
- abdominal **120**
- assistance **110**
- bleeding risk predictors 87
- endosonography **236**
- interventional risk **86**
- liver, indications **120**
- palliative **365**
- thoracic **120**

diagnostic microbiology **68**

diagnostic paracentesis **128**
– laboratory tests 134, **134**
– needles 136
diathermy devices 228, *232*, **232**
– gas generation 232
– wire guidance 232
diathermy rings 228, 233, **241**
diffuse large cell B-cell lymphomas (DLCL) 46
diffuse liver diseases 120, **120**
diffuse peritoneal adenomucinosis (DPAM) 133, *133*
digital flexor tendon injections *311*
dilators **27**
– EUS-guided cholangiodrainage 244
– fixed-diameter **228**, *230*
– interventional endosonography **228**, *230*
– materials 27
– percutaneous transhepatic cholangiodrainage 200, **206**
– peripancreatic fluid collection drainage **241**
– selection criteria 27
diloxanide furoate 78, 156–157
direct puncture, *see* trocar technique
Disoprivan, *see* propofol
disposable probe covers **83**
disseminated intravascular coagulation (consumption coagulopathy) 157
diuretics therapy 134
diverticulitis 155
documentation **33**, 225
dog tapeworm, *see* Echinococcus granulosus
double bubble sign 320
double line sign 171 172, *174*
double-pigtail stents 230, *231*
drain placement **103**, *112*
– assessment 22
drainage catheters **27**, *29*
– abscess drainage *146*, **146**
–– catheter properties **147**
–– catheter size **146**
–– trocar vs. Seldinger technique **146**
– coatings 28
– drainage hole arrangement 28
– liver cysts, percutaneous sclerotherapy 164
– materials 27
– paracentesis 136, *136*
– percutaneous transhepatic cholangiodrainage 200
– radiographic images, visibility on 28
– single- vs. multilumen 27
– thoracic interventions 263, *264*
drainage procedures **102**
– *See also* individual procedures
– chest 261
drainage systems **29**
drug-eluting stents (DES) 90
drying artifacts 55
duodenal perforation 249
dysontogenetic cysts, spleen 255

E

echinococcosis **168**
– alveolar 168–169, *170*
– calcifications 173
– classification systems 169
–– functional **171**
–– morphologic **171**
–– WHO, *see* WHO classification
– clinical manifestations **169**
– complications 169
– diagnosis **169**
–– pitfalls **173**
– epidemiology **168**
– honeycomb/rosette pattern 171–172
– imaging studies **169**
– interventional treatment **168**
– laboratory parameters **169**
– local ablative procedures **175**
– serology **169**
– staging **169**
– transitional stage 171
– treatment **173**, 175
Echinococcus 70, 157, 168, **168**
Echinococcus granulosus 168, **168**
– worldwide distribution 168, *168*
Echinococcus multilocularis (fox tapeworm) 168, **169**, *170*
echocardiography, pericardial fluid 334, *334*
EchoTip ultra EUS aspiration needle *228*
elastography 45
elderly patients 159, 301
ELISA, echinococcosis 169
embolization coils 248
embryonal tumors 42
emergency interventions **330**
– antisepsis **332**
– complications **332**
– contraindications **331**
– indications **330**
– materials/equipment 331, **331**
– percutaneous interventions and 330
– problems 332, **332**
– ultrasound for control purposes 331
– ultrasound technology **331**
emetine 78, 157
empyema **333**
– drainage 333, *334*
– fibrinolytic agent instillation 333
– rupture 132
– treatment 333
end-cutting needles **19**
endobronchial ultrasound-guided transbronchial needle aspiration (EBUS-TBNA) **101**
endocystectomy 174
endometrial hyperplasia 42
endorectal ultrasound 356
endoscopes **238**
endoscopic biopsy **40**
endoscopic retrograde cholangiography (ERC) **177**, 198, **356**
endoscopic retrograde cholangiopancreatography (ERCP) 121, 198, 206
endoscopic ultrasound-guided biopsy
– accidental sheath perforation 235, *235*
– advantages 224
– complications risk **237**
– contraindications **238**
– indications **234**
– specimen processing **235**, *236*
– suction **235**
– supplementary techniques **234**
– techniques **235**
endoscopic ultrasound-guided celiac plexus block (EUS-CPB) 102
endoscopic ultrasound-guided celiac plexus neurolysis (EUS-CPN) 102, 224
endoscopic ultrasound-guided cholangiodrainage (EUS-CD) 198, **243**, *245*
– access/drainage route 243
– antibiotic prophylaxis 244
– as rendezvous procedure 243
– complication rates 102
– complications 102, **246**, 249
– equipment **244**
– indications **244**
– intrahepatic bile duct puncture 244
– mini-rendezvous version 244
– palliative indications 244
– postinterventional care **246**
– preparation **244**
– results assessment **246**
– success rate 249
– technique **244**
– tract dilation 244
– treatment goals **244**
endoscopic ultrasound-guided drainage 224, 234
endoscopic ultrasound-guided fine needle aspiration (EUS-FNA) **101**
– aspiration 49
– benign pancreatic lesions 250
– complications **101**, 249–250
– contraindications **101**
– diagnostic yield-affecting factors 237
– false-positive rates 64
– gastrointestinal indications 236
– historical aspects 224
– impact of 224
– lesions sampled 237
– suction 235
endoscopic ultrasound-guided intravascular injection 345, *347–348*
endoscopic ultrasound-guided therapeutic interventions 238, **238**
– clinical trials 238
– complications **102**, 249, **249**
– contraindications **239**
– success rates 249
endoscopic ultrasound-guided transmural necrosectomy 249
endoscopic ultrasound-guided Trucut biopsy (EUS-TCB) 99, **101**
endoscopic ultrasound-guided tumor ablation with alcohol **247**
endoscopy unit **224**
endoscopy, diagnostic without EUS-FNA 249
endosonographic guidance 93
endosonographically guided drainage of the pancreatic duct (EUS-PD) **246**
– complications 102, **246**, 249
– indications **246**
– technique **246**
endosonographically guided vascular interventions **248**, **345**
– advantages/disadvantages **348**
– complications **248**, **348**
– contraindications **348**
– indications **248**, **345**
– materials **248**, **347**
– postprocedure care **248**, **348**
– results assessment **248**, **348**
– technique **248**
– treatment goals **248**, **345**
endosonography, interventional, *see* interventional endosonography
endovaginal ultrasound 356
endovascular therapies **337**
– materials **339**
– procedure **339**, *340*
Entamoeba histolytica 156
enterography *356*, **356**
epithelial neoplasms 42, 44, 60
equipment **13**, **35**
esophageal perforation 249
esophageal stricture 223
ethambutol 77
ethanol
– percutaneous injection, *see* percutaneous ethanol injection (PEI)
– percutaneous sclerotherapy 164, 166
evacuation procedures, thyroid 296, **296**
examination rooms **38**
examiner experience, complications and **86**
excisional biopsy **40**
extravascular contrast-enhanced ultrasound (EVCEUS) 336, 354
exudate, intra-abdominal **129**, *130*

F

false aneurysms, *see* pseudoaneurysms
febrile reaction, PAIR-induced **177**
female infertility tests 355
femoral artery puncture 337
femoral nerve block **323**, *324*, 327

femoropopliteal angioplasties, CDU-guided 339
fibrinolytic agents 333
fine needle aspiration biopsy (FNAB) 40, **49**, **138**
- abdomen **138**
- air drying 54–55, **55**
- ancillary tests **56**, *59*
- aspiration **49**
- chest wall lesions 264, *266*
- clinical data **63**
- cytologic diagnosis, final **63**
- cytomorphologic evaluation **58**
- cytopathology reporting **63**, 64
- diagnostic certainty **63**
- EUS-guided, *see* endoscopic ultrasound-guided fine needle aspiration (EUS-FNA)
- false-positive rates 64
- fixation **55**
- hepatic metastases **365**
- historical background 49, **138**
- interpretive errors 64
- local anesthesia 141
- lymph node metastases 126
- malignant effusions **366**
- needle movement **49**
- needle pass number 62–63
- needle path length **138**
- needle path obstructions **139**
- needle type used **138**
- pancreatic lesions 7, **365**
- requisition form data 63
- ROSE, *see* Rapid On-Site Evaluation (ROSE)
- sampling errors 40, 64
- sedation 141
- solid lesion aspirates **50**
-- cell blocks **54**
-- cytocentrifugation **54**
-- labeling **52**
-- material expulsion onto slide *51*, **51**
-- preparation errors **52**, *53*
-- pull-apart technique *51*, 52
-- smearing technique *51–52*
- specimen collection **49**
- specimen preparation **49**
-- centrifuging effusions **49**
-- fluid aspirates **49**
- spleen 255
- staining **55**
- subpleural lung lesions 266, *268*
- synonyms 40
- techniques **138**
-- specific needle types **141**
- thin-layer preparations 54, **54**
- thyroid **288**, **292**, *295*
- wet fixation 54–55, **55**, *56–57*
- working without ROSE **63**
fine needle aspiration cytology (FNAC), *see* fine needle aspiration biopsy (FNAB)
fine needles 15, **138**
finger interventions **309**
fistulotomes 233
flexor tendon tenosynovitis **309**, *311*
flip technique 52
flucloxacillin 80–81
fluconazole 80–81
fluid collections
- abdominal, *see* abdominal fluid collections
- chest wall 264
- nonpancreatic, treatment **242**
- peripancreatic, drainage, *see* peripancreatic fluid collections drainage
fluid color sign *261*, 264
flumazenil 36
fluorescence in situ hybridization (FISH) 58
focal liver lesion biopsy 16, **121**
- benign lesions **121**
- benign/malignant differentiation *122*
- liquid lesions **122**
- malignant lesions **121**
focal nodular hyperplasia (FNH) 121
focal renal lesions 124, *124*
focused assessment with sonography for trauma (FAST) 110, 330
follicular lymphomas 46
foreign language speakers 34
fox tapeworm (Echinococcus multilocularis) 168, **169**, *170*
Franseen needle 19, **142**
freehand biopsy technique **13**, 14, *14*, 138, *139*
Freka Pexact system 26, 215
fresh frozen plasma (FFP) 91
Frimberger drain **206**
funnel adapters 29
fusion imaging **359**, *360*

G

gallbladder drainage **159**
gallbladder hydrops rupture 132
gastrointestinal bleeding, nonvariceal 345, *348*
gastrointestinal hollow organs biopsy **100**
gastrointestinal non-Hodgkin lymphoma 46
gastrointestinal perforation **132**
gastrointestinal tumors 126
gastropexy 219, *219*, **220**, *221*
gastropexy systems 220, *221*
germ cell tumors 42, 44
German Societies for Pathology and Cytology Standardized Reporting in Extragenital Cytology 63–64
Gharbi cyst classification 171
Gianturco stent **210**
Giovannini set *232*, 240
glenohumeral joint interventions **307**, *310*
gloves, sterile 82
glucagon 220
glycogen storage diseases 120–121
goiter 290
gouty arthritis 81
gowns 82
Gram stain **69**, 70, *70–71*
Gram-negative pathogens 71
Gram-positive pathogens 71
gray-scale technology, history 3
guidewires **26**
- design 26, *27*
- diameters 26
- interventional endosonography **227**, *229*, **239**, 244, 246
- materials 26
- percutaneous sonographic gastrostomy **220**
- peripancreatic fluid collection drainage **240**
- PTCD 26, 200, 205, *205–206*
- selection 27
- surface coating 26
- tip configuration 26

H

hair coverings (caps) 83
hair removal 84
hand antisepsis **83**
- hygienic 83, 110
- surgical (surgical hand scrub) 83
hand interventions **309**
Hashimoto thyroiditis 288, *290*
heart failure, transudates **130**
hemangiomas 94, 121, 255
hematomas
- perirenal 95, 97, 99, 277
- subcapsular *97*
- thyroid biopsy complication 290
hematopoietic neoplasms 42, 44
hematoxylin and eosin (H&E) stain 55, *56–58*
- air-dried smears *53*, 55, *56*, *58*
hematuria *97*, 99
hemochromatosis 120–121
hemoperitoneum **130**, *131*, 332
hemorrhages, *see* bleeding complications
hemostasis, EUS-guided 248, 347
hemothorax *333*, **333**
heparin bridging **91**
hepatic adenoma 121
hepatic metastases
- diagnostic interventions **121**, *122*, **365**
- early detection benefits 364
- needle tract seeding **88**
- palliative staging 364
- prognosis 364
- surgical resection 364–365
hepatic porphyria 120–121
hepatitis, chronic 120–121
hepatocellular carcinoma (HCC)
- biopsy indications 122, *122*
- cirrhotic liver 122
- fusion imaging *361*, 362
- histologic confirmation **180**
- local ablative procedures 179, **180**
- needle tract seeding 88, **88**
- prognostic factors **180**
- recurrence 89
- treatment options 185
hepatosplenic candidiasis 255
hip joint interventions **307**, *308*, 313
histology **41**
- accessories 111, *111*
- classification (typing) **41**
- cytology vs. **40**
- error/misinterpretation sources **40**, 41
- grading 41
Hodgkin lymphoma 47
hormone growth factor receptor analysis **47**
Horner syndrome 318
human thrombin solution injection 95, *96*
hybrid wire 227
hydatid disease, *see* echinococcosis
hydatid sand 171
hydrodissection 92
hydronephrosis *97*, 99
hydrothorax 355
hydroxyethyl starch (HES) 334, *335*
hygiene management **82**
hyperthermic intraperitoneal chemotherapy (HIPEC) 135
hyperthyroidism exacerbation 301
hypoalbuminemia **130**
hysterosalpingo-contrast sonography (HyCoSy) 355

I

immunocytochemical markers 57, 60
implied consent **33**
in-plane technique, needle insertion **316**, *317*
incidentaloma 125
incisional biopsy **40**
indirect hemagglutination antibody test (IHAT) 169
infections **68**
- iatrogenic, musculoskeletal interventions 312
- necrotic tumor components **158**
- postinterventional **88**
- prevention **93**
- puncture site **316**
informed consent **32**
- *See also* individual procedures
- delegating **33**
- disclosure means **32**
- discussion **32**, **33**, 110, *110*
- documentation **33**
- emergencies 33
- indications **32**
- information disclosed **32**
- patients lacking capacity to consent **33**
- procedure explanation **32**
- process timing **33**
- risks/complications **32**

– special situations **33**
– waiving **34**
infraclavicular brachial plexus block **320**, *321*, 327
interferon gamma release test 77
internal jugular vein catheterization 335–336, *336*
international normalized ratio (INR) 87, 90
interscalene brachial plexus block **318**, *319*, 327
interventional endosonography **113**, **224**
– *See also* individual procedures
– antibiotic prophylaxis 234
– assistance **113**
– biopsy technique **235**
– complications **249**, 251
– cost-benefit analysis **224**
– diagnostic interventions **236**
– diagnostic yield-affecting factors 237
– established systems **225**
– historical aspects **224**
– interventional ultrasound and 10
– materials/equipment **224**, *225–226*
– medications **234**
– needle insertion rules **234**
– orientation **234**
– pancreatic biopsy 123
– patient monitoring 115
– patient positioning 234
– postinterventional care **250**
– procedure **234**
– sedation **234**
– specimen processing *236*
– techniques **225**
– therapeutic interventions **238**
interventional procedures **13**
– historical aspects **13**
interventional risk **86**
– factors influencing **86**
– target site and **86**
interventional urology **280**
intra-abdominal abscesses
– causative organisms 80
– drainage 10, 102, **333**
– treatment 80
– unknown cause 158
intra-abdominal fluid, *see* abdominal fluid collections
intraepithelial neoplasia 42
intraperitoneal chemotherapy **135**, 136
intraperitoneal hemorrhage *96*, 98
intraperitoneal tuberculosis 158
intrathecal injection 322
intrathoracic free fluid **333**
intravenous sedation 36
– complications prevention **92**
– personnel requirements 114
– venous access, difficult 111, *112*
invasive procedure classification 38
iodoquinol 156
isoniazid 77

J

Jagwire 227, *229*
joint effusion **81**

K

knee interventions **311**

L

laparoscopic cyst removal 167
large-bore catheter systems 29
lateral femoral cutaneous nerve block **326**, 327, *327*
lidocaine 36
linear array transducers 4, *7–8*, 275
liver abscess(es) **77**, 145
– biliary disease **155**
– biopsy indications 122
– microbiological testing **77**
– posttransplantation **158**, *159*
– sequelae 159, *160*
– unknown cause 158
liver biopsy 7, **95**
– bleeding risk predictors 87
– CEUS-guided 122
– complications *96*, 98, **98**
– historical aspects 2, *3*
– indications **120**
liver cysts
– biliary communication 164
– biopsy indications 122
– contraindications 163
– epidemiology **163**
– etiology **163**
– intracystic hemorrhage 164
– percutaneous sclerotherapy, *see* percutaneous sclerotherapy, cysts
– ruptured, ascites 132
– surgical interventions 163
– symptoms **163**
– treatment options **163**
liver disease, advanced 89
liver fibrosis 121
liver mass, microbiological testing **77**
liver metastases, *see* hepatic metastases
liver tumors *44*, **121**
liver, diagnostic interventions **120**
local ablative procedures **103**, **179**
– *See also* individual procedures
– adjacent organ damage prevention **92**
– alternatives **104**
– combination treatments 185
– complications **103**, **182**
– concepts **185**
– considerations **179**
– contraindications **103**, **180**, **187**
– curative intent 185
– echinococcosis **175**
– EUS-guided **247**
– follow-up care *182*, **182**
– general anesthesia 180
– hepatocellular carcinoma 179, **180**, **185**
– indications **179**, **186**
– liver tumors **185**
– materials/equipment *180*, **180**
– needle insertion **180**, *181*
– palliative 185, **367**
– practical aspects **180**
– preparations **180**
– prognostic factors **183**
– single vs. multiple sessions **179**
– suitable tumors **179**
– technique **180**
– thyroid gland 296, **296**
– treatment response monitoring *182*, **182**
local anesthesia **36**
– *See also* individual procedures
– complications prevention **92**
– therapeutic interventions 23
longitudinal endosonography 225, *225*, 226, *226*
low-molecular weight heparin (LMWH) 91, 250, 316
lower limb nerve blocks **322**
Luer lock connector 17, 27
lumbosacral plexus blocks **322**
Lunderquist wire 27, 151
lung biopsy **101**
lung cancer *44*, **88**
lung mobility *271*
Lyme disease 81
lymph node biopsy 45, **126**
lymph node metastases 45, 126, *126*
lymph node(s) 45, *45*
– histologic evaluation **43**, *45*
– immunocytochemistry *58*, *61*
lymphadenectomy 125–126
lymphadenopathy 74
– differential diagnosis 73
– infectious causes 45, 73
– investigations 43, *45*, **73**, 74–75
– serology 75–76
lymphoepithelial lesions 46
lymphomas 45
– biopsy indications 45, 126
– histology 42, **45**
– immunocytochemical markers 60
– mediastinal 269
– small cell tumors vs. 47, *48*
– splenic 255
lymphoreticular tumors 44

M

machine decontamination 85
macrohematuria 277
magnetic field-assisted needle tracking **362**
magnetic resonance imaging (MRI) **146**, **173**, **186**, **359**
Malecot catheter 28
Mallinckrodt system 215
MALT lymphomas 46, *47*
mantle cell lymphomas 46
materials, interventional **13**, **37**
May–Grünwald–Giemsa (MGG) stain *52*, 54–55, *56–57*
mebendazole 174
Medi-Globe appliances 225, 227
mediastinal biopsy **101**, **268**, *270*
mediastinal lymphadenopathy 74, 257
mediastinal masses 260, **268**, *270*
medications **35**
– *See also* individual drugs
– sedation **114**
medullary thyroid carcinoma *289*
Mendel–Mantoux skin test 77
Menghini biopsy 18
Menghini needle (Surecut needle) **18**, 120
meralgia paresthetica 327
meropenem 80
mesenchymal tumors 42, 60
mesenteric masses, biopsy **100**, 126
metal stents *231*, **231**
metastatic prostate cancer 281
Metro wire 227, *229*
metronidazole 77–78, 155–157
mezlocillin 155
microbiological specimens **68**
microbiological testing **68**
– differential diagnosis **73**
– guidelines **73**
– immediate examination of specimens **69**
– limitations **72**
– parasite detection **70**
– prerequisites **68**
– results turnaround time 72, **72**
– skin preparation **68**
– specimen collection **68**
– specimen labeling 69
– specimen receipt during off-hours **72**
– specimen submission to laboratory **68**, *69*
– specimen volume 68, **68**
– stains **69**
– techniques **69**
microhematuria 277
microsensors 362
microwave ablation (MWA) 103
midazolam 35, 114
minors, informed consent **33**
modified Bosniak classification, cystic renal lesions 165
molecular tests 58, **169**
monitoring, during procedures **37**
mortality rates **86**
motor vehicle operation 301
Munich drain *201*, **206**
muscle imaging **316**
musculoskeletal interventions **304**
– blind procedures 304
– complications/pitfalls **312**
– contraindications **304**
– indications **304**
– injection site preparation 305
– materials/equipment **304**, 305, *306*
– patient positioning 305

- postprocedure care **313**
- preparations **305**
- procedure **305**
- technique 304, *306*, **306**

mycobacteria 77

N

N-butylscopolamine 220
naloxone 36
nasogastric irrigation tubes 242
Navarre universal catheter 147
neck pain 299
necrosectomy 232, 249
necrotic metastases 148
necrotizing pancreatitis 131, *131*
needle applicators, RFA *189*, **189**
needle guide attachments **13**, 14, *14*, *140*
- long needle path length 138, *140*
- percutaneous renal biopsy 275

needle holder 153, *154*
needle knives 228, 232, **241**
needle tract seeding 9, **88**
- *See also* individual tumors
- clinical significance **89**
- endosonographic interventions 251
- incidence **88**
- malignant tumors **89**
- needle size in 16
- post-thoracic interventions 270
- prevention **92**
- radiofrequency ablation **192**, 193
- thyroid biopsy 290

needle(s) **15**
- color coding 15–16
- diameter designating systems 15
- EUS-guided vascular interventions 347
- interventional endosonography **225**
- interventional risk and **86**
- length **16**
- local ablative procedures 180
- materials 15
- musculoskeletal interventions 305
- paracentesis 136
- percutaneous renal biopsy 275
- peripancreatic fluid collection drainage **240**
- regional anesthesia *317*, **317**, 318
- retrieved specimen length 16
- selection 16
- size **16**, 23
- technology **15**
- therapeutic interventions 17, *10*, **23**, **238**
- thoracic interventions 262–263
- thyroid biopsy 290
- tip configurations **16**, 17, *17*, 23
- tracking 6, 16

nephropyelostomy *8*
nephrostomy sets *166*, 282, *283*
nerve imaging **316**
neuroectodermal tumors 42
neuroendocrine tumors 42, 44
neurologic deficit **316**
neurologic interventions **315**
neutral electrode *113*
Nimura dilator 27
Niti-S stent **212**
non-Hodgkin lymphoma (NHL) 45, *45*, 46, *48*, 255
nonalcoholic steatohepatitis (NASH) 120–121
nonsteroidal anti-inflammatory drugs (NSAIDs) 81, 250, 316
novel oral anticoagulants (NOACs) 90–91
nucleic acid amplification **71**
nurse-administered propofol sedation (NAPS) 111, 114

O

obstetrics and gynecology 7
obstructive jaundice, malignant 199, 208
obturator nerve block **323**, *324*, 327
off-plane needle tracking 362
one-second liver biopsy 18
one-stick technique, *see* trocar technique
operational requirements **38**
opioid antagonists 35–36
organizational requirements **38**
Otto needle 19, **142**, 180
out-of-plane technique, needle insertion *316*
oxygen desaturation, sedation-induced 115

P

pain, as complication **86**, 95
PAIR (puncture-aspiration-injection of alcohol-reaspiration)
- contraindications 147
- echinococcal liver cysts 10, **175–176**
-- follow-up **176**
-- indications/contraindications 176
-- technique *176*, **176**, *177*
- risks **177**
- side effects management **177**

palliative care **364**
- content/goals **364**
- oncologic follow-up **364**
- ultrasonography, role in **364**

palliative care team 367
palliative chemotherapy 365, *365*
palliative interventions 365, 366
- diagnostic **365**, 366
- therapeutic 366, **366**

palliative staging **364**
palliative treatment monitoring **364**
palliative tumor ablation **367**
palliative ultrasound 364, **367**
pancreatic abscess drainage **241**, *243*, 249
pancreatic biopsy **99**, 100, **123**
- endosonography in 123

pancreatic cancers
- biopsy indications 123, *123*
- needle tract seeding 89
- palliative interventions **365**

pancreatic cystic lesions
- biopsy 123, *124*
- diagnostic parameters 124
- EUS-guided ablation 249
- ruptured 132
- tumors vs. 123–124

pancreatic duct, dilated 7, *9*
pancreatic metastasis 123
pancreatic necrosis 243
pancreatic pseudocysts
- biopsy indications 123
- communication detection 357, *357*
- drainage 10, 29, **102**, **243**
-- EUS-guided 249
-- indications 240
-- large-bore metal stents 232
- EUS intervention timing 240
- puncture 7
- stent placement 241

pancreatitis **131**, **134**, **156**
pancreatitis-associated cystic lesions **357**
pancreatogenic abscess 131
Papanicolaou staining 54–55, **55**, *56–57*
- air-dried smears 55, *57*

papillary thyroid carcinoma *289*
paracentesis *136*
- bile leakage drainage (with irrigation) **135**, *136*
- complications **136**
- contraindications **136**
- diagnostic, *see* diagnostic paracentesis
- free abdominal fluid **128**
- how/where to aspirate **133**
- indications **134**
- local anesthesia 134
- materials **136**
- palliative **367**
- postprocedure care **136**
- ultrasound contrast agents 355

parasites **70**, 122
parenchymal liver diseases 120
parents, informed consent 33
parietal pleura *261*
paromomycin 78, 156–157
partial hepatectomy 185
partial thromboplastin time (PTT) 22, 90
Partington–Rochelle pancreaticojejunostomy 243
patent tract sign 96
pathology **40**
- antibody selection, undifferentiated tumors 45
- specific analysis **43**
- staging **41**
- tumor grading **43**, *44*

patient positioning **37**
patient-related risks 32
peel-away sheath **24**, *25*
percutaneous abscess drainage, *see* abscess drainage
percutaneous acetic acid injection (PAI) **179**
- ethanol injection vs. **179**
- hepatocellular carcinoma 103, 179
- indications 179
- liver tumors 103
- single vs. multiple sessions 179

percutaneous cholangioscopy (PTCS) 206
percutaneous decompression 21
percutaneous endoscopic gastrostomy (PEG) **215**
- advantages/disadvantages 216
- complications 217, 367
- head and neck tumors 217
- introducer method **216**, 217, 222
- palliative **367**
- pull method 215, **215**, 217, 222
- push method **216**, 217
- success rates 216

percutaneous ethanol injection (PEI) **179**
- acetic acid injection vs. **179**
- alcohol volume injected **181**
- echinococcosis 103
- hepatocellular carcinoma 17, 179, 185
- historical background 10
- indications 179
- informed consent 298
- liver tumors 103
- needle types *23*
- prognostic indicators 182
- radiofrequency ablation vs. **179**
- single vs. multiple sessions 179
- thyroid adenomas 290, 296, **298**, *299*
- thyroid cancers, recurrent 297
- thyroid cysts 297, *300*, **301**
- thyroid gland **296**
-- advantages/disadvantages 297
-- complications/pitfalls **299**, **301**
-- contraindications 297
-- dose 298
-- follow-up **301**
-- indications 297, **298**, **301**
-- postprocedure care **301**
-- procedure *298*, **298**, 299, *299*
-- results assessment 299, *299*
-- snowstorm cloud pattern 298, *298*
-- therapeutic goals 297
- thyroid nodules 296–297

percutaneous gallbladder drainage 103
percutaneous gastrostomy **215**
- *See also* individual types
- complications **216**, 217
- contraindications **215**
- fluoroscopy vs. sonographic guidance 217
- indications **215**

- materials/equipment **215**
- problems/strategies for solution 223
- sedation 217
- success rates **216**
- transillumination failure 223
- tube placement assessment 218
- types **215**, 216
- ultrasonography, role of **217**, *218*, 222

percutaneous laser ablation (PLA), thyroid gland **301**
percutaneous needle aspiration, prostatic abscess 281
percutaneous nephrostomy (PCN) **282**
- anesthesia **283**
- collecting system, inadequate dilation **284**
- complications **282**
- indications **282**
- materials/equipment *282*, **282**, *283*
- positioning **283**
- postoperative care **284**
- preparations **282**
- procedure **283**, *284*
- puncture **283**
- relative contraindications **282**
- technique **282**, *283*
- tube placement **283**

percutaneous pleural drainage **265**
percutaneous radiologic gastrostomy (PRG) 216, **216**, 217, *222*
percutaneous renal biopsy **99**
- access route 276
- alternatives **99**
- anesthesia 276
- as outpatient procedure 278
- asepsis 276
- bleeding risk predictors 87, 95, *97*
- clinical applications 7
- complications 99, **99**, **277**
- contraindications **99**, **274**
- indications **124**, **274**
- informed consent 275
- materials/equipment **275**, *276*, **278**
- mortality rate 277
- patient positioning 276
- postbiopsy care **278**
- preparations **275**
- procedure *276*, **276**, *277*
-- native biopsy **276**
-- renal allografts *277*, **277**

percutaneous sclerotherapy, cysts **163**
- alternative procedures **167**
- complications 164
- drain placement confirmation 164
- follow-up care **164**
- liver cysts **163**
-- cyst aspiration/drain insertion **164**
-- equipment/materials **163**
-- indications **163**
-- local anesthesia **163**
-- skin preparation **163**
-- technique **163**
- prognosis **164**
- recurrence rate 164
- renal cysts **164**
-- technique *166*, **166**
- sclerosing agents **163**, 164, **166**
- sclerosing time 164
- technique **164**, *165*

percutaneous sonographic gastrostomy (PSG) *219*, **219**, *221*
- advantages/disadvantages 216
- complications 217, 220, *222*
- contrast instillation 220, *222*
- drainage type **221**
- extragastric tube position 220, *223*
- gastropexy 219, *219*, 220, **220**, *221*
- infusion pump use 220
- materials *222*
- prophylactic antibiotics **220**
- spasmolytic agent use **220**
- success rates 216
- tube position checking 220

percutaneous thrombin injection, pseudoaneurysms 342
- advantages/disadvantages 347
- arteriovenous fistula and 343, *346*
- complications 343, 347
- contraindications 343
- dosage 343
- materials 342
- success rate 345
- technique **343**, *344–345*
- thrombin leakage 343

percutaneous transhepatic cholangiodrainage (PTCD) **103**, **198**
- additional treatment options **206**
- advantages 198
- aftercare **208**
- alternatives **103**
- attachment **207**
- bile assessment 203
- bile leakage 209, *211*
- biliary drainage setup **206**, *207*
- biliary stenting vs. external catheter drainage 201
- biliary tree puncture **203**
- blind fluoroscopic technique 203, *203*
- cholangiography **203**
- combined approach 201
- complications **103**, 132, 203, 208, **208**
-- management **208**
- contraindications **103**, **199**
- contrast media 203, 205, *206*, *209*, **209**, *210–211*
- dilation **206**
- drainage **202**
- drainage sets 200
- drains 202, **206**, 209
- endoprostheses comparison **208**, **210**
- endoscopic retrograde approach vs. **199**
- indications **198**, 199
- literature analysis **210**
- local anesthesia *202*, **202**
- materials/equipment **200**, *201–202*
- mortality rate 208
- needle insertion **202**
- needle orientation **202**
- needle placement **204**
- outpatient basis 209
- palliative 198, **366**
- patient positioning *202*, **202**
- procedure planning **205**
- puncture site/access route **202**
- sedation 201
- single-needle technique **203**
- special puncture sets 205
- stent placement **207**
- success rate **207**
- technique **103**, **201**, *204–205*
-- ultrasound-guided **203**
- two-needle technique **203**

percutaneous transhepatic cholangiography (PTC) 198, 209
percutaneous transluminal angioplasty (PTA) 338
percutaneous vascular interventions **335**
perianal fistula 356
pericardial effusion **79**
pericardial fluid
- drainage 334, *335*, **335**
- emergency interventions 330, **334**

pericardial tamponade 330, 334
pericardiocentesis *335*
pericystectomy 174
peridiverticulitis, abscess drainage 155
perilesional injection therapy, pseudoaneurysms **343**, 347
perinephritic abscess 80
peripancreatic fluid collections drainage **239**, *242*
- abscesses **241**
- anatomical considerations **239**
- complications **243**
- diagnostic workup **239**
- dissection (fenestration) 241, **241**
- EUS intervention timing **240**
- history aspects **239**
- indications **240**
- infected necrosis **241**
- needle handling rules **240**
- one-step systems **240**
- pathologic considerations **239**
- postinterventional care **243**
- procedure selection **240**
- prophylactic antibiotics 240
- stent insertion 240
- stent placement **241**
- surgical options **243**
- technique **240**
- transmural approach 240
- two-step drainage 240
- wire handling rules **240**

peripancreatic necrosis 240
peripheral vein catheterization 336, *338*
perirenal hematoma 95, *97*, 99, 277
peritoneal carcinomatosis **130**, **133**
- cytostatic therapy **135**
- palliative paracentesis **135**

peritoneal cavity *128*, **128**, **355**
peritoneal fluid collections, *see* ascites
peritoneal masses 126
peritoneum 128
- metastatic spread 133

peritonitis **79**
- abscess drainage **153**
- ascites **130**
- classification 79
- diagnosis **79**
- emergency interventions 332
- postinterventional **88**
- secondary 79
-- diagnosis 80
-- emergency interventions 332
-- risk stratification 80
-- treatment 80
- treatment **80**

personal protective equipment **82**
PET, ultrasound fusion **359**
pethidine 35
pheochromocytoma 125
phlegmonous inflammation 145, *145*
phrenic nerve palsy 318
pigtail catheters *24*, 28, *29*
- abscess drainage 147
- hemothorax 333
- interventional endosonography 230, *231*
- percutaneous nephrostomy 282, *285*
- percutaneous transhepatic cholangiodrainage 206

piperacillin 77, 79–81
plasmacytoma 264
plastic stents **230**, *231*
platelet concentrates 91
platelet counts
- bleeding risk prediction 87, 90
- therapeutic interventions 22

platelet function tests 87, 274
pleural biopsy **101**, 265
pleural drainage *267*
pleural effusion **78**
- causes 78
- diagnosis **78**
- differential diagnosis 78
- malignant 265, **265**
- swinging heart motion 334, *334*
- thoracentesis 264, *266*
- treatment **78**

pleural empyema 78, **265**
pleural mesothelioma **88**, 101
pleural sliding sign 282
pleural space interventions 261, *261*, **264**
pleurodesis **265**

Pneumocath catheter 29, *29*, *264*
pneumothorax
- drainage procedure **333**
- emergency interventions 330, **333**
- follow-up care 270
- motion artifact absence *271*, 282
- postbiopsy 101, **269**, *271*
- prevention **92**

point-of-care ultrasound 331
polidocanol 164
polycystic kidney disease 166
polymerase chain reaction (PCR) 58, 77–78
polyurethane 27–28
popliteal cyst puncture **311**, *312*
portable ultrasound 331, *367*, **367**
portal vein, gas in 157
portocaval shunt creation 248
postprocedure care
- complications detection **95**, *96*
- monitoring **37**

PPSB 91
precursor lesions 42
premedication **35**
preprocedure examination **37**
primary biliary cirrhosis (PBC) 120–121
probes, *see* ultrasound probes
procedure room **37–38**
- endoscopic ultrasound 224
- functional/design requirements **38**
- lighting conditions *109*, 113, *113*
- minor invasive procedures **38**
- musculoskeletal interventions 305

procedure-related risks 32
procoagulant therapy **94**
propofol 35–37, 114
- interventional endosonography 234
- monitoring requirements 115

prostate 280
- diseases **280**

prostate biopsy **281**
- antibiotic prophylaxis 281, *281*
- complications **281**
- indications **281**
- informed consent **281**
- preparation **281**
- systematic vs. targeted 281

prostate cancer **280**
- diagnosis **280**
- etiology **280**
- incidence **280**
- metastatic 281
- treatment **280**

prostate specific antigen (PSA) 281
prostatic abscess **281**
protective eyewear 03
prothrombin time 21, 87, 90
protozoan infections 157, **157**
pseudoaneurysms **341**
- arteriovenous fistula vs. 341
- complications **343**
- diagnosis *341*, **341**, *342*
- follow-up 345
- materials **342**
- therapeutic procedures **341**, *342*
-- advantages/disadvantages **343**

pseudoascites 133
pseudomyxoma peritonei **132**, *133*
psoas compartment block 322, **322**, *323*, 327
pulley ganglion injection *311*
pulmonary abscesses **268**, *269*
pulmonary hypertension 101, 180, 182
pulmonary lesions visualization 260
punch biopsy 40
puncture needles, PTCD 200
purulent material 72
purulent peritonitis 130, *130*
pyogenic liver abscess **154**, *160*
pyrazinamide 77

Q

Quantum TTC balloon dilators 229
Quick value (thromboplastin time) 21, 90

R

radiofrequency ablation (RFA)
- antibiotic prophylaxis **187**
- colorectal liver metastases 186
- complications 103, **193**
- contraindications **187**
- control **189**
- gas generation 193, *194*
- general anesthesia **187**
- hepatocellular carcinoma 185
- liver tumors **185**
-- clinical aftercare/follow-up **196**
-- glucose solution injections 187, 191, *191*
-- historical background 10
-- imaging modality selection **186**
-- indications **186**
-- intraoperative applicator use *193*
-- necrotic zone estimation 192, *192*
-- number of tumors **186**
-- postinterventional care **196**
-- preparations **187**
-- probe insertion *190*, **190**, *191*
-- recurrence 196
-- sequence *194*
-- specific systems **191**
-- technique **189**, *190*
-- track ablation **192**
-- treatment efficacy assessment *192*, **192**, *194*
-- treatment planning **187**
-- tumor location **186**
-- tumor size **186**
- local anesthesia **187**, *190*, **190**
- materials **187**, *188*
- monopolar vs. bipolar systems **188**
- multineedle systems 186
- multipolar systems **188**
- needle perfusion flow rate **189**
- palliative 367
- patient positioning 187, **189**, *190*, 196
- percutaneous ethanol injection vs. **179**
- principles *188*, **188**
- renal tumors 103
- sedation **187**
- system characteristics 188
- temperature measurement **189**
- thyroid gland **301**

radiofrequency generator *188*
radiography 2, **146**
radiotherapy, prophylactic 92
Rapid On-Site Evaluation (ROSE) **58**
- importance **59**
- rapid fixation/staining **59**, *62*
- working without **62**

receptors 60
recombinant coagulation factor VIIa 91
rectovaginal fistulas 357
refractory ascites 134
regional anesthesia **315**
- advantages 315
- contraindications **315**
- history/development **315**
- indications **315**
- lower limb **322**
- materials/equipment *317*, **317**
- needle insertion techniques **316**
- nerve/muscle imaging **317**
- out-of-plane vs. in-plane technique *316*, **316**, *317*
- ultrasound machines *317*, **317**
- upper limb **318**

renal allograft biopsy *277*, **277**
renal artery stenosis 339
renal biopsy, percutaneous, *see* see percutaneous renal biopsy
renal cysts
- classification 165, **165**
- differential diagnosis **165**
- epidemiology **165**
- minimally complex 165–166
- percutaneous sclerotherapy, *see* percutaneous sclerotherapy
- ruptured 132
- sonographic features 165

renal disease, advanced 89
rendezvous techniques 198, **199**, 206
respiratory depression, midazolam-induced 114
retroperitoneal lymphomas 138
retroperitoneoscopic renal exposure 167
rib metastases 264
rifampin 77
risky lesions **94**
Romanowsky stains **55**
rotator cuff interventions **309**, *310*

S

sacroiliac joint injections **312**, *313*
sacroiliitis 312
saphenous nerve block *326*, **326**, 327
sarcoma 126, *126*, 257
Schlottmann paracentesis needle 28
sciatic nerve block 322, *325*, **325**, 327
sclerosing cholangitis 164
scratch artifacts 52
sedation 35, **35**, **111**, **114**
- *See also* individual procedures
- antagonists 36
- assisting staff **111**, 114
- complications **115**
- discharge criteria 115
- intravenous, *see* intravenous sedation
- local ablative procedures 180
- medications **114**
- monitoring requirements **115**
- nonanesthesiologists, administration by 114
- oxygen administration 111, *112*
- oxygen desaturation 115
- personnel requirements **114**
- postprocedure care **115**
- radiofrequency ablation **187**
- recommendations 36

Seldinger technique 21, **24**
- abscess drainage **146**, **151**, *152*
- equipment 24, *24*, *146*, *166*
- modified version 24
- percutaneous transhepatic cholangiodrainage **206**
- trocar technique vs. 24

sepsis 88, **157**, 201
septic (pyogenic) abscess **157**
septic arthritis 81
serology **71**
- echinococcosis 70, **169**
- lymphadenopathy 75–76
- parasite detection 70
- pericardial effusion 79

setup requirements **37**
shadowing artifacts 181, 354
short beveled tip, biopsy needle 16, *17*
shoulder interventions **307**, *309*
shoulder pain, right 159
skin markings **37**
skin preparation, patient **83**
- microbiological testing 68

sliding lung sign 331
small cell tumors 47, *48*, *58*
smears **51**
Soehendra stent retriever 233, *234*
SonoTip ultra EUS aspiration needle *228*
Spannguide wire 27
spasmolytic agents **220**
specialized ambulatory palliative care (SAPV) 367
splenic abscesses **255**, *256*
splenic biopsy **100**, **123**, **256**
splenic cysts **167**, **255**
splenic drainage 256
splenic infarction **254**
splenic interventions **254**
- anatomical considerations **255**

- complications **257**
- contraindications **256**
- diffuse splenic changes **254**
- focal splenic changes **255**
- indications **256**
- postinterventional care **257**
- procedures **255**
- specific disorders **254**
- vaccinations, preinterventional **257**

splenic macroabscesses 255
splenic metastases **255**, 256
splenic microabscesses 255
splenic rupture **254**
splenic sarcoma 257
splenic tumors **255**, 256
splenomas 255
splenomegaly 254
spray fixatives 55
stains **69**
status post biliary-enteric anastomosis 187
stent angioplasty, renal artery stenosis 339
stent retrievers **233**, *234*
stents 244, *365*
- *See also* individual types

stool antigen test 78, 156
stopcocks, drains 29
Strecker stent **211**
subacute granulomatous thyroiditis 288, *289*
subcapsular hematoma, renal *97*, 99
subclavian vein 319, *320*
- catheterization 336, *337*

subcutaneous masses 126
subdiaphragmatic liver lesions 186
subphrenic abscess 158
subpleural lung lesions **265**
suction needles **17**, *18*
sulbactam 77, 80
sump syndrome 155
Super Stiff wire 227
super-stiff cyst access wire 227
superficial nerve blocks 316
supraclavicular brachial plexus block 315, **319**, *320*, 327
supraspinatus muscle interventions **309**, *310*
Surecut needle (Menghini needle) 6, **18**, 120
surgical masks 82
sutures
- diameter designating systems 153
- materials 153
- techniques *25*, **25**

swelling artifact 52
swinging heart motion 334, *334*
syringes 112, *113*

T

T-anchors (T-fasteners) 219, *219*, 220
T-fasteners (T-anchors) 219, *219*, 220
tandem needle biopsy technique 23
tandem trocar technique 23
Tannenbaum (Christmas tree) stents 230
tazobactam 77, 79–81
tele-ultrasound 110
Terumo guidewire 26, 227
tetracycline 78, 157
therapeutic interventions **20**
- *See also* individual interventions
- access routes **21**
- accessories **29**
- assisting staff's duties **111**
- bleeding risk predictors 87
- coagulation testing **21**
- complications **22**
- contraindications **21**, 22
- historical background **10**, **20**
- improper postoperative care 22
- indications **21**
- interventional endosonography **238**
- interventional risk **86**
- materials **20**
- needle techniques **23**
- palliative **366**
- patient preparation **21**
- special needle types *23*, **23**
- suture techniques *25*, **25**

thick-layer artifacts 52, *52–53*
thoracentesis **264**, *266–267*
- complication rates, ICU patients 332

thoracic inlet 260, *260*
thoracic interventions **260**
- *See also* individual interventions
- biopsy devices **262–263**
- complications/problems **269**
- contraindications **261**
- follow-up **270**
- indications **120**, **261**
- local anesthesia 264
- materials/equipment **261**, 263
- patient discharge 271
- patient positioning 264
- postprocedure care **269–270**
- preparations *260*, **263**, **269**
- procedure steps **269**
- specimen collection methods 260
- technique **264**, **269**
- ultrasound-guided, advantages **260**

thoracic tumors, imaging 262, *262*
thromboembolic prophylaxis, nerve blocks 316
thromboplastin time (Quick value) 21, 90
thymomas, mediastinal 269
thyroid abscess *290*, 296, **296**
thyroid adenomas 290, 296, **298**
thyroid adhesions 301
thyroid biopsy **288**
- antisepsis **292**
- aspirate preparation **293**
- complications **290**
- contraindications **288**
- drill technique **293**
- false-negative rates 294
- false-positives 294
- fine needle nonaspiration **293**
- indications **288**
- long-axis technique *290–292*, **292**
- materials/equipment **290**, *291*
- methods **288**
- patient positioning **291**
- pitfalls **294**
- preparation **291**
- problems **293**, 296
- procedure 288, **292**
- short-axis technique **292**, *293–294*
- target site selection **291**
- ultrasound technology **290**, *291*
- ultrasound vs. palpation-guided 288

thyroid cancer, sonographic criteria 288, *289*
thyroid cysts *293*, 296, **296**
- ablation 297, *300*, **301**

thyroid interventions **288**
- ablative procedures 296, **296**
- diagnostic **288**
- evacuation procedures 296, **296**
- therapeutic 288, **295**, 296

thyroid lymphomas 288, *290*
thyroid nodules 288, 297
tirofiban (Aggrastat) 36
tissue anchors 25, *26*
tissue characterization 3
Titan balloon dilators 230, *230*
transducers, biopsy, *see* biopsy transducers
transenteric biopsy route 140
transgastric biopsy route 140
transjugular liver biopsy 99, 121
transjugular parenchymal biopsy 93
transperineal prostatic biopsy 281, **282**
transrectal prostatic biopsy **102**, 281
- antibiotic prophylaxis 93
- complications 88, 102, **102**, 281

transrectal ultrasonography of the prostate (TRUS) **280**
transudate, intra-abdominal *129*, **129**
trocar technique 21, **23**
- abscess drainage *146*, **151**
- chest 263
- drains 23, *23–24*
- instrument set *146*, *166*
- Seldinger technique vs. 24

trocar tip, biopsy needle 16, *17*
Trucut needle 6, *19*, **19**, *20*
- automated systems 20
- biopsy technique 19, 140, *141*, **143**
- disadvantages 19, 143
- needle tract seeding 9
- percutaneous renal biopsy 275
- thoracic interventions 263

tuberculosis 75, **76**, **131**, *132*
tuberculosis PCR assay 77
tuberculous ascites 131, *132*
tuberculous pericarditis 79
tuberculous pleurisy 78
tumor ablation therapy, *see* see local ablative procedures
tumor(s), *see* individual types
- benign-malignant differentiation 41
- classification **41**
- grading **43**, *44*
- marker antibodies 44
- necrotic components, infections **158**
- needle tract seeding, *see* needle tract seeding
- tissue of origin 42
- WHO classification 43

U

Ultraflex stents 232
ultrasound (interventional)
- abscess drainage **144**
- alternatives **93**
- assistance, *see* assistance/assisting personnel
- clinical applications **7**
- emergency interventions **331**
- endosonography and 10
- historical background **2**
- later developments **10**
- liver tumors, local ablative procedures **186**
- optimal approach **93**
- outlook **10**
- procedures classification 109
- risks **9**
- routine clinical use **3**
- techniques, evolution **3**

ultrasound contrast agents (UCAs) **354**
- abscess drainage 149, *150*, *151*
- administration technique **354**
- approved indications **354**
- biliary tract **356**
- complications **354**
- contraindications **354**
- dilution 354
- enterography **356**
- extravascular use **354**
- nonphysiologic body cavities **356**
- physiologic body cavities **355**

ultrasound fistulography **356**
ultrasound gastroscope *226–227*
ultrasound gel **83**
ultrasound probes 109
- classification 84
- cleaning 84, 109
- covers **83**, 305–306
- decontamination **84**
- disinfection 84, 93
- for biopsies, *see* biopsy transducers
- hygiene **84**, 93

- sterilization 85, 93

ultrasound tracking 367

ultrasound-assisted percutaneous endoscopic gastrostomy (US-PEG) **218**, *219*, 222

ultrasound-guided compression therapy, pseudoaneurysms 341, *342*, **342**, 343, 347
- complications 343, 347
- materials 342

ultrasound-guided fine needle aspiration (US-FNA)
- complication rates 86
- historical aspects 49
- intra-abdominal free fluid 332
- mortality rates 86
- specimen collection **49**
- thyroid gland 288

ultrasound-guided forceps biopsy 265, *268*

ultrasound-guided punctures *2*, 3, *3*

ultrasound-guided regional anesthesia, *see* regional anesthesia

Uni-Core biopsy needle 19

uninformed consent 34

Union for International Cancer Control (UICC) tumor grading system 43

upper limb blocks **318**

urinary tract infections 88, 102

urine leak, intraperitoneal *132*, **132**

urinoma **132**

uterine cervix, epithelial changes 42

V

vaccinations **257**

vacuum syringe *113*

variceal bleeding, recurrent 345, *347*

vascular access **335**, *336*

vascular interventions
- EUS-guided, *see* endosonographically guided vascular interventions
- percutaneous **335**
- ultrasound-guided 330, **330**

vascular surgery, pseudoaneurysms 341, 347

vasovagal reactions **86**

vesicoenteric fistulas 357

vesicoureteral reflux **355**

Vidoson system 4, *6*

Vienna Congress **2**

Vim–Silverman needle 18

vitamin K 91

vitamin K antagonists (VKAs) 90

Vitesse needle 143

voiding sonography, vesicoureteral reflux 354, **355**

volume navigation **359**
- case reports/illustrative images *361*, **362**
- position marking **359**
- tracking **359**, *360*
- volume data set fusion **359**
-- archived ultrasound data **362**

von Meyenburg anomalies 163

W

WallFlex metal stent *231*, 232

Wallstent biliary endoprosthesis 208, **212**

water lily sign 171

white blood cell count, joint effusion 81

WHO classification
- cystic echinococcosis **171**, 172
-- group 1: active cysts **171**, *173–174*
-- group 2: involuting cysts 171, **172**, *175*
-- group 3: inactive cysts **172**, *175*
-- nonspecific cystic lesions 172
- tumors 43

Wills–Oglesby gastrostomy sets 215

Wilson disease 120–121

Y

Yamakawa drain **206**

Z

Ziehl–Neelsen stain **70**

Zilver stent 210